CANCER REGISTRY
MANAGEMENT
Principles & Practice

Second Edition

Editors

Carol L. Hutchison
Herman R. Menck
Mindy Burch
Roanne Gottschalk

National Cancer Registrars Association, Inc.
Alexandria, Virginia

KENDALL/HUNT PUBLISHING COMPANY
4050 Westmark Drive   Dubuque, Iowa 52002

Cover:
The survival graph is the outcome of cancer registry work. Cancer Registrars capture
a complete summary of patient history, diagnosis, treatment, and disease status
for every cancer patient in the United States, and other countries as well. Cancer
Registrars hope their work will lead to better treatments, and ultimately, a cure.

Copyright © 1997, 2004 by the National Cancer Registrars Association, Inc.

ISBN 0-7575-0192-3

Printed in the United States of America
10 9 8 7 6 5 4 3 2

CONTENTS

Chapter 11:
JOINT COMMISSION ON ACCREDITATION OF HEALTHCARE ORGANIZATIONS (JCAHO) 99
Catherine Gray

Chapter 12:
CASE ASCERTAINMENT 109
Fred F. Wacker

Chapter 13:
RAPID CASE ASCERTAINMENT 117
Carol Lowenstein

Chapter 14:
STANDARDS FOR DATA AND DATA MANAGEMENT 121
Jerri Linn Phillips
Carol Hahn Johnson

To all those people whose lives have been touched by cancer:

to our colleagues of the past, present, and future committed to cancer data management;

to all physicians, researchers, epidemiologists, and administrators who use our data to understand neoplasms, improve cancer treatment, increase survival, and improve long-term quality of life for cancer patients;

to all the patients we serve;

we dedicate this book.

PREFACE

The first edition of this book was written nearly five years ago and since then, many advances have been made in cancer data collection and reporting. The first edition was well received throughout the field and seemingly fulfilled its overall objective to provide technical and management issues defined in a comprehensive textbook. The first edition of this book was used by many new cancer registrars studying for their certification, college and university instructors teaching cancer registry classes, and hospitals starting new cancer programs.

Readers of the first edition will recognize several topics and subjects that were covered in the first book. These topics have been revisited with an intent to update, enhance, and enrich the original pretext of those subjects, as new material has been discovered and technologies improved. In all cases through this book, new axioms and approaches are delineated in the interest of providing the reader with the most effective strategies available in the essential responsibilities of a cancer registrar.

Additionally, a few new chapters have been added and new chapter sections have been introduced, addressing new critical areas of responsibility for the cancer registry or cancer program. The order of chapters was changed and grouped to reflect five main areas of cancer registry management:

- Introduction
- Administrative Operations
- Technical Operations
- Data Usage and Reporting
- Specialized Registries and Networking

As with the first edition of this book, the second edition can be used as a basis for all disease registries, but cancer registry issues are addressed specifically. The book addresses demands for registrars employed in hospitals, free-standing facilities and central registries. Both clinical and administrative aspects of the acquisition and dissemination of cancer information are addressed. This book is not intended to duplicate other reference material, but rather enhance their importance and connect them.

All chapters are concisely written, and most contain charts, tables, or illustrations that are universal, are critical to practice, and advance the cancer registry operation. Most chapters begin with an introduction and end with a brief summary, study questions, and a list of recent references including both texts and journals. Because some of the terms in the textbook are high technical in nature, a glossary is provided to clarify the usage within the text. Answers are provided to all chapter study questions in a separate appendix to facilitate the learning process.

This textbook, *Cancer Registry Management: Principles and Practice, Second Edition,* is the result of a collaborative effort by a volunteer team of many health professionals and the National Cancer Registrars Association. The editors, chapter authors, reviewers, and other contributors have received no payment or honoraria. If it may be called such, this is a labor of love for our profession.

Carol L. Hutchison, Herman R. Menck,
Mindy Burch, Roanne Gottschalk

ACKNOWLEDGMENTS

The Editors have many people to thank for their help in writing this book. First and foremost we must thank those individuals who were willing to author chapters and share their information and ideas to advance the cancer registry profession.

We wish to thank the members and Board of Directors of the National Cancer Registrars Association (NCRA) for your understanding and patience during the writing of this textbook. We are especially grateful for the ongoing encouragement, support and direction that NCRA President Donna Gress and Executive Director Lori Swain have provided to the entire team throughout this project. We hope that you will be proud of the finished product.

We are especially grateful to Licking Memorial Health Systems, Newark, OH, who understood the merit of this textbook and supported us throughout the project. Also, special thanks must be given to Cindy Evans and Janelle Osborn who diligently assisted in many ways. We would also like to thank Sara Edgerton and William Dugan, Jr., MD, of Community Cancer Care, Inc., Indianapolis, IN, for their support of this book. Many work hours, mailings, and telephone calls were contributed by both of these fine organizations.

The quality of this book is due to the many skillful reviewers who read the manuscripts for accuracy, consistency, and completeness, including the staff of the Commission on Cancer of the American College of Surgeons and other contributors as well. We thank you for your advice and wisdom.

Finally, we wish to thank our families, friends, and colleagues, who endured our temperaments during this enormous undertaking. We believe that it has been well worth the effort.

EDITORS AND CONTRIBUTORS

EDITORS:

Carol L. Hutchison, CTR
Licking Memorial Health Systems
Newark, Ohio

Herman R. Menck, MBA, CDP
Independent Consultant
Marina Del Ray, CA

Mindy Burch, CTR
Community Cancer Care, Inc.
Indianapolis, IN

Roanne Gottschalk, RN, BSN
Licking Memorial Health Systems
Newark, OH

CONTRIBUTORS:

Tim E. Aldrich, PhD, MPH, CTR
Independent Consultant
Louisville, KY

Patricia Babin, RHIT, CTR
Naval Hospital Pensacola
Pensacola, FL

Connie Bura
Cancer Programs, American College of Surgeons
Chicago, IL

M. Asa Carter, CTR
Cancer Program, American College of Surgeons
Chicago, IL

Karen I. Christie, MA, CTR, CCRA
Independent Consultant
Greenville, NC

Rosemarie E. Clive, LPN, CTR
Independent Consultant
Winter Park, FL

Gayle Greer Clutter, RT, CTR
National Program of Cancer Registries
Atlanta, GA

Barbara M. DeCoe, CTR, RHIT
St. Mary's Cancer Center
Grand Rapids, MI

Marilyn S. Desler, CTR
Legacy Good Samaritan Hospital & Medical
   Center
Portland, OR

Raye-Anne Dorn, CTR
Department of Veterans Affairs
Washington, DC

Thomas H. Faris, Esq., JD, CQA, CQM
IMPAC Medical Systems, Inc.
Mountain View, CA

Patrick L. Fitzgibbons, MD
SNOMED International
Winnetka, IL

April Fritz, BA, RHIT, CTR
National Cancer Institute/SEER Program
Bethesda, MD

Catherine R. Gray, BA, CTR, CCRP
Independent Consultant
Newton, MA

Donna M. Gress, RHIT, CTR
South Coast Medical Center
Laguna Beach, CA

Holly Howe, PhD
North American Association of Central Cancer
   Registries, Inc.
Springfield, IL

Suzanna Hoyler, BS, CTR
Washington Hospital Center
Washington, DC

Dianne Hultstrom, BS, RHIT, CTR
IMPAC Medical Systems
Acton, MA

Carol L. Hutchison, CTR
Licking Memorial Health Systems
Newark, OH

Mary D. Hutton, MPH, CTR, RN
National Program of Cancer Registries
Atlanta, GA

Ryan Intlekofer, RN, CTR
Research Assistant, University of Iowa
Iowa City, IA

Carol Hahn Johnson, BS, CTR
National Cancer Institute/SEER Program
Bethesda, MD

Carol Kosary, MA
National Cancer Institute, SEER Program
Bethesda, MD

Carol L. Lowenstein, MBA, CTR
Harvard School of Public Health
Boston, MA

Mary F. Kennedy, MPH
SNOMED International
Winnetka, IL

Karen Malnar, RN, CTR, CCRC
University of Oklahoma Health Science Center
Tulsa, OK

Daniel P. McKellar, MD, FACS
Cancer Program Surveyor
Dayton, OH

LeeAnn McKelvey, MAT
Independent Consultant
Salem, OR

Herman R. Menck, MBA, CDP
Independent Consultant
Marina Del Ray, CA

Marla Moloney, MD
Children's Hospital
Columbus, OH

Betty Nielsen, RHIT, CTR
49th Medical Group
Holloman AFB, NV

Jerri Linn Phillips, MA, CTR
Cancer Program, American College of Surgeons
Chicago, IL

Karen S. Phillips, BS, CTR
IMPAC Medical Systems, Inc.
St. Peters, MO

Richard Reiling, MD, FACS
Cancer Program Surveyor
Charlotte, NC

Frances E. Ross, BA, CTR
Kentucky Cancer Registry
Lexington, KY

Frederick B. Ruymann, MD
Children's Hospital
Columbus, OH

Andrew K. Stewart, MA
National Cancer Data Base, American College of
    Surgeons
Chicago, IL

Judy Tryon, CTR
William Beaumont Army Medical Center
El Paso, TX

Carol S. Venuti, RHIA, CTR
Massachusetts General Hospital
Boston, MA

Fred Wacker, PhD, CTR
CPC Network
Lubbock, TX

Scott W. Ward, CTR, CCRA
Independent Consultant
Houston, TX

Sue A. Watkins, RHIA, RHIT, CTR
Santa Barbara City College
Solvang, CA

Ted Williamson, MD, PhD, CTR
Salem Hospital, Radiation Oncology
Salem, OR

Lisa Wise, CTR
Children's Hospital
Columbus, OH

Barbara Zaranek, CTR
Dana-Farber Cancer Institute
Boston, MA

chapter

INTRODUCTION TO CANCER REGISTRIES

Rosemarie E. Clive
LPN, CTR

INTRODUCTION

Although the incidence and mortality of cancer have continued to decline, the disease affects the lives of millions of Americans whether they are patients, family, or friends. More than 16 million patients with cancer have been diagnosed in the United States since 1990. The American Cancer Society (ACS) estimated that 1.3 million new cancer patients would be diagnosed in 2002[1]. This projection did not include in situ cancers of most sites and basal and squamous cell carcinomas (cancers) of the skin. The skin cancers total an additional 1 million cases. The National Cancer Institute (NCI) estimated that in 1997, more than 8.9 million living Americans had a history of a cancer. Presently, cancer is the second leading cause of death, accounting for one out of every four deaths in the US, up from one out of five in 1999. Nearly 550,000 people die of cancer each year—more than 1500 per day. The 5-year relative survival of all cancers combined is 62%. [1]

This previously mentioned information is typical of that comprised of data from cancer registries merged with that from vital statistics. The cancer registry also collects more detailed information about the very complex disease, cancer. These data profile the patient, the particular cancer, the treatment, and the outcome of each patient's cancer. By combining the data on many patients with similar characteristics, information is provided for both medical and public health communities.

HISTORY OF CANCER REGISTRATION

Europe: Cancer was first documented as a cause of death in 1629 in the *Bills of Mortality,* which was produced annually in England. The first known systematic collection of information on cancer was the general census of cancer in London in 1728.[2] The first reliable cancer statistics appeared in mortality figures for the city of Verona in 1842.[3] Also in the 1840s, W. H. Walshe reviewed cancer occurrence in social categories he thought to be important.[4]

United States: In 1913, the fourth annual Congress of North American Surgeons charged the Cancer Campaign Committee with the collection of data on the use of radiation therapy in the management of gynecologic malignancies. The analysis demonstrated that surgery and radiation therapy were equally effective in the management of early stage cancers of the uterine cervix. Radiation therapy provided palliation and improved survival for women with late stage cancers of the uterine cervix and corpus. The project was a successful demonstration of the use of data collection methods to monitor and evaluate patterns of outcome.[5] Nearly a decade later, Dr. Ernest Codman established the first cancer registry to track the etiology, management, and survival of patients with sarcomas of the bone. This was followed in 1925 with specialized registries for cancers of the breast, mouth, tongue, colon, and thyroid.

The Commission on Cancer (CoC) of the American College of Surgeons (ACoS) initiated clinical surveys and approval of cancer clinics in the 1930's. Although the clinics used cancer registries to collect and report data, there was no formal requirement to maintain a registry. However, many clinicians and scientists appreciated the value of comprehensive data collection. Hospitals developed their own registries in response to both the demand of physicians and the mandates of regulatory agencies that were responsible for a growing number of centralized, population-based registries. Among the first central cancer registries was the population-based Connecticut Tumor Registry. The first hospital-based cancer registry was at Yale, New Haven. In 1942, the Danish Cancer Registry became the first program to register all cases of cancer for an entire nation.[6]

In 1956, the approval standards of the CoC were revised and the cancer registries were designated as mandatory components of Commission-approved cancer programs. The End Results Program began continuous collation of cancer registry data in the 1950s.[7,8,9,10] The effort was expanded following passage of the National Cancer Act in 1971 when the Surveillance, Epidemiology, and End Results Program (SEER) was established under the umbrella of the National Cancer Institute. The SEER program began recording population-based data on cancer in selected areas in order to answer important cancer research questions. Initially these areas represented approximately 11% of the US population.[11] Currently, the SEER Program covers approximately 14% of the US population (www.seer.cancer.gov).

Over the next two decades, additional states implemented population-based registries to collect and analyze incidence to support their cancer control and epidemiology programs. There was a corresponding increase in the number of hospital-based registries which collected the cancer data required by state registries along with other clinically focused data necessary for monitoring patterns of patient management, disease recurrence, and outcome.

Federal, state, and local leadership; clinicians; and the public expressed a growing need to expand the monitoring of cancer incidence and cancer control effort. The US Congress enacted Public Law 102-515 in October 1992; the Cancer Registries Amendment Act established the National Program of Cancer Registries (NPCR).[12] This legislation authorized the Centers for Disease Control and Prevention (CDC) to enhance centralized cancer registry operations in all states and to establish central cancer registries where they did not previously exist. The initial aims were to stimulate centralized data collection in states without population-based registries and assist existing state registries in broadening their capabilities. Minimum standards for completeness, timeliness, and quality were defined for all NPCR-supported central registries. Currently the NPCR supports state central registries representing approximately 93% of the US population (www.cdc.gov/cancer/NPCR). In selected states, there is a blending of the reporting effort between SEER and NPCR central registries. For example, metropolitan Detroit and Atlanta are SEER registries and provide data on one or more representative populations. The states of Michigan and Georgia are NPCR state central registries as they collect data on the entire population of those states. In November 2002, the National Cancer Institute and the Centers of Disease Control issued a joint report on cancer in the US.[13] The history of cancer information is summarized in Table 1-1.

CANCER REGISTRIES AND CANCER CONTROL

Cancer registries exist in a wide range of settings and function within varying organizational structures, including hospitals, diagnostic and treatment facilities, research centers, laboratories, and other cancer-related entities. They may be independent or part of a corporate group, publicly or government supported in the private sector. The expectations of these supporting entities differ. However, cancer registration is a quantifiable, organized process by which data are systematically collected. These specifics are

Table 1-1

History of Cancer Information

- 1629   Bills Of Mortality (England)
- 1728   General Cancer Census (London)
- 1842   Cancer Mortality Statistics (Verona)
- 1840s   Social Categories and Cancer (Walshe)
- 1913   Cancer Campaign Committee (ACoS), Chicago
- 1923   Bone Sarcoma Registry (Codman)
- 1930   Survey and Approval Cancer Clinics (ACoS)
- 1932   Connecticut State Cancer Registry
- 1932   Yale-New Haven Hospital first approved hospital cancer program
- 1942   Danish National Cancer Registry
- 1956   Commission on Cancer requires registry in CoC-approved programs
- 1950s   End Results Program initiates collection of regional data
- 1971   National Cancer Act
- 1973   Surveillance, Epidemiology, and End Results Program
- 1974   National Cancer Registration founded
- 1983   NCRA certification and recredentialing implemented
- 1989   National Cancer Data Base
- 1990   North American Association of Central Cancer Registries
- 1992   Cancer Registries Amendment Act
- 1992   National Program of Cancer Registries

included in the fundamental data set: 1) occurrence of cancer (incidence); 2) types of cancer (site, morphology, and behavior); 3) extent of disease at the time of diagnosis (stage); 4) kinds of treatment received by the patients; and 5) outcomes of treatment (survival). The registry unit is the on-site access to cancer data. The data from registries are reported to state central registries, such as those involved in the SEER program or the NPCR. Cancer registries in CoC-approved cancer programs are required to report their data to the National Cancer Data Base (NCDB).

A time- and labor-intensive effort, cancer registration begins with the identification of cancer patients (casefinding) who have been diagnosed or received medical care in hospitals, clinics, radiology departments, surgical facilities, doctors' offices, or other healthcare settings. Detailed information about the patient, the cancer, and its treatment is retrieved (abstracted) from a wide range of sources including health records, appointment logs, pathology and laboratory records, medical facility billing departments, administrative records, and other sources of cancer information. These data are obtained, stored, and analyzed under strict standards of patient confidentiality. At the registry unit level (hospital, clinic, treatment centers, etc.), the cancer registrars continue to monitor patients annually throughout their lifetimes (active follow-up). The data from annual follow-up identifies patients who have a recurrence of their initial cancer (primary) or who are diagnosed with another cancer. It also permits registries to record data about additional treatments, progression, or remission of disease, and the vital status of patients.

Cancer information is translated into an abbreviated or coded statement using standardized rules of data collection. The data are entered into computer software designed specifically for cancer registration. The software is available commercially or may be developed by the facility. A standard format for data fields, coding, edit checks, reports, and data transmission are part of all such software. The consistency and quality of the data are validated (editing) through a series of quality control methods including: 1) computerized edit checks; 2) visual review; 3) chart comparison; 4) cross-abstracting; and 5) editing at the state and national levels of the individual registry and the merged data. Each patient-cancer record must pass edits before it can be accessed for analysis or transmission to state and other reporting sources.

The ultimate goal of the analysis of cancer data is to prevent and control cancer, including the improvement of cancer patient care. The modern cancer registry is an important resource of information for healthcare providers, public health officials,

administrators and others and is widely used by clinicians, scientists, and health services investigators. Examples of the uses of cancer registry data in cancer control include, but are not limited to 1) assisting physicians in assessing the efficacy of diagnostic and therapeutic methods; 2) aiding in decision-making about unmet healthcare needs, physician recruitment, space needs, resource allocation, and health planning; and 3) responding to local needs concerning referral patterns, cancer trends, and development opportunities (Figure 1-1).

CANCER REGISTRAR EDUCATION

Education has a significant influence on the quality of cancer registry operations. The educational opportunities for cancer registrars have evolved slowly since the 1950s, from non-systematic and informal programs and scarce educational references and materials to today's organized, well documented, and technologically sophisticated programs as well as locally available formal education resources. Three organizations have led the effort to structure and make accessible educational programs designed for cancer registrars. These include the SEER program, the CoC, and the National Cancer Registrars Association (NCRA). Other groups have added to the range of educational opportunities for cancer registrars, such as the American Cancer Society (ACS), North American Association of Central Cancer Registries (NAACCR), state and regional registrar associations, and state central registries.

SEER: Historically, the SEER program has been the source of self-instructional manuals, coding, extent of disease, and recoding references. In 2001, SEER instituted an on-line educational outlet for new, intermediate, and experienced cancer registrars. The site (www.training.seer.cancer.gov) consists of modules designed for those entering the registry pro-

Figure 1-1
Cancer Registry Information

A traditional role of the registry has been to evaluate critical outcomes and the quality of medical care. This includes assessing treatment patterns, complications, cancer recurrence, re-treatment patterns, and survival, as well as providing access to, and use of, healthcare services and resources. In addition the registry's value as a source of information to identify patient subgroups for special research studies, the modern registry may collect data on co-morbid conditions, prognostic indicators, healthcare coverage, and patient eligibility and participation in clinical trials.

fession, and provides more technical instruction on major changes in registry coding, staging, and other aspects of data collection. In addition, SEER continues to provide numerous references related to cancer registration such as coding manuals, extent of disease guides, and recoding texts. Educational workshops and meetings are conducted for personnel of SEER registries and are open to others, when appropriate. The SEER Program has a SEER Inquiry System (SINQ) on the SEER website.

Commission on Cancer: The CoC has focused its educational programs on the needs of hospital-based cancer registries. In 2002, the *Facility Oncology Data Standards (FORDS)* was published and its content required to be implemented in Commission-approved program registries for all cancers diagnosed as of January 1, 2003. The text is a reference on cancer registry data requirements and data coding standards. Ongoing educational programs include patient care evaluation studies, scientific monographs, Speakers' Bureau, videoconferences, and an on-line FORDS self-instructional training module. The CoC provides instruction for qualified individuals on a variety of topics. The CoC-prepared faculty is prepared to address current educational needs of cancer registry personnel and other individuals or groups. In addition, the CoC offers similar educational opportunities regarding the American Joint Committee on Cancer (AJCC).

The Inquiry and Response System (IRS) was implemented in 1999 and is available on-line to support inquiries for interpretation or assistance in data collection as defined by the CoC or the AJCC standards. The CoC organizes seminars where information is presented about the survey process for cancer program approval.

The on-line CoC site can be accessed through *www.facs.org*, which is also the site for the *CoC Flash*, an archive of the email newsletter on Commission- and cancer-related topics.

The National Cancer Registrars Association (NCRA): This organization represents cancer registry professionals. The Association has directed its full energies and resources to the advancement of the registry profession and the enhancement of registrar visibility and position. NCRA continues its long-standing commitment to the education of cancer registrars. The NCRA Vision Statement (Figure 1-2), Mission Statement (Figure 1-3), and the NCRA Core Values (Figure 1-4) are vital and based upon

Figure 1-2
NCRA Vision Statement

NCRA VISION STATEMENT:
Serving professionals who provide data that make a difference in the war on cancer.

Figure 1-3
NCRA Mission Statement

NCRA MISSION STATEMENT:
To promote education, credentialing, and advocacy for cancer registry professionals.

Figure 1-4
NCRA Core Values

NCRA CORE VALUES:
Networking, Mentoring, and Making a Difference.

the original statements created at the organization's founding in 1974.

Major milestones of NCRA include the development of educational standards, a formal certification program,[14] mandatory continuing education,[15] a code of ethics,[16] and regional and annual national educational programs for cancer registrars. A process for approval of formal education programs is in place.[17] The Association publishes the peer-reviewed *Journal of Registry Management* and *The Connection,* a quarterly newsletter. The educational standards of NCRA address the fundamental functions of registries, including registry organization, operations, computer principles, medical sciences, data utilization, abstracting, coding, staging, communication skills, statistics, and epidemiology.

These educational standards are also reflected in the Association's certification program, which was introduced in 1983. Today, there are more than 3,400 Certified Tumor Registrars (CTRs). Interested candidates must possess specific qualifications to be eligible to sit for the examination. Those who successfully pass the examination are entitled to use the CTR credential, and are required to meet continuing education requirements to maintain that credential. In 1994, the certification process was transferred to an independent body, the National Board of Certification of Registrars, which in 2002 was reorganized as the Council on Certification. The Council is comprised of seven elected, voting members and other appointed non-voting members as needed to conduct the business of certification body. Inquiries about the CTR process can be sent to www/ctrexam@ncra-usa.org.

The annual meeting of NCRA offers programs designed to meet the educational needs of registrars (members and non-members) with varying levels of experience. In addition to plenary sessions, a comprehensive array of educational courses is offered. Additional resources are devoted to the needs of individual registrars through regional workshops and ongoing communication with state and regional cancer registrars associations. Numerous publications are directed at the educational interests and advancement of the registry professional. Regional and state registrar associations as well as special interest groups, such as veterans hospitals, military hospitals, research and trauma registries, software providers, and independent consulting firms, interface with NCRA to provide accessible and comprehensive education that matches the specific needs of the individual cancer registrar. These varied activities have enhanced the knowledge base and abilities of cancer registrars and have greatly improved the quality and sophistication of cancer registries.

CANCER REGISTRY DATA STANDARDIZATION

As the cancer registration process and the state and national reporting requirements have evolved, the critical need for uniformity and consistency have expanded. The North American Association of Central Cancer Registries (NAACCR) established national standards for completeness, timeliness, and quality of cancer registry data. Current versions of the standards are available on-line at www.naaccr.org.

Since all three standard-setting organizations (CoC, SEER, and National Program of Cancer Registries [NPCR]) represent varying registry interests, (hospital based [CoC-NCDB], population-based sampling [SEER-NCI], and population-based state central registries [NPCR-CDC]), the NAACCR initiated an effort to standardize and document in a single reference the requirements of all three groups. Since that initial effort, NAACCR has continued as the arbitrator for merged standards. Among the objectives of the standardization were: 1) to improve state-to-state comparability; 2) to enhance the representativeness of data; 3) to increase the data accuracy; 4) to make information more rapidly available; and 5) to reduce or eliminate conflicts in the data requirements and standards among the standard-setting organizations. Cancer registrars were the fulcrum of this initiative as they were and continue to be the instrument which collects cancer patient data.

CANCER REGISTRAR AND CANCER CONTROL

Cancer registries are an integral component of cancer control and the cancer registrar is an active member of the cancer team, preparing and presenting data for cancer conferences, grand rounds, tumor boards, and planning meetings. With the escalating demands of managed care organizations, insurers, and healthcare agencies to validate quality of care as a component of healthcare reform and contract negotiations, the registrar's role has expanded exponentially. Registrars provide the data that permits scientists, clinicians, health officials, and others to assess the needs, efficacy, and outcomes of cancer control initiatives, including cancer patient management. In addition to the value of the data to the individual institution, collection of cancer data at the point of service, e.g., hospital, clinic, doctor's office, laboratory, etc., is key to cost-effective monitoring of the frequency of occurrence and the pattern of diagnosis and treatment at local, state and national levels. Overall cancer registrars are the trustees of cancer data, ensuring its accuracy, completeness, and timely reporting while at the same time protecting the privacy of cancer patients. The registry network of information sources and the ability of the cancer registrar to integrate these disparate sources into a comprehensive data and information resource assist in the transfer of new knowledge into daily practice and in the conduct of special studies.

Registrars bridge the information gap caused by the shift from an inpatient to an outpatient care delivery system by retrieving complete information about patients and the management of their malignancies. Cancer registrars are irreplaceable, essential links between cancer care and rational cancer control. Cancer registrars are the lifeblood of cancer registries and the backbone of local, state, and national cancer surveillance and cancer control programs in the United States.

ONGOING REGISTRY AND REGISTRAR ISSUES

As registrars develop their education and experience, the medical profession and technology advance swiftly, requiring cancer registrars to continually hone their base of knowledge. Additionally, the scope and shape of the data requirements, staging, and coding are also affected by changing medical technology and science. The standard-setting organizations respond with revisions to their standards. This is an inevitable concern for cancer registrars, as with each alteration there is a learning curve, software changes, and additional tweaking that affect productivity and data quality in significant ways.

Implementing new standards is a major production. Documentation of the standards and case examples are part of the process. The standard-setting organization sends specifications to software providers in advance of going live with data collection. Revamped or new applications of registry software require reprogramming by the providers, along

with alpha and beta testing. Existing databases are converted to the new format and outliers dealt with appropriately. Standardized specifications and conversion tables are prepared. On a parallel track, changes in requirements are sent to the NAACCR Uniform Data Standards Committee and to a similar committee on the standardized data transmission format. A national educational effort is mounted to aid in the rapid transfer of information and deal with concerns and questions. This is and will be an ongoing issue for cancer registries.

Of greater concern is the financial pressure experienced by healthcare facilities and providers, who support the registry as part of their commitment to quality patient care or as a requirement of CoC-approval. Without this network of support, the ability to collect detailed, quality data to support local, state, and national needs would not likely be sustained. The registrar is often required to juggle increasing data collection and reporting burdens, with little or no staff. Add to this the ongoing issue of a limited understanding of the value and purpose of the cancer registry, and the registrar must struggle to do more and more with less and less.

This financial crunch also affects the registrar's ability to access and participate in educational programs designed to facilitate and improve data management or to maintain the CTR credential. The pendulum has swung back to the 1970s when "tumor" registrars were given time off but required to pay all education and membership costs. Modern registrars are more adequately compensated than the registrars of the seventies, but are often not given the time off to attend educational sessions. Creative ways to provide educational resources continue to spring up and include regional programs offered on Saturdays, teleconferencing, and web-accessible training.

Registrars are responsive to the demand of administrators, product line managers, surgeons, physicians, nurses, rehabilitation teams, social workers, investigators, public health and regulatory agencies, and accrediting organizations. The multiple-master complex is a real and frustrating condition for the registrar. On one hand, their employer demands that the registry give priority to their internal needs and to those required for CoC approval. Additional priorities often exist for research, marketing, and other special interests. The CoC requires an expanded data set beyond that needed in an incidence registry, including annual follow up, a minimum lost-to-follow-up rate, participation in patient care evaluation studies, and annual reporting to the NCDB. On the other hand, SEER and NPCR population-based central registries focus on incidence data and may have different data, coding, and staging standards than those of CoC or research programs. Getting caught in the crossfire can seriously impact the registrar's position. The combined efforts of NAACCR, CoC, NPCR, and SEER have reduced some of the disparities. Several states have instituted registrar-state committees or discussion groups to encourage cooperation and communication.

Recognition and compensation continue to be of concern to the registrar. Both issues have improved significantly over the past 20 years, but more needs to be done if registrars and the value of cancer registries are to be fully appreciated.

Many institutions have implemented various strategies to deal with backlogs in cancer registry abstracting and follow up. Often a contractor-abstractor is retained to catch up the workload. In other situations, overtime is authorized or additional non-registrar personnel are used. A consistent registry issue is designing a user-friendly, factual report on staffing needs. References to the CoC requirements, the *NCRA-CoC Staffing and Compensation Manual* (reference) may be shrugged off by employer and registrar alike, as too general and not specific for their situation. Comparisons may be made between the productivity of a contract abstractor with that of existing registry staff. Verbal responses as to the other duties conducted by registry staff may go unrecognized. In some instances, there may be internal productivity issues. Exploration of a more useful tool, including assessment of the depth and difficulty of institution-specific data collection should be considered as another variable in the staffing equation.

SUMMARY

The cancer registry and the cancer registrar fill a unique niche in cancer control. Building on the hospital-based registry unit, a network of standardized cancer data is captured and analyzed to expand what is known about cancer in all of its permutations. Without the support of hospitals, clinics, and other grass roots registries, the financial burden of this regional, state, and national data collection would exceed the resources available.

National standard-setting organizations continue efforts to reduce duplication of effort and minimize the differences in their respective requirements. Computerization of cancer registry data has broadened to permit the registrar to access other existing point-of-service data systems, reducing paper flow while improving completeness, accuracy, and timeliness of data collection.

Registrar educational opportunities expand to keep pace with advancing technology as budgetary and work demands escalate—a challenge for the future for registries and registrars.

Cancer registrars have a unique perspective about the occurrence and management of cancer in a given institution that no one else has. The cancer registrar is usually the only person to review detailed information on *every* cancer patient diagnosed and/or treated at a particular medical facility. As such, the cancer registrar could be considered an *expert* on cancer.

STUDY QUESTIONS

1. What is the ultimate goal of cancer registration?
2. List three methods of quality control of registry data.
3. What organizations have led the way in registrar education?
4. What are the major milestones of the National Cancer Registrars Association?
5. List four ongoing issues in cancer registration.

REFERENCES

1. CANCER *Facts and Figures*–2002. Atlanta, Ga: American Cancer Society; 2002.
2. Clemmensen J. Statistical studies in the aetiology of malignant neoplasms. *Acta Pathologica Microbiologica Scandinavica (Suppl)*. 1965; 1741: 2-3.
3. Stern R. Fatti statistici relativi alla malattie cancerose. *Giornali per Servire al Progressi della Patologica e della Terapeutica*. 1842; 2: 407-17.
4. Walshe WH. *The Nature and Treatment of Cancer*. London: Taylor and Walton; 1846.
5. Brennan MF, Clive RE, Winchester DP. *The CoC: Its Roots and Destiny*. Chicago, Ill: American College of Surgeons; 1994.
6. Jensen OM, Storm HH, and Jensen HS, *Cancer Registration in Denmark and the Study of Multiple Primary Cancers*. National Cancer Institute Monograph 68. Bethesda, Md: National Cancer Institute; 1985: pp. 245-51.

7. Axtell LM, Asire AJ, Myers M, eds. *Cancer Patient Survival.* DHEW Publication NIH 77-992. Bethesda, Md: National Cancer Institute; 1975.

8. Cutler SJ, Young JL Jr., eds. *Third National Cancer Survey: Incidence Data.* National Cancer Institute Monograph 41. Bethesda, Md: National Cancer Institute; 1975.

9. Dorn HF. Illness from cancer in the United States. *Public Health Report 59.* 1944: 33-48, 65-77, 97-115.

10. Dorn HF, Cutler SJ. *Morbidity from Cancer in the United States,* parts I and II. Washington, DC: US Department of Health, Education, and Welfare and Public Health Service; 1959.

11. Ries, L, Pollack ES, Young JL Jr. *Cancer Patient Survival: Surveillance, Epidemiology, and End Results Program,* 1973-79. National Cancer Institute Monograph 70(4). Bethesda, Md: National Cancer Institute; 1983: 693-707.

12. Cancer Registries Amendment Act, Public Law 102-515. *Congressional Record* 138, 106 STAT 3372-3377; 1992.

13. Garguillo P, Edwards BK, et al, eds. *United States Cancer Statistics: 1999 Incidence.* Bethesda, Md: Centers for Disease Control, Atlanta, Ga and National Cancer Institute; 2002.

14. Council on Certification of Cancer Registrars. *Handbook for Candidates, Certification Examination for Cancer Registrars.* In press: National Cancer Registrars Association 2003.

15. National Cancer Registrars Association (NCRA). *Continuing Education Requirements,* revised edition, Alexandria, Va: NCRA; 2002.

16. National Cancer Registrars Association (NCRA). *Guide to the Interpretation of the Code of Ethics,* revised edition. Alexandria, Va: NCRA; 2002.

17. National Cancer Registrars Association (NCRA). *Essentials for Formal Education.* Alexandria, Va: NCRA; 2001.

chapter
2

THE NATIONAL CANCER REGISTRARS ASSOCIATION, INC.

Ryan Intlekofer
RN, CTR

INTRODUCTION

The National Cancer Registrars Association, Inc. (NCRA) is a nonprofit professional association for cancer registrars. NCRA promotes accurate, timely data and advances professional development. The purpose of NCRA is to provide educational opportunities for continuous learning; advance knowledge of all new technologies that influence cancer data; establish standards on education; promote the value of the certified registry professional; and support professional standards and ethics (Table 2-1).[1] There currently are over 3,500 national and international members of NCRA. The NCRA annual budget is approximately 1,000,000 dollars.

HISTORY

The National Cancer Registrars Association, Inc. was chartered in May 1974 and incorporated in October 1976. Prior to that time, registrars worked with little support in the field. Based on what was seen as a real need to expand the profession and commitment to providing adequate education and training for registrars, a dedicated group of cancer registry professionals held the first meeting of the National Tumor Registrars Association (NTRA) in Dallas, Texas in May 1974. An integral part of that early vision was to develop educational standards for registrars and design a certification process. In 1983, the first credentialing process was implemented, and the credential Certified Tumor Registrar (CTR[TM]) was bestowed on those who met the qualifications and passed the credentialing examination. Since that time the association has experienced continued growth and change. In 1992, the association underwent a name change to the National Cancer Registrars Association, Inc., and in May 2001, NCRA hired paid staff and established its own headquarters office for the first time.

Table 2-1
NCRA Vision, Core Values, and Mission Statement

- Vision: Serving professionals who provide data that make a difference in the war on cancer.
- Core Values: Networking, Mentoring, and Making a Difference.
- Mission: To promote education, credentialing, and advocacy for cancer registry professionals.

MEMBERSHIP

As a multidisciplinary organization, membership is open to all individuals involved in cancer registry activities. Membership is by individual status, not organizational affiliation. The membership year is the calendar year, January 1 through December 31. All memberships are on an individual basis and cannot be transferred from one individual to another. NCRA maintains eight membership categories: Active, Associate, Student, Sustaining, Honorary Life, Honorary, Inactive and International (see Table 2-2).

GOVERNANCE

Board of Directors

A 12-member volunteer board of directors is elected from the membership to provide governance for NCRA. These include officers who are president, vice president, secretary, treasurer, president-elect, and immediate past president. The remainder of the board is comprised of six regional directors, one junior director, and one senior director from each region—East, Midwest and West. Eligibility requirements and duties of each office are outlined in the corporation bylaws. Election is done by mail ballot.

The president-elect, vice-president, secretary, and junior regional director are elected for a term of one year. Every other year the treasurer is elected for a term of two years. Upon expiration of the president-elect's term, he or she will become president for a term of one year. Upon expiration of the junior regional director's term, he or she will become the senior regional director for a term of one year. Upon expiration of the president's term, he or she will serve as immediate past president for one year and will chair the Governance Planning and Evaluation Committee.

Representatives

The Council on Certification consists of an administrator and six representatives. These are elected positions to administer and manage NCRA's certification program.

To be eligible for the office of the Council on Certification Representative, the active CTR certificant shall have a minimum of three years experience as a Certified Tumor Registrar (CTR[TM]) and shall not hold employment in any educational services related field that provides education to future regis-

Table 2-2
NCRA Membership Categories

- Active: An active member shall be a Certified Tumor Registrar or a person whose primary occupation is involved with any or all facets of cancer registry work. An active member in good standing shall be entitled to all membership privileges including the right to vote, hold office, and chair or serve on a committee.
- Associate: An associate member shall be any person interested in the purpose of the corporation who does not meet the qualifications of any other membership category. A Certified Tumor Registrar who is no longer active in the field may apply for associate membership. An associate member shall not vote, hold office, or chair a committee, but may serve on a committee.
- Student: A student member shall be a person who is enrolled in a college level curriculum and is interested in the purpose of the corporation, but who does not meet the qualifications for active membership. A student member shall be eligible for this classification for no more than five years from the date the member first joined in this category. A student member shall not vote, hold office, or chair a committee, but may serve on a committee.
- Sustaining: A sustaining member shall be any person, institution, or organization interested in promoting the purpose of the corporation. A sustaining member shall not vote, hold office, or chair or serve on a committee.
- Honorary Life: Past presidents shall become honorary life members at age 60. They shall retain all privileges of active membership without payment of dues or annual conference registration fees. An honorary life member shall not hold any other class of membership in the corporation.
- Honorary: Persons other than past presidents who have made a significant contribution to the profession of Cancer Registry Administration or have rendered distinguished service in the profession or its related fields may be elected to honorary membership by a unanimous vote of the corporation's active members present and voting, after recommendation by the Board of Directors. Honorary members shall be exempt from dues. Honorary members shall not vote, hold office, or chair or serve on a committee. Honorary members shall not hold any other class of membership in the corporation.
- Inactive: An individual who previously qualified as an active member but is no longer in the work force is eligible to be an inactive member. An inactive member shall not vote, hold office, or chair a committee, but may serve on a committee. This category includes retirees, unemployed persons, and persons on extended leave from their job.
- International: Any person who is not a resident of a North American country may elect to be an international member. Persons residing outside of North America are not restricted to this membership classification. International members shall not vote, hold office, or chair a committee, but may serve on a committee.[2]

---

trars. Elected members of the Council on Certification serve a term of not more than two years and may not serve more than two consecutive terms; they do not have to hold membership in NCRA.

COMMITTEES

NCRA has multiple committees to assist in the delivery and management of various association activities. Currently, NCRA has 17 active committees. Their description and functions are given in Table 2-3.

SPECIAL INTEREST GROUPS

Registrars function in varying fields of practice; because of this diversity in membership, NCRA supports special interest groups to provide technical expertise and networking opportunities. These groups include: Hospital Registrars, Central Registrars, Federal Registrars, Pediatric Registrars, Registry Management/Clinical Trials, and Contract Registry Services. The special interest groups are given time at the NCRA annual conference to meet, select leadership, and network. The annual conference program

Table 2-3
NCRA Committees

- **Annual Conference Program Committee:** Responsible for the educational program content and arrangements for Annual Conference educational activities.
- **Awards:** Responsible to manage the selection and delivery process for the awards program to recognize individuals and their contributions in specific areas. Awards are given in the areas of education, literary, and outstanding performance of a new professional and to recognize distinguished members.
- **Continuing Education:** Administers the continuing education requirements to maintain the Certified Tumor Registrar (CTR^{TM}) credential.
- **Continuing Education Program Recognition:** Reviews submitted educational programs for validity and the enhancement of knowledge of the cancer registry professional. If it is determined that a program meets the requirements established, a clock hour value is assigned to that activity.
- **Communications:** Responsible for the NCRA publications: The *Journal of Registry Management,* the official NCRA journal, and *The Connection,* the official NCRA newsletter.
- **Education:** Identifies the ongoing educational needs of NCRA, and then makes recommendations to the Board of Directors in order to establish or enhance new and current programs and coordinates existing continuing educational programs. Subcommittees include: Alternative Methods and Educational Materials. The Alternative Methods of earning continuing education credit is responsible to develop high quality, meaningful, affordable, and easily accessed educational programs whereby the CTR^{TM} can earn CE credit hours through approved methods of self-study.
- **The Educational Materials Committee:** Responsible for development and marketing of new educational products, and for assuring that current products marketed by NCRA contain up to date information.
- **Ethics:** Reviews complaints regarding violations of the Code of Ethics of NCRA. The committee may recommend action to be taken by the Board of Directors.
- **Finance:** Chaired by the Treasurer, this committee maintains the fiscal stability of NCRA by monitoring and directing the flow of NCRA funds.
- **Formal Education:** Responsible for all formal education activities, to enhance NCRA's relationship with colleges offering cancer registry education and to ensure that standards are met. Also assists in the expansion and development of new college programs.
- **Governance Planning and Evaluation Committee:** Offers advice to the President and Board of Directors, monitors the strategic plan, and administers the NCRA annual conference scholarship fund.
- **Legislative:** Monitors legislative and regulatory initiatives in an effort to keep the membership informed of potential changes that may affect cancer registries and registrars.
- **Membership:** Oversees all membership promotion and service activities.
- Nominating: Responsible for preparation of the ballots for elected officers and representatives serving on the Council on Certification. The committee chair is appointed by the President, the other members are elected and include two members from each of three regions.
- **Public Relations:** Responsible for promotions, products, and projects that relate to NCRA's public image.
- **Website:** Oversees NCRA's web page and web presence.

---

committee strives to offer educational topics of interest related to all of these fields of practice.

LIAISONS

NCRA has formal liaisons with the American Joint Committee on Cancer, College of American Pathologists, Commission on Cancer of the American College of Surgeons, National Coordinating Council for Cancer Surveillance, and North American Association of Central Cancer Registries.

Special appointments may be made to promote NCRA or to represent NCRA members regarding special issues at specific meetings or events of to other organizations. These organizations may include: American Cancer Society, American Health and Information Management Association, Association of Cancer Executives, Association of

Clinical Oncology Administrators, Association of Community Cancer Centers, Joint Commission on Accreditation of Healthcare Organizations, and American Society of Clinical Oncologists.

ACCOMPLISHMENTS

NCRA sponsors an annual conference and regional workshops offering educational sessions designed to improve registrars' knowledge and professional expertise. The annual conference also provides an excellent networking opportunity. The regional workshops assist registrars who cannot attend the annual conference by allowing them to maintain their skills locally. The Regional Directors offer a mechanism whereby local and state associations are kept informed of activity on a national level and any local concerns are communicated back to the NCRA board for discussion and action if needed. Members are given updated information through the quarterly publication of the association newsletter, *The Connection,* and by more frequently via NCRA's website and broadcast emailing. NCRA has seven educational publications in print, and two revisions are underway.

The *Journal of Registry Management (JRM),* a scientific journal, is published quarterly by NCRA. In addition to registry management and scientific articles, the *JRM* includes another feature to improve data quality: This is the Continuing Education Quiz, which provides an easy way to maintain continuing education credit. NCRA has 10 approved programs providing formal education in cancer registry science.

The CTR^{TM} remains a standard of quality in the registry profession. The NCRA Council on Certification administers this examination process. Candidates must meet eligibility requirements that include a combination of experience in the cancer registry field and educational background. After a candidate successfully passes the certification examination, the CTR^{TM} credential is awarded. These registrars have demonstrated that they have met or exceeded the standard level of experience and knowledge required for effective performance. To maintain the CTR^{TM}, continuing educational requirements must be met. This requirement provides assurance that the registrar's knowledge and skills are continuously monitored and maintained. Governance of the credentialing process was changed with the establishment of a Council on Certification in 2002.

As mentioned above, in May 2001, NCRA hired paid staff and established a corporate office to enhance the significant volunteer effort that has been the true foundation of NCRA for 29 years.

FUTURE PLANS

In the late 1990s, NCRA's leadership made the decision that NCRA needed to change to achieve its mission. The operational structure in place at that time did not support the significant needs of the cancer registry field. NCRA had a wealth of knowledge, information, and commitment from its volunteer members, but remained unable to move forward to advance the field. To maximize the volunteer effort, NCRA moved from a management firm to hiring an Executive Director and paid staff to provide support. To further clarify NCRA's vision, a consultant was contracted to work with NCRA stakeholders to develop a business model which was implemented in 2003. Through the use of an email survey, the membership at large provided input into the process and five key areas of focus were identified. These areas included education, administration, certification, communication, and advocacy. The following goals have been established and initiated (Table 2-4).

Table 2-4
NCRA Strategic Plan Goals

Goal 1—Education: To offer comprehensive educational opportunities in a variety of media to support those in the field and to encourage entrance into the field. (Scope will include the annual meeting, regional workshops, formal education, continuing advanced education, publications, and structure).

Goal 2—Administration: To have an efficient and effective infrastructure. (Scope will include the office, Board of Directors, committees, SIG leaders, and liaisons)

Goal 3—Certification: To provide and maintain varying cancer registry credentials.

Goal 4—Communication: To maintain global communication and to foster and encourage the sharing of information.

Goal 5—Advocacy: To identify issues, assess their validity, and engage in a process to educate and affect opinion.

SUMMARY

NCRA is the professional association for the entire cancer registry field. NCRA's considerable strengths include diversity, volunteerism, staff, dedicated members, mentors, financial security, and past history, all which significantly position the association to attain the goals set out in this aggressive strategic plan. The strength of the association strengthens the members and in turn provides them with the skills and tools necessary to continue the fight against cancer.

STUDY QUESTIONS

1. List five of NCRA's committees.
2. Identify two different features the *Journal of Registry Management* provides the membership.
3. What requirements must be met before a person is allowed to take the certification exam?
4. What five goals were identified in the strategic planning process?

REFERENCES

1. The Cancer Registry and The Registrar. National Cancer Registrars Association, Inc.
2. Bylaws. National Cancer Registrars Association, Inc.

chapter **3**

THE NATIONAL PROGRAM OF CANCER REGISTRIES

Mary D. Hutton
RN, MPH, CTR

Gayle Greer Clutter
RT, CTR

PURPOSE

The National Program of Cancer Registries (NPCR) is a program of the Centers for Disease Control and Prevention (CDC) that provides funds and technical assistance to improve cancer registration and cancer surveillance throughout the United States. NPCR's goal is to build state and national capacity to: monitor the burden of cancer including the disparity among various subgroups in the population; provide data for research; evaluate cancer control activities; and plan for future healthcare needs.

BACKGROUND

In 1921, the American College of Surgeons introduced to the United States the concept of the cancer registry with the establishment of a bone sarcoma registry that was later expanded to include other types of cancer. This initiative resulted in the publication of the first standards for the evaluation of cancer clinics and registries. It also initiated clinical surveys and an approvals process for cancer clinics, and was in part responsible for the establishment of centralized, population-based cancer registries. The Connecticut Cancer Registry, which began in 1941 and registered cases back to 1935, was the first population-based central cancer registry that is still in continuous existence today.[1]

In subsequent decades, the field of cancer registration expanded and benefited from the support of many organizations and programs such as the National Cancer Institute's Surveillance, Epidemiology, and End Results Program (SEER), which began in 1973; the North American Association of Central Cancer Registries (NAACCR); the National Cancer Registrars Association, Inc. (NCRA); and the National Cancer Data Base (NCDB), which is jointly sponsored by the Commission on Cancer of the American College of Surgeons and the American Cancer Society. As recently as 1993, however, even though approximately 40 states had a central cancer registry, the data items and record layouts in most states were not standardized and few states had data of sufficient completeness and quality to use for planning and evaluating cancer control activities.[2]

NPCR BASICS

Public Law 102-515

In October 1992, in order to address the need for cancer incidence data for planning and evaluating

cancer control activities, Congress passed Public Law 102-515 (PL 102-515).[3] PL 102-515 is known as the Cancer Registries Amendment Act. From its beginnings, this law enjoyed strong grassroots support from cancer survivors and members of the registry profession. In fact, cancer registry professionals assisted in drafting and reviewing the law. The Cancer Registries Amendment Act became a major milestone for cancer registration in the United States.

This law established the NPCR and authorized CDC to:

1) Provide funds and technical assistance to improve or enhance existing statewide central cancer registries, or plan and implement statewide central cancer registries where they did not already exist;
2) Set standards for data completeness, timeliness, and quality;
3) Develop model laws and regulations for states and territories;
4) Establish a set of required data items and a uniform reporting format;
5) Provide training and support related to central registry operations.

In 1998 Congress passed additional legislation to reauthorize the program.[4]

State Laws and Regulations

Underlying the ability to continually collect population-based cancer data is the need for appropriate state laws and regulations. Therefore, PL 102-515 required that each NPCR-funded central registry be supported by a state law that authorizes the registry and regulations that provide for:

1) Complete case reporting from all facilities diagnosing or treating cancer;
2) Complete case reporting from all practitioners diagnosing or treating cancer;
3) Access to appropriate medical records;
4) A uniform set of data elements in a uniform format;
5) Protection of patient confidentiality;
6) Access to data by researchers;
7) Authorization to conduct research;
8) Protection from liability for individuals who abide by the law.

The required set of state laws and regulations provides a strong foundation for each NPCR registry and assures that the data can legally be collected and made available for program planning, evaluation, and research.

Reportable Cancers

PL 102-515 defined reportable cancer as "each form of in situ and invasive cancer (with the exception of basal cell and squamous cell carcinoma of the skin)."[3] Subsequently, in 1993, pre-invasive cervical cancer was excluded following recommendations made by a NAACCR workgroup.[5] One reason for this exclusion was a long-standing lack of agreement among experts in cancer pathology as to the exact definition of cancer in situ of the cervix as distinguished from pre-invasive conditions equivalent to or on a continuum with it. In 2002, Congress passed the Benign Brain Tumor Cancer Registries Amendment Act (PL 107-260), which added benign brain-related tumors to the list of cancers to be reported to the registries.[6]

Program Standards

NPCR's program standards (Table 3-1) are based on the requirements of PL 102-515.[3] To the extent

Table 3-1
Overview of NPCR Program Standards

Legislative	• The state has a law authorizing a statewide cancer registry.
Authority	• The state has legislation and regulations in support of all criteria specified in PL 102-515.
Data Content and Format	• The information collected or derived on cancer cases includes all data elements required by NPCR. • Data codes are consistent with those prescribed by NPCR. • The state registry uses a standardized, NPCR-recommended data exchange record layout for exchange of data.
Completeness	• Within 12 months of the close of the diagnosis year, 90% of expected, unduplicated cases of reportable cancer occurring in a state's residents are available to be counted as incident cases at the central cancer registry. • Within 24 months of the close of the diagnosis year, 95% of expected, unduplicated cases of reportable cancer occurring in a state's residents are available to be counted as incident cases at the central cancer registry. • Within 24 months of the close of the diagnosis year, the state has performed death clearance and followback, and 3% or fewer of the cases in the database are reported by death certificate only. • Within 24 months of the close of the diagnosis year, 1 (or fewer) duplicate cases per 1,000 are present in the database.
Timeliness	• Because NPCR completeness standards include a time requirement, standards for timeliness are the same as those for completeness.
Quality	• Within 12 months of the close of the diagnosis year, 97% of the cases pass an NPCR-prescribed set of standard data edits. • Within 24 months of the close of the diagnosis year, 99% of the cases pass an NPCR-prescribed set of standard data edits.
Annual Report	• Within 12 months of the close of the diagnosis year the state produces an annual report with data that are at least 90% complete. The report can be in either hardcopy or electronic format. Minimum content should include site-specific age-adjusted incidence and mortality rates by sex, race, and ethnicity for selected cancer sites as appropriate.
Data Use	• The central cancer registry, health department, or designee use registry data for planning and evaluation of cancer control objectives. • Within 24 months of the close of the diagnosis year, an analytic data set that meets NPCR standards for data completeness and quality is available for research purposes.

possible, NPCR adopted standards already established by the SEER Program or recommended by NAACCR. However, there are several standards that are unique to NPCR. NPCR-funded states, the District of Columbia, and territories (referred to in the rest of this chapter as "NPCR states") are required to meet program standards. Each state's progress in meeting the standards is reviewed at least annually.

Reporting Areas

In 1994, 37 states were the first to participate in NPCR. By 1997 and through the present, 45 states, the District of Columbia, and 3 territories have been participating in the program (Figure 3-1). NPCR registries cover 96% of the U.S. population. NCI's SEER Program funds cancer registration in the 5 states not participating in NPCR and also provides supplemental funds to 4 NPCR states. In addition, SEER funds 6 large metropolitan areas within NPCR states. These metropolitan areas report data to both SEER and the state registry. The SEER program covers 26% of the U.S. population. For more information, see the SEER chapter.

NPCR Cancer Surveillance System

In 2001, for the first time, CDC received state data (with personal identifiers removed) for entry into the

NPCR Cancer Surveillance System (NPCR-CSS). The NPCR-CSS processes and evaluates the data and provides feedback to state registries on their completeness and quality. In addition, NPCR-CSS disseminates the data in the form of reports that track national and regional progress in reducing the burden of cancer. *United States Cancer Statistics* is one such report (www.cdc.gov/cancer/npcr/uscs/).[7] *United States Cancer Statistics* was first published in November 2002 and is updated annually. CDC's NPCR-CSS is currently developing public-use and restricted-access data files for release with appropriate safeguards for protecting confidentiality.

NPCR ACTIVITIES

Funding, Technical Assistance, and Training

A major task of NPCR is providing funds to state and territorial health departments. These funds supplement funds provided by the state health department: each state must contribute 1 dollar for every 3 NPCR dollars they receive. In addition, each state must continue to fund the registry with state dollars at the same level at which it was funded during the year before the state first received NPCR funds. These requirements reduce the likelihood that state support of the registry will be reduced, even in times

Figure 3-1

State and Metropolitan Area Cancer Registries by Current Federal Funding Source, 2003.

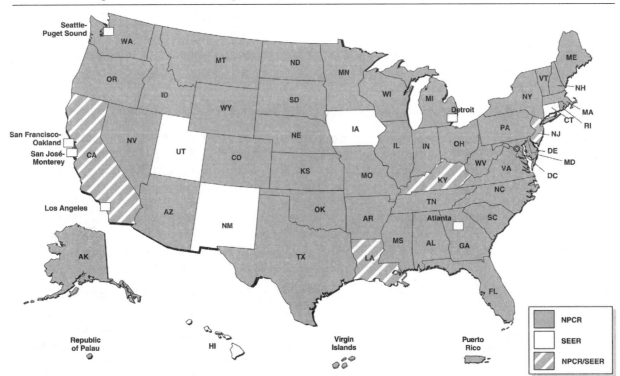

of scarce resources. Between 1994 and 2002, the average annual NPCR award made to each state health department or its designee was $386,394. The central registry uses these funds to meet NPCR standards for data completeness, timeliness, and quality and to improve cancer registration throughout the state. CDC also provides funds to national organizations, such as NCRA, NAACCR, and the College of American Pathologists. Examples of projects that have received funds from CDC are NAACCR's annual certification of registries that have high quality data and NCRA's annual meeting.

CDC's NPCR staff members have a wide range of professional experience and include certified cancer registrars, nurses, physicians, health scientists such as epidemiologists, specialists in information technology and program evaluation, computer programmers, data analysts, and business administration professionals. Staff members provide guidance to grantees and others regarding program standards and funding requirements and carry out a broad range of special projects, some of which are described below. CDC's NPCR staff members also provide technical assistance directly to funded registries through site visits and consultations and indirectly through participation in NAACCR and NCRA committees.

NPCR has responded to the educational needs of its funded programs by sponsoring a series of national and regional workshops on topics such as death clearance. Topics selected for these workshops result from needs identified through audits, consultation with state registries and NAACCR committees, NPCR program evaluation results, and assessment of central registry data that are submitted to CDC. Recently sponsored events include the "East" and "West" basic registry training institutes provided by NAACCR. CDC also provides funds to national organizations such as NAACCR and NCRA for developing their own training programs and educational materials consistent with NPCR's goals and objectives. NPCR-sponsored training materials have been used as references in the central registry and as resources for hospitals submitting cancer data. In addition, CDC supports organizational websites where educational materials can be found, such as the NAACCR website, www.naaccr.org.

Quality Assurance

High quality data are essential for achievement of NPCR's goals. Therefore, quality assurance is a critical priority for NPCR. Recognizing that all aspects of a registry's operations impact data quality, NPCR requires funded registries to comply with established data quality standards such as the standardized data items and codes that are agreed upon by NAACCR members.[5,8] NPCR central registries are required to have periodic external audits that are funded by CDC through a contract. The audits provide information about the completeness and quality of data from a randomly selected group of reporting facilities in the state. Additionally, NPCR staff members evaluate the quality of data that state registries submit annually to the NPCR-CSS and provide feedback to states in data evaluation reports.

Computer Software

CDC has developed a number of software applications to improve data quality, all of which are available at no charge to the cancer registry community. One such product is EDITS. EDITS is a software application that can be used by cancer registries to apply automated edits to a dataset. Automated edits allow the computer to check the validity of certain data items. For example, if a patient was diagnosed with cancer in 1998 and their birthdate is recorded as 1999, an edit error would be produced because the combination of these responses is not logical. The EDITS software package can apply edits at the reporting facility or at the central registry or elsewhere, and can be run either interactively at the point of data collection or in batch mode after the data are collected.

The automated edits that are most often used by cancer registries were initially developed by the SEER program in another form and later incorporated into the EDITS system. NAACCR maintains standardized edits based on requirements of SEER, CDC, and the American College of Surgeons. The American College of Surgeons' National Cancer Data Base uses EDITS to validate data submissions from facilities. NAACCR and CDC have used EDITS to evaluate data submitted by central registries to their Calls for Data. EDITS, and the standardized edits maintained by NAACCR, are widely used in cancer registry software products. EDITS software has other uses in addition to applying automated edits; it has been used to create record layouts, specify algorithms, logic and documentation, and maintain look-up tables. More information on EDITS can be found at www.cdc.gov/cancer/edits.htm. The standardized edits maintained by NAACCR can be found at www.NAACCR.org.

Another software application developed and supported by CDC is a suite of software programs known as *Registry Plus. Registry Plus* applications include:

- *Abstract Plus,* a program used to produce electronic abstracts of cancer cases for submission to state central registries;
- *Registry Plus Online Help,* a stand-alone HTML Help application that contains the text of standard coding manuals including the Commission on Cancer's FORDS, the NAACCR data dictionary, the SEER code manual and EOD manual, and ICD-O-3. These help files can be used alone without other executable programs;
- *GenEDITS Lite,* a Visual Basic program offering a modern and simple graphical interface for use with EDITS that is used in numerous locations throughout the United States.
- *Prep Plus, CRS Plus, and Registry Plus Utilities* which are used for managing data in central cancer registries;
- *Link Plus* (now in the later stages of development) which will assist with linking cancer registry records to other data sources.

More information on CDC software applications for managing cancer data is available at: www.cdc.gov/cancer/npcr.

Annual Call for Data

Central registries supported by NPCR submit cancer incidence data (with personal identifiers removed) to NPCR-CSS each year. Since 2000, this data submission has occurred during the month of January. After CDC receives the data, they are processed through standardized edit programs and reviewed for completeness and quality; NPCR then produces a set of data evaluation reports for each state. CDC uses the cancer incidence data to review and report on the burden of cancer in the nation, and to provide aggregate data to national organizations and for public use. National organizations that use these data include the American Cancer Society for its regional cancer control planning activities, and the National Cancer Institute, for the State Cancer Profiles Project www.statecancerprofiles.cancer.gov/, which is a collaborative project with CDC. NPCR is currently developing procedures for releasing web-accessible public-use data and confidential data for researchers.

Publications

United States Cancer Statistics is a publication coauthored by CDC and NCI in collaboration with NAACCR. The first edition of this report, entitled *United States Cancer Statistics: 1999 Incidence (USCS),* was published in November 2002.[7] Annual updates are anticipated. The report summarizes the incidence of cancer for the United States and by state and U.S. census region, by site, race (white, black, all races), and sex for the 1999 diagnosis year. Cancer incidence data on more than 1 million cancer cases from central cancer registries in 37 states, 6 SEER metropolitan areas, and the District of Columbia (areas representing more than 78% of the U.S. population) met the quality criteria required for inclusion in this volume. It is anticipated that coverage of the U.S. population will increase in future years as data from more central registries meet the required data quality criteria. Planning for future editions is in progress, and it is expected that future editions will include topics such as childhood cancer, cancer among other racial and ethnic groups, and cancer mortality. Hard copies of the 2002 publication are available from NPCR, or it can be viewed on the Web at www.cdc.gov/cancer/npcr/uscs/.

NPCR does not publish a program manual. Program requirements are described in the program's announcement of funds. In addition, to the extent which is possible, NPCR requires compliance with previously established registry standards, such as those developed by SEER or recommended by NAACCR. NPCR staff members have prepared publications on a number of topics, including a recent review of the implications of collecting birthplace of cancer patients[9] and a comparison of cancer incidence in the total geographic areas covered by SEER and NPCR registries.[10]

Research

Data from the central cancer registry provide an important resource for research. Because the central cancer registry collects data on all cases of cancer occurring in the state, the data are population-based. Population-based data have an advantage for research because they can be used to make decisions about all similar at-risk persons in the population or in a well-defined subgroup of that population, such as a minority group or a group living in a medically underserved region of the state.[11] Most NPCR-funded state registries with high quality data make the data available for research. In addition, CDC collaborates with state registries and researchers to conduct research projects designed to improve cancer registry methods and data quality and to enhance cancer treatment and survival (Table 3-2).

Evaluation of State and National Progress

CDC evaluates the progress of funded states each year by means of the NPCR program evaluation. States have made substantial progress since 1994 in meeting the program objectives and standards, as shown by an analysis of states' progress from 1994 to 1999.[12] In 1994, 41 (80%) states had a population-based central cancer registry and in 1999 that number had increased to 50 (98%). In 1994, the percentage of states that had a law authorizing formation of the cancer registry was 39 (85%), and in 1999 this increased to 44 (96%). However, in 1994, only 15 (33%) of the states had legislation authorizing the registry and regulations that supported all eight requirements specified by PL 102-515; by 1999 this had increased to 38 (83%).

Table 3-2
Selected National Program of Cancer Registries Research Activities

---

- **Patterns of Care Study: Prostate, Colon, Breast, and Ovarian Cancers:** NPCR is conducting four studies to compare the quality of treatment and stage data reported to 10 NPCR registries with re-abstracted data from the corresponding medical record. These studies also will use population-based samples to estimate the proportion of patients in each state who received the recommended standard of care. In addition, patterns of care for localized prostate and breast cancer and stage III colon cancer will be described according to patient and disease characteristics, comorbid conditions, and insurance coverage. For ovarian cancer, both outcome and staging will be assessed according to physician specialty.

- **The CONCORD Study:** The CONCORD study will measure and explore differences in cancer survival among cancer patients in Europe, Canada, and the United States. The study focuses on breast, prostate, and colorectal cancers. Population-based cancer registries in 17 NPCR-supported programs, 6 Canadian provinces, and 16 European countries are participating. The study will explore the extent to which international differences in cancer survival can be attributed to differences in tumor biology, disease definition, stage at diagnosis, treatment, healthcare systems, or other factors. Results of Phase I of the CONCORD study are anticipated in 2003.

- **New York State Cancer Registry—Feasibility Study of Cancer Survival:** Most population-based cancer registries in the United States do not have the resources needed to conduct active follow-up on cancer cases, resulting in little information about cancer survival. This study assesses whether the use of administrative databases to augment follow-up provides the necessary data for conducting survival analyses. Costs for linkages are also being assessed. Results from this project are expected in spring 2003.

- **Strategies for Implementing Pathology Protocols—Reporting Colon and Rectum Cancers:** The College of American Pathology developed and published Standardized Reporting Protocols in 1998 to help the surgical pathologist achieve completeness, accuracy, and uniformity in collecting and reporting pathology-related tumor data. CDC has funded two state registries (California and Ohio) to work with selected pathology laboratories to evaluate the use of structured data entry for pathology reports for cancers of the colon and rectum that are submitted to cancer registries.

- **Data Linkage with the Indian Health Service:** Previously documented misclassification of American Indians and Alaska Natives in cancer registry data affects cancer statistics for these populations, as well as program planning for cancer prevention and control efforts. The Indian Health Service (IHS) and CDC are conducting a one-year data linkage project to help registries more accurately describe the burden of cancer among these populations. Data from 25 state registries in the NPCR will be linked with data from the IHS patient registration records to improve the classification of American Indian/Alaska Native races in the registries. Preliminary results are anticipated in late 2003.

Another area of significant change can be noted in the collection of uniform data elements in a standardized format. In 1994, only four (9%) states collected information for all of the NPCR required data elements. This number increased to 32 (70%) by 1999. In 1994, 17 states (37%) used the NAACCR data exchange record layout for importing and exporting data, which increased to 45 (98%) by 1999. Other program areas that demonstrated improvements over the five-year period were the number of states performing death clearance, using automated data edits, conducting casefinding and reabstracting audits, and having an independent audit of the state central cancer registry.[12] NPCR added objectives for data use in preparation for its second 5-year project period and improvements are being seen now in that area as well.

Another indication of progress in cancer registration in NPCR states can be seen in results of the NACCR registry certification program. In 1997, when NAACCR began its registry certification program with an evaluation of 1995 incidence data, 9 NPCR registries and all 10 SEER registries were certified. Six years later, when NAACCR evaluated the 2000 incidence in 2003, 32 NPCR registries, 4 NPCR/SEER registries, and all 10 SEER registries were certified (www.naaccr.org).

PUBLIC HEALTH SURVEILLANCE OF CANCER

CDC carries out its mandate to monitor the nation's health by conducting and sponsoring a wide range of activities, one of which is public health surveillance. Public health surveillance has been defined as "the ongoing systematic collection, analysis, and interpretation of health data essential to the planning, implementation, and evaluation of public health practice, closely integrated with the timely dissemination of these data to those who need to know. The final link in the surveillance chain is the application of these data to prevention and control."[13] Cancer is the second leading cause of death in the United States, and its costs and burden are expected to increase in the twenty-first century with the growth and aging of the population. State health departments increasingly are spending public funds to control cancer. The local, state, and national burden of cancer needs to be monitored so that limited resources can be applied effectively to cancer prevention and control activities. Cancer is currently a reportable disease in

almost all states, and reporting of cancer cases to the state cancer registry is mandated by state law in nearly all states. State registries in turn report the data to CDC through the NPCR-CSS.

The data submitted to central cancer registries by reporting facilities are crucial to the prevention and control of cancer in the United States. Local and state health departments, national organizations, and CDC use the data to determine the need for cancer-related health services in the community and to design and evaluate cancer screening, treatment, and control activities. An example of a community cancer control program is the National Breast and Cervical Cancer Early Detection Program.[14] This CDC program assists state health departments to increase services, especially to women age 40 years or older, including those in poor or underserved segments of the U.S. population, to have routine mammograms and Papanicolaou (Pap) smears with appropriate treatment if cancer or its precursors are detected. Health departments use data from the central cancer registry to monitor, for example, the proportion of breast and cervical cancers occurring in early or in situ stages along with mortality from these cancers, in order to plan for future services. This is an example of how public health surveillance data are used to benefit the U.S. population.

THE REGISTRY PROFESSION AND NPCR

NPCR and Cancer Registration

Many organizations and individuals have contributed to the progress seen in cancer registration since NPCR began; however, NPCR's impact is clear. One reason for NPCR's success is its strong basis in law, a law which cancer registrars helped to develop. NPCR's requirement for national standardization of data items and formats has facilitated comparison of cancer occurrence and treatment from location to location. Standardization is needed for regional and national analyses. Such analyses are important because possible risk factors or environmental exposures are not likely to honor geographical boundaries.

Additionally, NPCR's emphasis on making central cancer registries statewide and population-based with complete case ascertainment improves the representativeness of cancer data so that it better reflects the population, provides more stable estimates of cancer incidence for racial and ethnic minorities, and facilitates research. NPCR's requirements for quality control of data collection and processing foster the accuracy of cancer data for research and disease surveillance; and NPCR's support for timely and efficient reporting of data without compromising completeness or quality makes cancer information more readily available to those who need to know such as the public, researchers, clinicians, public health officials, and policymakers.

NPCR and Cancer Registrars

NPCR activities have resulted in increased use of hospital cancer registry data, and this in turn benefits the registry profession. In the past, the major focus for hospital cancer registry data use was to evaluate cancer care at one facility. Later, hospitals began to contribute their data to the Commission on Cancer's national patient care evaluation studies and to the National Cancer Data Base. Today, hospital data are also submitted to the central registry, and the central registry data in turn are used to create national databases such as those for SEER, NPCR, and NAACCR.

Recently, the prestigious Institute of Medicine of the National Academy of Sciences recommended the use of population-based central cancer registry data as a sampling frame for selecting patients for studies on the quality of cancer patient care, referring to the central registries as "powerful tools for assessing quality of care."[11] The scope and the use of hospital cancer registry data have expanded tremendously from the support of one facility to the support of cancer control efforts for the entire country. This increased utilization highlights the importance of hospital-based cancer registry programs and supports the need for their continuation. Additionally, use of registry data within the state and nationally brings visibility to the cancer registry profession and emphasizes the need for highly skilled professionals who can collect and process high quality data. While hospital cancer registries remain the major employer for cancer registrars, increased government funding through NPCR has resulted in increased employment opportunities at state central registries and in national organizations.

NPCR acknowledges the importance of the certified tumor registrar (CTR) credential for assuring high quality data and fostering efficient central cancer registry operations. NPCR funding is used by many state cancer registries for activities directed at increasing the number of CTRs in the state and for providing incentives and rewards for registrars within the state. Examples of these activities include the following:

- Many central cancer registries use NPCR funds to provide basic training locally for registrars who would otherwise not be able to attend state or national training programs. The central registry may also provide scholarships to hospital registrars to attend state or national educational programs;
- Central cancer registry staff members in some states provide technical support by answering abstracting and coding questions or providing statistical assistance for developing annual reports;
- Because of the need for timely data, central cancer registries may help hospital registrars obtain help to get the job done. For example, central registries in some states have alerted hospital administrators to the need for more staff or provided temporary hands-on help with case identification and record abstraction;
- Routine management reports from the central cancer registry on completeness and timeliness provide useful feedback to hospital cancer registries. These reports can be used to develop work plans or document staffing needs;
- Quality assurance activities conducted by the central cancer registry provide an outside, independent confirmation of the quality of the hospital registry data and help identify training needs. Quality assurance reports from the central cancer registry also may be used to meet the Commission on Cancer's quality assurance requirements;
- Central registries can provide hospital registries with comparison data for annual reports, follow-up information, and responses to requests for special reports.

CONCLUSION

NPCR is a federally funded program with the goal of improving cancer registration in the United States and ultimately reducing suffering and death from cancer. NPCR is an important member of the cancer registry community but it cannot function without the involvement of its critical partners. While

NPCR enhances the work of cancer registrars and cancer registries, it depends upon the contributions made each day by individual registrars for its success.

STUDY QUESTIONS

1. What is the goal of the National Program of Cancer Registries (NPCR)?
2. List three programs of NPCR?
3. How is high quality data achieved for NPCR goals?
4. What publication is coauthored by CDC and NCI in collaboration with NAACCR?

REFERENCES

1. Garfinkel L. History of US central cancer registries. In Menck H, Smart C, eds. *Central Cancer Registries: Design Management, and Use, Appendix A.* Chur (Switzerland): Harwood Academic Publishers; 1994: 303-9.
2. Centers for Disease Control and Prevention (CDC). State cancer registries: status of authorizing legislation and enabling regulations—United States, October 1993. *MMWR.* 1994;43(4):71-75.
3. Cancer Registries Amendment Act, Pub. L. 102-515, 106 Stat. 3372 (Oct. 24, 1992). Available at: www.cdc.gov/cancer/npcr/npcrpdfs/publaw.pdf.
4. Women's Health Research and Prevention Act, Pub. L. 105-340, 112 Stat. 3191-4 [Sec. 202] (Oct. 31, 1998).
5. Standards for Case Inclusion and Reportability. In Hultstrom D, ed. *Standards for Cancer Registries:* vol. II: *Data Standards and Data Dictionary,* version 10. 7th ed. Springfield, Ill: North American Association of Central Cancer Registries; 2002.
6. Benign Brain Tumor Cancer Registries Amendment Act, Pub. L. 107-260, 116 Stat. 1743 [access 42 USC 208e] (Oct. 29, 2002).
7. U.S. Cancer Statistics Working Group. U.S. Cancer Statistics: 1999 Incidence. Atlanta, Ga: Department of Health and Human Services, Centers for Disease Control and Prevention and National Cancer Institute; 2002. Available at: *http://www.cdc.gov/cancer/npcr/uscs/.*
8. North American Association of Central Cancer Registries (NAACCR). *Standards for Cancer Registries:* vol. III: *Standards for Completeness, Quality, Analysis and Management of Data.* Springfield, Ill: NAACCR; 2000.
9. Clutter GG, Hall HI, Gerlach K. Birthplace data: an important piece of the cancer puzzle. *Journal of Registry Management.* 2002;29(4):108-16.
10. Wingo PA, Jamison PM, Hiatt RA, et al. Building the infrastructure for nationwide cancer surveillance and control – a comparison between The National Program of Cancer Registries (NPCR) and The Surveillance, Epidemiology, and End Results (SEER) Program (United States). *Cancer Causes and Control.* 2003; 14:175-193.
11. Institute of Medicine. *Enhancing Data Systems to Improve the Quality of Cancer Care.* Washington, DC: National Academy Press; 2000.
12. Hutton MD, Simpson LD, Miller DS, Weir HK, McDavid K, Hall HI. Progress toward nationwide cancer surveillance: an evaluation of the National Program of Cancer Registries, 1994–1999. *Journal of Registry Management.* 2001;28(3):113-120.
13. Thacker SB, Berkelman RL. Public health surveillance in the United States. *Epidemiol Rev.* 1988;10:164-90.
14. Henson RM, Wyatt SW, Lee NC. The National Breast and Cervical Cancer Early Detection Program: a comprehensive public health response to two major health issues for women. *J Public Health Management Practice.* 1996;2(2):36-47.

chapter 4

HEALTH INFORMATION PRIVACY AND SECURITY

Thomas H. Faris
Esq, JD, CQA, CQM

INTRODUCTION

Need to Protect Confidential Information

"Have you ever been diagnosed with a sexually transmitted disease?" "Have you ever experienced high blood pressure?" "Do you drink alcohol or use illegal drugs?" Patients peruse the waiting room, making a quick "double take" to ensure that no one is looking at their answers. But, what happens after the new patient information is handed over to the receptionist? Who has access to the medical records that include all of your physician's notes about your most personal conditions, feelings, traits, and problems? What do they do with the information and who are "they" anyway? Medical records can contain the most highly personal and sensitive information about a person.

Enter the Computer Age. Handheld computers, the Internet, email communication, and the use of personal computers enable people unknown to you to store nearly limitless amounts of data, perform timely searches and reports, and distribute large quantities of information to a wide audience in practically no time. The healthcare industry is now able to make patient records and image data instantaneously available at multiple locations, as well as provide summary analysis of multiple patient, facility, or regional studies with very little effort. Information is power.

Junk mail, credit card offers, email spam, telemarketing—how do they find us? Marketing firms exist in today's business world solely for the purpose of accumulating and selling information about individuals. Your name, address, and information about your spending habits, property interests, creditworthiness, political affiliation, or health conditions are routinely sold without your slightest awareness. The best information gathering services are able to accumulate information about millions of people using highly focused research efforts. This information is of great value to those looking for someone to buy their products, creating a product to sell, or determining how to relate their advertising to their "market." Information is money.

Health Information and Cancer Registry

Cancer registries necessarily deal with significant amounts of confidential information, including patient identification information and detailed medical histories. Cancer registry personnel routinely collect, evaluate, interpret, and disclose patient health information. It is critical that registrars be very familiar with what comprises confidential health information; the regulations and laws applicable to the access to, usage, and disclosure of confidential information; and the processes and technologies necessary for protecting the privacy and security of this information.

NOTABLE INCIDENTS

The following are actual events that demonstrate the relevance of privacy and security protections in health information management:

- A hospital employee's child copied patient contact information from hospital records and "jokingly" notified the patients that they were diagnosed with HIV.
- A county health board member, who was a banker, reviewed patient information under his control to determine which of his customers were diagnosed with cancer. He recalled their mortgages for immediate payment.
- A health information website mistakenly posted the names, addresses, and telephone numbers of thousands of users who requested drug and alcohol addiction information.
- A pharmacy clerk's son informed a prescription holder's children that their father had AIDS.[1]
- A hospitalized patient discovered that over 200 hospital employees had accessed her health information.
- The purchaser of a used computer discovered that it contained detailed prescription and identification records kept by the pharmacy that previously owned the computer.
- An auction bidder attempted to purchase a health practice's medical records for the purpose of, among other things, selling the information back to the patients.[2]

INITIAL LEGAL PROTECTION

The initial protection of confidential patient information was developed on a state-by-state basis. State statutes and regulations have been sporadically adopted, spanning many decades, disciplines of applicability, and scopes of coverage. The Health Privacy Project sponsored by the Institute for Health Care Research and Policy of Georgetown University conducted a detailed comparative analysis of all state statutes seeking to protect the privacy of patient health information. The project highlighted the following trends:

- State privacy legislation is predominantly enacted on an entity basis. Statutes typically regulate the activity of specific types of entities; therefore, different entities are subject to different levels and types of controls.
- Only two states have even attempted to enact comprehensive privacy law. Almost all states seek to implement privacy protections within other larger statutes, resulting in piecemeal protection based upon ancillary topics.
- State statutes infer a duty to maintain confidentiality. Although penalties for specified breaches are provided, the explicit duty to keep information confidential is, most often, conspicuously absent.
- The statutes that are in place today have not remained current with technological advancements or healthcare industry standards.[3]

Such a piecemeal system for the protection of confidential patient health information causes many problems. Treatment, billing, and general healthcare operations may be spread across a number of states, resulting in complex law-to-be-applied questions. Patient information is subject to differing levels and types of protection, depending upon where treatment was provided or healthcare operations are performed. Clearly, comprehensive federal protection is necessary to provide uniform and fair health information management privacy and security practices.

CURRENT DRIVERS OF PRIVACY AND SECURITY PROTECTION

HIPAA

The Health Insurance Portability and Accountability Act (HIPAA) of 1996 was enacted by Congress to answer the pleas of the healthcare industry to simplify and reduce the skyrocketing costs of healthcare administration. The industry and government agreed that requiring standardized health transactions and coding standards would decrease administrative overhead. HIPAA promotes "good business" for the healthcare industry by pursuing the most effective and efficient use of modern information technology. HIPAA also calls for the implementation

of common sense privacy and security protection of the personal patient information reflected in the data to temper the risks posed by the powerful information technology. This portion of HIPAA is entitled *Administrative Simplification.*

The Department of Health and Human Services (DHHS) defines the purposes of the Administrative Simplification rule as follows:

1) To protect and enhance the rights of consumers by providing them access to their health information and controlling the inappropriate use of that information;
2) To improve the quality of healthcare in the US by restoring trust in the healthcare system among consumers, healthcare professionals, and the multitude of organizations and individuals committed to the delivery of care;
3) To improve the efficiency and effectiveness of healthcare delivery by creating a national framework for health privacy protection that builds on efforts by states, health systems, and individual organizations and individuals.[4]

The Security and Electronic Signature Standard ("Security") and the Privacy of Individually Identifiable Health Information Standard ("Privacy") comprise a team of regulations intended to protect patient health information. Privacy defines the permissible means of access to, usage, and disclosure of the applicable patient information, while Security governs the operational and technical mechanisms necessary to protect this information.

Specific HIPAA requirements are discussed in detail at the end of this chapter.

Several other federal enactments have recently been implemented to protect confidential data in other areas, including:

- The Gramm-Leach-Bliley Act—Protects consumers of financial institutions from unknown or deceptive use of their personal financial information and provides the opportunity to opt out of certain disclosure practices.
- The Privacy Act (of 1974)—Protects the individually identifiable information held by the federal government from inappropriate use or disclosure.
- The Public Health Service Act—Protects information obtained during drug or alcohol related

treatment at federally-funded facilities from inappropriate use or disclosure.

Industry Standards

Trade and professional associations consist of learned professionals who evaluate and resolve issues that affect their industry. Ethical canons are typically pledged that promote the development of "best practices" for the industry, including minimal standards of quality assurance, development and operational methodologies, and product acceptability. Association participants represent many years of experience in the field and can provide intimate insight into the values and perils associated with particular processes, technologies, and product requirements. They contend, and the federal government quite often accepts, that legitimate self-regulation by industry standards reasonably ensures adequate results for consumers, mitigates unreasonable risks and side-effects, and levels the playing field for competitors.

Healthcare industry participation in the development of privacy and security standards is of the utmost importance. Existing associations have been developing applicable standards for many years. Privacy and security technology continuously advances; however, it is not usually practical or efficient to use the newest technology. Cutting edge privacy and security devices, tools, and processes are often expensive, unwieldy, unpredictable, and failure-prone. Also, information system applications have traditionally been developed in near isolation. Privacy and security vulnerabilities are identifiable as the information travels between these information management systems, technologies, and processes. Cooperation within the industry is necessary to mitigate these identifiable gaps. Industry associations analyze these issues, based upon their experience and tribulations, and identify minimal compliance standards to be satisfied by all applicable industry participants.

Duty of Care

Regardless of the existence of specific state law, a patient will be able seek legal compensation for healthcare organization security and privacy breaches on the basis of civil negligence theory. A patient will be able to legally recover damages if the healthcare organization caused unprivileged access, use, or disclosure of protected information by failing to perform a duty to use reasonable care in the exercise of

information security or privacy. This legal action is based upon a party's negligence. Intentional disclosure or distribution is not necessary.

The key issue for legal consideration is whether a duty of care exists for the healthcare organization to provide adequate security and privacy. A duty of care is a socially defined standard of care for the protection of others against unreasonable risks. A standard of care arises from foreseeability of injury to a third party and a reasonable expectation that the responsible party would prevent that harm.[5] Standards of care are very often based upon standard business practices, providing clear indication of which actions are considered reasonable by the industry. An organization can create an unreasonable risk of harm to a person by failing to provide protections that are common to the same industry.

Furthermore, common business practice does tend to indicate that a standard of care exists, but it is not always necessary to substantiate that the standard of care exists. The famous T.J. Hooper case (T.J. Hooper, et al. v. Northern Barge Corp., et al.) provides legal precedent that a standard of care may exist even when current common business practice does not dictate that it exists.[6] The T.J. Hooper was a tugboat that lost its barge and cargo during a storm. The captain indicated that he would not have ventured into the storm if he knew that the storm was coming, but did not have a radio receiver to notify him of the impending storm. Very few tugboats at that time were equipped with radio receivers, as it was very new technology. The court found that the owner of the tugboat had a duty of care to provide the receiver to prevent unreasonable risk to the cargo owner's property.

Indeed in most cases reasonable prudence is in fact common prudence; but strictly it is never its measure; a whole profession may have unduly lagged in the adoption of new and available devices. It [the industry] may never set its own tests, however persuasive be its usages. Courts must in the end say what is required; there are precautions so imperative that even their universal disregard will not excuse their omission.[7]

The requirement for adequate information security and privacy in the healthcare industry is becoming unquestionable. Numerous standards, as well as plenty of state and federal legislation, make it clear that carefully protecting confidential information that is entrusted for healthcare purposes is prudent. While there will be plenty of argument reserved for what levels of protection are to be considered reasonable, there is no doubt that the failure to provide reasonable privacy and security protection is actionable.

Patient Interests

Patients want nothing less than complete privacy and security applied to all of their medical information, but the complexity and reality of the modern healthcare system complicates the realization of their expectations. Many patients' rights advocacy groups and vocal patients express the concern that the patient should have full control of their medical information; however, this position is not fully compatible with the provision of quality healthcare.

Gone are the days in which a doctor keeps each patient's record in a single folder, hidden from all potentially prying eyes. We no longer pay with eggs, or even the whole chicken, if complex treatment is required. Payment is a complex network of health insurance claims, authorizations, coordination of benefits analysis, co-pays, billing agencies, collection agencies, and public programs. The family doctor has become a multi-physician network with shared administrative resources. Referrals to specialists are very common to diagnose and treat particular disorders. Support organizations play significant roles in accumulating, transferring, and coding health information for numerous operational purposes. Data are collected to identify disease trends, evaluate treatment effectiveness, assure the quality of healthcare operations, and many other healthcare improvement purposes. Society's interest in maintaining order requires that certain suspected abuses and dangers be reported to public officials. In short, patient health information may pass through many hands as it travels the well-beaten paths of the healthcare system.

Healthcare organizations must realize that the complexity of the healthcare system does not lessen the need to adequately protect confidential information while still providing patients with quality healthcare. In fact, many medical advances increase patient interest in a tighter grip on the data: the breakdown of the human genome, hereditary predictability, statistical inferences based upon physical characteristics, and better early detection methods and technologies. The intended or unintended release of confidential health information can easily result in serious ramifications that irrevocably affect patients' lives.

Some patients, worried about the potential distribution of their information and the growing risk of privacy breaches, are taking impractical steps to protect their confidential information. Some patients pay cash for insurance-covered care instead of permitting their information to travel the course of medical billing. Many patients withhold, alter, or request their doctors to refrain from recording pertinent information in their records. Others refuse recommended tests or treatment altogether.[8] Current and accurate information is necessary to achieve correct diagnoses and treatment of the illnesses and diseases that afflict those seeking healthcare. Organizations that foster practices that discourage the intended free flow of information between doctor and patient interfere with the healing process to which the healthcare industry is committed.

IDENTIFYING CONFIDENTIAL INFORMATION

Although this chapter focuses on the confidentiality of *patient-related health information,* there are several distinct types and levels of confidential information associated with healthcare organizations. *Webster's II New College Dictionary* defines *confidential* as "1. Communicated or effected secretly. 2. Entrusted with the confidence of another. 3. Denoting intimacy or confidence."[9]

The Health Insurance Portability and Accountability Act (HIPAA) protects *individually identifiable health information,* which refers to any information related to the condition of the patient, treatment, or billing that reasonably identifies the patient. Information is individually identifiable if it explicitly identifies the patient by name, identifier, address, social security number, phone number, or similar information; or if the content provides some information that permits reasonable deduction of the patient's identity.[10] Health information legislation and regulation, such as HIPAA, typically protects information that connects patient identification with other health information. Healthcare organizations must protect the privacy and security of individually identifiable health information to comply with the law.

Health organizations also compile significant quantities of information about the organization, its employees, and business partners that must be adequately protected. All business entities collect information regarding employees that is likely protected by federal and/or state law, such as employees' personal and salary information. The law does not require the same protection of organization planning, financial, and performance data; however, an organization will compile and maintain significant information that it would probably not intend to subject to public review. Business partners will also provide information to the organization that they would not like to place into public view. In fact, non-disclosure agreements may require an organization to take affirmative steps to maintain the privacy and security of the information. The organization must identify internal organization, employee, and business partner data and ensure that necessary privacy and security controls are implemented to adequately protect the information.

Organizations must also consider and apply adequate protections to accumulated data that represent work product, research results, or other information of potential value. Despite the unlikelihood that an organization would be legally bound to protect proprietary information that the organization creates, analyzes, and maintains, the organization could lose all potential value of this information asset if the information were ever inappropriately disclosed or disseminated. It is in the best interest of any organization to ensure that its proprietary information is kept private and secure.

All organizations must conduct analyses of all information under their control to determine what must be considered *confidential*. Applicable standards and regulations immediately classify certain data as confidential as a matter of law. An organization must continue reviewing its information to determine what other collected, created, and maintained information must or should be protected from unintended access, use, or disclosure, based upon personal, business, or proprietary interests. An organization must determine and establish sufficient and appropriate privacy and security controls to protect all of the confidential information received, maintained, or transferred by the organization.

PRIVACY VS. SECURITY

Perhaps the only issue in competition with the rivalry created by the famous "chicken or the egg" question is the ability to separate the concepts of information privacy and security. Together, privacy and security form a team of protections that prevent

unintended access, use, and disclosure of confidential information. It is difficult to examine either of the concepts separately, without overlapping the other. Privacy generally refers to the requirements of restricting access, use, and disclosure of confidential information to parties with privilege to the information; however, security's operational and technical protections are the tools that ensure implementation and maintenance of these requirements. Security is often the methodology by which privacy or confidentiality is attained. Many protections, therefore, may be considered privacy and/or security. *Webster's II New College Dictionary* does little to clarify the distinction: privacy comprises "seclusion or isolation from the view of, or from contact with, others," while security is defined as "the degree to which a program or device is safe from unauthorized use."[9] Regardless, we can consider these two information management necessities as co-concepts, working in calculated unison to protect confidential information from unintended access, use, and disclosure. The descriptions below reflect the predominant role of the defined protection, admitting that the roles may often be complicated and reversible.

PRIVACY

Health information privacy prevents the unreasonable offense of a patient's interest in restricting unnecessary knowledge of personal information provided by the patient to assist diagnosis or treatment, or derived during medical care in furtherance of those healthcare objectives. Although it has been made clear that no absolute constitutional right to privacy exists, law is being established providing that individuals generally have the right to determine the use and disclosure of intimate or personal information. Patients provide information to medical practitioners and allow the collection of health-related information for the purpose of identifying and treating their medical afflictions. Privacy protections are aimed at meeting confidentiality expectations for data provided or accumulated to that end.

The following privacy practices define typical elements necessary to reasonably protect the privacy of confidential information. Cognizance of these elements pertains to privacy issues to be considered when handling confidential information within many different types of organizations, not limited to the healthcare industry and HIPAA. These are general considerations and may or may not be legally required in specific circumstances, depending on the type of confidential information, specific regulatory context, and type of organization. Specific healthcare privacy requirements are enumerated in the HIPAA section at the end of this chapter.

Notification of Privacy Practices

An organization must provide the individual with a notification of the organization's information handling practices and policies prior to any access, use, or disclosure of confidential information. The notification must be clearly identifiable as a "Notification of Privacy Practices" and be written in a language and format that individuals can read and understand. An organization may choose the method of providing the notification, but must carefully communicate the notification in a manner that the individual will receive, recognize, and have the opportunity to review. The notification must provide contact information for the receipt of questions and complaints. HIPAA requires healthcare providers to secure a signed receipt of the notification from the patient prior to or at the time of treatment, payment, or healthcare operations.

The notification must clearly and simply describe the specific access, uses, and disclosures that the organization plans to or may potentially undertake. The notification must also clearly identify any mandatory disclosures that the particular organization may have a legal duty to provide, such as reporting suspected abuses, business records under order of court subpoena, information for law enforcement purposes, reporting evidence of fraud, etc. Examples should be provided to clarify the types of access, use, or disclosure that may apply. Although it may be impracticable to illustrate every potential use or disclosure, the notification must ensure that the individual is reasonably aware of where his or her data may travel and the types of people who may have access to it.

The notification must also enumerate any applicable individual rights, such as access to review the confidential information, ability to object to or amend, regulatory protections, the grievance process provided by administrative agencies, and the ability to opt out, if applicable.

INDIVIDUAL RIGHT OF CONTROL

The issue of who owns a patient's medical record has been puzzling doctors' offices and patients alike for many decades. The current consensus appears to reflect that a doctor's office owns the actual record as a necessary and standard business record; however, the patient holds an important interest that can restrict a doctor's ability to access, use, and disclose the information contained within that business record. The same holds true for most other industries that rely upon the confidential information of others. The confidential information is necessary for effective pursuit of the organizations' objectives in furtherance of the interest of the individual. The individual must contribute or permit the accumulation of certain private or personal information. In exchange, the individual is typically provided with assurances of confidential practices and certain other identified rights to maintain a degree of control over the actual use and disclosure of the confidential information. Other industries follow similar precedent.

Ability to Deny Use

The primary privacy right of individuals is to deny any and all use of their confidential information by an organization; however, the ramification of this denial is typically the individual's inability to receive the services of the organization. In the healthcare world, this leaves the patient without diagnosis and treatment. In the banking world, the consumer is unable to use a credit card or open an account. The basis for this protection is the fact that the consumer is not forced into the relationship and openly agrees to permit the stated regular use and disclosure of their confidential information by participation in the business relationship. Clearly, the ability to deny all use and access alone does not provide any protection to those who must enter into service arrangements with particular organizations.

The government often recognizes the difficulty inherent to adhesion situations, in which individuals have no significant choice but to select from a limited number of organizations for a substantially necessary service (i.e., medical treatment at a hospital), and mandates legal limits to industry's use and disclosure of the confidential information. Regardless of any regulatory requirements, organizations do require standard practices of multiple uses and disclosures of confidential information, up to and including routine disclosures to other third parties, in furtherance of their business objectives. The individual's only means of preventing all use and disclosure of their confidential information is to deny all use by withholding all personal information and refusing to enter into the business relationship with the organization.

Ability to Opt Out of Certain Uses or Disclosures

(Not applicable to healthcare organizations)

Organizations can often find great value in the use and disclosure of accumulated confidential information, including promotion of other services and products, sale of individual information for mailing lists or other "partners," the accumulation of generalized knowledge, and indirectly related research. These data uses enable an organization to generate additional revenue from confidential information collected throughout its normal course of business; however, they are clearly outside of the scope of service requested by and provided to the individual. In many cases, an organization must not only notify individuals of these practices, but also enable them to specifically "opt out" or deny the additional uses of their personal information. The fact that an individual does not opt out of a particular notified practice does not permit the organization to use or disclose confidential information in any manner prohibited by law.

Authorization

HIPAA privacy requirements do not permit healthcare facilities to use or disclose individually identifiable information even if the individual does not opt out. Rather, the healthcare facility must procure a signed authorization from the patient permitting any access to or disclosure of any individually identifiable health information for any purpose beyond treatment, payment, and healthcare operations. The authorization must clearly identify the applicable confidential information, who may use or disclose the information, and a description of the use or disclosure.

Organizational Control of Confidential Information

The organization must take affirmative steps to ensure that the privacy of the confidential information is adequately protected from inappropriate access, use, or disclosure.

Minimum Necessary

Organizations must follow reasonable standards for using only the minimum amount of information necessary when pursuing permissible uses and disclosures of confidential information. This requirement to use only the minimum necessary to accomplish the intended objective pertains to all uses and disclosures of confidential information, regardless of who is to use or receive disclosure of the information, or the intended use of the information. (Exception: The minimum necessary requirement does not apply to healthcare facilities for the purpose of providing treatment to patients.) The minimum necessary standard is not intended to impose an overly strict standard to scrutinize all uses and disclosures of confidential information. The organization should use professional judgment and establish applicable policies and procedures to define the minimum necessary for routine uses and disclosures.

Privileged Use

As prescribed by the actual requirements of the organization and applicable law and regulation, the organization should establish a documented system of procedures and policies that provide for all routine privileged use and disclosure of confidential information. The management system requirements should clearly demonstrate all legally and ethically acceptable uses and disclosures of confidential information within the organization, including identification of which employees may access the confidential information, the particular portions of information that may be accessed, and the specific purposes for which the information may be used. Organizational privacy management personnel must take steps to ensure that all access, use, and disclosure of information is appropriately privileged.

Privileged Disclosure

Organizations must ensure that all disclosures of confidential information to third parties are legally permissible. Disclosures necessary to support the operation of the organization, the needs of the individual, or those that the organization is legally bound to provide are typically permissible, while uses that are solely intended for the benefit of the organization will probably require notice and authorization by the patient and the individual's ability to opt out. Applicable regulations may provide a list of permissive or mandatory disclosures that the organization may consider privileged as a matter of law. Privileged disclosures should be described in detailed written procedures for consistent application and foolproof employee decision-making.

Disclosure Accounting

An organization must maintain records that track confidential information disclosures made by the organization. The accounting need not typically include information regarding regular internal uses and disclosures related to providing requested services to the individual. The disclosure accounting must include the date, destination, purpose, and description of all information subject to disclosure. The disclosure tracking records must be provided to internal auditing personnel to ensure compliance with internal procedures and policies, to regulatory auditors as part of regulatory inspections, and to requesting individuals to notify them of the full distribution of their confidential information.

Current and Accurate Information

The organization must take reasonable steps to ensure that all confidential information remains sufficiently current and accurate to prevent any inappropriate detriment to the individual.

Minimum Necessary Maintained

An organization must maintain the minimum amount of information required to fulfill the expectations of the individual and support its business operations. It is unethical and often illegal to collect and maintain amounts and types of information beyond what is needed in the course of business, especially when the information is collected and maintained solely for the purpose of profiting from the individual's confidential information.

Disposal at Termination of Need

The organization must not maintain confidential information once the business need has terminated. Confidential information about individuals must not be held as speculative property, waiting for a commercial value to be found for it. An organization must take steps to identify when confidential information is no longer required and return or destroy the information. Businesses may be required to maintain certain business records for minimal regulatory retention periods; however, the privilege to access, use, or disclose information at some point does not vest a perpetual ownership interest in that confidential information.

Individual Ability to Review

Many regulations, including HIPAA, provide the individual with the right to review records maintained about them. Individuals may be irrevocably harmed by the use or distribution of false or inaccurate information about them. The ability to review provides the individual with the ability to understand precisely what information an organization has accumulated about them and to evaluate the accuracy of that information.

This right does not provide the individual with a virtual search warrant to enter the organization's premises to demand an inspection any information in the business records that may pertain to them. The organization must define acceptable means for providing the contents of the applicable records to the individual, including the means of filing the request, reasonable timelines for supplying the information (within regulatory requirements), format for information delivery, and cost to be charged for the disclosure.

Individual Ability to Correct

Individuals must have the ability to address any believed inaccuracies in the records maintained about them, especially if the records will be used in a manner that may unduly affect their well-being. An organization must establish a formal process to incorporate an individual's requested corrections. The process may permit the correction of or amendment to the confidential record to clearly note the individual's contention with the maintained information. Organizations that do not agree with the request of the individual must at least document the individual's objection to the decision not to correct or amend the information. Future users of the confidential information must be made aware of the individual's contention with the record.

Culture of Confidentiality

Organizations that routinely deal with confidential information must establish a culture of confidentiality to reasonably sustain the privacy and security of the information. The consideration for confidentiality must permeate regular business activities to the extent that it is not simply a precaution to follow but is ingrained into the fabric of the organization's routine operational practices, policies, strategic objectives, and priorities.

Policies and Procedures

An organization should establish internal procedures as part of their operational management system to appropriately document intended usage of confidential information and restrict all improper access, use, and disclosure. The operational management system provides organizational management with appropriate direction for managing the organization by concisely stating particular information control requirements. Policies and procedures related to privacy and security efforts may be integrated into existing operational procedures that already govern the operation of the organization. Requirements specific to privacy protections, such as training, internal audits, document control, and other elements discussed in this chapter, can easily be integrated into existing operational procedures handling those matters. Operational policies and procedures provide a clear and consistent means of communicating specific requirements as well as avail employees of the opportunity to reference the information at a later date.

Employees

All employees must be made aware of the importance of maintaining the privacy of confidential information. Training must be provided to all employees when they begin work at the organization, stressing that all activities, responsibilities, and decisions must consider what is in the best interest of maintaining the privacy of confidential information. Employee managers must consider the effectiveness and appropriateness of their employees' efforts in maintaining privacy during employee reviews, including compliance with all applicable procedures. Internal auditing must review all required activities to ensure successful implementation. Employees must be held strictly accountable and appropriately disciplined for any breach of privacy caused by their inappropriate actions or failure to follow procedures.

Control of Associates

Organizations must take reasonable steps to protect the confidential information that they must pass to business associates, and ensure that it remain reasonably protected. An organization cannot and should not control the operations of an associate to ensure that privacy breaches do not occur; however, the organization should contractually require that privacy protection equivalent to the organization's stan-

dards be applied to the confidential information. An organization must ensure that privacy breaches caused by the business associate be communicated to the organization and mitigated or cured, if possible. The organization must terminate the contract and cease doing business with the associate if the associate fails to address a breach or maintains inadequate privacy protection.

Adequate Security

In clear overlap of the two information protection considerations, privacy requires an organization to establish adequate information security. The requirements listed above can only be met if operational, physical, and technical security measures are in place to support the privacy efforts. Attempts to keep information private are fruitless if no boundaries are in place to prevent others from freely accessing or disclosing the information.

Use of De-Identified Information

Although organizations cannot commercially profit from distributing individuals' confidential information without their express permission, an organization may be permitted to remove the identifying information from the data to utilize the lessons learned, examine the case study, or draw statistical inferences by aggregating remaining information. Below are some potential commercial uses involving de-identified confidential information.

No Identification Captured

No privacy concern typically exists if the information does not contain individually identifiable information and cannot otherwise be used to link the information to a particular individual. An organization can use this information without further regard to privacy.

Removal of Identification

The organization that routinely handles or maintains individually identifiable information as part of its standard business practices may wish to utilize portions of the information for other commercial purposes. The privacy concern becomes moot if the organization takes steps to remove all individually identifying information and reasonable inferences from the data.

Coding / Encryption

Rather than fully removing identifying information from the data, the organization may encode or encrypt the identifying information to prevent any unintended recipients from interpreting or understanding this information. The de-identified information could then be re-identified at a later point when a legitimate and privileged business need arises.

Aggregation with De-Identified Results

Privilege may exist to aggregate individually identifiable information, even though the result of the aggregation may not include the confidential identification information. For instance, HIPAA permits the aggregation of individually identifiable information from many healthcare provider facilities for the purpose of quality assurance comparison of operations. The individually identifiable information may play a significant role in performing the aggregation and comparison, such as eliminating duplicate cases; however, the final reports or conclusions cannot disseminate any individually identifiable information.

Complaint Handling Process

All organizations must provide the ability for individuals to file complaints regarding alleged privacy and security breaches. Organizational representatives must be appointed to receive such complaints and ensure timely, independent, and adequate investigation of the individual's claim. The representative must have sufficient responsibility and authority to provide redress to the complainant, take reasonable steps to cure or mitigate any actual breach, improve the privacy and security system to prevent similar events in the future, and ensure necessary disciplinary action is taken against any culpable employees.

SECURITY

Information security is a comprehensive system of affirmative actions taken to protect the confidentiality, integrity, and availability of an organization's electronic data, work product, information systems, and other related intellectual and physical property. The affirmative actions must reflect operational policies and procedures, physical safeguards, and technical security devices.

- Confidentiality—Protection of entrusted information from unauthorized use, access, or disclosure.
- Integrity—Preservation of the specific nature, character, and content of the information.
- Availability—Ability to access, use, or disclose the information as intended in an effective and efficient time, place, and manner.

The following practices and mechanisms provide a high-level overview of the typical elements necessary to reasonably protect the security of confidential information. Although the considerations are not solely applicable to the security of health information, implementation of these requirements should nonetheless be considered minimally acceptable security protection for individually identifiable health information. Specific healthcare security requirements are enumerated in the HIPAA section at the end of this chapter. At the time of this writing, the HIPAA Security rule is still in draft form.

Operational Policies and Procedures

Organizations must establish formal operational procedures and policies to provide security guidance and instruction to all applicable personnel and to ensure that all pertinent functions are consistently performed in accordance with the organization's security needs.

Security Management Planning

Organizational security management must evaluate the flow of confidential data throughout the organization and identify all unreasonable security vulnerabilities. This data flow analysis must consider all inputs, internal uses, data resting points, transmissions, external disclosures, and third party access points to identify all potential security weaknesses. Security management must determine which vulnerabilities are considered unacceptable and establish appropriate security protections or mitigations to reduce the vulnerabilities to reasonable levels. The results of the security vulnerability analysis shall be formulated into a security management plan and translated into specific organizational requirements, as defined below. Organizations must routinely review both the vulnerability analysis and security management plan to ensure that they remain effective as the operation evolves.

Security Configuration Management

The security management plan must be translated into specific requirements for implementation and maintenance. Security management must clearly specify the entire security system, including technical requirements and data flow modeling. Procedures must be established to control all changes to the security specifications, including validation of the effectiveness of any planned changes.

Management Responsibility

Organizational management must ensure that adequate authority and responsibility are delegated to effect the implementation and maintenance of the security management plan. They must appoint a security officer, with executive responsibility, and provide him or her with full authority and responsibility to oversee the entire security system, establish policy and procedures to provide reasonable security protection, and respond to security breach incidents and other significant issues. The security officer must routinely report on the status of the organization's security efforts to executive organization management to review the suitability and effectiveness of the security management plan. The executive managers must identify, evaluate, and resolve deficiencies in operations or the security management plan to ensure that confidential information is maintained and used in a reasonably secure environment. The organization shall ensure that adequate resources are dedicated to implement and maintain the security management plan.

Information Handling Procedures

Similar to and perhaps in conjunction with privacy procedures, information handling procedures shall establish appropriate controls over the handling and control of confidential information during all pertinent operations. Procedures should detail confidential information handling requirements during the entire flow of information throughout the organization. Specific designation of personnel and limited amounts of data for use must be specified, as well as any security vulnerability mitigations deemed appropriate by the security management plan. The information handling procedures must consistently secure the handling of confidential information as long as it is used or controlled by the organization.

Access Controls

Security management must create operational procedures to identify which particular employees or classes of employees may have access to defined confidential information. The procedure must define operational steps to ensure that access rights are correctly assigned and exercised.

Personal Authorization Controls

Security management must procedurally define actions to be undertaken to verify the identity and authority of employees before granting access to, use of, or disclosure of confidential information. This will include new employee rights assignment procedures, grants of access to particular buildings and areas, key distribution, release of information authority, and supervision of visitors and contractors. Records must be maintained of all approved grants of access.

Information Technology Use Policies

Security management must recognize the security risks inherent in the use of certain technologies and proceduralize appropriate controls. E-mail and Internet use provides substantial risk, with direct ingress and egress from the outside world into the organization's network. Uncontrolled disclosures could potentially contain confidential information. Uncontrolled incoming files could contain viruses, worms, or trojans. Procedures must be established to ensure appropriate controlled use of these and other similar communication technologies.

Employee Training

Employees must be aware of potential vulnerabilities and the organization's means of controlling those vulnerabilities. Employees must receive training upon hire and routinely thereafter to ensure that they can consistently fulfill all security requirements that apply to their responsibilities. Training elements must include a description of:

- The organization's security vulnerabilities.
- The employee's responsibility for mitigating those vulnerabilities.
- All security requirements that pertain to employee job functions.
- Social engineering—a type of attack where the employee is subjected to trickery by another person and persuaded to inappropriately provide

information to breach security. Tips to recognize, avoid, and report social engineering attempts.

- The identification of confidential information and the controls necessary to protect the confidentiality, integrity, and availability of that information.
- Applicable laws and regulations.
- Incident reporting and response procedures.
- Disciplinary procedures for failure to follow established procedures and policies and directions of the security officer.

Employees must receive sufficient training to ensure their full awareness of performing their security requirements and the importance of those requirements. Security culturing efforts are also necessary to ensure that employees perform their security responsibilities with diligence. Management must demonstrate complete and consistent support for the security management plan and security management. Employees must be made aware of the priority of security and the fact that they will be held accountable for their security responsibilities.

Disciplinary Action

Security management must establish policies and procedures to appropriately discipline employees for any breach of security caused by their inappropriate actions or failure to follow procedures. Disciplinary action procedures must be clearly defined and consistently applied across the organization. Management discretion must be removed from the process to ensure that the message is very clear that the protection of security and privacy of confidential information is a top organizational priority. Disciplinary action must apply to all levels of the organization.

Employee Termination

Human resources and information services must immediately terminate all access rights and abilities of employees who have left the organization, including the removal of all computerized and physical access rights and passwords, collection of keys or tokens, and the return of all equipment held by the employee. An organization must take immediate steps to ensure that the terminated employee retains no ability to access confidential information or systems.

Vendor/Associate Control

Security management must ensure that third parties receiving access to confidential information adequately protect the security of that information. Organizations must ensure that partners or associates intended to receive distributions of confidential information legally agree to provide security protections equivalent to the organization. See the discussion of Control of Associates in the Privacy section above for more information.

The organization must ensure that any business partners that may have electronic or physical access to confidential information located within the organization's facilities do not pose an unreasonable security risk to the confidential information. The vulnerability analysis must consider potential third party access, use, and disclosure when identifying security management plan requirements. Care must be taken to supervise and control the access of necessary partners and contractors, such as after-hours maintenance, network administration, vendor technical support, and temporary office personnel.

Internal Auditing

The organization must take affirmative steps to evaluate the sufficiency and effectiveness of all security measures established under the security management plan. Internal operational audits must be performed to determine whether security-based operational procedures are being correctly and effectively implemented. Internal auditors must review operational records, speak with responsible employees, and observe process activities to ensure intended awareness of employees and effectiveness of security requirements. Audit results must be made available to security and executive management to determine whether additional or improved action should be taken.

Security management may also find value in having external personnel attempt to breach the organization's security system. Attempted attacks on operational systems, physical safeguards, and security technology can yield valuable improvement information about the effectiveness of security efforts and any continuing vulnerabilities.

Contingency/Disaster Recovery Planning

Security management must identify potential events that could interfere with the organization's business operations and establish a plan for continuing operations for each contingent event. A vulnerability analysis must be performed to indicate what potential disasters, failures, or other events could reasonably be expected to occur and interfere with business operations. Plans must be created that include steps to ensure that information necessary for business continuation is routinely archived, protected, and easily accessible for timely restoration in case of a disaster. The organization must be able to restore the information and re-establish necessary business operations, as the plan deems necessary.

Incident Handling

Formal processes must be established to report, investigate, and resolve incidents that may reflect security breaches. See the Complaint Handling Process description in the Privacy section of this chapter.

Compliance Certification

Business partners, regulatory authorities, and consumers require assurance that an organization is in full compliance with security requirements and is able to adequately protect the confidentiality, integrity, and availability of confidential information. The organization must employ either internal or external review authority to reliably determine and certify that adequate security is effectively implemented.

Physical Safeguards

Appropriate physical safeguards must be established to prevent unreasonable threats to an organization's buildings, equipment, and media, as deemed appropriate by the security vulnerability analysis. The organization must consider physical threats, such as disaster, physical or electronic break-in, theft, and careless or intentional physical access to confidential information. Physical safeguards shall be implemented in layered coordination with each other and with other security requirements to protect information from identified threats. It is important to remember that these safeguards are intended to protect against both external and internal threats, as the interest to be protected is the controlled access to confidential information.

Locks

An individual cannot improperly access, use, or disclose confidential information if he or she cannot get

to it. Buildings, rooms, file cabinets, and even workstations can be locked to prevent access by anyone who does not hold a key, token, or access code. The most critical areas, such as a network administration control room, shall typically have the most restrictive locking systems—possibly within a locked cage in a keypad controlled room within a facility accessible only by pass card or key fob.

Physical Barriers

Walls, fences, doors, and shaded glass may be used to provide additional layers of security protection. For instance, the walls or shaded windows between the reception area and the administrative office prevent bored patients from incidentally eavesdropping upon patient-related office conversations or viewing open medical records on the desk. Also, record casing could be used to provide fire resistance to critical business information. Physical barriers apply a layer of protection between the information and the person or danger to be kept away.

Monitoring

As no security is invulnerable, security management must be notified when security breaches are attempted. Intrusion alarms will directly alert security management, law enforcement personnel, or whomever the organization deems appropriate in case of a break-in or unauthorized entry. Alarms can trigger actions to investigate breaches or attempted breaches, make security management aware of the disclosure of accessed information, and provide a deterrent to prevent continuation of the security breach attempt. Smoke and other detectors must be installed to provide awareness of conditions that may be hazardous to equipment, personnel, or information. Well-lit areas ensure that suspicious or inappropriate activity does not escape unnoticed. Video monitoring permits the supervision of multiple areas with less attention. Also, video monitoring provides a deterrent, as the attacker will fear being caught because he or she is being watched at that time and/or recorded. Security guards may be utilized to provide focused surveillance of areas requiring more intense protection. Monitoring provides timely awareness of the occurrence of activities in identified areas of concern.

Visitor Control

Visitors represent potential customers, job candidates, personal friends, business partners, and sales people—and no one wants to upset a coworker or manager by harassing his or her visitors. In fact, they can often wander facilities unchallenged, especially if they are dressed in formal attire or provide the impression that they know where they are going.

Visitors inherently have no access right to any of the organization's information. Security management policy must provide definite controls over the ability of visitors to have any access to any secure locations or information. In fact, visitors should be required to sign a visitors' log, wear a name badge, have an escort at all times, and be confronted if they are found roaming the building unattended.

Control of Media

Information from heavily secured networks can still be copied to diskettes and CDs, which provide few or none of the protections performed by the network. Employees can take work home or leave it in their cars and expose it to all kinds of security risks. Archive tapes that are necessary to recover systems when disasters strike can potentially permit anyone who swipes a tape to replicate an organization's stored data. An organization's vulnerability analysis must identify which uses of media, information transfer, storage requirements, and work processes represent reasonable practices. Procedures should be established to detail all media use, storage, and disposal practices.

Control of Equipment

Information system equipment is the gateway into an organization's computer network. Network security can be defeated if an administrative access terminal is left unprotected. Employee workstations will necessarily be placed in an open work environment, so they must be subject to username and password protection and timeout after periods of inactivity.

New technology offers great advances in efficiency and effectiveness, but often carries its own security quandaries. Here are some examples and security considerations:

- Laptop computers—Laptops are often and easily stolen. They can hold large quantities of confidential information, which is often unprotected and accessible just by turning on the computer. "Remembered" dial-in's and passwords can per-

mit purported privileged access to a protected network with a single click.
- Wireless devices—A wireless device connects to a host network via a wireless transmitter and receiver. It connects into an independent access point into the network; however, other wireless devices can just as easily tap into the network's wireless connection. The lack of access controls will result in full access to the network. Also, wireless communications can be captured and easily read if not encrypted.
- Personal Digital Assistants (PDA's)—PDA's can be subject to all of the concerns above, but typically offer less CPU processing power and storage space. Therefore, security protections that could mitigate the above vulnerabilities often interfere with the speed and efficiency of operation of the device.

During vulnerability analysis, an organization must carefully consider how devices will be used and define appropriate control procedures and technical protections.

Corporate Security Culturing

There exists a fine line between adequate security control and the appearance of going overboard. Security vulnerability mitigations can be burdensome, time consuming, and confusing. Procedures may often seem overly strict and a waste of time. Therefore, it is essential for all employees to fully understand and support an organization's security efforts. Employees must be trained not only on the security protections, but also about why each protection is necessary. Whenever possible, employees should be permitted to participate in the evaluation, implementation, and maintenance of security requirements. Employee support is necessary to fully recognize vulnerabilities and identify and report actual or potential security breaches.

An organization must not destroy employee trust by using security mechanisms to unnecessarily monitor or punish employee performance. An employer will quickly turn into "big brother" if network audit trails are used as employee timecards or production gauges, if area monitors are used to watch general employee behavior, or if employee communications are overly monitored or scrutinized. Security is intended to protect privacy, not permit its invasion.

Technical Security Mechanisms

Security technology must be implemented to protect information stored on a computer network or otherwise electronically communicated from unauthorized access, use, or distribution. An organization's security vulnerability analysis must consider all potential points of access of electronic information, including the following four access concerns:

- Network—Network access must not be permitted without valid login.
- Network File Structure—User and user group rights must be assigned based upon the need and privilege to access information.
- Application—Applications typically permit the assignment of either user group or function to recognize access privileges.
- Communications—Communication methods must not permit receipt or review of any confidential communications by any unintended parties.

Firewalls

A firewall is the front-line perimeter protection that separates a network from the world on the other end of a communication connection. There are many variations of firewalls, but they all primarily control two functions: 1) the control of the specific information that comes into the network through the firewall, and 2) the control of the information that exits the network through the firewall. These controls effect the most basic access control into and out of the protected network.

Firewalls can protect the network in a number of ways. The easiest way to think of it is as a gatekeeper. Security management programs the firewall to permit or reject passage of certain types of traffic that pass through it. Typically, it is programmed to support security policies that have been enacted by the organization. The difficulty with firewall operation is that each permitted communication weakens the protection value of the firewall. The firewall is opened to permit incoming and outgoing transmission for e-mail, Internet use, authenticated interactive session logins, and many other uses. Incorrectly or loosely configured firewalls provide very little protection to the network.

Intrusion Detection

Nearly all entities attached to the Internet receive some sort of malicious attack: scans to find communication openings left open in the firewall, attempts to crack or guess passwords to enter the network via an existing user account, trojan programs that enter the network attached to email or another validly transferred files and then open a port in the firewall from inside, or attempts to interfere with communications by hitting the site with repeated information requests. Intrusion detection applications review firewall logs or other communication data to identify suspected attack attempts. The detection system alerts security management of the attempted breach of access control protection.

Alarms

Alarms notify security management of suspicious access control activity that may represent a security breach or attempted breach in progress. Intrusion detection systems send an alarm when external breach attempts or other abnormal conditions are suspected by the application. Alarm systems also review internal access activities or attempted access activities to identify suspicious activities. For instance, repeated login failures, attempts to access multiple unauthorized network locations, repeated access of a particular record by many employees, or one employee accessing many records. The alarm provides security management an early detection notice of a breach or potential breach to allow time to apprehend the perpetrators and mitigate or prevent the damage caused by the incident.

Access Control

Access controls protect information resources by restricting access to particular users or classes of users. Firewalls are the first line of organization access controls, preventing unauthorized network access. Lower level access controls are implemented within the network and within applications that maintain and control confidential information. Access rights may be restricted on a user level or to defined user function(s). This may be implemented by network access to particular organizational groups, classifications or levels of employees, or employees charged with defined functions.

User Authentication

Network and application administration must verify that users are who they purport to be before access is granted. Authentication may take the form of password or personal identification number (PIN) entry, biometric evaluation (i.e., fingerprint, voice recognition, or retinal scan), or electronic or physical token. Authentication information must be kept personal and confidential to remain effective, so passwords and PIN's must be subject to standard protections: minimal length, routine change, and timeout after a number of failed attempts.

Audit Trail

Audit trails track the details of substantial user accesses, changes, and decisions related to confidential information. The audit trail provides a mechanism for the review of access activities, as well as material to be examined for suspicious access, use, or disclosure activities as part of a security audit.

Encryption

Confidential information transmitted across an open network, such as the Internet or widely accessible network, must be transmitted in a manner that cannot be intercepted and understood by unintended recipients. In short, all emails, electronic data interchange (EDI) transmissions, and similar transfers must be subject to reasonably unbreakable encipherment or encryption, unless they are transmitted across a dedicated communications line.

Virus Protection

Viruses can be introduced into an organization's network by nearly any transmission from the outside world: email, downloaded files, or diskettes brought to work. All files brought into the network should be scanned upon incoming transmission. Also, security management must routinely perform up-to-date virus scanning of the entire network and all connected workstations. Viruses must be detected and neutralized before they are permitted to cause damage to information or applications stored within the organization's network. Virus incidents must also be considered within an organization's incident handling procedure.

SUMMARY

Protecting confidential health information is everyone's job. Organizations in the healthcare industry hold some of the most personal and private information about an individual. Medical information can provide an understanding of what kind of lifestyle an individual has led, how long he or she is likely to live, and what ails and aches he or she currently suffers. We all want retain the privacy of our confidential information, it is in the best interest of the patient, and now it is legally required.

Confronted with the need to determine what would be considered adequate privacy and security, healthcare organizations must look to numerous developing industry standards, federal and state regulations that state that "reasonable" protections must be applied, and an industry history of checkered performance. It is now within an organization's grasp to evaluate its own operations and practices to determine what privacy and security risks are reasonable and which must be mitigated. The bottom line is that "adequate protection" means "reasonable protection," based upon the abilities of current technology, current industry practices, and what the organization determines to be reasonable under the circumstances.

Privacy and security standard development is not unique to the health information industry. It is affecting nearly all information-based industries. Organizations will find it in their best interest to create dynamic systems that remain current with the industry standard protections—not the state of the art, but what provides the best protection of confidential information without undue effort or cost to the organization.

SUMMARY OF HEALTH INSURANCE PORTABILITY AND ACCOUNTABILITY ACT (HIPAA) REGULATORY REQUIREMENTS

This section includes a summary of the requirements of the HIPAA Privacy and Security Regulations. It provides a general overview only and does not reflect many specific exclusions, conditions, and other requirements included within the detailed regulations. This is included solely to provide a general understanding of the HIPAA regulations and does not reflect legal opinion or advice.

Table 4-1
Privacy of Individually Identifiable Health Information

Uses and disclosures of protected health information	Permitted disclosures:	To the individual. For treatment, payment, or healthcare operations. Pursuant to and authorization by the individual. Incident to other requirements or permissive disclosures identified by this regulation. To business associates that perform privileged operations in the name of the covered entity.
	Minimum necessary applies. Minimum necessary does not apply to:	Healthcare provider for treatment. Disclosures made to the individual. Uses or disclosures made pursuant to an authorization. Disclosures made to the Secretary for inspection. Uses or disclosures that are required by law.
	Applies to records of deceased patients. Personal representatives:	Various rules for use of personal representatives appointed or otherwise identified to legally represent the individual.
	Uses and disclosures must be consistent with notice or privacy practice. Disclosures may be protected for defined whistleblowers and workforce member crime victims.	
Uses and disclosures: Organizational requirements:	Rules apply only to the healthcare component(s) of entities that pursue other non-covered operations.	"Covered entity refers only to the healthcare component of the covered entity. "Protected health information" refers to the information under control of the healthcare component. Protected information must not be access or used by or disclosed to non-covered portions.
	Business associate contracts	Covered Entity is responsible for breaches of Business Associate if known and did not terminate relationship or notify the Secretary. Legal Business Associate agreement must be executed, specifying permitted uses, safeguard requirements, incident reporting, and other mandated requirements.
Uses or disclosures to carry out treatment, payment, or healthcare operations:	Access, use, and disclosure permitted for treatment, payment, or healthcare operations:	For a Covered Entity's own treatment, payment, or healthcare operations. For treatment activities of any other healthcare provider. For the payment activities of the entity that receives the information.

Table 4-1
Continued

		For provided healthcare operations activities of the entity that receives the information.
		Within organized healthcare arrangement.
Uses and disclosures for which an authorization is required:	Unless otherwise provided within the rule (above and below), all access, use, and disclosure must be pursuant to individual authorization.	Special requirements for psychotherapy notes and marketing purposes.
	Valid authorizations:	Within dates of effectiveness.
		Contains all required elements: information to be disclosed, who will make and receive the disclosure, purpose, expiration date, and signature.
		Not revoked by individual.
		May not be a condition of treatment.
Uses and disclosures requiring an opportunity for the individual to agree or to object:	Permits access, use, and disclosure for:	Facility directories.
		Involvement in the individual's care and notification purposes (i.e., family, under defined circumstances).
Uses and disclosures for which an authorization or opportunity to agree or object is not required:	Permits access, use, and disclosure for:	Requirements of law.
		Public health activities.
		Victims of abuse, neglect or domestic violence.
		Health oversight activities.
		Defined judicial and administrative proceedings.
		Defined law enforcement purposes.
		Decedent handling requirements.
		Limited research purposes.
		Aversion of a serious threat to health or safety.
		Specialized government functions (as defined).
		Workers' compensation claims.
Other requirements relating to uses and disclosures of protected health information:	De-identified information is not subject to legal protection.	
	Minimum necessary uses of protected health information:	Identify employees permitted to access minimum necessary individually identifiable information.
		Reasonably limit access to minimum necessary.
		Procedures must provide for routine uses, others must be individually reviewed.
		Minimum necessary does not apply to information used for treatment purposes.

Table 4-1
Continued

Notice for protected health information:	Uses and disclosures for fundraising: An individual has a right to adequate notice of privacy practices	Covered Entities can use information for their own fundraising purposes. Standard title for recognition. Description of permitted uses and disclosures. Statement that individual signature will be required for additional uses and disclosures. Enumeration of patient rights. Enumeration of Covered Entity's duties. Complaint handling process. Identification of Covered Entity contact. Effective Date. Individual must sign to acknowledge receipt prior to initial treatment.
Rights to request privacy protection for protected health information:	Individual has right to request additional restrictions. The Covered Entity need not agree to the additional restriction.	
Access of individuals to protected health information:	An individual has a right of access to inspect and obtain a copy of protected health information.	
	Unreviewable grounds for denial:	Psychotherapy notes. Information prepared for legal proceeding. Prohibited by CLIA. Correctional institution discretion for inmates. Individual agreement under course of research. Under the Privacy Act. Obtained from another for under confidentiality.
	Unreviewable grounds for denial:	Physical endangerment of the individual or another.
Amendment of protected health information:	Individual right to amend:	Individual has right to request amendment to record. Covered Entity can deny amendment. Covered Entity must either amend the record or permit the individual to add a statement of disagreement to the record.
Accounting of disclosures of protected health information	Individual has a right to an accounting of disclosures, except for disclosures:	To carry out treatment, payment and healthcare operations To the individuals. For treatment, payment, or healthcare operations. Pursuant to an authorization signed by the individual. For the facility's directory. National security or intelligence purposes

Table 4-1
Continued

	Content of the accounting:	Disclosures made by Covered Entity during last six years. Date of the disclosure. Identity of recipient of the disclosure. Content of disclosure. Statement of purpose. Can describe routine disclosure, instead of itemization.
Administrative requirements:	Administrative protections must be established:	Designation of privacy officer. Designation of recipient of complaints. Privacy Training must be provided to entire workforce. Adequate security to protect information. Complaint handling process. Disciplinary action process. Incident handling and requirement to mitigate.

Table 4-2
Security Standard (Draft at the time of this writing)[12]

Administrative procedures:	Certification	
	Chain of Trust Partner Agreement	
	Contingency Plan	Applications and data criticality analysis. Data backup plan. Disaster recovery plan. Emergency mode operation plan. Testing and revision.
	Formal Mechanism for Processing Records	
	Information Access Control	Access authorization. Access establishment. Access modification.
	Internal Audit Personal Security	Assure supervision of maintenance personnel by authorized, knowledgeable person. Maintenance of record of access authorizations. Operating and, in some cases, maintenance personnel have proper access authorization. Personnel clearance procedure. Personnel security policy/procedure. System users, including maintenance personnel, trained in security.
	Security Configuration Management	Documentation. Hardware/software installation and maintenance review and testing for security features.

Table 4-2
Continued

		Inventory.
		Security testing.
		Virus checking.
	Security Incident Procedures	Report procedures.
		Response procedures.
	Security Management Process	Risk analysis.
		Risk management.
		Sanction policy.
		Security policy.
	Termination Procedures	Combination locks changed.
		Removal from access lists.
		Removal of user account(s).
		Turn in keys, token, or cards that allow access.
	Training	Awareness training for all personnel (including mgt.).
		Periodic security reminders
		User education concerning virus protection.
		User education in importance of monitoring log in success/failure, and how to report discrepancies.
		User education in password management.
Physical Safeguards	Assigned Security Responsibility	
	Media Controls	Access control.
		Accountability (tracking).
		Data backup.
		Data storage.
		Disposal.
	Physical Access Controls	Disaster recovery.
		Emergency mode operation.
		Equipment control (in and out).
		Facility security plan.
		Access authorization before granting physical access.
		Maintenance records.
		Need-to-know procedures for personnel access.
		Sign-in for visitors and escort.
		Testing and revision.
	Policy/Guideline on Workstation Use	
	Secure Workstation Location	
	Security Awareness Training	
Technical Security Services	Access Control	Procedure for emergency access.
		One of three access types:
		• Context-based access,
		• Role-based access, or
		• User-based access.

Table 4-1
Continued

	Audit Controls	
	Authorization Control	Role-based access or User-based access.
	Data Authentication	
	Entity Authentication	Automatic logoff. Unique user identification.

		One of five authentication types:
		    Biometric,
		    Password,
		    PIN,
		    Telephone callback, or
		    Token.

Technical Security
    Mechanisms
	Communications and
	    Network Controls
		Message authentication.
		Integrity controls.

	Communications or Network Controls	Access controls or encryption.
	Additional Network Controls	Alarm. Audit trail. Entity authentication. Event reporting.

STUDY QUESTIONS

1. Why is there a need to protect confidential information?
2. What is the Health Insurance Portability and Accountability Act (HIPAA)?
3. Who owns the patient medical record?
4. What steps must be established in order to safeguard confidential information?
5. The four areas of access for electronic information that must be analyzed for protection of confidential information?

REFERENCES

1. Health Privacy Project. *Medical Privacy Stories.* Georgetown: Institute for Health Care Research and Policy, Georgetown University; 2002: 1-7.
2. 65 Fed. Reg. 82467 (December 28, 2000).
3. Pritts J, Goldman J, Hudson Z, Berenson A, Hadley E. *The State of Health Privacy: An Uneven Terrain—A Comprehensive Survey of State Health Privacy Statutes.* Georgetown: Health Privacy Project, Institute for Health Care Research and Policy, Georgetown University; 1999: 8-9.
4. 65 Fed. Reg. 82463 (December 28, 2000).
5. Kenneally E. "The byte stops here: duty and liability for negligent Internet security." *Computer Security Journal.* 2000; XVI(2): 3-6.
6. Salaverry P. "From boats to bytes: establishing a Y2K standard of care. *Texas Lawyer.* February 8, 1999; 14(46): 25.
7. In re Eastern Transp. Co.; New England Coal & Coke Co. v. Northern Barge Corporation; H. N. Hartwell & Son, Inc., v. Same. 60 F. 2d 737, 740 (2nd Cir. 1932)
8. 65 Fed. Reg. 82468 (December 28, 2000).
9. Severynse M, editor. *Webster's II New College Dictionary.* Boston, Mass: Houghton Mifflin Company; 1995: 236, 880, 998.
10. *Privacy of Individually Identifiable Health Information.* 45 CFR 164:501.
11. *Privacy of Individually Identifiable Health Information.* 45 CFR 164. 102-534.
12. 65 Fed. Reg. 43269-43271 (August 12, 1998).

chapter 5

LEGAL AND ETHICAL ASPECTS OF CANCER DATA

Sue Watkins
RHIA, RHIT, CTR

INTRODUCTION

This chapter addresses both the legal and ethical issues that must be considered in hospital and population-based cancer programs. The legal aspects encompass requirements and principles related to data collection, maintenance, and security; release of information; and use of confidential and aggregate (non-confidential) data. Ethical issues include professional conduct and adherence to professional codes of ethics.

LEGAL ASPECTS

There are numerous rules and regulations that define the legal aspects of cancer registry data. These include state and national laws, regulations from governmental and nongovernmental agencies, and institutional policies. The phrase *legal aspects* generally implies circumstances relating to the law. *Law* is a term that encompasses common law, statutory law, and regulations of administrative agencies (administrative law).

- Common Law: Body of principles that has evolved and continues to evolve and expand from court decisions. Many of the legal principles and rules applied by courts in the United States have their origins in English common law.[1]
- Statutory Law: Law that is prescribed by legislative enactments.
- Administrative Law: issued by administrative agencies to direct the enacted laws of the federal and state governments. It controls the administrative actions of government. Administrative agencies have legislative, judicial, and executive functions. They have the authority to formulate rules and regulations necessary to carry out the intent of the law.

The laws pertaining to cancer registries and patient information are designed to protect patient privacy while allowing the data to be used for important research and surveillance activities. State and federal laws are usually quite specific in their requirements for the content and use of the data.

Two powerful federal administrative agencies of importance to cancer registries are the National Cancer Institute (NCI) and the Centers for Disease Control and Prevention (CDC). The National Cancer Act of 1971 mandated the collection, analy-

sis, and dissemination of data for use in the prevention, diagnosis, and treatment of cancer. This mandate led to the establishment of the Surveillance, Epidemiology, and End Results (SEER) Program, an ongoing project of the National Cancer Institute, which is an agency of the US Department of Health and Human Services. The SEER Program operates population-based cancer registries in various geographic areas of the country covering approximately 14% of the US population. (See Chapter 33.)

In October 1992, Congress established a National Program of Cancer Registries (NPCR) by enacting Public Law 102-515, The Cancer Registries Amendment Act. Through this legislation, authority was given to the Centers for Disease Control and Prevention to do the following:

- Provide funds to states and territories to enhance existing population-based cancer registries;
- Plan and implement registries where they do not exist;
- Develop model legislation and regulations for states to enhance viability of registry operations;
- Set standards for completeness, timeliness, and quality;
- Provide training.

Both NCI and CDC work closely with the Commission on Cancer (CoC) of the American College of Surgeons. Although not a federal agency, the CoC has operated a voluntary system of approval for hospital cancer programs since 1932. Standards have been established for these approved programs, including a requirement for a hospital cancer registry and policy statements about protecting patient confidentiality and release of information.

The Privacy Act of 1974 grants individuals the right to:

- Find out what information is collected about them by the government;
- See and have a copy of that information;
- Correct or amend their information;
- Exercise control over disclosure of that information.

The Health Insurance Portability and Accountability Act of 1996 (HIPAA) addresses confidentiality by requiring covered entities by law to maintain the privacy of individual's information. Authorizations for disclosure of patient information are required by law under HIPAA. Cancer surveillance data is an exception to this rule if it is required by state law. HIPAA is covered in Chapter 4.

State laws regarding confidentiality vary; some are very specific and others are worded in a more general manner. The North American Association of Central Cancer Registries (NAACCR) has distributed standards for confidentiality and disclosure of data and for what legislation and regulations should specify. These standards are being used by CDC in the implementation of the National Program of Cancer Registries. Copies of the appropriate law governing the registry's area of coverage can be obtained by contacting legal counsel or the population-based registry serving the geographic area of interest.

Institutional rules and regulations governing confidentiality and release of information must be observed. In addition to abiding by state and federal laws, it is important for registry professionals to be aware of institutional regulations. Policies and procedures can be implemented by institutional review boards or other committees established to review confidentiality and ethics. These policies can extend from medical facilities to the central cancer registries to which they report their cancer patient data.

The cancer registry professional plays a key role in ensuring that legal requirements are met by all those involved in the collection, maintenance, and use of cancer information. This responsibility includes being knowledgeable about governmental and institutional policies and procedures concerning the data, and ensuring that they are communicated, understood, and followed.

Confidentiality

Cancer data are highly confidential, and one of the most important responsibilities of cancer registry professionals is to safeguard the confidentiality of cancer patient information. Improper disclosure of these data could result in emotional, psychological, and financial harm to the patients and their families. The standard of confidentiality maintained by cancer registries is similar to that of the doctor-patient relationship, and it extends indefinitely, even after the patient is deceased. Although patient confidentiality is of paramount importance, it is also critical that cancer registries implement policies to protect the privacy of physicians and healthcare facilities. The terms *confidentiality* and *privacy* are often used interchangeably in reference to medical information.

Definition of Confidential Data

Confidential is defined in *Webster's New World Dictionary, Second College Edition,* as "told in trust, imparted in secret; entrusted with private or secret matters."[2] The American Health Information Management Association, in its 1993 position paper on disclosure, makes a distinction between confidential and non-confidential information. Researchers using medical information often distinguish between aggregate data, which are combined without patient identifiers, and confidential data. Although the legislation and regulations under which the cancer registry operates may only define patient-specific data as confidential (for example name, address, phone number, and social security number), registries should also treat any information that specifically identifies a healthcare professional or an institution as confidential.

Personnel Policies and Procedures

All cancer registry staff must be responsible for the confidentiality of all patient information encountered during the collection, maintenance, and dissemination of cancer data. NAACCR standards recommend that the registry staff "sign, as part of their employment agreement, a declaration that they will not release confidential information to unauthorized persons."[3] All cancer registrars must sign a confidentiality agreement annually as a reminder of the importance of this issue. A sample confidentiality pledge is shown in Figure 5-1.

Registry staff training should include a comprehensive session concerning the confidentiality of the data. Fictitious names or anonymous data sets should be used in training and demonstrations of the computer system used in registry operations.

Nonregistry staff who request access to registry data should also sign confidentiality agreements. Nonregistry staff must agree to adhere to the same confidentiality policies as practiced by registry staff.

Release of Cancer Registry Data

The use of registry data is fundamental to the success of the registry. Release of cancer data for clinical purposes, research, and administrative planning is central to the utility of the registry. In order to ensure that information is only disclosed to authorized parties, policies and procedures for release of cancer registry data must be developed and instituted.

Figure 5-1
Sample Confidentiality Pledge

Confidentiality Pledge

I understand and accept the legal and moral responsibility of maintaining the confidentiality of all data and information collected and processed by the (*facility name*) cancer registry. I also understand my role in ensuring the right to privacy of persons and institutions cooperating with the cancer registry data collection activities. Furthermore, I understand that the (*facility name*) has policies that protect the patients' rights to every consideration of their privacy regarding their medical information. I understand that I must not reveal any confidential information to anyone except those individuals authorized to receive such information, such as another staff member or the original reporting source. I also understand that failure to adhere to this policy may result in disciplinary action up to and including automatic dismissal without further notice.

I have read and understand (*facility name*)'s confidentiality policy and procedures and pledge to act in accordance with these policies and procedures.

Signature Date

Supervisor Date

Confidential information about cancer patients, care providers, and healthcare facilities must not be released for purposes other than those specified by the registry unless all parties concerned provide written authorization and agree in writing to adhere to all confidentiality policies.

Confidential cancer registry data should never be made available for uses such as businesses trying to market a product to cancer patients, healthcare institutions trying to recruit new patients, or insurance companies or employers that are trying to determine the medical status of a patient. Under no circumstances should confidential information be published or made available to the general public. Inquiries from the press should be referred to an administrator or another staff member who has been delegated the authority to respond.

Information should not be given to individual patients about themselves, except when required by law. Requests from patients for specific registry information should be referred to the attending physician; the physician should be notified of the patient's request and the action taken by the registry staff.

The cancer registry may permit the release of confidential data to other treating hospitals in their own state, or other states, for the purpose of patient follow-up. Policies and procedures should be instituted that include a case-sharing agreement among multiple facilities and a central registry, if appropriate. Approval of the policies and procedures from the institution and the hospital cancer committee is recommended.

Data Security

Measures must be taken to ensure the physical security of confidential data stored on paper, microfilm, microfiche, and electronic media. Suitable locks and alarm systems should be installed to control access to the registry. Fireproof, lockable file cabinets should be considered for filing hard-copy abstracts, computer printouts, and other reports.

HIPAA security provisions include administrative provisions, physical safeguards, technical safeguards, and network and communications safeguards. Computers used for cancer registry data must be controlled by electronic and physical measures to enhance the security of the data. Electronic or technical controls include use of passwords (access controls), automatic logging of all attempts to enter a computer system (audit controls), and different levels of data access, such as read-only files.

Data Transmission

Confidential data must not be transmitted by any means—mail, telephone, or electronic without explicit authorization from administration. Authorization may be granted for use in follow-up activities, for the transfer of data to a central registry, and for other appropriate activities. Cancer registries should consider the use of registered mail, overnight mail, or courier service for delivering confidential data and should consider separating patients' names from other data for transmission. Use of double envelopes, with confidential data in a separate envelope stamped or marked *confidential* and placed in the mailing envelope, is suggested for registries sending data via regular mail. A return address using the words *Cancer Registry,* or other similar term, should not be used on envelopes containing materials or requests for information that are sent to patients.

Computerized data should be encrypted to ensure confidentiality. Encryption of data (a process of encoding textual material and converting it to scrambled data that must be decoded in order to be understood) must be used for data transmitted over public networks or communication systems.

Physical safeguards include the protection of computer systems from natural and environmental hazards and intrusion. In addition to the physical access controls discussed above, policies and procedures should be written that address the physical safeguards necessary to minimize or eliminate the possibility of unauthorized access to information at workstations. For example, the facility might require users to log off the computer system when they are not using it or to turn computer terminals away from public view.

Remote access to data by physicians, registrars performing off-site data collection, and others may require additional security measures. The use of notebook computers for off-site data collection necessitates specific policies and procedures for maintaining database security and restricting unauthorized access.

Policies should also be developed and implemented for the disposal of confidential data. The use of shredders or incinerators is common in hospitals. Paper abstracts, computer printouts, copies of pathology reports, and other materials should all be stored or disposed of properly. Care must be taken not to leave these documents lying where unauthorized persons may have an opportunity to read them.

ETHICAL ASPECTS

Ethics, or moral philosophy, is the branch of philosophy concerned with conduct and character. Medical, or biomedical ethics, deal with moral decisions in medicine. For some, ethics means following the "letter of the law." Others regard ethics as a statement of acceptable behavior found in a code of conduct or regulations developed by a professional organization. The ethical conduct of cancer registry professionals is of major importance in ensuring the integrity of cancer data and the cancer registry profession. The National Cancer Registrars Association adopted a professional code of ethics and published a *Guide to the Interpretation of the Code of Ethics* (reprinted in Appendix I of this book), in 1986. The NCRA Code of Ethics was revised in 1995 and 2002 and addresses the issues listed in Table 5-1.

In general, the members agree to conduct themselves in the practice of the profession "so as to bring honor and dignity to [themselves,] the cancer registry profession, and the Association."

Table 5-1

Issues Addressed in the National Cancer Registrars Association Code of Ethics

- Cancer registrar practice and standards of conduct
- Confidentiality
- Cooperation with other health professions and organizations to promote quality of healthcare programs and the advancement of medical care
- Discharge of entrusted professional duties and responsibilities
- Preservation and security of cancer registry records and the information contained therein
- Disclosure of sensitive information acquired during employment or fulfillment of contracted services
- Compensation for professional services
- Professionalism
- Increasing the profession's body of systematic knowledge and individual professional competency
- Participation in the development and strengthening of professional work force
- Honorable discharge of association responsibilities

The comprehensiveness of the issues covered in the NCRA *Code of Ethics* demonstrates the importance of these ethical concerns. The NCRA publication was used as a guide for the rest of this section; it is not reprinted in full.

Cancer registrar practice and standards of conduct address everything from serving employers in an honest and ethical manner to declining favors that might influence decisions and avoiding commercialization of one's position. In today's healthcare environment, many registry professionals are finding new career opportunities. Numerous medical facilities are using consulting and abstracting services and outsourcing other registry activities. Ethical issues encompass the appropriate use of credentials and honesty and integrity in the promotion and delivery of services. A breach of ethics by one registry professional may have a negative impact on the entire profession.

Registry professionals also have an ethical obligation to recognize, encourage, and support other members of the profession.

Confidentiality has already been addressed in this chapter, but an example provided in the NCRA *Code of Ethics* is appropriate here. With regard to the release of confidential information, it is unethical to "provide lists of patients' names for marketing research or other commercial use." Such practice is not a proper function of a health institution, and these lists should not be released by a cancer registry professional without the proper authorization.

Cooperation with other health professions and organizations to promote quality of healthcare programs and the advancement of medical care is an essential factor in the cancer registry profession's greater aim of improving health services and supporting research relevant to cancer patients. Respecting, cooperating, and working with other health professionals will foster good relationships, which will benefit both professions and, ultimately, the cancer patient.

Discharge of entrusted professional duties and responsibilities is the ethical conduct expected of the cancer registry professional. It is unethical to accept a position or contract for services for which one is inadequately prepared. It is also unethical to vacate a position without adequate notice or to fail to complete an assignment without ensuring that the work that was entrusted will be completed in a satisfactory manner. It is further incumbent on the cancer registry professional to render a truthful accounting of the status of the work for which he or she is responsible.

The cancer registry professional should strive consistently to uphold professional standards for producing complete, accurate, and timely information to meet the health and related needs of the cancer patient. In addition, it would be unethical to participate in any improper preparation, alteration, or suppression of medical or health records.

It is the responsibility of the cancer registry professional—consultant, supervisor, employee, advisor, or other—to advise the employer or client if, in the registrar's professional judgment, there is the danger of making errors of commission or omission.

Compensation for professional services should be accepted only in accordance with services actually performed. It is unethical for the cancer registry professional to place material gain ahead of service. Primary importance should be placed on providing a high standard of professional service; financial considerations are secondary to this objective.

The cancer registry professional should endeavor to avoid a conflict of interest by providing full disclosure to the employer, client, or professional organization of any interest in any provider of services or products.

Professionalism requires one to represent truthfully and accurately professional credentials, education, and experience in any official transaction or notice, including other positions held and any possible conflict of interest. Misrepresentation of one's professional qualifications or experience is unethical. A statement of any other positions of possible duality of interest in the health or health-related fields, either remunerative or non-remunerative in nature, should be made available on request of the employer. Examples of possible duality of interest are outside consultation services, committee appointments, advisory positions, elected offices, business enterprise interests, and the like.

Increasing the profession's body of systematic knowledge and individual professional competency through continued self-improvement and application of current advancements to the conduct of cancer registry practice is an ethical goal. The attainment and preservation of professional status are accomplished through the mastery and competent handling of cancer registry activities and the continual development of new knowledge and skills.

Dissemination of new developments or changes in methods or procedures should be shared with other cancer registry professionals in a timely manner for the purpose of increasing the knowledge and skills of the profession.

Participation in the development and strengthening of the professional work force is the responsibility of all cancer registry professionals. The future of the profession is dependent on the affirmative and responsible endeavors of professionals to recruit and train other cancer registry specialists. Providing training and clinical experience to students, participating in career fairs, and writing for professional publications are all ethical undertakings that meet these objectives.

Honorable discharge of association responsibilities is expected of every cancer registry professional who accepts an appointed or elected position. Examples include the execution of one's obligation to the profession with integrity, discretion, and conscientious performance of the duties and responsibilities of the office or assignment accepted. Preserving the confidentiality of privileged information obtained through this association is one's ethical duty.

Breaches of ethical conduct are very serious. The NCRA has established an ethics committee charged with the responsibility of receiving, investigating, and handling written complaints of unethical behavior or alleged violations. The complaint procedure can be obtained from the chairperson of the NCRA Ethics Committee.

STUDY QUESTIONS

1. The National Cancer Act of 1971 led to the establishment of what organization? For what purpose?
2. Public Law 102-515, The Cancer Registries Amendment Act, established what program? For what purpose?
3. Define the term *confidential data* and explain its importance in cancer registry operations.
4. List three inappropriate releases of cancer registry data.
5. List three measures used for data security.

REFERENCES

1. Pozgar GD. *Legal Aspects of Health Care Administration,* 8th ed., Md: Aspen Publications; 2002
2. Guralink DB, ed. *Webster's New World Dictionary,* 2nd ed. New York, NY: Simon & Schuster; 1982.
3. Seiffert J, ed. *Standards for Cancer Registries,* vol. III: *Standards for Completeness, Quality, Analysis, and Management of Data.* Sacramento, Calif: North American Association of Central Cancer Registries; 1994.

BIBLIOGRAPHY

Cofer J, ed. *Health Information Management,* 10th ed. Chicago, Ill: American Health Information Management Association; 1994.

Flight M. *Law, Liability, and Ethics for Medical Office Personnel,* 2nd ed. Albany, NY: Delmar Publishers, Inc.; 1993.

National Cancer Registrars Association. *Guide to the Interpretation of the Code of Ethics.* Lenexa, Kan: National Cancer Registrars Association; 2002.

Menck H, Smart C, eds. *Central Cancer Registries, Design Management, and Use.* Langhorne, Penn: Harwood Academic Publishers; 1994.

Pozgar GE. *Legal Aspects of Health Care Administration,* 8th ed, Apsen Publications; 2000.

Seiffert J, ed. *Standards for Cancer Registries, Vol. III: Standards for Completeness, Quality, Analysis, and Management of Data.* Sacramento, Calif: North American Association of Central Cancer Registries; 1994.

Watkins S, ed. *Tumor Registry Management Manual,* 4th ed. Santa Barbara, Calif: Cancer Registrars Association of California; 1992.

chapter **6**

CANCER REGISTRY PERSONNEL, OFFICE SPACE, AND EQUIPMENT

Barbara M. DeCoe
CTR, RHIT

Scott W. Ward
CTR, CCRA

INTRODUCTION

A significant amount of early preplanning must take place prior to establishing a hospital-based cancer registry. This chapter provides an overview of areas and issues to be evaluated and some mechanisms that can assist in quantifying them. After the registry objectives are defined, the major goals are to establish the workload, determine the staffing requirements, and provide the necessary tools and space to accomplish the operations. Refer to the chapter in this textbook regarding Cancer Registry Management for further information about planning a registry.

ESTABLISHING THE CASELOAD

To establish the personnel, equipment, and space needs of the registry, the number of cases accessioned into the registry annually must be determined. For more information on determining the annual caseload, refer to the Case Ascertainment chapter in this textbook. Some projections can be made, however, by using the annual disease index or diagnosis index in the Health Information Management Department. Counting the number of discharges with a primary or secondary diagnosis of ICD-9CM codes 140-195 and 199-208 can give an estimate of the caseload. The important thing to remember is that the registry staff must collect cases according to various standards established by the Commission on Cancer of the American College of Surgeons, state cancer registries, etc. These organizations periodically add or delete cancer sites or types to be collected; therefore, the caseload may change periodically. Likewise, the pathology department is a valuable resource for identification of cases and may be able to generate a list of all cancer diagnoses at your institution for a given time period. The number of cancer cases can also be estimated by counting the total number of beds for medical and surgical patients. Additional statistics can be obtained from hospital administration for the percentage of oncology patients that have occupied beds in the past. Applying the percentage of bed occupancy to the total number of hospital beds can provide an estimated number of cancer cases accessioned.

Factors that affect the number of staff needed in the registry for abstraction activities include completeness of the health records to be reviewed, the amount of data to be collected, registry computerization and whether the registry will function under Commission on Cancer Guidelines.[1] Also, determine if there are any other areas of data collection that may involve or be included with the cancer registry such as the collection of AIDS cases, a trauma registry, or centralized registry where these other types of data are collected. A time-and-motion study[2] is recommended to better define staffing needs and is shown in Table 6-1.

It is important to remember that no follow-up activities will be necessary the first year. It is not until the second year that the cases in the registry from the previous year are due for annual follow-up which is discussed in another chapter of this textbook. Provisions for staffing to conduct follow-up must be projected for the year following the first year of abstracting. Four major tasks that affect staffing for follow-up are listed in Table 6-2.[2]

Once these factors have been reviewed, another time-and-motion study can be performed to determine the personnel needed for each task.[2] A time-and-motion study for follow-up is shown in Table 6-3.

Table 6-1

Performing a Time-and-Motion Study for Abstracting

1. Identify a series of cases to be abstracted.
2. Note the amount of time it takes to obtain the health records, abstract the cases, obtain missing information, refile the records, and create and file all registry documents.
3. Calculate per-case and per-year statistics, using the following formulas:

$$\textit{total time for abstracting} = \text{minutes per case number of cases abstracted}$$

$$\text{Number of cases abstracted annually} \times \text{minutes per case} = \text{minutes per year}$$

Example: The national averages are 40 minutes per abstract and 604 abstracts per year, or approximately 4 abstracts per working day.[2]

Table 6-2

Factors Affecting Staffing for Follow-Up

1. Letter generation
   — typed or handwritten
   — computerized
2. Number of cases
3. Type of population being followed
4. Longevity of the registry

Additional registry activities that affect staffing and should be considered are participation in studies, quality improvement activities, cancer conference preparation and attendance, quality management and studies, improvements, and production of the annual report. Each of these activities requires staff time that should be taken into account.[1]

WORK SPACE

After staffing has been determined, the work space required for efficient operation must be allocated. Whether the registry is a part of a larger department or independent, a well designed and quiet environment is necessary. It is important to think about office space early, taking into consideration not only the workload, but proximity to necessary resources, available storage, and special needs such as security of information and conference area availability. It is best to evaluate past growth and provide a growth projection in addition to establishing current needs. This will help ensure long-term space stability. Table 6-4 shows factors to consider in planning the registry office.

Office needs must be well documented, with growth projections in place, in order to include all resources in budget projections. Refer to the chapter

Table 6-3

Time-and-Motion Study for Follow-Up

1. Identify all cases to be followed for the selected month, using follow-up tickler cards or a computer-generated control listing.
2. Record the amount of time needed to check cases against the health records department's master file, generate and mail letters, post updated information to the abstracts, and perform secondary follow-up of the remaining cases. Because these processes are carried out in several phases, this time-and-motion study may take several weeks of intermittent effort.
3. Calculate per-case and per-year statistics, using the following formulas:

$$\frac{\text{total time for follow-up}}{\text{number of cases followed}} = \text{minutes per case}$$

Number of living patients in registry × minutes per case = minutes per year

Example: The national averages are 19 minutes for follow-up with 2,875 cases under active follow-up, or approximately 240 cases per month.

Table 6-4

Factors to Consider in Planning the Registry Office

1. Overall needs of the registry
2. Physical facilities available
3. Location of the registry in relation to other departments:
   physicians
   patient services areas
4. Special function areas:
   cancer registry activities private (work) conversations
   storage of confidential documents
   files and supplies
5. Computer equipment and other furnishings necessary for work done by registry staff including a computer work station for each employee with access to Internet connections.

of this textbook that discusses the Cancer Registry Budget for more information on how to translate the plan for organizing a registry into costs to include in the operating budget.

Next, it is important to meet with the facility's development or engineering department to determine the best way to design the office environment. Factors that should be discussed are sound, layout, temperature, humidity, and lighting. The overall image of the registry must also be considered. The department should be pleasing in appearance, not only for staff working there, but for other hospital staff, patients, and visitors.

In establishing the physical portion of the office structure, certain standards must be met. Tweedy suggests office design standards as shown in Table 6-5.[3]

To meet today's standards and mandates, the office must be wheelchair accessible and usable. Equipment must be within easy reach for registry personnel. For example, if two employees share the same responsibilities, placing their desks facing each other affords better communication and easier access to common resources. It can also decrease telephone expenses, enabling them to share an extension.

The amount of office space that is allocated to the registry will determine the type of office furniture that can be selected. If space is limited, an L-shaped desk with extension should be considered. An extension that is flexible and can be installed on either side of the work area provides additional work space. Most registrars spend their day working at a computer or desk and need a chair that is not only comfort-

able but ergonomically correct and adjustable. Even if funding is modest, careful consideration should be given to providing adequate office chairs.

Security is a major consideration when purchasing storage and filing systems. The need to maintain confidentiality of registry information is primary. The type of storage and filing system will depend on the amount of space that is available and whether or not the registry is computerized, manual or a combination of both. Registries that maintain paper abstracts require a significant amount of storage and filing space compared to those with a computerized system requiring less paper. High-density filing and storage units may be desirable, even if the initial cost is greater. Furniture systems are available in a variety of styles and colors that can add visual appeal to the registry environment. In addition, this type of furniture can be used to divide work space and provide privacy for staff.

Another concept in office design is modular furniture. One of the benefits of modular furniture is its mobility. Relocation or restructuring is simpler if modular furniture is used. It is also very practical in the event of staff increases and expansion, and it provides some degree of privacy. One disadvantage is the sacrifice of some space, because modular office furniture is larger than standard office furniture. The benefits and the disadvantages must be weighed for all design types in order to select the best possible configuration and remain within the budget.

The most important pieces of registry equipment are the computer and printer. Other chapters

Table 6-5
Office Design Standards

- Each employee should have ample work space which can accommodate a computerized work station; a minimum standard is approximately 60 square feet of work space per employee.
- Arrange desks facing each other with approximately 2 1/2 to 3 feet between desks.
- Main walkways and aisles should not be less than 44 inches wide—67 inches wide is preferable. Three feet of space for the chair and for walking behind the desk is considered a minimum standard.
- Main aisles with file cabinets that open toward desks or other furniture should measure 43 to 67 inches wide when the file drawers are open. Secondary aisles should measure 28 to 36 inches when file drawers are open.
- Large, open spaces are preferable to dividing the area into smaller rooms. Open spaces make communications easier and provide better light and ventilation.
- Take advantage of outside light whenever possible. When partitions are installed around a workstation used by several employees, two exits should be provided.
- Paperwork flow distance should be minimized with simple and direct routing where possible.
- Remove all unused equipment.

in this textbook provide suggestions that are helpful in selecting the hardware and software. Other office equipment that can be considered if the registry is an independent department include a copier, facsimile machine, and modems for transmitting and receiving data and electronic communications.

SUMMARY

The physical organization of the registry is very important. When the layout is being planned, the first step should be to determine the annual caseload and follow-up requirements and other necessary tasks in order to make reasonable assessments about other aspects of the organization plan. Personnel, office space, and equipment are all determined by the amount of work to be accomplished on a yearly basis. Whether used for a cancer registry or other disease registry, the information presented in this chapter can assist in the decision-making process.

Proper organization and efficient structuring can help the department operate smoothly. If adequate research is not done, the registry is likely to have problems from the start. Spending less does not always save money in the long run when selecting personnel, equipment, and office space. In the current atmosphere of financial constraints, when hospitals and healthcare facilities are moving to cut costs, it might be wise to invest a little more initially to minimize the disruption of later, perhaps frequent, changes to staff and equipment.

STUDY QUESTIONS

1. How can the registrar project the number of cases that will be accessioned into the registry over a year?
2. How is the staffing required for abstracting registry cases calculated?
3. List the factors that affect the number of staff required for follow-up.
4. What is the most important key factor in meeting today's standards in office design?

REFERENCES

1. Commission on Cancer. *Standards of the Commission on Cancer, vol. 1: Cancer Program Standards.* Chicago, Ill: American College of Surgeons; 1996.
2. National Cancer Registrars Association and Commission on Cancer of the American College of Surgeons. *Registry Staffing Manual.* Alexandria, Va: National Cancer Registrars Association; 1989.
3. Tweedy DB. *Office Space Planning and Management: A Manager's Guide to Techniques and Standards.* Westport, Conn: Quorum Books; 1986.

chapter

CANCER REGISTRY BUDGET

Sue Watkins
RHIA, RHIT, CTR

INTRODUCTION

To operate a cancer registry efficiently, managers must plan and control the acquisition and use of their department's resources.[1] To obtain financial information quickly about these two important activities, planning and controlling, management relies on budgeting.

Budgeting is the process of planning future activities and expressing those plans in a formal manner in terms of cost. The budget is a vital ingredient in the planning and control system that permits management to monitor and direct registry activities. Budgetary control is the use of the budget to regulate and guide activities requiring and using resources for the development of new services, expanding or contracting services, increasing revenues, or decreasing operating expenses. Table 7-1 describes three different types of budgets.

THE ROLE OF THE CANCER REGISTRAR IN THE BUDGET PROCESS

The role of the cancer registrar in the budget process varies with the organization and size of the facility, the registry size, and the scope of responsibility assigned to the cancer registrar. The cancer registrar's level of responsibility in the budgetary process ranges from complete preparation and total control to monitoring the budget and providing justification for variations. Some registrars are even responsible for submitting budget requests to a larger department of which the cancer registry is only a subdepartment. According to the National Cancer Registrars Association, Inc. (NCRA) *Registry Staffing Manual,* there is a direct correlation between the time devoted to budget planning and the reporting structure of the registry. When the registry is not autonomous, budget development may only involve providing input on registry needs; however, in an autonomous registry, more time is required for budget planning and preparation, as well as for monitoring the budget. Regardless of the level of responsibility, each cancer registrar plays a role. Understanding the budgetary process provides cancer registrars with valuable tools for present and future professional performance. Budget objectives vary, as can be seen in Table 7-2.

Participation in the budget process allows cancer registry staff, in concert with the cancer committee, to set goals and long-range plans for the department and the cancer program that are in line with the institution's goals, to accept fiscal responsibility for the department's performance, and to coordinate activities with other departments.

BUDGET COMPONENTS APPLICABLE TO CANCER REGISTRY FUNCTIONS

The three types of budget components applicable to cancer registry functions are expense, capital, and revenue. Expense budgets encompass the allocation of expenditures for personnel, supplies, office equipment, postage, maintenance, and so forth. Capital budgets are used to plan and purchase major equipment (usually valued at over $500, with a life expectancy of two or more years). Revenue budgets forecast income from sources such as patient fees, grants, service contracts with other facilities, donations, and fund-raising activities.

Cost components of budgets can be fixed, variable or semivariable, direct or indirect. All of these

Table 7-1
Types of Budgets

- *Traditional*: based on past experience plus forecasts to account for inflation and other variables
- *Program*: planning built around identifiable projects that must be accomplished
- *Zero-based*: a resource allocation method that requires budget makers to examine every expenditure during each budget period and justify the expenditure in light of current needs

Table 7-2
Budget Objectives

- *A basic plan* through which expenditures for all purposes and revenues from all sources can be forecasted and displayed
- *A statement on the objectives* of the registry and cancer program, expressed in quantitative terms
- *An estimate of future needs* arranged in an organized manner, covering some or all of the activities of the cancer program for a defined period of time
- *Pre-established standards* against which actual operations are compared
- *Motivation* of all individuals by creating a climate of cost consciousness

components are found in cancer registry budgets and are explained in Table 7-3.

PLANNING AND BUDGET CYCLES

The budget cycle includes five steps: preparation, presentation, adoption, administration, and monitoring (Table 7-4). Reports designed for use in preparing and monitoring the budget typically include budget performance reports, which depict the budget, actual income and expenditures, and the variance between the two. These reports often show the current reporting period and the year-to-date figures. Year-to-date cumulative figures are often more significant than monthly figures when comparing budgeted and actual expenses. For example, the year-to-date actual expenses tend to smooth out some of the variances caused by "one-time-only" events, such as attendance at an annual meeting. Variances exceeding a certain percentage often require an explanation or reason for their occurrence. An example of a monthly budget control report is shown in Figure 7-1.

Analysis reports are useful in comparing program costs against a specific unit of measure, such as the number of cancer cases. For example, a simple analysis of a cancer program budget of $50,000 with 1,000 annual new cancer cases would reveal a cost per case of $50.

Budgets are usually prepared for a fiscal year or any consecutive 12-month period, which may or may not coincide with the calendar year. Budget planning normally begins several months prior to the new fiscal year. The fiscal, or accounting, department usually coordinates this activity. Information on past budget performance and present budget status, guidelines for forecasting future revenues and expenditures, timelines, worksheets, and basic instructions are customarily provided to the planners. Instructions on reading fiscal reports, which are sometimes difficult to interpret, should also be available.

Financial control does not end with successful budget preparation. Monitoring ongoing expenses and revenues is also important. The budget is a plan. When the actual does not match the plan, a variety of

Table 7-3
Budget Terms

- *Fixed:* costs usually related to a time period and tending to remain unchanged when the volume of activity changes. An example is equipment depreciation.
- *Variable:* costs that change in response to changes in the volume of activity. Examples include staffing and supplies.
- *Semivariable or mixed:* costs that include both fixed and variable components. Semivariable costs increase or decrease with changes in activity but are directly proportional to changes in operating volume. Examples include full-time staff, who are paid regardless of the volume of cancer cases, compared with part-time or temporary help, who work only when the volume is high or the department is behind.
- *Direct:* costs that originate in and are directly charged against the department's budget. Examples include personnel and depreciation expenses of the equipment used solely by a specific department.
- *Indirect:* costs that are general in nature and benefit several departments or services. Examples include electricity, building maintenance, accounting, and Human Resource services.

Table 7-4
Five Steps of the Budget Cycle

1. *Preparation* of the budget: meeting with administrator or budget director, identifying department or program, space, personnel, and equipment needs. New items require justification-costs versus benefits, which may not be monetary (for example, prestige, improved patient care, or physician recruitment).
2. *Presentation* of budget documents: submission to required individuals. Registrars should be prepared to meet with those in authority and respond to questions.
3. *Adoption, or approval,* of the budget for implementation: approval to incur expenditures.
4. *Administration, or execution,* of the budget: spending monies and implementing budget plan.
5. *Monitoring* budget performance: use of control documents to monitor revenues and expenditures in relation to budget.

Figure 7-1
Sample Registry Budget Control Report

COMMUNITY HOSPITAL
Monthly Budget Control Report
March, 2004

Accounts	Current Month				Year to Date			
	Budget	Actual	Variance $	%	Budget	Actual	Variance $	%
1. Personnel								
Wages								
Fringe benefits								
2. Services and Supplies								
Office/Computer								
Postage								
Reproduction								
Maintenance								
Rental/Lease								
Communication								
Books/Dues/Sub								
Training/Education								
Travel								

Total Expenses

Variance $ = Actual minus Budget

Variance % = $\frac{\text{Variance \$}}{\text{budget}} \times 100$

Please comment if any line item or total variance is > 5% or > $500.

Comments

---

actions can be taken. In most organizations, monthly reports detailing revenues and expenses are provided. In addition, reports are generated that compare monthly and year-to-date actual results with the budget. These reports should be reviewed each month to ensure that there are no errors in assigning revenues or expenses to the correct budgets and to monitor actual results from the plan. It is important to understand what caused the variation or variance from the budget. Was it a one-time occurrence or will the variance continue? What actions are necessary to modify future results in order to achieve the overall targets? It is important to stay within the budget, but if justified, expenses may exceed the budget as it is important to complete the objectives set for the registry and the cancer program.

Planning for the cancer program budget should involve the cancer committee. Long- and short-range goals must be reviewed to assess the accomplishments of the program and to determine what resources are needed to meet future objectives. Key individuals should be involved in the planning process, particularly those that may be affected. Goals for the cancer committee to consider could include approval of the cancer program by the Commission on Cancer; computerization of the cancer database; increased use of registry data; development of patient management guidelines; community outreach activities such as education, prevention, and screening; and increased frequency of and attendance at cancer conferences.

OPERATING BUDGET

The operating budget consists of revenues and expenses, as shown in Figure 7-2. Table 7-5 lists examples of the line items traditionally found in cancer registry budgets.

Figure 7-2
Sample Registry Operating Budget

COMMUNITY HOSPITAL
Anywhere, USA

Department: Cancer Registry   **Fiscal Year: 2003**

Revenues

Ladies Auxiliary donation	$5,000
Memorial Hospital contract	30,000
Total Revenue:	**$35,000**

Expenses

Personnel

Wages	70,000
Fringe benefits (25%)	27,500

Services and Supplies

Office and computer supplies @ 200 per month	2,400
Postage: 3,000 pieces @ 37¢	1,110
Reproduction (outside, annual report)	5,000
Maintenance contracts: computers, copier	1,000
Rental/Lease: copy machine	1,200
Communication/Telephone @ $80 per month	960
Books, dues, and subscribtions	500
Training and education (registration fees)	1,000
Travel (local, state and national conferences): 2 persons @ $2,000 ea	4,000
Total expenses:	**$104,760**
Department Profit (Loss):	**$(69,670)**

Note: Budget based on direct costs for computerized registry, 2.5 FTEs, 550 cases per year at Community Hospital, 250 cases per year at Memorial Hospital, three years of follow-up at Community Hospital, no follow-up at Memorial Hospital (new program).

Table 7-5
Traditional Items Found in Cancer Registry Budgets

Revenue
- *Revenue* or income sources for cancer registries have usually been limited to donations, grants, and fund-raising activities. Healthcare reform, mandated by government legislation or by local market forces, has become a reality. Mergers and acquisitions of hospitals, clinics, physician groups, medical laboratories, and other patient care services have resulted in new opportunities for cancer program income. Mergers and acquisitions often result in one hospital managing another. It is not uncommon for one cancer registry to assume the operation of another, either through direct administration or through a fee-for-service contract. As more states develop central cancer registries with mandated statewide reporting, other opportunities will become available for contracting services to hospitals without cancer registries.

Expenses
- *Personnel:* generally the largest component of a cancer registry budget. Salaries and fringe benefits make up the personnel budget. The budget for salaries should include anticipated merit and cost-of-living increases. Fringe benefits consist of paid time off (vacations, holidays, and sick leave), state disability, social security, workers' compensation, FICA, retirement, and insurance. The personnel department can provide relevant information for budget planning.
- *Communications:* telephone, facsimile, modem lines
- *Supplies:* staples, pens, pencils, paper, letterhead, envelopes, paper clips, graphic aids, and other consumable materials
- *Postage:* first- and third-class postage, overnight mail
- *Books, subscriptions, dues:* reference materials and membership dues in professional organizations
- *Printing and duplicating:* letterhead, cancer conference bulletins, newsletters, annual report
- *Data processing:* software or upgrades, data-processing fees, network access fees
- *Equipment maintenance:* maintenance contracts on computer hardware, copy machines, and other office equipment
- *Travel:* transportation, lodging, per diems for program and professional development
- *Training:* registration fees for educational programs
- *Small tools:* nonconsumable equipment (that does not meet capital budget minimum criteria)
- *Other expenses:* food and services for cancer committee meetings, cancer conferences, cancer registry week celebrations, and miscellaneous expenses such as bottled water, audio visual supplies, depreciation

CAPITAL BUDGET

Capital budgets are used for the purchase of major equipment. The definition of major equipment varies from one facility to another. One facility may define it as any piece of equipment with a cost exceeding $300 and having a three-year life expectancy. Another may define it as equipment with a cost exceeding $500. Some facilities change their definitions from one year to the next. The fiscal department should be contacted to obtain the current definition for a particular facility. As a general rule, specific forms are required for requesting capital budget items. These forms are provided by the fiscal department. A sample form for the capital budget is shown in Figure 7-3.

SUMMARY

Historically, hospital cancer registries have been susceptible to cost-saving reductions, and even eliminations in times of fiscal crisis. Cancer registry staff should be cognizant of opportunities to generate income and be fiscally responsible at all times. Cancer registry budgets should be compatible with overall institutional budget goals. Each member of the registry staff should be conscious of the positive impact of careful fiscal management. Many of the goals of the overall cancer program will be reflected in the fiscal planning of the cancer registry budget. By working together to develop short- and long-range goals for the cancer program and the registry, the efforts of the cancer committee and registry staff will benefit the hospital and the cancer patients.

Figure 7-3
Sample Capital Budget Request Form

COMMUNITY HOSPITAL
Capital Budget Request

Department:

Contact: **Phone #**

Quantity	Cost Each	Total $	Name/Description of Item and Request Justification

Approved: _____ In full _____ Only as noted _____ No

Comments:

Signature: _____ **Date:**_____

STUDY QUESTIONS

1. Identify and describe two budget objectives.
2. Define fixed, variable, and semivariable cost components of budgets.
3. Contrast direct and indirect costs.
4. Describe the five steps of the budget cycle.
5. Name and describe one of the three types of budgets presented in the chapter.

REFERENCES

1. Watkins S, MacKinnon J, Price W. *Budgets and Staffing.* In: Menck H, Smart C, eds. *Central Cancer*

Registries: Design, Management and Use. Chur, Switzerland: Harwood Academic Publishers; 1994.

BIBLIOGRAPHY

Cofer J, ed. *Health Information Management,* 10th ed. Chicago, Ill: American Health Information Management Association; 1994

Johns M. ed. *Health Information Management Technology: An Applied Approach.* American Health Information Management Association; 2002.

National Cancer Registrars Association and Commission on Cancer of the American College of Surgeons. *Registry Staffing Manual.* Lenexa, Kan: National Cancer Registrars Association; 1989.

Ward WJ. *Health Care Budgeting and Financial Management for Non-Financial Managers.* Westport, Conn: Auburn House; 1994.

Watkins S, ed. *Tumor Registry Management Manual,* 4th ed. Santa Barbara, Calif: Cancer Registrars Association of California; 1992.

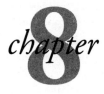

chapter 8

CANCER REGISTRY MANAGEMENT

Carol S. Venuti
RHIA, CTR

Barbara Zaranek
CTR

INTRODUCTION

Cancer registry supervisors have varying educational backgrounds and management styles. Successful management requires careful planning, direction, and control of staff and operations. This chapter addresses several management components that must be in place before the cancer registry begins to collect data. Unless otherwise specified, the term *supervisor* refers to any individual directly responsible for overseeing daily cancer registry operations.

CANCER REGISTRY PLANNING

The first step in the planning process is to define registry objectives. Once objectives are defined, personnel, space, and equipment needs can be determined. The *Standards of the Commission on Cancer* and the *Facility Oncology Registry Data Standards* (FORDS), provide a basis for objective development by outlining all requirements that must be met to maintain approval.[1] If cancer reporting is a requirement in your state, attention must also be paid to those requirements. Medical and administrative staff may contribute suggestions for additional objectives, depending on the goals of the institution.

Although the majority of registry data are utilized by medical staff to evaluate cancer caseloads, treatment, and survival, administrators are increasingly using registry data for resource planning and referral pattern identification. In managed care settings, registry data may be used to identify service areas, physician recruitment opportunities, service usage, hospice needs, resource usage, or payment sources.[2] As a result, the registry may need to modify objectives to meet changing institutional goals. Once defined, objectives provide a basis for developing registry staff position descriptions.

CANCER REGISTRY POSITION DESCRIPTIONS

Cancer registry position descriptions should be specific enough to outline all job responsibilities yet flexible enough to allow for staff and cancer program growth.[3] Many facilities have specific formats for position descriptions. Although the formats may differ, position descriptions in all facilities should contain similar information. The 1989 *Registry Staffing Manual* published by the National Cancer Registrars Association (NCRA) recommends that the position description include requirements or comments regarding 14 areas of responsibility, as shown in Table 8-1.

Computer proficiency is an absolute must in today's cancer registry world. The cancer registrar should have a knowledge regarding database management in addition to experience using word processing, presentation programs, and spreadsheets.

In smaller registries, one person may be responsible for all functions, in which case one position description covers all responsibilities. However, larger registries may require the development of several specialized position descriptions (for example, cancer program manager, who handles administrative and staffing issues; abstractors, who abstract and code the data; follow-up person, who conducts all follow-up activities; or another for the person who is responsible for reporting data statistics). Specialized position descriptions may be more efficient and cost effective and cover a broader range of expertise and services.[3]

Cancer registry responsibilities may change with yearly caseloads or as cancer program responsibilities

Table 8-1
Details to Be Included in Position Descriptions

- Responsibility for cancer program management
- Responsibility for information management
- Responsibility for information retention and retrieval
- Responsibility for personnel administration
- Responsibility for registry statistics
- Responsibility for legal and ethical perspectives (including release of information)
- Responsibility for quality assurance
- Responsibility for diagnosis, stage, and treatment coding; classifying; and indexing
- Educational or technical qualifications including knowledge of the disease process, diagnostic methods and procedures, composition of the health record, data interpretation, and statistical and analytical skills
- Hours of work
- Responsibility for interactions with medical and administrative staff
- Responsibility for intradepartmental and interdepartmental relationships
- Required memberships, if any
- Physical requirements, if applicable

change. As a result, position descriptions should be reviewed and revised annually. Once cancer registry responsibilities are defined, staffing and workload distributions can be determined.

OFFICE MANAGEMENT

Planning is required to ensure that registry staffing meets the requirements of the Commission on Cancer (CoC) of the American College of Surgeons. Several factors affect registry staffing, including yearly caseload, data usage, longevity of the database, managerial and administrative responsibilities, computerization, and cancer program functions.[2] Institutions may hire part-time or full-time staff or consultants to perform registry and cancer program functions. The hours of cancer registry operations can vary; for example, five days a week, eight hours per day, or four days a week, ten hours per day. However, staff should be available during normal business hours to accommodate study requests from medical and administrative staff. Staffing hours may also vary in order to facilitate follow-up calls to patients, outside institutions, or physicians' offices. Methods for task distribution vary from registry to registry.

The possibility of distributing and sharing responsibilities is greater in larger registries.[3] Some registries delegate specific responsibilities to each staff member, whereas others distribute all responsibilities equally among all staff members. Abstracting responsibilities might be distributed by cancer site, alphabet, or medical record number. For example, a particular staff member may be responsible for abstracting and following all patients with breast cancer or all patients with a last name beginning with the letters A through D, and so on. Varying staff or their responsibilities allows the supervisor to achieve goals while providing staff with the opportunity to expand their knowledge and skills.

Once data collection begins, continuous monitoring is required to ensure compliance with the CoC, the State Registry, and other requirements. For example, if concurrent abstracting is not done, abstracting should be initiated between four and six months after diagnosis and the follow-up percentage must be maintained at or above 90%.[4] When backlogs occur, rearranging responsibilities to meet deadlines may be necessary. The development of

productivity standards will assist the supervisor in monitoring compliance.

PRODUCTIVITY STANDARDS

Productivity standards should clearly define departmental and individual staff expectations, as well as performance and evaluation methods. The NCRA *Registry Staffing Manual* outlines specific productivity standards and suggestions for conducting time-and-motion studies for casefinding, abstracting, and follow-up. Conducting time-and-motion studies within the department can help to establish internal productivity standards or validate existing standards. Another resource for productivity standards is the NCRA *Cancer Registry Staffing & Compensation Manual* which summarizes the results of a survey taken in August 2000. This manual presents a methodology for determining staffing levels based on average productivity reported by the survey participants.[5]

Productivity standards provide a basis for performance evaluations by allowing measurement of job performance. In addition, productivity standards data can be used to justify the need for additional staff or equipment.[2] For more information on standard calculations, refer to Chapter 6 of this textbook, Cancer Registry Personnel, Office Space, and Equipment.

POLICY AND PROCEDURE MANUAL

Every registry within a CoC-approved cancer program must develop and maintain a procedure manual that documents each phase of cancer registry operations. This manual promotes smooth operation of the registry and serves as a training reference for new staff.[2] A complete and current procedure manual outlines operational and departmental expectations. In addition, an updated manual can help registry staff keep current regarding changes in the profession. Table 8-2 contains a list of items that are recommended to be included in the policy and procedure manual.

In addition to a procedure manual, computerized registries must also maintain an operations manual that addresses the items listed in Table 8-3.[1]

The cancer committee must be involved with the development of the policy and procedure manual. Once developed, it should be reviewed and

Table 8-2
Cancer Registry Procedure Manual

The cancer registry procedure manual includes, but is not limited to:

- Abstracting
- Case accessions
- Case eligibility
- Casefinding
- Coding references
- Confidentiality and release of information
- Dates of implementation or changes in policies or registry operations
- Follow-up
- Job descriptions
- Maintaining and using the suspense system
- Quality control of registry data
- Reference date
- Reporting requirements and mechanisms
- Retention of documents
- Staging systems

Areas of program activity include, but are not limited to:

- Cancer committee meetings
- Cancer conference activities
- Cancer program objectives
- Policy for American Joint Committee on Cancer (AJCC) staging
- Studies of quality and quality improvement system

---

revised at least once a year. The procedure manual must be updated as procedures change to maintain current documentation.

REFERENCE DATE

To ensure a valid statistical database, the Commission on Cancer (CoC) of the American College of Surgeons requires that a start date be established for the registry before data collection begins. This date is known as the reference date. It should be set as January 1 of a given year. Once this date is established, all cases diagnosed and/or treated at the facility on or after this date must be entered into the registry. Registries in cancer programs seeking approval from the CoC must first accrue two years of data with one year of successful follow-up.

Table 8-3
Items to Be Included in a Computerized Registry Operations Manual

- Instructions for initiation and termination of computer operations
- Instructions for completing routine tasks
- Description of potential problems and resolutions
- Documentation of edit checks
- Backup and data-loss prevention procedures
- Disaster recovery plan
- Security procedures
- Data submission to central registry

The original reference date must be maintained unless one of the items in Table 8-4 occurs.

Requests to change the reference date must be submitted to the CoC in writing. Requests are considered and approved by the CoC Administration.

REPORTABLE LIST

The CoC requires the cancer registry to collect information on malignancies diagnosed and/or treated at the hospital. There are some exceptions and the current Facility Oncology Registry Data Standards (FORDS) 1 should be reviewed for reportable and non-reportable cases. It should be noted that some state registries require certain cases to be reported that are not required by the CoC. The cancer committee is responsible for developing a reportable list that identifies all types of cases to be included in the cancer registry database. The reportable list identifies malignancies with a behavior code (fifth digit) of 2 or 3 as identified in the *International Classification of Diseases for Oncology*, 3rd edition (ICD-O-3)[1] State Registry regulations may require the reporting of additional neoplasms. In addition, the reportable list identifies reportable-by-agreement benign or borderline disease processes not required by the CoC or state registries. These reportable-by-agreement cases may be institution specific and mandated by the institution's cancer committee. Ultimately, the reportable list includes malignant cases, reportable-by-agreement and diagnoses to be entered into the cancer registry database as well as nonreportable cases (diagnoses that should not be included).

Table 8-4
Reasons for Possible Change of Reference Date

- Changes in population or census
- Inconsistencies or lapses in the database
- High lost-to-follow-up rate
- Changes in data acquisition methods
- Lack of staffing for an extended period

The reportable list should be reviewed annually by the cancer committee to determine the addition or deletion of reportable cases. Cancer committee minutes should reflect reportable list approval, annual reviews, changes, and effective collection dates.[2] When developing or changing the reportable list, it is important to remember that collecting additional reportable-by-agreement cases may necessitate additional staffing due to increased case load and related activities.

CANCER REGISTRY ORGANIZATION

Cancer registry supervisory responsibilities vary depending on the size of the cancer program. In large cancer programs, supervisors may spend more time monitoring and coordinating cancer program activities and staff. Supervisors in smaller cancer programs may spend most of their time overseeing and performing registry functions.

The department responsible for overseeing the cancer registry varies by institution. For example, the registry may be a part of the medical oncology, radiation oncology, pathology, quality improvement services, health information management, or another appropriate department. In most instances, the registry supervisor reports to the director, assistant director, or administrator of the department. Inevitably, cancer registry operations are affected by the goals of the department overseeing it. For example, registry staff within the health information management (HIM) department may be used for coding, chart analysis, or chart retrieval when HIM backlogs or staffing shortages occur. Therefore, the administrator responsible for the cancer registry must be educated regarding registry purposes and functions. This is vital to ensure that adequate staffing and time are devoted to registry operations. Additionally, the cancer committee is ultimately responsible for overseeing cancer registry operations. Therefore, educat-

ing cancer committee members regarding the functions of the registry is also essential to ensure their support and guidance.

SUMMARY

Although the backgrounds of registry supervisors vary, overall responsibilities remain the same. The cancer registry supervisor oversees daily operations of the cancer registry. On a monthly basis, responsibilities may include coordinating and overseeing the institution's cancer program compliance with approval requirements. The percentage of time spent on these responsibilities varies depending on the size of the cancer program.

The first step in cancer registry planning is the development of objectives. Once these are established, position descriptions, staffing, and workload distributions can be determined to meet CoC requirements for cancer program approval. The development of productivity standards facilitates compliance monitoring.

The development of a policy and procedure manual ensures that functions are performed consistently throughout the registry. In addition, establishing the reference date and reportable list provides a basis for data collection consistency by establishing the start date for collection and specifying which cases will be collected.

STUDY QUESTIONS

1. List the uses of registry data.
2. Identify and describe at least six areas of responsibility that position descriptions should address.
3. What are the benefits of delegating shared cancer registry responsibilities?
4. List eight of the items that should be included in the policy and procedure manual.
5. List the conditions under which a registry's reference date can be changed.

REFERENCES

1. Commission on Cancer. *Facility Oncology Registry Data Standards* (FORDS). Chicago, Ill: American College of Surgeons; 2002.
2. Watkins S, ed. *Tumor Registry Manual,* 4th ed. Santa Barbara, Calif: California Cancer Registrars Association; 1992.

3. Clutter G, Fritz A, Hannouch G, et al. *Registry Staffing Manual.* Alexandria, Va: National Cancer Registrars Association; 1989.

4. Commission on Cancer. *Cancer Program Standards 2004.* Chicago, Ill: American College of Surgeons; 2003.

5. National Cancer Registrars Association and The Commission on Cancer of the American College of Surgeons. *Cancer Registry Staffing and Compensation Manual: Results of a Survey Conducted for the National Cancer Registrar's Association,* Alexandria, Va: National Cancer Registrar's Association; 2001.

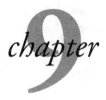

chapter

THE AMERICAN COLLEGE OF SURGEONS COMMISSION ON CANCER

Connie Bura

HISTORICAL OVERVIEW

The Commission on Cancer of the American College of Surgeons (ACoS) is a consortium of professional organizations dedicated to reducing the morbidity and mortality of cancer through education, standard-setting, and the monitoring of quality care.

The Commission on Cancer, as it is known today, was initially formed in 1922 and was named the Cancer Campaign Committee. The committee's early efforts focused on the study of the use of radium treatment for uterine cancers. In the 1930s, the Commission teamed up with the already established American Cancer Society to pursue a cooperative venture concerned with establishing standards for cancer clinics. This era marked the birth of the Commission's Approvals Program and hospital cancer programs have been surveyed and approved now for more than 70 years.

In 1930, the committee was renamed the Committee on the Treatment of Malignant Disease. Standards were published that year under the title Organization of Service for the Diagnosis and Treatment of Cancer. The standards were centered around the evaluation of cancer clinics and registries. In 1940, the committee was renamed the Committee on Cancer and, in 1947, a grassroots program to identify a surgeon at the hospital level who would promote and oversee the programs of the Committee on Cancer was instituted. This Cancer Liaison Program continues today. In 1954, the standards for cancer programs were updated to include mandates for a multidisciplinary cancer committee, tumor boards, and methods of monitoring and reporting end results. The requirements for an approved cancer program were expanded in 1956 to include a cancer registry, which incorporated diagnostic, staging, treatment, and annual lifetime follow-up for all cancer patients. Since then, the Committee on Cancer has been a key supporter of hospital-based cancer registries. In recognition of the increasingly multidisciplinary nature of cancer care, the committee was expanded in 1965 to include members from a variety of professional organizations involved in the care of the cancer patient and was renamed the Commission on Cancer (CoC).

Today, the multidisciplinary CoC sets standards for quality, multidisciplinary cancer care delivered primarily in hospital settings; surveys hospitals to assess compliance with those standards; collects standardized quality data from its approved hospitals to measure treatment patterns of care and outcomes; and uses these data to evaluate hospital provider performance and develop educational interventions to improve cancer care outcomes at the national and local level.

COC STRUCTURE

The CoC includes 100 members from the ACoS and 39 national, professional organizations that reflect the full spectrum of cancer care. These participating member organizations are listed in Table 9-1. The CoC has evolved to play a major role in the development of standards for cancer data collection and for cancer programs with a process for program monitoring and approval. The CoC remains active in the education of surgeons and registrars, as well as in the collection of data on national patterns of cancer care. These activities are reflected in the organizational structure, which includes 3 standing committees, 13 disease site teams, and 3 subcommittees (Figure 9-1). American Cancer Society (ACS) members are elected to the CoC for a six-year term, and representatives from member organizations are also elected for a six-year term. Committee chairs serve for three years, and the chair of the Commission serves for two years. The executive committee includes the commission chair, the chair-elect, the chairs of the standing committees and nominating committee, a cancer program surveyor, as well as representatives from seven member organizations: the American Cancer Society, American College of Radiology, American Joint Committee on Cancer, American Society of Clinical Oncology, American Society of Therapeutic Radiology and Oncology, College of American Pathologists, and Oncology Nursing Society.

THE APPROVALS PROGRAM

The Committee on Approvals administers the activities of the Approvals Program which is designed to ensure that the structure and processes necessary for quality cancer care are in place. In 2003, the CoC released its current standards for cancer programs, *Cancer Program Standards, 2004*.[1] The 36 standards included in *Cancer Program Standards, 2004* are all mandatory, form the basis for the approval award, and are organized into eight major areas. These standards continue to promote and support the four historic cornerstones of the Approvals Program:

Table 9-1
Member Organizations of the CoC

American Academy of Hospice and Palliative Medicine	American Urological Association
American Academy of Pediatrics	Association of American Cancer Institutes
American Association for Cancer Education, Inc.	Association of Cancer Executives
American Cancer Society, Inc.	Association of Community Cancer Centers
American College of Obstetricians And Gynecologists	Association of Oncology Social Workers
American College of Oncology Administrators	Canadian Society of Surgical Oncology
American College of Physicians	Centers for Disease Control, Division of Cancer
American College of Radiology	Prevention and Control
American College of Surgeons	College of American Pathologists
American Dietetic Association, Oncology Nutrition	Department of Defense
Dietetic Practice Group	Department of Veterans Affairs
American Head and Neck Society	International Union Against Cancer
American Hospital Association	National Cancer Institute—SEER Program
American Joint Committee on Cancer	National Cancer Institute—Outcomes Research Branch
American Medical Association	National Cancer Registrars Association, Inc.
American Pediatric Surgical Association	National Surgical Adjuvant Breast and Bowel Project
American Society for Psychosocial and Behavioral	North American Association of Central Cancer Registries
Oncology	Oncology Nursing Society
American Society of Clinical Oncology	Society of Gynecologic Oncologists
American Society of Colon and Rectal Surgeons	Society of Surgical Oncology
American Society for Therapeutic Radiology and	Society of Thoracic Surgeons
Oncology	

Figure 9-1
CoC Current Structure

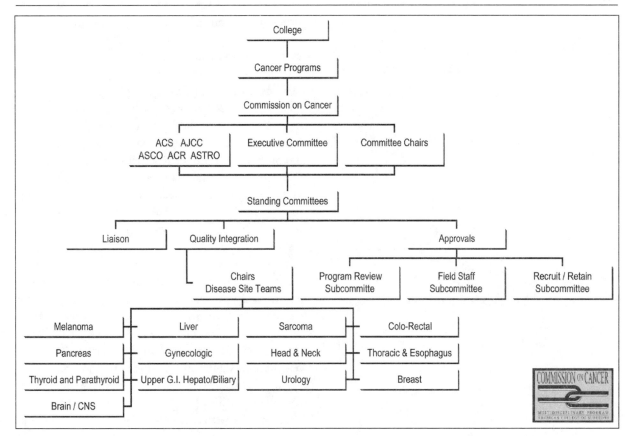

multidisciplinary cancer conferences, a multidisciplinary cancer committee, a program of quality improvement and outcome assessment, and a cancer registry. *Cancer Program Standards, 2004* became effective in January, 2004 for participating hospital cancer programs. These new standards provide a more flexible approach to cancer program management and take into account the various types and sizes of hospitals with category-specific requirements defined for many standards. These requirements are designed to recognize the type of facility, services provided, and cases accessioned.

The eight areas of program evaluation include institutional and programmatic resources cancer committee leadership, cancer data management and cancer registry operations, clinical management, research, community outreach, professional education and staff support, and quality improvement (Table 9-2). Examples of new standards include the requirement that case abstracting is performed or supervised by a Certified Tumor Registrar (CTR). The CoC believes that in order to positively impact cancer patient care, the facility must ensure that case abstracting is performed or supervised by a CTR. Successful operation of the cancer registry requires credentialed staff who are trained and knowledgeable in all aspects of oncology data collection and case abstracting. All cancer programs approved by the CoC must comply with this standard by 2006. Programs surveyed prior to that date are asked to demonstrate that they are working towards compliance with this standard and will be required to show documentation of recruitment efforts and/or plans for current staff certification. All participating programs will continue to meet the current requirement for AJCC staging to be assigned by the managing

Table 9-2
Cancer Program Standards:
Eight Areas of Evaluation

- Institutional and Programmatic Resources
- Cancer Committee Leadership
- Cancer Data Management and Cancer Registry Operations
- Clinical Management
- Research
- Community Outreach
- Professional Education and Staff Support
- Quality Improvement

---

physician and recorded in the medical record, however, as of 2005, programs are required to implement the use of a staging form in the medical record to document staging by the managing physician.

CoC-approved cancer programs are required to annually submit data to the National Cancer Data Base (NCDB); this allows regular assessment of national patterns of care and creates benchmarks for outcomes comparisons. The new standards require that cases submitted to the NCDB for the most recent accession year requested meet the established quality criteria included in the annual Call for Data. Accurate data are necessary for the meaningful comparison of treatment and patient outcomes. These data form the basis for the feedback provided to cancer programs. As part of its annual Call for Data, the NCDB documents the conditions that will cause the cases submitted to the NCDB to be rejected. Standardized, nationally accepted data edits are applied to all analytic cases submitted. The reporting registry is notified of the problematic cases through an edit report. Problematic cases identified in the edit report are required to be corrected and resubmitted to the NCDB for the most current accession year by September 1 of the year following the most recent Call for Data.

Facilities participating in the CoC Approvals Program are concerned with the continuum of care from prevention and early detection, pretreatment evaluation, and staging, to optimal treatment, rehabilitation, surveillance for recurrent disease, support services, and end-of-life care. CoC approval is granted only to those facilities that have voluntarily committed to provide the best in cancer diagnosis and treatment and are able to comply with the CoC's established standards. Participation in the Approvals Program is voluntary. The success of a cancer program depends on the leadership of a multidisciplinary cancer committee. The committee is responsible for planning, initiating, stimulating, and assessing all cancer-related activities at the facility. Because quality of care requires a serious commitment to the necessity and value of the cancer program, facilities are surveyed only at the written request of a member of the their administrative or professional staff. This request should be made when the cancer committee is confident that the CoC cancer program standards have been met. Prior to initial survey, the institution must demonstrate one year of compliance with the standards, have accrued two years of data with one year of successful follow-up,

Table 9-3
Requirements for a Cancer Program to be Considered for Approval

Hospitals, freestanding treatment facilities, and healthcare networks are eligible to participate in the CoC Approvals Program. Each facility ensures that patients have access to the full scope of services required to diagnose, treat, rehabilitate, and support patients with cancer and their families. Prevention and early detection services are made available to the community. Services are provided on-site, by referral, or coordinated with other facilities or local agencies.

Five elements are key to the success of a Commission-approved cancer program:

1. The clinical services provide state-of-the-art pretreatment evaluation, staging, treatment, and clinical follow-up for cancer patients seen at the facility for primary, secondary, tertiary, or quaternary care.
2. The cancer committee leads the program through setting goals, monitoring activity, and evaluating patient outcomes and improving care.
3. The cancer conferences provide a forum for patient consultation and contribute to physician education.
4. The quality improvement program is the mechanism for evaluating and improving patient outcomes.
5. The cancer registry and database is the basis for monitoring the quality of care.

and have met the requirements for consideration for approval (Table 9-3).

The assessment of cancer programs is carried out by staff-trained, volunteer physician surveyors and is overseen by the CoC technical staff, and the Program Review and Field Staff Subcommittees of the Committee on Approvals. Each cancer program must undergo a rigorous evaluation and review of its performance and compliance with the CoC standards every three years. When the survey visit is scheduled, time must be allotted on the agenda for the surveyor to meet with the administrator, cancer committee chair, cancer registrar, and the cancer liaison physician, as well as other members of the facility's cancer team. The surveyor reviews documentation of cancer committee meetings, cancer conferences, and quality management processes and improvements. The visit also includes a review of documentation that supports the cancer program's compliance with the standards, including the Web-enabled CoC Survey Application Record (SAR) completed by the facility prior to the survey. At the conclusion of the survey, the surveyor may have recommendations to align the program with current standards.

A quantitative rating system, consistent with that used by the Joint Commission on Accreditation of Healthcare Organizations (JCAHO), is in place to ensure objectivity and consistency among reviewers (Table 9-4). To ensure consistent interpretation of compliance with the 36 standards, the rating system includes criteria for compliance with each standard; and a compliance rating is assigned by the facility, the

surveyor, and the CoC technical staff. Commendation ratings have been established for nine of the 36 standards, or 25% of all standards. Commendations received for individual standards will be acknowledged in the Approved Cancer Program Performance Report that is provided to the program following the survey. A program that receives a commendation rating in all nine defined areas along with a compliance rating for all other (27) standards will earn the CoC Outstanding Achievement Award. Awards will be granted to each program upon completion of the survey and evaluation of compliance with the established criteria. This award will be in place until the next survey. The purpose of the CoC Outstanding Achievement Award is to: recognize cancer programs that strive for excellence in providing quality care to the cancer patient; motivate other programs to work towards improving their care, and foster communication between award programs and other programs to share best practices,

Table 9-4
System for Rating Compliance with CoC Cancer Program Standards

1+ - Commendation
1 - Compliance
5 - Noncompliance
8 - Not Applicable

Criteria for rating compliance were developed for each individual standard.

serve as a resource, and act as a "champion" for the CoC Approvals Program. Cancer programs receiving this award will receive a letter of recognition from the CoC chair addressed to the CEO/administrator; a specifically designed press release, marketing information and special certificate; CoC publicity via the CoC *Flash* email newsletter and CoC Website, and acknowledgement in a public forum including the CoC Annual Meeting. An Award Matrix (Table 9-5) is used to assign approval awards on the basis of compliance with the 36 mandatory standards.

The Committee on Approvals recognizes that the cancer services available at a facility will vary depending on its size and scope. Therefore, approval is given in different categories. Each facility is assigned to a cancer program category by the CoC staff. The type of facility or organization, services provided, and cases accessioned are considered when making category assignments. The CoC has defined nine cancer program categories and describes the requirements for each as they relate to specific standards. A sample of program categories includes those institutions funded by the National Cancer Institute (NCI) as cancer centers, defined as NCI-designated centers; teaching facilities, defined as facilities with at least 4 residency programs; comprehensive community, facilities that see more than 650 analytic cancer cases annually and provide a full range of cancer services; and community hospitals, which see a smaller number of cases annually. The Network Cancer Program category reflects the sharing of cancer treatment and data resources among hospitals in healthcare networks. Additional categories exist that allow participation by facilities that provide only specialized elements of cancer care.

At present, there are more than 1,400 CoC-approved cancer programs in the United States and Puerto Rico. Of these, 39% are community programs, 35% are comprehensive community programs, and 23% are either NCI-designated or teaching programs. Approved programs are widely distributed throughout the United States as illustrated in Figure 9-2, and a public list is available on the Cancer Programs page of the American College of Surgeons website (www.facs.org).

Data from the approvals process are used to generate Approved Cancer Program Performance Reports comparable with the hospital performance reports issued by the JCAHO. These reports allow cancer programs to compare their ratings for mandatory standards with approved programs in their state, their award category, and nationally. The reports also facilitate the identification of areas for program improvement.

Today, CoC-approved cancer programs are credited with diagnosing and treating 80% of all newly diagnosed cancer patients nationally. The Approvals Program is recognized by other national healthcare organizations, including the JCAHO, as having established performance measures for high-quality cancer care. An approved program provides a forum for interdisciplinary communication and interaction. It ensures that multidisciplinary, integrated, and comprehensive oncology services are being offered to patients, and approval demonstrates to the community that the institution is willing to commit the resources necessary to provide the very best cancer care. CoC-approved cancer programs benefit from free marketing by partnering with the CoC and American Cancer Society (ACS) in the Facility

Table 9-5
Approval Award Matrix

	Full Approval (Three Years)	Three-Year Approval with Contingency	Non-Approval	Approval Deferred*
36 Standards	No deficiencies	One to seven deficiency(ies) (up to 19% of standards)	Eight or more deficiencies (22% or more of standards). Requires recommendation by the Program Review Subcommittee and confirmation by the Committee on Approvals	One deficiency (2% of standards)

*Valid only for new programs.

Figure 9-2
U.S. Distribution of CoC-Approved Cancer Programs

AK	2	KS	12	NY	73
AL	23	KY	25	OH	85
AR	11	LA	31	OK	19
AZ	9	MA	48	OR	18
CA	125	MD	35	PA	75
CO	21	ME	11	PR	4
CT	24	MI	37	RI	10
DC	8	MN	16	SC	17
DE	7	MO	31	SD	6
FL	65	MS	13	TN	31
GA	37	MT	3	TX	70
HI	8	NC	34	UT	7
IA	13	ND	6	VA	43
ID	7	NE	12	VT	5
IL	92	NH	10	WA	41
IN	35	NJ	54	WI	27
		NM	7	WV	13
		NV	3	WY	0

9/03

Information Profile System (FIPS)—a voluntary information sharing effort of resources and services and cancer experience for the Society's Website and National Call Center. Participation by approved programs in the NCDB provides the facility with benchmark reports containing national aggregate data and individual facility data to assess patterns of care and outcomes relative to national norms.

THE NATIONAL CANCER DATA BASE

The NCDB is a nationwide oncology outcomes database for over 1,400 facilities in 50 states. The NCDB was founded as a joint project of the CoC and the ACS in 1988. Currently, the NCDB collects data on approximately 850,000 (70%) of all incident cancer diagnoses annually, and includes detailed information on over 13 million cancer patients in the U.S. representing 60 different cancer sites. The NCDB has undergone a number of changes since its inception and is now recognized as the world's largest clinical database, providing vitally important patterns of care information upon which

quality improvement can be leveraged at the point of delivery of cancer care in the US. Information is collected on an annual basis on patient demographics, diagnostic methods, AJCC stage, treatment, and mortality; this allows for the definition of current patterns of care and changes over time. Submission of data to the NCDB has been a requirement for approved cancer programs since 1996. Each year, the NCDB issues a Call for Data to all CoC-approved cancer programs. The Call for Data collects data items required by the CoC Approvals Program. Original data collection commenced with 1985 diagnoses and now provides 15 years of follow-up on over 2 million patients with gastrointestinal tumors, almost 2 million breast cancer patients, 1.5 million cases of prostate carcinoma, and 1.4 million cases of non-small cell lung cancer. Relatively uncommon cancers have accumulated in impressive numbers. For example, the database now contains 140,000 cases of carcinoma of the thyroid and over 15,000 cases of male breast cancer.

A central advisory panel guides and assists in the prioritization of the work conducted by the NCDB staff. The Quality Integration Committee (QIC) is concerned with, and represents the CoC in matters addressing the progress and direction of research and continuing education as it pertains to improving the care of cancer patients. The QIC directs and oversees the activities of 13 Disease Site Teams (DSTs) that were formed in order to better meet the national demand for ongoing assessment of the quality of cancer care by conducting research using NCDB resources; developing focused studies; collaborating with national agencies in cancer care initiatives; designing educational interventions, and evaluating quality of cancer registry data. These teams consist of approximately 10 members apiece, and focus on breast, colorectal, gynecologic oncology, head and neck, liver, melanoma, pancreas, sarcoma, thoracic oncology, thyroid and parathyroid, upper GI, urology, and brain/central nervous system tumors. The DSTs are multidisciplinary in membership with national representation in surgical oncology, medical oncology, radiation oncology, pathology, and radiology. Utilizing the expertise of the DSTs, the CoC designs and conducts at least two special studies annually. Hypothesis-based special studies are designed to evaluate patient care, set benchmarks, and provide feedback to improve patient care in cancer programs. Based on study criteria, select approved programs will participate in each study.

With respect to quality improvement, a number of opportunities using NCDB data are available. Web-based benchmark report applications, available from the Cancer Programs page of the American College of Surgeons website (www.facs.org), have been developed to promote access to NCDB data by the general public, researchers, and clinicians. The benchmark reports were initially designed to facilitate public use. Subsequent development has included the Hospital Comparison Benchmark Reports that have been designed specifically for use by CoC-approved cancer programs as a tool by which to evaluate and compare the cancer care delivered to patients diagnosed and/or treated at their facility. These reports are provided as a direct benefit of their CoC approval status. When CoC-approved cancer programs are surveyed every three years, surveyors will address whether facilities have taken steps to improve the quality of care delivered to their patient populations. The CoC cancer program standards require the cancer committee at each approved facility to analyze patient outcomes and disseminate the

results of the analysis, complete and document studies that measure quality and outcomes, and implement two improvements that directly affect cancer patient care. The CoC has developed a predetermined set of indicators from the NCDB Hospital Comparison Benchmark Reports for use at the time of survey as needed. Surveyors will access information for 3 or 4 specifically define quality indicators that can be discussed with the cancer committee during the survey visit. This discussion should result in a set of actions initiated by the cancer committee to further evaluate and improve its program's performance in a specific area by the time of the next survey. Some examples of these reports would include stage distribution for a particular site to target early detection initiatives, variations in treatment patterns for a particular site and stage of disease, patterns of local and regional recurrence, and variations in long-term outcomes for patients receiving treatment at a particular facility.

EDUCATIONAL PROGRAMS

In 2001, the American College of Surgeons (ACoS) established a Division of Education to reorganize and centralize all educational programs delivered by the ACoS into one area of responsibility. In light of this decision, the CoC eliminated the Committee on Education. The CoC leadership, with input from the DSTs, works with staff in the division to develop educational initiatives directed toward surgeons. This includes selecting content and speakers for a cancer-focused postgraduate course held during the Clinical Congress of the ACoS, as well as for a disease-site symposium held at the same venue targeted to general surgeons. The symposium highlights data from the NCDB or CoC special studies.

The CoC plays a major role in educating hospital-based cancer registrars by offering programs related to understanding the Approvals Program standards; preparing for survey; learning the CoC's required data set; using NCDB data and benchmark reports; staging of cancer by physicians and cancer registrars; providing educational interventions based on NCDB data, and promoting best practices. The CoC Speakers Bureau facilitates the delivery of these CoC-focused training programs to the cancer registrar community. Each year the CoC trains a dozen or more individuals to serve as CoC-trained speakers. Volunteer speakers are selected on the basis of their cancer registry knowledge and experience, activities within the cancer registry profession, and instructional or speaking experience. The CoC also conducts an annual training program for the Approvals Program surveyors and independent cancer program consultants to increase the quality of their on-site review.

CANCER LIAISON PROGRAM

The Committee on Cancer Liaison administers the activities of the Cancer Liaison Physician network. This nationwide network of more than 1,600 physician-volunteers provides leadership for local hospital cancer programs and supports the programs and initiatives of both the CoC and American Cancer Society. These physicians serve as the link between the CoC and hospitals with approved cancer programs or those hospitals that are working toward approval. Physicians who accept the role as cancer liaison physician for their facility are required to: have a strong commitment to the success of the cancer program and the quality of care provided to patients with cancer, be an active member of the cancer committee, participate in cancer conferences, and have an interest in working with and volunteering for the local American Cancer Society on cancer control initiatives. These individuals are appointed by their respective hospital cancer committee and their term of appointment is three years with eligibility to serve an unlimited number of three year terms based upon performance. Currently, 60% of cancer liaison physicians are surgeons; with 40% representing other specialties.

The State Chair physician network was formulated to direct the activities of the local cancer liaison physicians in each state. The primary areas of responsibility for the 65 state chairs include: communicating regularly with their liaison physicians, coordinating a meeting of the cancer liaison physicians in their state, promoting participation in CoC and ACS programs at the local level, and participating in collaborative activities in the state. These include serving on the American College of Surgeons chapter council in their state, working with the division staff of the ACS, serving on the team coordinating the state cancer plan, and making presentations about the CoC and its programs at state-based cancer meetings.

The specific duties of the cancer liaison physician include: spearheading community outreach initiatives, developing and strengthening relationships with the local ACS, and using data to identify areas for cancer program improvement. The CoC's cancer program standards define a role for the cancer liaison physician as the community outreach coordinator. In this role, the cancer liaison physician is responsible for coordinating supportive services on-site or with local agencies such as the ACS, coordinating two prevention or early detection programs annually, and working with the cancer committee to monitor community outreach activities. To ensure the cancer liaison physician's success as the community outreach coordinator, the CoC has been working closely with the ACS divisions in a joint effort to provide resources and tools that will facilitate both entities in reaching their mutual goals and objectives. Interventions have been designed which CoC-approved cancer programs can implement in partnership with the ACS to meet the community outreach standards. Cancer liaison physicians are encouraged to work with the local ACS cancer control staff to explore this activity, as well as invite the ACS cancer control staff to become a regular participant at cancer committee meetings to report on ACS activities and discuss areas of collaboration. Cancer liaison physicians are also required to use data to identify areas for cancer program improvement. This effort is facilitated through cancer liaison physician use of the NCDB Hospital Comparison Benchmark Reports to identify areas for improvement in care, and to illustrate cancer program successes. Evaluation tools are in place to measure performance of both state chairs and cancer liaison physicians, to ensure that orientation programs have been upgraded, and to guarantee that quarterly communications are disseminated about current CoC activities for sharing with hospital cancer committees.

STANDARDS

In 1999, the CoC launched the Web-based Inquiry and Response (I & R) System. This system provides uniform and consistent interpretation of CoC cancer program and data standards, and promotes quality data abstracting. Users can access the database on-line and search by category (AJCC TNM cancer staging, CoC cancer program standards, registry operations and data standards, CoC special studies, etc.) or by key words (e.g., breast, physician staging). They can submit a new question at any time during the search. Users can also fax or email questions to the CoC. Members of the I & R technical staff team, composed of certified tumor registrars, are randomly assigned to review, research, and respond to inquiries. Answers that can be supported by reference to CoC publications or other standard sources are entered into the database. More difficult queries and proposed answers are presented at weekly I&R team meetings for discussion and consensus answers. When necessary, questions are referred to external sources. For example, questions regarding histology are referred to the SEER Program professionals, and questions regarding AJCC staging are referred to physicians who serve as AJCC curators for individual cancer sites. All queries and responses are reviewed for quality before being transferred to the I & R database on the ACS Website. A communication from the I & R team is sent to each user. Currently, the database houses more than 5,000 questions and answers. Data from the I & R system is routinely referenced and incorporated into CoC training programs, and is used to identify standards or staging rubrics that lack clarity or consistency for consideration in the development of future versions of CoC standards manuals and the AJCC TNM *Cancer Staging Manual.*

Registry data management is an essential element of each CoC-approved cancer program. The CoC's data standards ensure consistent and accurate hospital cancer registry data that support the meaningful evaluation of patient diagnosis and treatment. All CoC-approved cancer programs use the data standards defined by the CoC appropriate for the year of diagnosis for that case. Cancer registries may be required to comply with additional mandates pertaining to case and data reporting established by the federal or state government, or by the facility's cancer committee. In 2002, the CoC published the *Facility Oncology Registry Data Standards (FORDS)*[2] Manual required for use by all CoC-approved cancer programs beginning with cases diagnosed January 1, 2003. The *FORDS* Manual includes more complete treatment data, data on comorbid conditions, and enhanced staging data.

FUTURE DIRECTIONS

The CoC is currently structured to better meet the national demand for the ongoing assessment of quality cancer care. The CoC has broadened multidisciplinary participation in its activities with formation of the disease site teams, has increased responsiveness to internal and external requests from other organizations through the revision of its cancer program and data standards, developed tools promoting access to the NCDB data, and enhanced educational offerings targeted to key constituent groups. Finally, the CoC has achieved a high level of program integration by incorporating the NCDB into the Approvals Program standards and survey process.

The CoC hopes to raise awareness among patients, physicians, and health plans of the quality standards for CoC-approved cancer programs. The new approach of measuring quality outcomes will focus CoC educational efforts on areas in which clinical practice is not compatible with the best available evidence. Physician liaisons will be the key advocates of this program by helping to initiate change at the local level. The established strengths and infrastructure of the CoC support the schema for an integrated approach to quality improvement. NCDB data will continue to be used to identify variations in care. The Quality Integration Committee will determine whether there is compelling evidence to support a particular pattern of care. If there is, a focused educational intervention will be undertaken. The Committee on Approvals will determine whether this pattern of care is significant enough to be incorporated as a quality standard for cancer program approval. Changes in care as a result of this standard will be monitored with the NCDB data. This integrated quality improvement approach is illustrated in Figure 9-3.

STUDY QUESTIONS

1. What is the goal of the Commission on Cancer?
2. How many CoC-approved cancer programs are there in the US?
3. *The Cancer Program Standards, 2004* focus on eight areas of evaluation. List five.
4. List a benefit of cancer program approval.

Figure 9-3
CoC Integrated Quality Improvement Approach

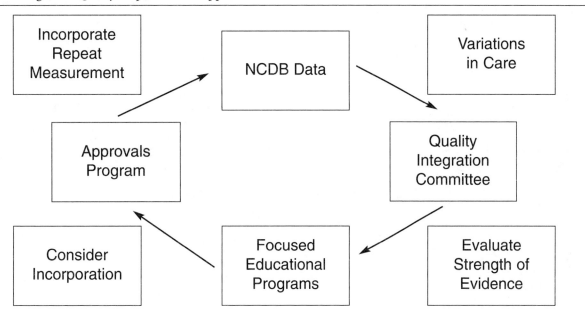

5. What are the three eligibility requirements that must be met before a cancer program can be considered for survey?
6. Give an example of a new CoC cancer program standard.
7. What percentage of newly diagnosed cancer patients are accessioned annually into the NCDB?
8. Name an activity of the Disease Site Teams (DSTs).
9. What do CoC-approved cancer programs use the NCDB Hospital Comparison Benchmark Reports for?
10. What are the specific duties of the cancer liaison physician?

REFERENCES

1. Commission on Cancer. *Cancer Program Standards, 2004.* Chicago, Ill: American College of Surgeons; 2003.
2. Commission on Cancer. *Facility Oncology Registry Data Standards (FORDS).* Chicago, Ill: American College of Surgeons; 2002.

BIBLIOGRAPHY

Davis L. *Fellowship of Surgeons: A History of the American College of Surgeons.* Chicago, Ill: American College of Surgeons; 1988.
Brennan, MF, Clive RE, Winchester DR. The CoC: its roots and destiny. *American College of Surgeons Bulletin.* 1994; 79: 14-21.

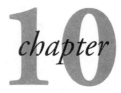

CANCER PROGRAM SURVEY AND APPROVAL PROCESS OF THE AMERICAN COLLEGE OF SURGEONS COMMISSION ON CANCER

M. Asa Carter
CTR

Daniel P. McKellar
MD, FACS

Richard Reiling
MD, FACS

INTRODUCTION AND BACKGROUND

In an effort to standardize clinical cancer care, the American College of Surgeons (ACoS) Committee on the Treatment of Malignant Diseases published minimum standards for cancer clinics and recommended the formation of cancer clinics in general hospitals. These minimum requirements for cancer program approval were first published in 1930. The early requirements were the model for the current multidisciplinary approach to cancer care that has become the standard in the United States for both Commission on Cancer (CoC)-approved and non-approved facilities.

Initial pilot test surveys of cancer clinics were performed in 1931 by one surgeon employed by the ACoS, and one National Cancer Institute (NCI) employee who was made available as part of an NCI grant to the ACoS.

The first listing of the 140 approved cancer clinics was published in the ACoS Bulletin in 1933. At that time, approval was granted to 70% (140/200) of the surveyed cancer clinics. By 1955, 693 clinics had gained approval.

In 1965, the multidisciplinary Commission on Cancer replaced the Committee on the Treatment of Malignant Diseases. Currently, the surveyor team has grown to 39 volunteer physicians representing the full scope of diagnostic and treatment specialties and two Certified Tumor Registrars.

The purpose and format of the survey has changed dramatically to keep pace with the advances in healthcare organization, operation, and technology. The Commission on Cancer surveys individual hospitals, integrated programs, freestanding facilities, and healthcare networks. The survey format and activity remains consistent, but the process may be tailored to accommodate complex facilities or relationships. For example, the survey of a Network Cancer Program always involves more than one surveyor and a visit to each site in the network.

The survey is designed to be both educational and evaluative. An interactive exchange with equal contributions from the surveyor(s) and program team is essential to successful completion of the survey. This open format both assesses compliance with the standards and provides the program with an opportunity to benefit from the surveyors experience so that future program activity can be enhanced. The survey process focuses on discussions with the multidisciplinary team to understand how:

- Clinical care is provided
- Data collection accuracy is assured
- Quality of care and patient outcomes are evaluated and improved

PREPARING FOR A SURVEY

Each cancer program is expected to maintain compliance with the standards at all times, including between surveys. Through the setting and monitoring of annual goals and the work of the four coordinators, the cancer committee assures the program's compliance with the standards and the program's readiness for survey at any time.

Notification

At the beginning of November, the CoC provides an initial survey notification to the cancer registrar for each program due for survey during the next calendar year. The notification includes information about the target time frame for the survey, how to access the Web-enabled Survey Application Record (SAR), the fee for survey, and how to request a survey extension.

This notification is shared with the cancer committee so that survey preparation can begin.

Pre-Survey Assessment

Using the documentation of program activity, the cancer committee performs an assessment of the programs compliance with the standards and readiness for survey. Early assessment enables the cancer committee to confirm that the program is meeting the standards or provides an opportunity to address deficiencies and implement changes that will improve compliance.

The cancer committee identifies one team member to be the key contact for the survey. The key contact coordinates the arrangements and preparations for the on-site visit (Table 10-1). In smaller facilities, the cancer registrar is most often designated to be the key contact. Larger facilities or networks may assign this responsibility to the Cancer Program Administrator or a physician member of the cancer committee.

Confirming the Survey Date

Survey dates and schedules are planned well in advance so that all cancer program team members

Table 10-1
Responsibilities of the Key Contact

- Negotiates with the surveyor and committee members to identify a survey dates and schedules
- Provides information about the surveyor(s) to the cancer committee using the surveyor profiles
- Coordinates development of the survey agenda
- Coordinates meeting rooms and facility tours
- Reviews and updates the SAR
- Plans for and assembles documentation of program activity

are able to participate in the visit, to limit the disruption to patient care, and to be sensitive to the needs of the surveyor(s). This involves multiple concerns and requires the coordination of surveyor(s) schedules, team member availability, tumor board/cancer conference dates, other survey activities, as well as surveyor(s) travel plans. Every effort is made to accommodate both the surveyor(s) and facility.

Most surveyors will make initial contact with the cancer registrar approximately six months before the target time frame for the survey. The cancer registrar provides the key contact information to the surveyor so the negotiation process can begin. As part of a network cancer program survey, one of the assigned surveyors is responsible for working with the key contact to negotiate the survey date and agenda.

The CoC provides a survey confirmation notice to both the program and the surveyor once the date and time for survey is confirmed.

Setting the Agenda

The on-site visit comprises a comprehensive review of all areas of the cancer program and requires one full day, a minimum of six hours, to complete. Two or more days are required for surveys of Network Cancer Programs.

The agenda is customized for each program but, each on-site visit includes:

- Discussion of program activity with the key members of the cancer program team, including the four cancer program coordinators
- Review of documentation

- Facility tour (inpatient medical oncology unit or functional equivalent)
- Participation in a cancer conference
- Meeting with the cancer registrar
- Quality control review of patient medical records and cancer registry abstracts
- Summation conference

Other items may be added to the agenda by either the surveyor(s) or program in advance of the on-site visit. Additional items will depend on the program scope.

The agenda should be provided to all members of the cancer program team in advance of the survey as a guide for survey preparation.

Completing the SAR

The Web-enabled Survey Application Record (SAR) is a primary source of program information. The SAR provides a summary of demographic information, resources and services, and description of annual cancer program activity for the facility. Information recorded in the SAR is used by both the surveyor(s) and CoC staff to evaluate and rate the program's compliance with the standards at the time of survey; therefore, complete information is required so that an accurate assessment and approval award are assured.

Each CoC-approved program updates selected areas of the SAR annually (Table 10-2). The cancer committee can use the annual updates to document and monitor program activity between surveys.

All information on the SAR is reviewed and updated prior to the survey. In preparation for survey, the program staff record a numeric rating of the program's compliance with each standard during the time between surveys. This self assessment can be used by both the cancer program team and the surveyor(s) to guide discussions during the on-site visit.

The SAR update is completed at least 14 days prior to the scheduled survey date to allow the surveyor(s) adequate preparation time. If the SAR is not updated, the survey will be based on incomplete information which will affect the survey outcome and approval award.

Surveyor(s) Preparation

Documentation of program activity is provided to the surveyor at least 14 days prior to the survey date. *Commission on Cancer, Cancer Program Standards*

Table 10-2
Areas of SAR Annual Updates

The numbers in parentheses ( ) indicate the corresponding cancer program standards.

- Cancer committee membership (2.2)
- Cancer committee coordinators (2.3)
- Cancer committee meetings and attendance (2.4)
- Cancer program goals (2.5)
- Cancer conference frequency and format (2.6)
- Cancer conference multidisciplinary requirement (2.7)
- Prospective and total case presentations at cancer conference (2.8)
- Outcomes analysis and dissemination of results (2.11)
- Registry staffing and CTR abstracting or supervision (3.1)
- Abstracting currency (3.3)
- Radiation oncology services (4.1)
- Inpatient medical oncology unit and staffing (4.2)
- Compliance with AJCC staging by the physician (4.3)
- Oncology nurses, ONS certified nurses, and competency evaluation (4.4)
- Nursing leadership of the inpatient medical oncology unit or functional equivalent (4.5)
- Compliance with CAP guidelines and other guidelines at the facility (4.6)
- Rehabilitation services (4.7)
- Clinical trial information (5.1)
- Clinical trial accruals (5.2)
- Supportive services (6.1)
- Prevention and early detection programs (6.2)
- Cancer-related educational activities (7.1)
- Annual cancer registrar educational activities (7.2)
- Studies of quality and outcomes (8.1)
- Patient care improvements (8.2)

2004, pages 6 and 7, lists the materials that are to be provided in advance of the on-site visit. Duplicate sets of documentation are provided to each surveyor assigned to perform a Network Cancer Program survey.

The documentation is needed to support the information and rating of compliance reported through the SAR. All documentation of the cancer program activity is thoroughly reviewed by the surveyor prior to the on-site visit. Additionally, the surveyor(s) may review information provided on the facility website which can provide a snapshot of the facility as a whole and the community served.

Prior to the on-site visit the surveyor(s) may begin to assign a rating of compliance to some standards when the documentation clearly shows the standard has been met.

COMPLETING THE ON-SITE VISIT

Discussion of Program Activity

A discussion of program activity with all members of the cancer program team is essential to understanding the programs organization, strengths, and opportunities for improvement. All team members are encouraged to describe their achievements and challenges, as well as plans and goals for their area of responsibility.

The four coordinators present information about the key areas of program activity to which they are assigned. The cancer conference coordinator describes the committee's process to establish the annual cancer conference goals. A discussion of the monitoring activity and findings, and the methods to address areas that fall below the established goals enables the surveyor(s) to confirm that the cancer conference activity is meeting the standards. The coordinator for the quality of cancer registry data shares information about the development and implementation of the cancer registry quality control plan. The areas of cancer registry operation targeted for evaluation, findings, and plans to address areas for improvement are highlighted during the discussion.

The annual submission of data to the National Cancer Data Base (NCDB) and the methods to ensure the quality of the data submitted are also discussed. The coordinator also reports on the quality of the data submitted to the NCDB at the most recent Call for Data, the NCDB edit report, and plans to review, correct, and resubmit the data to meet the requirements for standard 3.7: *Cases submitted to the NCDB for the most recent accession year requested meet the established quality criteria included in the annual Call for Data.*

The quality improvement coordinator describes the completed studies of quality and outcomes, and shares the plans for future studies. The process to identify topics and study development are also discussed with the surveyor(s). The coordinator reviews past annual improvements to cancer care and identifies improvements planned for the current year.

The community outreach coordinator (Cancer Liaison Physician) shares information about the screening and prevention activities completed since the last survey and plans for future programs and the monitoring and assessment methods used to evaluate the current programs.

Review of Additional Documentation

As part of the on-site visit, the surveyor(s) reviews additional documentation demonstrating the full scope of the cancer program activity. This may be accomplished during the meeting with the cancer program team or as a separate activity. A listing of additional documentation can be found on pages 6 and 7 of *Commission on Cancer, Cancer Program Standards 2004.*

Facility Tour

A tour of the facility enables the surveyor(s) to observe the care settings and staff interaction with patients. The surveyor(s) may review policies and procedures or interview staff during the tour.

The inpatient medical oncology unit, or functional equivalent must be part of the facility tour. The program may choose to include other areas such as the outpatient infusion center, oncology clinic, radiation oncology department, pathology department, pharmacy, or patient library. The scope of the tour is established during the development of the survey agenda.

Participation in a Cancer Conference

Observing the multidisciplinary participation and discussion of treatment options during the conference assists the surveyor(s) in evaluating and rating the team approach to the provision of patient care.

If a cancer conference is not held on the day of the survey, programs may provide a videotaped cancer conference to the surveyor(s) in advance of the on-site visit.

Meeting with the Cancer Registrar and Quality Control Review

Time spent with the cancer registrar allows for an exchange of information and suggestions to improve registry operations. The meeting includes an evaluation of the cancer registry standards (i.e. abstracting performed or supervised by a Certified Tumor Registrar [CTR] and follow-up rates) as well as cancer registry operations, such as the policy and procedure manual, suspense list, and data request log. The quality of the abstracted data recorded in the cancer registry database is compared to the information found in the patient medical records.

At least 25 medical records are reviewed to evaluate the completeness of physician staging, presence of the scientifically validated data elements in pathology reports, and completeness of treatment information recorded on the cancer registry abstract. The surveyor(s) may evaluate additional data items such as the date abstracted and follow-up information. As part of a network survey, 25 medical records from each network location are evaluated.

The review findings are shared with the cancer program team and the CoC to provide documentation of the surveyor(s) ratings for standards 4.3: *AJCC staging is assigned by the managing physician and recorded on a staging form in the medical record on 90% of eligible annual analytic cases*, and 4.6: *The guidelines for patient management and treatment currently required by the CoC are followed.*

Summation Conference

At a final conference following the complete evaluation of the cancer program, the surveyor(s) provides an oral summary of the findings of the evaluation to the cancer committee and other members of the cancer program team.

The interactive format of this meeting allows the surveyor(s) to acknowledge program strengths and identify the areas where program activity falls below the requirement (deficiency). The cancer program team has an opportunity to respond to the identified deficiency(ies) and provide additional documentation or information to resolve the ratings before the conclusion of the on-site visit.

The surveyor(s) will offer suggestions for improving current program activity, describe ways to resolve the identified deficiencies, and share information on important CoC initiatives and upcoming activities.

The surveyor(s) may also suggest that areas of the SAR be modified to offer more accurate or complete information about program activity.

POST-SURVEY ACTIVITY

Facility

The facility is allowed to make changes to the SAR during the 72 hours following the survey. Information that presents a more accurate picture of the program and clarifies services offered by the facility are added to the SAR by the cancer registrar or the key contact for survey preparation.

Within the two weeks following the survey, the cancer program team meets to discuss the survey experience and complete the on-line post-survey evaluation form.

The post-survey evaluation collects information about the survey scheduling process, customer support provided by members of the CoC Cancer Programs staff, as well as details about the surveyor(s) performance on-site. Completion of this evaluation is a required part of the survey and assists the development of educational programs for surveyors and Independent Cancer Program Consultants, enhances the survey process, and suggests overall improvements to the Approvals Program of the Commission on Cancer.

Surveyor(s)

Once the SAR is closed for changes to the facility, the surveyor(s) records comments about each standard and rates compliance based on the discussions and findings of the on-site visit. The surveyor(s) completes the program assessment within the two weeks after the survey. The Network Cancer Program surveyors discuss their findings, and agree to and record one rating of compliance for each standard.

All materials provided by the facility to the surveyor(s) in advance of and during the on-site visit are forwarded to CoC Cancer Program staff as part of the survey documentation.

THE APPROVALS PROCESS

Approval Awards

An Approval Award is granted to each program surveyed by the Commission on Cancer. The awards range from Full Approval to Non-approval. To be approved by the CoC, a program must be in compliance with at least 29 (80%) of the standards set forth in *Commission on Cancer, Cancer Program Standards 2004*.

Programs with fewer than eight deficiencies receive a Three-year with Contingency award and are expected to resolve the deficiencies within one year. A program that is not currently approved (new program) and is identified to have a deficiency in one standard will receive the Approval Deferred status. This status allows the program to make corrections to the identified deficiency and receive approval without a resurvey.

Programs that receive Non-approval are encouraged to make corrections to program activity and reapply for a survey at a future time. Historically, very few programs receive Non-approval.

Technical Review

Each survey is evaluated by a technical staff member of the Approvals and Standards Section at the CoC. The SAR, the facility and surveyor ratings with comments, and all program documentation submitted by the surveyor(s) are included in the technical review of the cancer program survey. This independent review ensures that the Commission on Cancer standards are accurately and consistently applied to all cancer programs.

When a compliance question surfaces during the technical review, the CoC Cancer Program Specialist may contact the facility for clarification, and may also confer with the surveyor(s) to confirm a non-compliance rating.

The Cancer Program Specialist records comments and assigns a rating for each standard in a special designated area of the SAR. An Approval Award is assigned to the program by the Cancer Program Specialist based on the consensus between the surveyor(s) and technical staff rating.

The survey may also be referred to the Program Review Subcommittee of the Committee on Approvals for review and confirmation of the approval award. Annually, the Program Review Subcommittee identifies and monitors several standards and other related issues. The Program Review Subcommittee also evaluates the survey information for all programs recommended for Non-approval. Non-approval awards are confirmed by the Committee on Approvals at either the annual committee meeting or by conference call.

Approved Cancer Program Performance Report

Within 12 weeks of the on-site visit, survey results and approval awards are available through the Web-enabled Approved Cancer Program Performance Report (Performance Report). The individualized Performance Report is prepared by the Cancer Program Specialist after confirmation of the approval award. Each Performance Report:

- Documents the approval award
- Identifies the deficient standards
- Provides a summary of the deficiency(ies) and the expected compliance
- Identifies the contingency period and the date documentation of compliance is due
- Acknowledges the commendation(s)
- Provides comparison data by state, category, and overall for all programs surveyed in the period

Following the review of the Web-enabled Approved Cancer Program Performance Report the facility cancer program team is allowed 30 days to ask for a review of any area on the Performance Report or given the opportunity to provide additional narrative comments before the report is finalized.

Program Recognition

The CoC recognizes each approved program by including the facility contact information in the searchable database on the Cancer Programs page of the American College of Surgeons website. The CoC also partners with the American Cancer Society (ACS) to provide to the public on the ACS website facility specific information on all approved programs

Following survey, each CoC-approved program is provided with a press kit and free marketing materials that can be used to promote the facility cancer program. Information describing the facility's CoC-approval status can be shared with facility staff and the community by placing notices or advertisements in local newspapers and magazines, including the approval status in reports or brochures, or posting information on the facility intranet or website.

CONCLUSION

The voluntary group of CoC-approved cancer programs provide care to 80% of newly diagnosed can-cer patients each year while representing only 25% of the acute care hospitals in the United States and Puerto Rico.

The facility demonstrates a commitment to provide high quality cancer care because of its voluntary participation in an objective external evaluation of the facility's cancer program as measured against the standards of the Commission on Cancer. The Commission on Cancer approval status recognizes the facility's achievement of the provision of high quality care.

STUDY QUESTIONS

1. Outline the responsibilities of the key contact for survey preparation.
2. Describe three uses for the SAR.
3. Discuss three reasons to involve all members of the cancer program team in the on-site visit.
4. Identify four ways that a facility can market its approved program.

REFERENCES

1. American College of Surgeons Archives, Commission on Cancer, letter from Thomas S. Cullen to Franklin H. Martin, 11/26/1932 including a copy of letter to Joseph C. Bloodgood (10/26/1928).
2. *Commission on Cancer, Cancer Program Standards 2004.* Chicago: American College of Surgeons; 2003.
3. *Commission on Cancer, Components of a Commission on Cancer Survey.* Chicago: American College of Surgeons website; 2004. Available at: www.facs.org/cancer.index.html.
4. *Commission on Cancer, SAR Training Guide.* Chicago: American College of Surgeons website; 2004.
5. *Commission on Cancer, Instructions to Complete the Application for Cancer Program Approval.* Chicago: American College of Surgeons; 2001.

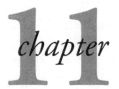

JOINT COMMISSION ON ACCREDITATION OF HEALTHCARE ORGANIZATIONS (JCAHO)

Catherine Gray
BA, CTR, CCRP

HISTORY OF THE JOINT COMMISSION

The conception of the Joint Commission on Accreditation of Healthcare Organizations (JCAHO) began with Dr. Ernest Codman in the early 1900s. Doctor Codman (who also formed the first cancer registry, a bone sarcoma registry at Massachusetts General Hospital) had a simple idea. He felt that every patient's health should be followed long enough to determine whether the treatment had been effective, and if not, why not. Dr. Codman believed corrective action, if necessary, should be taken to ensure that effective treatment was provided. This idea of service to the patient is the backbone of the Joint Commission's hospital accreditation program. Dr. Codman shared these ideas with Dr. Edward Martin in 1910, and, together with other physicians, they later founded the American College of Surgeons (ACoS).[1]

In 1912, at the Third Clinical Congress of Surgeons of North America, a proposal was made to establish an American College of Surgeons (ACoS). Part of the proposal was to include a hospital standardization program as part of the ACoS. This was suggested by Dr. Edward Martin and proposed by Dr. Allen Kanauel. Hospital standardization was one of the first activities of the newly formed organization. In October 1917, 300 fellows from the Committees on Standards from every state in the United States and every province in Canada met with 60 leading hospital superintendents to discuss hospital standardization. Today, the JCAHO continues to formulate policy by gathering informed and capable healthcare professionals to deliberate hospital standards.[1] After this Conference on Hospital Standardization, the ACOS formally established the Hospital Standardization Program, which was field tested with poor results. Of the 692 hospitals surveyed in the United States and Canada, only 89 hospitals met the standards, and most of the countries' most prestigious institutions did not qualify. These results further emphasized the need for standardization, and national support grew for the program.[1]

In December 1919, the college's board of regents approved five standards, which became known as the minimum standard (Table 11-1). These principles were considered necessary to ensure the proper care of patients in any hospital and were the beginning of the accreditation process as we know it today. The request for accreditation was, and continues to be, considered voluntary.[1]

The American College of Surgeons continued to administer the accreditation program until after World War II. It was at this time that the emergence of many medical specialties and the increasing complexity of healthcare dictated the need to establish an independent, nonprofit association. The ACoS joined with the American College of Physicians, the American Hospital Association, the American Medical Association, and the Canadian Medical Association to form the Joint Commission on Accreditation of Hospitals (JCAH), which actively began issuing accreditation to hospitals in 1953. The Canadian Medical Association formed its own hospital accreditation system in 1959, whereupon it withdrew from the JCAH.[1]

The next major milestone in the JCAHO's history was reached in 1966, when the JCAH was faced with competition from state government licensing boards and the federal government's requirements to participate in the Medicare program. The JCAH, concerned that they could become obsolete, changed their focus from ensuring the minimal acceptable level of hospital care to establishing the optimal achievable level of care. This resulted in the publication of the *1970 Accreditation Manual for Hospitals.* What had originated as five minimum standards was now a 152-page manual of updated standards.

The 1960s also saw the scope of the accreditation process increase to accredit other healthcare facilities such as psychiatric facilities and long-term care facilities. In the mid-1980s, in order to accommodate this increased scope, the name of the organization was changed by replacing the word Hospitals with Healthcare Organizations. The JCAHO continues to add healthcare facilities to their survey process as they are established, for instance, adding hospices in the 1980s,[1] which are now surveyed under the home care program. The current accreditation programs include hospitals, home care, long-term care, ambulatory care, healthcare networks, pathology and clinical laboratories, and behavioral healthcare. In 2000, there were 18,000 healthcare organizations and programs accredited by the JCAHO in the United States, including 4,800 hospitals.

The JCAHO has had ties to the government since the 1960s, when hospitals in compliance with JCAHO requirements were also deemed by the government to be in compliance with the requirements of the Medicare/Medicaid program and as meeting many states' requirements for licensure. Currently,

Table 11-1
The Minimum Standard

1. That physicians and surgeons privileged to practice in the hospital be organized as a definite group or staff. Such organization has nothing to do with the question as to whether the hospital is 'open' or 'closed,' nor need it affect the various existing types of staff organization. The word STAFF is here defined as the group of doctors who practice in the hospital inclusive of all groups such as the "regular staff," "the visiting staff," and the "associate staff."
2. That membership upon the staff be restricted to physicians and surgeons who are (a) full graduates of medicine in good standing and legally licensed to practice in their respective states or provinces, (b) competent in their respective fields, and (c) worthy in character and in matters of professional ethics; that in this latter connection the practice of the division of fees, under any guise whatever, be prohibited.
3. That the staff initiate and, with the approval of the governing board of the hospital, adopt rules, regulations, and policies governing the professional work of the hospital; that these rules, regulations, and policies specifically provide:
   (a) That staff meetings be held at least once each month. (In large hospitals the departments may choose to meet separately.)
   (b) That the staff review and analyze at regular intervals their clinical experience in the various departments of the hospital, such as medicine, surgery, obstetrics, and the other specialties; the clinical records of patients, free and pay, should be the basis for such review and analyses.
4. That accurate and complete records be written for all patients and filed in an accessible manner in the hospital—a complete case record being one which includes identification data, complaint, personal and family history, history of present illness, physical examination; special examination such as consultations, clinical laboratory, X-ray and other examinations; provisional or working diagnosis; condition on discharge; follow-up; and, in case of death, gross and microscopical pathological findings; progress notes; final diagnosis; condition on discharge; follow-up and, in case of death, autopsy findings.
5. That diagnostic and therapeutic facilities under competent supervision be available for the study, diagnosis, and treatment of patients; these to include, at least (a) a clinical laboratory providing chemical, bacteriological, serological, and pathological services; (b) an X-ray department providing radiographic and fluoroscopic services.

Reprinted with permission from the American College of Surgeons.

JCAHO accreditation fulfills licensure requirements for at least one regulatory entity in each of the 50 states. Despite these links with government requirements, the JCAHO remains committed to a voluntary accreditation process.

QUALITY ASSURANCE

Quality assurance was a formal approach to one of the original minimum standards. In the 1970s, hospitals were required to regularly review and evaluate their care of patients. However, reviews were informal, may have been biased, and were dependent on a reviewer's ability to judge care. Quality assurance research led to the development of more structured and objective patient care assessment. Two common principles evolved from this research: objective and valid criteria

for measuring quality of care must be established, and review procedures must be systematic.

The audit, which is retrospective, became a recognized tool to assess quality of care. Ongoing monitoring was conducted by required medical staff monitoring through surgical case review (indications and validation of diagnosis), pharmacy and therapeutics review (selection, distribution and handling, and administering drugs and diagnostic tests), blood usage review (appropriateness of transfusions), and health records review (documentation). Standards were also established for reviews of medical and support staff departments in the areas of safety management, infection control, and utilization. Also, hospitals were asked to consider the results of these retrospective and ongoing audits when verifying credentials and assigning staff privileges to physicians.[1]

Unfortunately, hospitals became overly focused on producing paper trails of formal audits for the sole purpose of passing JCAHO accreditation surveys, instead of focusing on the quality of care they were providing to the patients. In 1979, to counter this unforeseen problem, the JCAHO determined that there should be evidence of a well-defined, organized program to enhance patient care through the ongoing objective assessment of important aspects of patient care and the correction of identified problems. The three parts of the quality assurance process included implicit peer-based discussions; retrospective, time-limited audits; and ongoing monitoring using well-chosen process and outcome indicators.[1]

PERFORMANCE IMPROVEMENT

Discussion of performance improvement cannot begin without a review of the JCAHO's Agenda for Change, which was launched in 1987. The Agenda for Change was the JCAHO's response to critics who felt that the JCAHO was more concerned with policy documentation and minutiae in hospital manuals than with the actual quality of the care delivered. Critics charged that "good writers fared better than good providers."[2]

This was happening simultaneously with industry's development of Total Quality Management (TQM) and Continuous Quality Improvement (CQI). Total Quality Management is an organizational environment in which 100 percent quality is pursued. Principles include communication, empowerment, participation, continuous improvement, and customer-centered focus. Continuous Quality Improvement is the uninterrupted process of evaluating outcomes and the processes to achieve the goals of Total Quality Management. CQI theorists W. Edwards Deming and Joseph M. Juran stated, "Every process produces information on the basis of which the process can be improved."[3]

Both TQM and CQI "stress the importance of leadership, organizational culture, preeminence of external and internal customers' needs, goal-driven design of new products and services, broad deployment of measurement systems, data-driven performance assessment, and systematic redesign of important organizational functions or processes."[4] As industries developed systems for maintaining and improving the quality of services provided to the public while controlling costs, the public began to demand the same accountability for its healthcare services. JCAHO adopted many of the principles of TQM and CQI in drafting the Agenda for Change.[5]

AGENDA FOR CHANGE

The Agenda for Change was a result of a new movement in healthcare in the 1980s, which was a response to the dramatic rise in healthcare costs. This movement demanded greater efficiency in the delivery of services and insisted on objective evidence of the effectiveness of care. The public was demanding that the costs and quality of healthcare be balanced. At this same time the JCAHO was realizing that their focus should change from examining an institution's capabilities to deliver quality care to monitoring an institution's performance of healthcare delivery and evaluating the actual improvements achieved in the results.

The Agenda for Change was a response to these concerns, and marked the first time that improving performance would be a goal of the accreditation process. The JCAHO's Agenda for Change has four underlying concepts:

1. Patient outcomes are influenced by all of the activities of a healthcare organization.
2. Continuous improvement in the quality of care should be a priority of healthcare organizations.
3. The JCAHO should focus on those activities of healthcare organizations that are most important to the quality of care.
4. Traditional assessments of compliance with standards should be complemented by the accredited organization's collection, analysis, and feedback of data that reflect their actual performance in undertaking key activities.[6]

Because one of the goals of the Agenda for Change was to improve outcomes, the JCAHO stopped dictating to hospitals criteria that must be fulfilled. Instead, they expected hospitals to creatively use the JCAHO performance expectations to improve patient results. The JCAHO also began to view the institutions as using a multidisciplinary approach to patient care. "The new survey process moves away from the evaluation of specific departments and services. It focuses on assessing, across an organization, performance of important patient-focused and organizational functions that support quality patient care, rather than evaluating activities that may have been conducted primarily to 'pass' the survey."[7] The Agenda for Change revolutionized the JCAHO survey process. "Old standards were revised and new standards developed to emphasize evaluation of hospital performance aimed at continuously improving the outcomes of patient care."[7]

The three major initiatives were:

1. Redesign of the JCAHO standards to stress the entire organization's effectiveness in patient services
2. Redesign of the survey process to provide more interactive consultative services
3. Development of a national performance measurement system, commonly known as the Indicator Measurement System (IMSystem)[7]

With the goal being to evaluate an organization's performance improvement efforts and results, the survey process now includes a review of hospital documents, an interview with hospital leaders, a review of patient care and administrative units to see if practices reflect policies, and a review of the performance improvement activities, with an emphasis on determining multidisciplinary involvement in performance improvement. Then the surveyors report on their findings and recommendations to the JCAHO staff.[2](pp 5-9)

During the interview with hospital leaders, the surveyors seek to ensure that the leaders have developed a performance improvement plan that identifies priorities for improvement, have communicated the plan to staff throughout the organization, have provided a framework for reaching these goals, and have shown that they are teaching and directing the staff. Interviews with staff members and patients in the clinical and administrative areas are used to determine whether all staff members are working together to improve performance in areas identified by the leaders in their performance improvement plan.[2](pp 5-9) In the past, the emphasis was on finding individuals whose performance was unsatisfactory, and either correcting that performance or eliminating those individuals. The current focus is on systems, and improvement efforts should now concentrate on fixing and improving systems.

FRAMEWORK FOR IMPROVING PERFORMANCE

A large part of the Agenda for Change consists of the Framework for Improving Performance. The cycle for continuous performance improvement, illustrated in Figure 11-1, includes four elements: design, measurement, assessment, and improvement or innovation.[5](p59) A hospital must have a model for

Figure 11-1
Critical Aspects of a Health Care Organization's Internal Environment

Leadership
- mission
- vision
- priorities
- resources

Management of Human Resources
- education
- competence

Management of Information
- planning
- aggregate data
- comparative data
- knowledge-based data

Improving Organization Performance
- collaboration
- process thinking

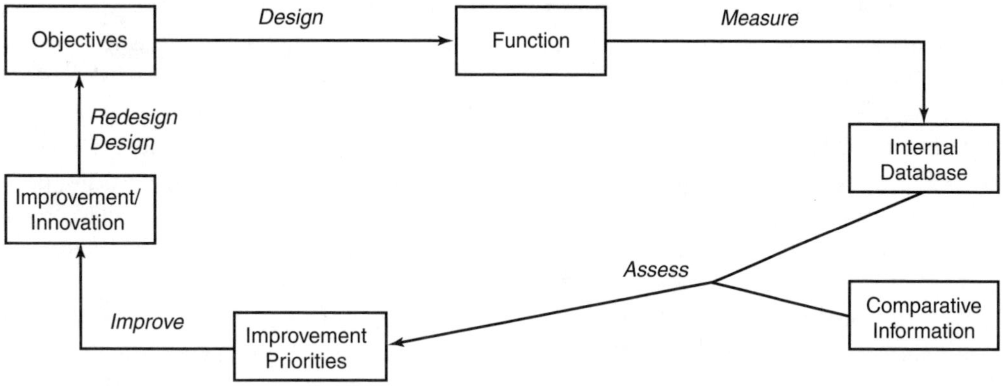

Reprinted with permission by the Joint Commission on Accreditation of Healthcare Organizations, *Comprehensive Accreditation Manual for Hospitals.* Chicago: The Commission, 1995, p. 36.

performance improvement in use, but it does not necessarily have to use the JCAHO's Framework for Improving Performance. However, in a hospital's performance improvement plan, the model on which it is based must be identified. (A common model used by many hospitals is the *plan, do, check, and act* model, or PDCA.)

Organizations should incorporate the needs and expectations of patients and staff when designing specific objectives for ascertaining quality of care. The procedures that will achieve those objectives are instituted, and data are collected systematically on preselected performance measures (originally called clinical indicators). The internal data are then assessed in reference to an external comparative database.

The assessment includes reviewing current data in addition to examining prior patterns of performance. The performance improvement cycle has no beginning or end. It is an ongoing process that may be entered at any point.[7(p33)] The accreditation surveyors look for positive responses to three critical questions: Has the organization developed a framework for improving care? Is the cycle being followed well? Is the cycle itself being continuously improved?

Clinical practice guidelines and critical pathways can be used to assess the organization's data. Clinical practice guidelines are outlines of strategies for patient management that describe a range of acceptable ways to diagnose, manage, or prevent specific diseases and conditions. The practice guidelines have been developed by a consensus of experts in the specified field. Critical pathways are descriptions of key elements in the process of care that should be accomplished in order to achieve maximum quality at minimum cost.

Critical pathways define the optimal sequence and timing of functions performed by physicians, nurses, and other staff for a particular diagnosis. Variations from the guidelines, or from the institution's desired performance targets, create improvement opportunities. These opportunities result in the redesign of an existing function or the innovative design of a new approach to meet or surpass the expectations and needs of the patients.

Deciding what to improve can often be difficult, but priority should be given to problems whose solution will result in the greatest improvement in patient care. High-risk, high-volume, problem-prone areas, in addition to high-impact clinical services (such as surgical procedures) and high-cost

functions, should be assigned high priority. Collected data should include measures in both high-priority areas. Likewise, when hospital cancer committee members plan the two evaluation priority studies required yearly by the Commission on Cancer (CoC) of the ACoS, they should also include measures in both high priority areas. For example, choose one of the top five sites at a hospital to meet the high volume criteria, or choose esophagogastrectomies to evaluate as both a high-impact clinical service and a high-cost function.

In addition to the performance improvement cycle, the JCAHO developed performance measures and a computerized system to evaluate an organization's performance with more accuracy and consistency than has been possible in the past.

PERFORMANCE MEASUREMENT SYSTEMS

According to the Joint Commission, a performance measurement system is an inter-related set of outcomes measures, process measures, or both, that supports internal comparisons of organizations' performance over time and external comparisons of performance among organizations at comparable times. Performance measurement activities serve as the basis for internal quality improvement activities in healthcare organizations. Also, the JCAHO staff will begin to use performance data to focus the accreditation process on clinical care issues and make it more immediately relevant to health professionals."[8]

A performance measure is a quantitative measure of an aspect of patient care that can be used as a guide to monitor and evaluate the quality and appropriateness of healthcare delivery. These measures serve as the data collection components of a performance measurement system. Performance measures are not direct measures of quality, but screens or flags in a performance measurement system to indicate which areas require more detailed analysis. The measures should incorporate data on processes or outcomes, using existing data elements whenever possible, with an emphasis on sparse collection of data. Measures should have known reliability and validity.[9]

As part of the Agenda for Change, the JCAHO developed the Indicator Measurement System (IMSystem®) in order to provide hospitals with internal and external benchmarking capabilities.

Internal benchmarking is the process of reviewing performance on critical measures of patient care quality. External benchmarking is the process of comparing performance on critical measures of patient care quality against others or the "best" in the industry. Internal benchmarks help a hospital improve its own performance over time; external benchmarks help hospitals assess where they are in comparison to others, based on industry standards. By developing a performance measurement system, the JCAHO wanted to measure the results of care (outcomes). Performance measurement data would allow the JCAHO to give hospital-specific information, upon request, to the public[2](p2-3) and to enhance the JCAHO's survey process by allowing intracycle monitoring through this clinical indicator-based performance measurement system.[9](p9)

According to the Joint Commission, the original intent of the their performance measurement system, when fully implemented, was to:

- continually collect objective performance data from each participating accredited healthcare organization;
- aggregate, risk adjust (as necessary), and analyze performance data;
- provide comparative performance data to participating accredited healthcare organizations for use in internal performance improvement activities;
- identify trends and patterns in the performance of individual participating accredited healthcare organizations that may call for more focused attention by those organizations[7](p30)

The actual performance measures created at the JCAHO were developed in consultation with groups of experts who worked in the field to which each measure pertained and who had been nominated by national organizations and professional societies at the request of the JCAHO. The original 25 performance measures were as follows: 1 to 5 were perioperative indicators, 6 to 10 involved obstetrics, 11 to 15 involved cardiovascular care, 16 to 20 were the oncology indicators, and 21 to 25 were the trauma indicators. The oncology performance measures were chosen from the high volume sites of breast, colon/rectum, and lung cancer. The qualifying patients were inpatients with a diagnosis of one of these cancers. The oncology performance measures were designed to be collected retrospectively, whereas the majority of indicators for the other disciplines were collected both prospectively and retrospectively.

The original five oncology performance measures examined were 1) the availability of data for diagnosis and staging, 2) the use of staging by managing physicians, 3) the use of tests critical for the prognosis and clinical management of female breast cancer, 4) the effectiveness of preoperative diagnosis and staging for patients with lung cancer and 5) the comprehensiveness of diagnostic workup of patients with colon cancer.

The JCAHO's Performance Measurement Initiative was finalized in 1994 with the publication of the final performance measures for their own performance measurement software system called the IMSystem®. However, in 1995 the Performance Measurement Initiative underwent another major change. The JCAHO announced its intention "to include a group of acceptable measurement systems in its accreditation process under a single performance measurement umbrella." An important objective of this plan was to preserve the element of choice for the accredited organization by allowing it to select the approved measurement system that best met its needs. Within each system, further choice was available to the accredited organization in permitting it to select the specific indicators that were most applicable to the patient care services it provided.[8]

The revised approach was more flexible and complete. It incorporated performance measurement systems developed by other organizations in addition to the IMSystem® developed at the JCAHO. Hospitals were offered a menu of performance measures so that each healthcare organization could choose a performance system relevant to its' needs.[10] The JCAHO did this in response to requests for inclusion of other measures and measurement systems developed by other entities as part of the accreditation process so that hospitals could have a choice as to which system to use for outcome measures.

The revised Performance Measurement Initiative was finalized In 1997, when the Joint Commission announced ORYX®: The Next Evolution in Accreditation. ORYX® was the name of the Joint Commission's initiative to integrate performance measures into the accreditation process. It was a term different from any other currently used in healthcare, reflecting the magnitude of the anticipated changes in the Joint Commission's accreditation process in the years ahead. For trivia buffs, oryx is defined in the dictionary as a kind of gazelle. Initially there were 60 performance measures accepted, some of which were the performance measures created by the JCAHO for their own system, including the oncology performance measures outlined earlier in this chapter.

In 1997, hospitals were required to notify the JCAHO which two performance measures they would be using. By 1998, hospitals had to be enrolled in at least one performance measurement system chosen from the list of acceptable performance measurement systems. (The IMSystem was sold in 1998.) Data collection on two measures representing at least 20% of the organization's patient population had to be instituted. The requirement went up incrementally: in 1999 four measures had to be chosen which represented at least 40% of the organization's patient population, and in 2000, six measures, representing 60% of the organization's population, had to be collected and data on these measures submitted to the JCAHO. This requirement was originally conceived to continue to increase every year, but it has now been capped at six measures.

The JCAHO has continuous performance data that will help identify performance trends and provide a database resource. However, it has not yet been determined how indicator rates will affect a hospital's final accreditation status. Some possibilities being considered are that performance improvement data could be used to determine the length of time between surveys, or an organization may be queried as to how the indicator data are being utilized internally to improve performance.

With the advent of the ORYX® initiative, hospitals could choose from over 200 performance measurement systems that were reviewed by the JCAHO staff and deemed acceptable. From these acceptable systems, an organization could choose among 8,000 performance measures to fulfill a hospital's internal measurement goals and their JCAHO ORYX® requirements. While the hospital staff appreciated this flexibility, it became a challenge for the JCAHO staff, as there was a lack of standardization across measurement systems. Although many ORYX® measures may appear to be similar, valid comparisons can be made only between healthcare organizations using the same measures that are designed and collected based on standard specifications. The availability of over 8,000 disparate

ORYX® measures may also limit the size of some comparison groups and hinder statistically valid data analyses. To address these challenges, standardized sets of valid, reliable, and evidence-based "core" measures were implemented by the Joint Commission for use within the ORYX initiative.

The process to select the Core Performance Measures was similar to the process used to create the ORYX® initiative. The JCAHO defines a core measure set as a "unique grouping of performance measures carefully selected to provide, when viewed together, a robust picture of the care provided in a given area". Five initial core measurement areas were selected and approved by the Executive Committee of the JCAHO. These measures are: Acute myocardial infarction (including coronary artery disease), heart failure, community acquired pneumonia, pregnancy and related conditions (including newborn and maternal care), and surgical procedures and complications. The last core measure, surgical procedures and complications, will be delayed in their implementation to ensure that duplication of data collection efforts does not occur, since the Centers for Medicare and Medicaid Services (CMS) (formerly the Healthcare Financing Administration) are also identifying measures related to surgery.

Currently, accredited hospitals are expected to begin data collection on the first sets of the ORYX® core performance measures. The various software systems that provided the acceptable measurement systems to hospitals to fulfill their original ORYX® requirements have all been given the computer specifications to enable them to include these core measures into their existing performance measurement software systems. By June, 2002, hospitals selected core measure sets based on the healthcare services they provide. If the hospital serves patient populations with conditions that correspond with two or more core measure sets, the hospital shall select two of the initial four sets and submit data via their selected measurement system. The hospital will no longer be required to collect and transmit data on their non-core measures.

At the time of surveys, the JCAHO surveyors will examine how an organization uses the core measures in their performance improvement activities. It is the intent of the JCAHO to eventually utilize a hospital's core measure data to help focus the survey evaluation activities.

In the future, additional sets of core measures will be identified and implemented based on input from the healthcare community and various public interest groups. Sets of core measures related to oncology may be established in the future, but there are no plans for that at this time.

SUMMARY

A thorough understanding of the Joint Commission's ORYX® initiative and its performance improvement standards is critical to the cancer registry profession. The American College of Surgeons Commission on Cancer Approvals Program surveys institutions for compliance with standards that cover eight areas of evaluation. Standards for quality improvement, detailed in section 8 of *Cancer Program Standards 2004*,[11] are easier for cancer registrars to comply with once they understand the principles of performance improvement outlined by the JCAHO in their survey process.

Finally, as the Joint Commission has stated, a department can no longer operate in isolation, but must join the multidisciplinary efforts of hospital-wide performance improvement initiatives. All performance improvement activities completed by the Cancer Committee to fulfill the eighth CoC standard should be included in the hospital-wide performance improvement activities. Cancer registrars must join these efforts and become recognized as members of the healthcare team.

STUDY QUESTIONS

1. Describe Total Quality Management (TQM).
2. What is the uninterrupted process of evaluating outcomes and the processes to achieve the goals of Total Quality Management?
3. What indicates that priorities for improvement have been communicated to the staff throughout the organization with a framework provided for reaching goals?
4. What do critical pathways define?

REFERENCES

1. Roberts JS, Coale JG, Redman RR. A history of the Joint Commission on Accreditation of Hospitals. *Journal of the American Medical Association.* 1987; 258(7); 936-40.
2. Veatch R. Hospital accreditation in 1994: The Joint Commission applies TQM to the survey process. *Quality Letter for Healthcare Leaders* 1994; 6(4):3.
3. Berwick DM. Continuous improvement as an ideal in health care. *New England Journal of Medicine.* 1989; 320: 54.
4. Anonymous. A framework for improving the performance of health care organizations. *Joint Commission Perspectives.* 1993; 13(6):A2.
5. Schyve PM, Kamowski DB. Information management and quality improvement: The Joint Commission's perspective. *Quality Management in Health Care.* 1994; 2(4): 54-62.
6. Joint Commission on Accreditation of Healthcare Organizations. The Joint Commission's agenda for change: stimulating continuous improvement in the quality of health care. In *Trauma, Oncology and Cardiovascular Indicators Beta Phase Training Manual and Software User's Guide.* Oakbrook Terrace, Ill: The Commission; 1991: 3-1-3-17.
7. Joint Commission on Accreditation of Healthcare Organizations. *Comprehensive Accreditation Manual for Hospitals.* Oakbrook Terrace, Ill: The Commission; 1995: 29.
8. Brown A. "Joint Commission Announces Evaluation Framework for Performance Measurement Systems." News release from the Joint Commission on Accreditation of Healthcare Organizations; January 1996.
9. National Cancer Registrars Association, Inc. NCRA Oncology Indicators Workshop Handouts. Lenexa, Kan: The Association; 1992: 9, 10.
10. Seidenfeld J, Harold L, Loeb J. From the Joint Commission on Accreditation of Healthcare Organizations of New Tool Request for Indicators. *Journal of the American Medical Association.* 1995; 273(9): 69.
11. Commission on Cancer. *Cancer Program Standards, 2004.* Chicago, Ill: American College of Surgeons; 2003.

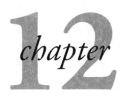

CASE ASCERTAINMENT

Fred F. Wacker
PhD, CTR

INTRODUCTION

Case ascertainment is the systematic process used to identify all cases eligible to be included in the registry database. All registries must perform case ascertainment, including hospital-specific and central or population-based registries. Although these registries may use different source documents, the procedures involved in their case ascertainment cycles are similar.

Most governing agencies (the Commission on Cancer CoC of the American College of Surgeons ACos and regional or state registries) typically only require in situ (ICD-O[1] behavior code 2) or malignant (ICD-O behavior code 3) cases to be included in the registry. However, hospital cancer committees may require the registry to include other or interesting cases not required by the governing agencies. These could include benign, borderline, or uncertain cases. Examples include benign brain tumors or carcinoid tumors of the appendix. The data set and policy as to whether patient follow-up is done must be determined by the cancer committee, as described in Chapter 8 of this textbook, Cancer Registry Management. The case ascertainment cycle would be the same for these cases as for the cases required by the governing agencies. Table 12-1 summarizes the case ascertainment cycle.

The criteria for eligible cases in a registry depend upon the governing agencies of the registry. Along with state-specific reportable cases, registries participating in the Approvals Program of the CoC must use the reportable list defined by the CoC.[2] Again, see Chapter 8 for a definition of the reportable list.

DETERMINING REPORTING METHODS

There are three types of casefinding methods used by registries: active, passive, and a combination of the two. In active casefinding procedures, registry personnel screen the source documents (including disease indices, pathology reports, etc.). The advantage of active casefinding procedures is that the case ascertainment is typically more thorough and accurate, because the registry personnel have extensive training in terminology that identifies reportable cases. The disadvantage of active case ascertainment is the financial cost. Review of each casefinding source requires additional processing time by the registry staff. The registry may lack the staff and financial resources necessary to allow registry personnel to actively review all potential casefinding sources.

With passive casefinding, or self-reporting, the registry relies on other healthcare professionals to notify the registrar of potentially reportable cases. The advantages of passive reporting include the decrease in the registry's casefinding labor cost and the sharing by nonregistry departments (pathology, admitting, and radiation oncology) of the burden of reporting. The disadvantage of passive casefinding is that nonregistry staff is not as familiar with reporting terminology and rules, so incomplete ascertainment typically occurs. For example, nonregistry staff could miss the collection of cases with diagnostic terms that may not sound cancerous (such as linitis plastica or Waldenstrom's macroglobulinemia).

Today, a combination of active and passive reporting is the most commonly used system in registries. The registrar must identify the critical casefinding sources that require active review by the registrar, decide the amount of passive case identification that should be performed, and determine which departments can provide high-quality casefinding information. An effective combination of active and passive casefinding reporting methods ensures more complete case ascertainment and reduces labor costs to the registry.

IDENTIFYING SOURCE DOCUMENTS

In a hospital, registry source documents can include the items shown in Table 12-2. The source documents may vary in individual institutions.

No single review alone can identify all cancer cases diagnosed or treated in a hospital. Reliance on multiple sources is necessary to obtain a complete description of the patient's cancer experience; for example, review of reports from diagnostic tests, surgery reports, pathology reports, and treatment summaries.

Table 12-1
Case Ascertainment Cycle

- Identifying source documents
- Determining reporting methods (active, passive, or a combination)
- Linking the identified cases
- Monitoring completeness of casefinding

Table 12-2
Case Ascertainment Source Documents

- Admission and discharge documents
- Disease indices
- Surgery schedules
- Pathology reports
- Cytology reports
- Nuclear medicine documents
- Radiation oncology logs
- Medical oncology logs
- Autopsy documents
- Admission and discharge reports

ADMISSION AND DISCHARGE REPORTS

Daily or weekly review of all inpatient and outpatient admissions and discharges facilitates quick ascertainment of cases presenting with a clinical diagnosis of cancer or discharged with a clinical or pathological diagnosis of cancer. Figure 12-1 is an example of an admission/discharge report. In this example, the lung cancer should be evaluated for inclusion in the registry.

Disease Indices

Once a month, the registry should request the previous month's disease index from the Health Information Management Department, which may provide this report in hard-copy format or electronically. When requesting the disease index, the registrar should specify the cancer codes used by the

Health Information Management Department to identify inpatient and outpatient visits. Use of the cancer-screening list of ICD-9-CM codes for casefinding will narrow the requested search to appropriate, registry-reportable cases. If the cancer committee wants additional types of cases included in the registry, the appropriate diagnostic codes for these case types should be added to the screening list. The registrar must determine what the hospital-specific guidelines are for coding certain diagnoses to ensure the accuracy of the codes used to identify cancer cases in the hospital. For example, it may be the coding policy of the hospital to code a re-excision performed as definitive treatment for a melanoma primary to a V10 code (personal history of malignant neoplasm) if there was no residual disease in the pathology specimen, rather than code 172.9 (melanoma of skin). In such a situation, both codes must be included in a review to identify all coded melanoma cases from the disease index. Figure 12-2 is an example disease index that should be reviewed for eligible cases.

Surgery Schedules

Surgery schedules (see the example in Figure 12-3) provide an additional source of casefinding. The accuracy of this source depends on appropriate documentation of orders and diagnoses at the time of surgery. This schedule should be reviewed daily or weekly. Any surgeries or diagnoses that indicate possible cancer cases should be reviewed for possible inclusion in the registry. The purpose of this type of review is to identify all cases that are reportable according to the registry reportable list.

Figure 12-1
Sample Admission/Discharge Report

			Admission/Discharge Date XX/XX/XXXX				
Name	*Health Record #*	*Department*	*Room*	*Payor*	*Date*	*Dx*
Admissions Lname, Fname	XXXXX	Med Onc	201-B	BC	XX/XX/XXXX	Lung cancer
Discharges Lname, Fname	XXXXX	OB	104-B	Pri	XX/XX/XXXX	Vaginal Delivery

Figure 12-2
Disease Index

Patient Name	Medical Record #	DX	DX Description	Dis Date	Service
DOE, JOHN	1234	185	PROSTATE CANCER	11/30/2004	INPT
DOE, JOHN	1234	600	PROSTATE HYPERPLASIA	12/15/2004	URO
DOE, JOHN	1234	185	PROSTATE CANCER	1/25/2005	RAD ONC
DOE, JANE	5678	1809	CERVICAL CANCER	10/15/2004	PATH
DOE, JANE	5678	2809	BLOOD LOSS ANEMIA	11/15/2004	LAB
DOE, JANE	5678	1809	CERVICAL CANCER	11/28/2004	HEM ONC

Figure 12-3
Example Surgery Schedule

		Surgery Schedule XX/XX/XXXX		
Date	Patient Name	Diagnosis	Surgery	Physician
XX/XX/XX	Lname, Fname	Rt colon CA	Colectomy	Dr. D. Smith

Pathology Reports

Typically, more than 90% of all cancers are histologically confirmed. Reviewing all pathology reports is essential to complete cancer reporting. If the pathology department is computerized and each report contains an ICD-O histology and behavior code, a computerized list of diagnoses with behavior codes of 2 (in situ) and 3 (malignant, primary) can be generated. A separate list of all diagnoses with behavior codes of 0 (benign) and 1 (uncertain and unknown behavior) should also be printed to allow review of these reports.

If the Pathology Department is not computerized or does not use ICD-O codes to code histology, the registrar must manually review each pathology report. Some cancer registrars arrange with the Pathology Department to automatically have copies of all pathology reports sent to the registry for review so that the registrar can determine which are reportable. This is an example of passive casefinding, which is not optimal.

Both computerized and manual methods of reviewing pathology reports must include a way to track reports to ensure that each report has been included in the registrar's review. A copy of the pathology report may not be in the file at the time of the registrar's review. Occasionally, slides are submitted for outside consultation and review, and pathologists require additional time to draft a final report for a pathology specimen. An example of a pathology tracking log is shown in Figure 12-4.

Cytology Reports

Cytology reports can be reviewed in a manner similar to that described for pathology reports. Cytology laboratories may maintain hard copy reports or computerized lists for the registrar's review. All reports must be reviewed to ensure complete ascertainment of all cytology cases. Figure 12-5 shows an example of a hard copy cytology report.

Nuclear Medicine Logs

The Nuclear Medicine Department is another area in which case ascertainment should be performed. For example, treatment of thyroid cancers with radioactive isotopes is a procedure performed in the Nuclear Medicine Department. Review of the treatment log is recommended to identify potential cases.

Figure 12-4
Example Pathology Screening Log

Pathology Screening Log

Date of Review	Pathology Log # Reviewed From	Pathology Log # Reviewed To	Missing Pathology Reports	Person Completing the Review
12-6-2004	11-1-2004	12-2-2004	2004-9994	CLH

Figure 12-5
Sample Cytology Report

Cytology Report

Specimen: Bone marrow aspirate right, iliac crest
Collected: XX/XX/XX   Received: XX/XX/XX   Specimen No: XX–XXXXX
Clinical Information: Breast primary
Microscopic Diagnosis:
Bone marrow aspirate showing adenocarcinoma consistent with breast primary
Comment:

Patient: Lname, Fname
              DOB xx/xx/xx
              Unit #:21000000

Figure 12-6
Sample Radiation Therapy Log

Radiation Therapy Log

Date	Patient	Diagnosis	Referring Physician
XX/XX/XX	Lname, Fname	Adenocarcinoma, prostate	D. Smith

Radiation Oncology Logs

For a facility with a Radiation Oncology Department, a review of the patient log (see the example in Figure 12-6) helps ensure complete ascertainment of all cases. Most radiation oncology logs include a diagnosis to help in appropriate identification of cases. This log should be reviewed for new cases. Some facilities may include radiation oncology visits in their disease index rather than a manual log. In this instance it is important to have the disease index generated with service codes. It is also a good system for collecting follow-up information on patients returning for three-, six-, and twelve-month follow-up. Some facilities send copies of consultation and treatment summary reports to registries in referring institutions.

Medical Oncology Logs

Patients receive chemotherapy either as inpatients, or in an ambulatory setting, a freestanding facility, or a physician's office. The registry staff must establish a policy and procedure for identifying patients who receive chemotherapy at any facility affiliated with the institution. The registrar should identify the inpatient unit (oncology-dedicated or the functional equivalent) that provides most oncology services and then request that a log be maintained to identify new patients. As in the radiation oncology logs, these encounters may be included with the disease index and identified by a service code. A method of obtaining the same information must be developed for ambulatory facilities or offices associated with the institution. A patient log similar to the one used in the radiation oncology department can be used for outpatient settings.

A review of medical oncology lists or logs should be completed at least once a month. As does the radiation oncology log, the medical oncology list or log serves as an excellent tool for collecting current follow-up information.

Autopsy Reports

Some facilities maintain autopsy or necropsy reports in the Pathology Department. These autopsy reports can be ascertained at the time of pathology review, although they are typically filed separately from the other pathology reports. For facilities that do not perform autopsies, these reports may be located in the Health Information Management Department. A system should be developed between the Health Information Management Department and the registrar to ensure that all autopsies are flagged for review by the registrar.

LINKING IDENTIFIED CASES

After identifying a potential case for the registry from a casefinding source, the registrar processes the case into either the suspense file, the master patient index file, or the history file of nonreportable cases.

The suspense file contains information on cases that are potentially reportable. This file should be reviewed monthly to ensure that cases are completed promptly. Cases entered into the suspense file but later determined not to be reportable are moved to the history file of nonreportable cases. Reportable cases are eventually moved to the master patient index file.

When entering a case into the suspense file, registry personnel should include data elements required by the governing body. Hospitals participating in the approvals process by the Commission on Cancer of the American College of Surgeons must include the patient name, patient identifier, date of diagnosis or date of first contact, and primary site.[2] A registrar may want to include information on the record to indicate the casefinding source. During the review of source document information, the registrar may discover that the patient is already in the registry's patient index file for the same primary cancer. If the source document indicates that this is a new primary, the case should be added to the suspense file so that the patient's health record can be reviewed to complete the documentation on the newly identified subsequent primary. If, after review of the health record documentation, the registrar determines a case to be either a history case (that is, the health record indicates that the malignancy was diagnosed prior to the registry's reference date) or a nonreportable case (for example, if the health record does not support the malignant disease code found on the hospital's disease index), the case should be maintained in the history file of nonreportable cases to prevent repeated pulling and review of the same health record. A sample format of a form for the history file is shown in Figure 12-7.

Registries that cannot maintain the history file of nonreportable cases in their computerized registry systems can use a separate database, spreadsheet, or word processing program. These programs allow the

Figure 12-7
Sample Format for History File of Nonreportable Cases

History/Nonreportable Cases						
Name	Date of Birth	SS#	Health Record #	Diagnosis	Date	Reason for Not Including the Case in the Registry
J. Smith	9-21-32	999-99-9999	888888	Adenoca	11-2-2004	Consult only

registrar to search the file by name, health record number, or social security number.

MONITORING COMPLETENESS OF CASEFINDING

Quality control procedures must be implemented to ensure complete reporting of all reportable cases. This quality control function should be performed semiannually at a minimum to allow for immediate correction of identified under-reported areas. If the number of reportable cases in the database has

dropped by midyear, the registrar should verify that all sources of case ascertainment have been reviewed. A monitoring log can help in this process but is not required. An example of a monitoring log is shown in Figure 12-8.

Other examples of quality control procedures for case ascertainment include comparing monthly cases in previous years with the current period. See Figure 12-9 for an example of a case-completeness log by month and year of diagnosis. Again, this type of log can be useful, but is not required.

Figure 12-8
Sample Casefinding Completeness Log

Casefinding Completeness Log—20XX

	Jan	Feb	Mar	Apr	May	Jun	Jul	Aug	Sep	Oct	Nov	Dec
Adm & Dis												
Dis Index												
Surg Schedule												
Path												
Cyto												
Nucl Med												
Rad Onc												
Med Onc												
Autopsy												
Other												

Figure 12-9
Sample Casefinding Completeness Log by Month and Year of Diagnosis

Casefinding Completeness Log by Month and Year of Diagnosis

Month	Number of Cases, 2003	Number of Cases, 2004
January	60	85
February	50	60
March	65	72
April	58	50
May	52	61
June	61	64
July	45	57
August	32	62
September	65	72
October	62	78
November	70	80
December	40	62

Figure 12-10
Sample Casefinding Completeness Log by Site and Year of Diagnosis

Casefinding Completeness Log by Site and Year of Diagnosis		
Site	*2003*	*2004*
Breast	91	104
Prostate	85	61
Melanoma	26	11
Lymphoma	25	24
Cervix	18	2

In the example in Figure 12-9, the decrease in cases in July and August 1995 might correlate with a primary physician taking an extended vacation. The decrease in cases for December 1995 and the increase in January 1996 may be due to a specialty group of physicians leaving the institution in December and the arrival of a new group in January. Fluctuations like those shown in Figure 12-9 should be reviewed and justified when differences are identified to ensure that casefinding is complete. The easiest way to accomplish this task is to request the disease indices again for the month in question so that patterns that deviate from previous months can be reviewed.

On a hospital and regional level, comparison of sites by the year of diagnosis can be helpful. Figure 12-10 shows an example of an evaluation form used for this purpose. This type of evaluation can show a decrease in outpatient visits, possible lack of coding or change in coding mechanism, use of a different laboratory for outpatient visits, physician change in facility preference, or patient movement to an outpatient physician office setting.

On a regional and state level, comparison of facilities by year could identify increases or decreases in cases. Increases may be due to the opening of a new cancer center or a different marketing approach. Decreases can be attributed to a facility closing, loss of an industry, or physicians leaving the area. Although these increases or decreases may be explainable, the reasons should be determined. In the example of a new cancer center opening, cases from neighboring or smaller facilities would decrease slightly. Using casefinding completeness logs and regularly monitoring case ascertainment enable the registrar to identify potential problems quickly and resolve true problems with immediate action.

SUMMARY

Ascertainment of cases is an important part of the registry. A system to monitor prospective cases must be in place in different areas of an institution. The completeness of case ascertainment must be monitored for quality control purposes.

In computerized registries, the logs described in this chapter can be electronically generated.

Each registry must determine the benefits and requirements of each log according to required standards, governing body requirements, or available resources.

STUDY QUESTIONS

1. Describe the activities involved in the case ascertainment cycle.
2. What factors should be considered in identifying the type of case ascertainment sources to be used by the registry?
3. Describe the difference between active and passive case ascertainment.
4. What is a suspense file?
5. What are the benefits of maintaining a history file of nonreportable cases?

REFERENCES

1. Fritz A, Percy, C, Jack A, et al. In *International Classification of Diseases for Oncology*, 3rd ed., U. S. interim Version 2000. Geneva, Switzerland: World Health Organization; 2000.
2. Commission on Cancer. *Facility Oncology Registry Data Standards*. Chicago, Ill: American College of Surgeons; 2003.

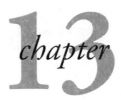

RAPID CASE ASCERTAINMENT

Carol Lowenstein
MBA, CTR

INTRODUCTION

The goal of rapid case ascertainment is to support and facilitate epidemiologic and clinical research by providing the rapid identification of cases eligible for studies requiring case identification shortly after diagnosis. Central cancer registry data have routinely been utilized for epidemiologic studies, particularly large population based studies. For those studies allowing for the utilization of cases diagnosed more than six months ago, hospital, central, and state-level data can be utilized. However, many studies require cases be identified shortly after diagnosis in order to provide researchers with immediate patient access.

For malignancies associated with high morbidity or mortality, such as lung, pancreatic, or ovarian cancer, it is particularly important to identify cases immediately after diagnosis so as not to lose the ability to interview patients directly. This can result in the loss of inclusion of potential cases or necessitate a reliance on next-of-kin interviews, which could bias the outcome of the study and lead to misleading results.[1] When dealing with younger, frequently mobile patients, there can be logistical problems associated with locating patients after diagnosis. As time goes on, it is also more difficult for patients to precisely recall elements of their lifestyle that might have changed after diagnosis and treatment, such as alcohol consumption and smoking history. The ability to collect blood and tissue samples is also greatly enhanced via the use of rapid case ascertainment.[2] Recent interest in the association of genetic issues surrounding the early detection, diagnosis, and treatment of cancer has greatly increased the demand for rapid access to study eligible cases.[3]

METHODS OF CASE ASCERTAINMENT

Rapid case ascertainment can occur in several ways: mandated reporting of cases within the first few weeks of diagnosis by hospitals to the central registry,[4] central registry personnel traveling into the field to collect cases for specific studies, and automated reporting of filtered pathology reports directly to the central registry.

Some central registries utilize a two-phase reporting requirement wherein an initial report containing patient demographics tumor site and histology is sent by the reporting facility to the central registry within six weeks of the initial date of diagnosis. This is followed by a full abstract to be reported within the usual six-month time frame following initial diagnosis. This system provides researchers access to cancers of all sites throughout the population covered by the central registry thus making it conducive to population-based studies.

Many central registries, particularly those associated with academic institutions, have rapid case ascertainment (RCA) units that are available on an ad hoc basis to perform casefinding for special studies. In these instances, cancer registrars from the RCA visit pathology and medical record departments on a circuit-riding basis to identify cases needed for special studies. Utilizing this method, cases can be identified within a very short time period following diagnosis. In addition, RCA staff can collect data required by individual researchers that may fall outside the confines of the standard central registry abstract, such as specimen numbers, first language spoken by the patient, or date of next clinic appointment. This situation is ideal for those studies requiring case identification and subsequent patient contact within days of diagnosis. Some RCA units also provide assistance to researchers with institutional review board approval and pathology specimen retrieval.[5] Working in concert with central registry staff, the RCA is also used as a resource for researchers by providing potential case numbers for study planning and grant-preparation purposes.[6]

New technology in the area of electronic pathology reporting has led to an increased interest and use of this method for overall central registry casefinding and rapid case ascertainment for special studies.[7] Electronic pathology reporting systems are based on the ability to scan text documents for key terms to determine reportability. Utilizing this method, central registries use the Search Term List[8] compiled by the North American Association of Central Cancer Registries to automatically screen pathology reports for the presence of terms indicating a positive diagnosis of cancer. Pathology reports containing reportable terms are then released to the central registry. Aside from rapid case identification, electronic path reporting also greatly reduces the amount of manual review of pathology reports. It also increases the degree of patient confidentiality in that only those cases meeting reporting requirements are made available to the central registry.[7] Establishing an electronic pathology reporting system does require a great deal of coordination and cooperation between reporting facilities and the central registry but the potential benefits are far reaching.

COST

The cost of the rapid case methods varies greatly. The two-phase system is relatively inexpensive in that a small amount of data is being gathered and reported through an existing mechanism, namely hospital to central registry. The initial rapid report is merely a subset of the greater data set and therefore does not require an additional effort on the part of hospital registries. There may be a slight amount of additional processing at the central registry to link subsequent reports to those reported in the rapid phase; this cost however is minimal.

The establishment and maintenance of a RCA unit bears a significant ongoing cost in that trained personnel are needed to perform accurate case review. The process of reviewing numerous pathology reports to find those meeting stringent eligibility requirements can be time consuming and labor intensive. In addition, some studies require the RCA circuit rider to cover large geographic areas thus increasing the amount of time required to complete the task. As a result, most RCA units charge on a fee-for-service basis, billing researchers for each case identified.[5,6]

Electronic pathology reporting systems bear a substantial up-front cost in personnel, software, and equipment. However, when these one-time costs are compared to the ongoing costs involved in maintaining an RCA unit, the impact diminishes and the cost per case found is reduced.[7]

CONFIDENTIALITY

Rapid case ascertainment must be performed under the same confidentiality mandates as all other activities conducted within hospital and central registries. Studies utilizing rapid case data must possess institutional review board (IRB) approval. In some states, approval is available under a statewide IRB and approval is then accepted at most hospitals in the state. Other states require IRB approval from each institution from which data will be obtained. Rapid case staff must carefully review the protocol and terms of approval prior to initiating casefinding activities to ensure IRB compliance.

SUMMARY

Rapid case ascertainment contributes greatly to the advancement of epidemiologic and clinical studies in all areas of cancer research. It provides a substantial economy of scale to researchers who would otherwise need to hire and train personnel to identify cases for each study that they initiate. The increased desire to examine genetic material and the ability of electronic pathology reporting combine to increase both the demand and potential usefulness of rapid case ascertainment.

STUDY QUESTIONS

1. Why is rapid case ascertainment important?
2. Describe how rapid case ascertainment occurs.
3. Describe the costs involved with rapid case ascertainment.

REFERENCES

1. Holly EA, Guatman M, Bracci PM. Comparison of interviewed and non interviewed non-Hodgkin lymphoma (NHL) patients in the San Francisco Bay area. *Annals of Epidemiology.* 2002; 12(6): 419-25.
2. Aldrich TE, Vann D, Moorman PG, Newman D. Rapid reporting of cancer incidence in a population-based study of breast cancer: one constructive use of a central cancer registry. *Breast Cancer Research and Treatment.* 1995; 35 (1): 61-4.
3. Results of the NCI Progress Review Groups National Cancer Institute. Available at: http://prg.cancer.org.
4. New Hampshire State Cancer Registry website.
5. Yale Cancer Center Rapid Case Ascertainment website. Available at: http://info.med.yale.edu.ycc/rs02j.htm.
6. Dana-Farber/Harvard Cancer Center website. Available at: http://www.dfhcc.harvard.edu/core.facilities.
7. Deapen D, Menck, HR, Ervin, IL, Leventhal M, Niland JC. Experience in developing E-Path cancer reporting for rapid case ascertainment. *Journal of Registry Management.* 2002; 29:44-51.
8. North American Association of Central Cancer Registries. Path Lab Committee Search Term List. Available at www.naaccr.org/Standards/pathlabcom.html

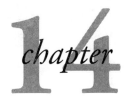

chapter 14

STANDARDS FOR DATA AND DATA MANAGEMENT

Jerri Linn Phillips
MA, CTR

Carol Hahn Johnson
BS, CTR

INTRODUCTION

Registry data collected in the absence of shared standards contribute little beyond anecdotal detail toward case management or cancer control. Shared standards ensure clarity of communication, protect the integrity of data when they are pooled or compared across multiple sources, and focus attention on key aspects of cancer care or cancer control.

Data collected by a cancer registry should be useful on several levels. First, the cancer registry is a source of personal and medical information necessary for planning and evaluating the individual patient's case management. Second, registry data provide administrative information for facility planners, cancer committees, and practitioners. Third, the data are used by government and private agencies for developing and evaluating cancer control programs after population-based registries consolidate individual reports. Fourth, registries provide a rich source of data for investigative cancer research.

Except for individual case reports, all uses of cancer registry data involve compilations of data in statistical summaries. The interpretation of compiled data requires uniformity of definitions and collection procedures for data elements and consistent use of codes. Consequently, even if universal standards do not exist, most registries institute local guidelines to meet their immediate needs for data consistency.

Interest in shared or uniform registry standards for data collection and management grew with the increasingly varied use of registry data, stimulated by adoption of computerized registry data systems. Contemporary standards for registry data and data management emphasize standardization of the data. That is, for items characteristically collected by cancer registries, the same codes and code definitions are applied, data are coded by the same rules and edited and updated according to the same guidelines. When standard rules for case inclusion or exclusion and standard grouping procedures are also followed, the resulting incidence, survival, and response rates have the same meaning no matter where they were produced. For registry data to be used optimally, uniform standards are necessary.

Historically, registry standards addressed diagnostic codes and general registry operations. The field of oncology data collection has continued to grow, especially since the advent of widespread computerization of registries. Clinical, epidemiological, and surveillance groups, as well as organizations evaluating data quality, became increasingly interested in pooling or consolidating registry data. Data are pooled when records from multiple sources are combined into a single, large database, each record representing a unique case. Data that are compiled separately are compared for presentation in a single publication. When multiple records applying to a single case are included, the data are consolidated to form a single, more complete record.

Central registries including the National Cancer Data Base (NCDB), the North American Association of Central Cancer Registries (NAACCR), the Surveillance, Epidemiology, and End Results Program (SEER), the National Program of Cancer Registries (NPCR), state or province registries, and other joint projects, collect data submitted electronically from multiple source registries. Without shared data-coding standards, the submitted data had to be reformatted and interpreted, as the hospital registries used different codes, coding rules, data sets, and software. Central registry administrators were among the first to realize the inconsistencies of data content, among contributing registries despite what had previously seemed to be shared codes and procedures.

This chapter describes the major standard-setting organizations and their spheres of interest and contributions to registry standards, and then outlines the areas where shared standards are being developed. It is beyond the scope of this textbook to reiterate individual standards. Registries should obtain current information directly from the governing bodies that affect their operations.

THE STANDARD SETTERS

Standards are rules set by authority. They reflect the organizational data needs of standard setters, including the need for consistency among groups. The standards that apply to cancer registries today evolved over the last half-century. It is no accident that the history of oncology data standards is closely linked to the groups that shaped their development. The standard setters identified in this section established the principles of cancer registration and continue to influence cancer data and registry operations. Their goals help determine what registries collect and how the data are processed and ultimately used. Within their spheres of responsibility, they are also the primary authorities with which to address questions on data and data management.

Three organizations were involved in the development of standard codes for describing the cancer itself. The World Health Organization (WHO), the American Cancer Society (ACS), and the American Joint Committee on Cancer (AJCC) developed standard codes for topography, morphology, and extent of tumor spread.

Three additional organizations shaped standards for facility and population-based registries. The Commission on Cancer (CoC) defined the role of the facility registry in cancer management. The National Cancer Institute's (NCI) Surveillance, Epidemiology, and End Results (SEER) Program developed procedures for central registry monitoring of data quality, and the National Program of Cancer Registries (NPCR), administered by the Centers for Disease Control and Prevention (CDC), added inducements for population-based central registries to adhere to guidelines.

The final two organizations overlap the others in time and purpose. Although all standard-setting agencies sponsor training programs, the National Cancer Registrars Association (NCRA) develops training programs specifically for registrars. The North American Association of Central Cancer Registries (NAACCR) promotes the development of standards shared by member central registries and the standard setters that sponsor it.

The World Health Organization (WHO)

After the United Nations was established, the World Health Organization became the organization responsible for publishing disease codes. The *International Statistical Classification of Diseases and Related Health Problems,* 10th revision (ICD-10),[1-3] is the most recent edition in a series that began in 1893. It forms the basis for the *International Classification of Diseases for Oncology, 3rd Edition* (ICD-O-3), the worldwide standard cancer diagnosis coding system. See Chapter 9 of this text, Coding of Neoplasms, for further information on coding cancer diagnoses. The cancer chapter was fully revised in ICD-10, and the topography codes are distinctly different from the earlier versions. ICD-10 can be purchased on diskette, complete with a file for use in coding software.

The ICD-10 disease codes for cancer are primarily topographical, though special codes that com-

bine topographic and morphologic characteristics of some cancers were added as the series evolved. The ICD-0 manuals provide registries with topography codes, from the ICD disease code tradition, and morphology codes developed from codes originally published by the American Cancer Society.

The American Cancer Society (ACS)

The American Cancer Society published the *Manual of Tumor Nomenclature and Coding* (MOTNAC) in 1951.[4] That early document served as the basis for a series of refinements in cancer morphology codes, including the *Systematized Nomenclature of Pathology (SNOP)*[5]; the *Systematized Nomenclature of Medicine (SNOMED),* published by the College of American Pathologists;[6] and the *International Classification of Diseases for Oncology* (ICD-O-3),[7] published by the World Health Organization.

The American Cancer Society supports cancer prevention and access to care, and sponsors research and training activities, working closely with other major standard setting groups.

The American Joint Committee on Cancer (AJCC)

The American Joint Committee on Cancer has guided the development, implementation, and use of the TNM (Tumor-Node-Metastasis) cancer prognostic system in America since 1959. The clinically oriented TNM staging scheme was developed by the AJCC in cooperation with the TNM committee of the International Union Against Cancer (UICC) and is used worldwide for prognostic staging of cancers.

The AJCC regularly updates its staging standards to incorporate advances in prognostic technology.[8] Current work concerns the development of prognostic indices based on molecular markers that assess the rate at which tumors grow. AJCC is committed to improving the predictive accuracy of the TNM system and making the system accessible and useful to the practicing clinician.

The Commission on Cancer (CoC) approvals program requires physicians to assign AJCC staging for all sites having defined staging schemes.

The Commission on Cancer (CoC) of the American College of Surgeons

The 1912 Clinical Congress of Surgeons of North America proposed the "standardization of surgeons," which resulted in the formation of the American College of Surgeons in 1913. Their second proposal was for the "standardization of hospitals," which led to the founding of the Joint Commission on Accreditation of Hospitals in 1918 (now called the Joint Commission on Accreditation of Healthcare Organizations [JCAHO]). The Board of Regents appointed the Cancer Campaign Committee (now known as the Commission on Cancer) in 1913. That committee started the process of outcome analysis of cancer cases based on stage and treatment.[9-14] CoC-approved programs are required to maintain a cancer registry which collects minimally all the data items published in Facility Oncology Data Standards (FORDS).[15] For further detailed information regarding these standard-setting organizations, see Chapter 9 of this textbook, The American College of Surgeons Commission on Cancer and the Approvals Program, and Chapter 11, Joint Commission on Accreditation of Healthcare Organizations.

The National Cancer Data Base (NCDB)

A joint effort by the American Cancer Society and the American College of Surgeons, the National Cancer Data Base (NCDB) collects data from computerized hospital cancer registries for use in evaluating cancer trends and in analytic research. Data submission to the NCDB, required for CoC-approved cancer programs since 1996, reinforces the importance of standard code definitions. For detailed information regarding the NCDB, see Chapter 31.

The Surveillance, Epidemiology, and End Results Program (SEER)

The SEER Program was established under the National Cancer Program by the National Cancer Act of 1971; data collection began in January 1973. SEER requires its constituent central registries to adhere to SEER's data standards. The SEER standards formed the basis for many central registry data standards today.[16-20] See Chapter 33 of this textbook, The Surveillance, Epidemiology, and End Results Program, for further detailed information.

The National Program of Cancer Registries (NPCR)

The Cancer Registries Amendment Act (Public Law 102-515), enacted by Congress in 1992, authorized the Centers for Disease Control and Prevention (CDC) to administer the NPCR. The intent of the federal law was to improve cancer control by encouraging development of state-level population-based central registries whose data would conform to uniform standards. NPCR provides planning grants to states without central registries and grants to enhance existing state population-based cancer registries.

National Cancer Registrars Association (NCRA)

This organization, formerly the National Tumor Registrars Association, was founded in 1974. NCRA plays a vital part in the professional development of cancer registrars. NCRA develops and maintains a variety of programs for training cancer registrars. The first certification exam for cancer registrars was offered by NCRA in 1983. NCRA provides ongoing training for cancer registry staff and mechanisms for communication between registry staff and other standard-setting organizations through its publications, annual conferences, workshops, and continuing-education credit program.

The North American Association of Central Cancer Registries (NAACCR)

NAACCR was established in 1987 to meet the needs of central cancer registries. Central registries in the United States and Canada use NAACCR as a forum to resolve problems, establish shared standards, and improve the quality and consistency of central registry operations. NAACCR took on the challenge of coordinating standards developed by other groups, developing standard codes and procedures not addressed by any single organization, and evaluating the quality of central registry data with respect to use of the data for cancer control.[21-26] See Chapter 32 of this textbook, The North American Association of Central Cancer Registries, of this textbook for further detailed information.

The Uniform Data Standards Committee (UDSC) of NAACCR

The UDSC compiles coding, editing, and data exchange standards, including remaining unresolved issues, which are published and disseminated by NAACCR. The work of UDSC built on earlier joint efforts of CoC and SEER, under the auspices of NCRA, to find ways to coordinate disparate codes and data sets.

By agreement of the participants, items under consideration for change by the standard setters that define data elements collected by registries are reviewed by the UDSC committee. Consideration of a proposed change includes the logical structure of the code (will it do what is intended?), continuity with past data (can the new code be collapsed for comparison with earlier codes?), reason for the change (for example, it may be needed because of technological developments or to correct an existing inconsistency), and underlying theory. Most proposals are resolved by adoption of the new standard (or retention of the old one) by all.

Apparent persisting inconsistencies in codes often reflect differences in underlying theory. That is, codes that might appear to measure the same thing do not, and they may differ in respects that remain important to the participating organizations. An example is the distinct codes that measure cancer spread at diagnosis, described in Figure 14-1.

THE SCOPE OF STANDARDS FOR DATA AND DATA MANAGEMENT

Shared registry data standards are undergoing rapid development. This section describes the scope of shared registry standards that already exist, are being developed, or are likely to be developed in the next few years.

Data Sets

Data sets are lists of data elements that must be collected to meet the minimal requirements of the group's goals, often with an additional list of elements that are recommended for the most effective operation. Required data sets are not the same for all standard setters. Data sets specified by different organizations are understandably different. For example, the underlying interest of the CoC is the quality of case management and medical care provided by the medical facility. Detailed information is

Figure 14-1

Example of Distinct but Similar-Appearing Code Structures: Measuring Disease Spread

The tumor (T), node (N), and metastasis (M) system, developed by the International Union Against Cancer and first established in US hospital registries by the American Joint Committee on Cancer, is based on site-specific prognostic indicators. It is updated with advances in prognostic knowledge and new approaches to treatment.

A second system, summary staging, codes cancer spread in anatomic terms with respect to the primary site organ. Summary codes classify the disease as in situ, localized, regional, distant, or unstaged. The code language is the same for every site. For the most part, categories do not change with advances in medical science. The first Summary Staging manual was published in 1977 and the first major revision to categories was published in 2000. Summary Staging is most widely used by population-based registries to track screening and early diagnosis in large demographic groups over time. It is not possible to convert all TNM codes to summary staging, and summary staging cannot be converted to TNM codes or AJCC stage groups.

The Surveillance, Epidemiology, and End Results (SEER) Program uses a ten-digit site-specific coding scheme for extent of disease (EOD). This coding scheme is designed to collapse into different stage groupings, including summary stage and a variation of the AJCC stage groups.

While the varied code structures satisfactorily meet the respective needs for which they were designed, many registrars have had to independently code multiple measures of tumor spread. Consequently, the affected standard setters devised an aptly-named approach, Collaborative Staging, which is modeled after SEER EOD. Collaborative staging breaks the information needed to code all AJCC T, N, M and Stage Group, SEER EOD, and SEER Summary Staging in discrete components which can then be combined electronically to generate those various measures.

collected on patients' prognostic and risk factors, treatments, and short- and long-term outcomes. The NPCR data set was specified to meet cancer control and surveillance goals, goals which require timely diagnosis and reporting of cases and information on demographic factors, first course of treatment, and mortality. SEER's data incorporate the goal of epidemiological research analysis. Each program includes items that indicate data quality with respect to its own data uses. Many of the data needs for these and other programs are similar, and the required data sets naturally overlap.

Most hospital registries are required to meet the standards for more than one organization and may also collect additional elements to meet internal needs. Most registries in hospitals or other medical facilities are required to meet the data standards of both the CoC and a state central registry. The CoC data set, in turn, includes items necessary to code TNM categories and other items required by its member organizations. Most state registries must meet data requirements set by SEER, NPCR, and state legislative mandate, in addition to those they themselves set internally. State registries that also function as central registries of hospitals collect the full CoC data set. Most states require at least some data elements beyond the set required by CoC, and most states do not use all CoC-required elements.

Code Categories

Given the overlap in data sets and central registry dependence on the hospital as the primary source of data, there is a great need for consistent data standards. Data elements having the same name or intent should mean the same thing in every registry that collects them. When they do not, comparisons of data across registries can be seriously misinterpreted.

It is useful to distinguish between categories (for example, race categories), and the codes assigned to them (01-99). Standard codes are necessary for reporting or exchanging data and are often more convenient to use internally. It is technically not necessary that they be used for internal storage in a registry. Standard categories must be retained in the registry structure, however, and conversion to and from standard codes must be built into routine computer operations. Because the assignment of categories must be similar for codes to indicate the same thing, it is not sufficient to convert nonstandard categories into standard codes.

Coding standards specify not only what codes to apply to "known" categories but also distinguish categories such as "not available in the record," "not appropriate to this case," or "not collected by this registry." The format of the code standardizes various detailed matters for the computerized record (for example, mixed or uppercase letters, left or right justification, numeric with leading blanks or numbers with a zero fill, blanks permitted or not).

Rules for Code Assignment

Simply defining code categories does not ensure data consistency. Both technical and nontechnical elements must follow coding rules for category assignment. For example, how exactly does an abstractor select among multiple references to morphology in a record? When does first-course therapy begin and end? Where does a transient live? The need for uniform coding rules is well recognized by registries and standard setters, and more progress in this area is likely to be achieved over the next several years.

Data Edits

Automated data edits are designed to identify potential problems internal to the data, and flag conditions that require review by the abstractor or coder. Single-item edits identify codes entered for an item that are not allowable. Inter-item edits test the logical effects of coding rules or natural relationships. For example, squamous cell carcinoma commonly develops in the lung but is not expected to develop in the pleura; an automated edit can question or flag a case coded as squamous cell carcinoma of the pleura. Depending on how the edit is implemented by the registry software, the software may prohibit saving that combination of codes, allow the registrar to set an override flag if necessary, or simply print an edit report for review later.

Differently edited data are not statistically comparable. This is an especially difficult concept to grasp because it challenges a widely accepted axiom, "the more editing the better." Consider, for example, the standard sex-primary site edit which checks that females do not have prostate or testis cancers and males do not have cancers of the uterus, cervix, vagina, or vulva. That edit is not the same as an edit which checks that only males have prostate or testis cancer and only females have cancers of the uterus, cervix, vagina, or vulva because the standard code for sex allows for options other than male and female and patients who fall into those categories may have one or another of these reproductive cancers.

The SEER Program developed the first standard edits for registry data. Through the leadership of NAACCR, edit standards have been compiled for data elements within and across standard data sets. When edits are adopted, any updated or modified data in the registry should be reedited with the same checks. Further information on computer edits can be found in Chapter 22, Computer Principles.

Case Consolidation

The logic of case consolidation is closely related to both code category assignment and data editing. When data from multiple sources pertaining to the same person or tumor are combined, inevitable discrepancies between information on file and new data appear. Some discrepancies represent new information (for example, a more detailed morphology), some are erroneous (a misspelled name). Consolidation rules determine which data inconsistencies can be resolved automatically and when to assign precedence of one category over another. Shared standards for case consolidation are likely to be developed in the coming years, as our understanding of this process evolves.

Cases to Be Covered by New or Changed Standards

Even though an important consideration in the use of standard code categories and procedures is continuity over time, introduction of new or revised codes is sometimes necessary. It is now accepted practice when introducing changes in data standards to specify a date of implementation for the new code. Data collected with outdated codes are often no more useful than old data. For example, to be useful, the AJCC prognostic stage groups require updating as medical technologies advance. Old AJCC stage grouping lacks the prognostic value of the revised codes.

Administrative Items

Standard administrative codes identify a code version or flag exceptions to standard edits. Pooled data collected from multiple sources over a period of years require some method of identifying which codes were applied to those data. Sometimes codes are revised by splitting old code values into multiple new ones and adding new categories, but occasionally old codes take on new meaning. Both types of code change affect data distribution, and redefined codes obviously affect code interpretation.

Standard administrative items permit communication about the nature of the data in a form that can be interpreted by a computer program. Although administrative items are not an obvious component of a data set that serves the needs of any particular standard setter, they are valuable parts of shared or exchanged data. The registry software can add some administrative items as cases are entered; others can be added automatically when data are written to exchange records. However, others, such as edit override flags, must be added by the registrar in those rare circumstances when they apply.

Data Management Procedures

Standards for data management procedures for hospitals and population-based registries developed largely independently, and have been defined by different standard setters. However, the scope of operations covered is similar: staff training and qualifications, case inclusion, case ascertainment, procedures for adding new cases to the permanent data set, rules for updating or changing data on file, follow-up, data exchange, and data analysis and publication.

Hospital registry operational requirements are defined by the COC approvals program as part of its *Cancer Program Standards*. State central registry standards are defined in *Standards for Cancer Registries, vol. III: Standards for Completeness, Quality, Analysis, and Management of Data* by NAACCR. Specific standards are also defined by SEER and NPCR.

Differences in data management standards reflect differences in registry operation and, for the most part, are not contradictory. For example, population-based central registry case ascertainment standards require coverage of all facilities that care for cancer patients in the geographic region, whereas registries in individual facilities must check the records of all services in the facility in which cancer patients may be identified.

However, registrars usually must comply with more than one standard for case inclusion. CoC specifications for facility registries identify the types of cases for which the facility, or its staff, have care responsibility. Many states require reporting of cases specifically excluded from CoC coverage, because central registries use this information to form a consolidated record for the patient from all sources. Hospitals also sometimes choose to collect data for cases not required by CoC or state laws. Benign tumors, preleukemic conditions, and similar diagnoses may be included by local standard.

SUMMARY

Cancer data standards may be established by the registry, a governing organization, or by mutual agreement among standard setters. Most registries must meet standards set by more than one governing organization. The absence of shared standards can make pooling or consolidation of data from multiple sources both time- and cost-intensive and can compromise data quality. Shared standards evolve as registry data uses expand, as computerization becomes more readily available, and as oncologic knowledge grows. In the future, registrars must be aware of changes in standards that affect their work. All aspects of registry operations affect data quality and consistency, from registry software to staff, and all must be addressed in the implementation of shared standards.

STUDY QUESTIONS

1. Define the term *standard*.
2. List three functions of shared standards.
3. In one or two sentences, describe the role of each of the following organizations for cancer registry standards:
   a. American Cancer Society (ACS)
   b. American Joint Committee on Cancer (AJCC)
   c. Commission on Cancer (COC)
   d. National Cancer Registrars Association (NCRA)
   e. National Program of Cancer Registries (NPCR)
   f. North American Association of Central Cancer Registries (NAACCR)
   g. Surveillance, Epidemiology and End Results (SEER)
   h. World Health Organization (WHO)

REFERENCES

1. *International Statistical Classification of Diseases and Related Health Problems,* 10th revision, vol. 1: Tabular List. Geneva: World Health Organization, 1992.
2. *International Statistical Classification of Diseases and Related Health Problems,* 10th revision, vol. 2: Instruction Manual. Geneva: World Health Organization, 1993.
3. *International Statistical Classification of Diseases and Related Health Problems,* 10th revision, diskette version. Geneva: World Health Organization, 1994.
4. *Manual of Tumor Nomenclature and Coding.* New York: American Cancer Society, 1951.
5. *Systematized Nomenclature of Pathology,* Chicago: College of American Pathologists, 1965.
6. Cote, R. A. (ed.), *Systematized Nomenclature of Medicine.* Skokie, IL: College of American Pathologists, 1977.
7. Fritz, A., C. Percy, A. Jack, K. Shanmugaratnum, L. Sobin, D. M. Parkin, S. Whelan (eds.), *International Classification of Diseases for Oncology,* 3rd ed. Geneva: World Health Organization, 2000.
8. Greene F.L., Updates to Staging System Reflect Advances in Imaging, Understanding. *Journal of the National Cancer Institute* 2002; 22: 1664-1666.
9. *Manual for Staging of Cancer,* 1978 (2nd printing). Chicago: American Joint Committee for Cancer Staging and End Results Reporting, 1978.
10. *Manual for Staging of Cancer,* 2nd ed. Philadelphia: J.B. Lippincott, 1983.
11. *Manual for Staging of Cancer,* 3rd ed. Philadelphia: J.B. Lippincott, 1988.
12. Beahrs, O.H., D.E. Henson, R.V.P. Hutter, B.J. Kennedy (eds.), *Manual for Staging of Cancer,* 4th ed. Philadelphia: J.B. Lippincott Company, 1992.
13. Fleming, I.D., J.S. Cooper, D.E. Henson, R.V.P. Hutter, B.J. Kennedy, G.P. Murphy, B. O'Sullivan, S.H. Sobin, J.W. Yarbro (eds.), *AJCC Cancer Staging Manual,* 5th ed. New York: Lippincott-Raven, 1997.
14. Greene, F. L., D. L. Page, I. D. Fleming, A. G. Fritz, C. M. Balch, D. G. Haller, M. Morrow (eds.), *AJCC Cancer Staging Manual,* 6th ed. New York: Springer, 2002.
15. *Facility Oncology Registry Data Standards,* Chicago, IL: American College of Surgeons, 2002.
16. *Comparative Staging Guide for Cancer, Major Cancer Sites,* Version 1.1. Bethesda, MD: National Institutes of Health, National Cancer Institute, 1993.
17. *SEER Extent of Disease—1988, Codes and Coding Instructions,* 2nd ed. Bethesda, MD: National Institutes of Health, National Cancer Institute, 1992. NIH pub. no. 92-2313.
18. Summary Staging Guide. Bethesda, MD: National Institutes of Health, 1977 (Reprinted 2001), NIH pub no. 01-2313.
19. Young JL Jr, Roffers SD, Ries LAG, Fritz AG, Hurlbut AA (eds). SEER Summary Staging

Manual—2000: Codes and Coding Instructions, National Cancer Institute, Bethesda, MD, 2001. NIH Pub. No. 01-4969

20. *SEER Program Code Manual,* rev. ed. Bethesda, MD: National Institutes of Health, National Cancer Institute, 1992. NIH pub. no. 92-1999.

21. Gordon, Barry (ed.) *Standards for Cancer Registries, Version 5.0, vol. 1: Data Exchange Standards and Record Description.* Np: North American Association of Central Cancer Registries, 1996.

22. Menck, Herman, and Jennifer Seiffert (eds.), *Standards for Cancer Registries. vol. 2: Data Standards and Data Dictionary,* 7th edition. Np: North American Association of Central Cancer Registries, 1995.

23. Hultstrom, Dianne (ed.) *Standards for Cancer Registries. vol 2: Data Standards and Data Dictionary.* North American Association of Central Cancer Registries, 2002.

24. Seiffert, Jennifer (ed.), *Standards for Cancer Registries, vol. 3: Standards for Completeness, Quality, Analysis, and Management of Data.* Np: North American Association of Central Cancer Registries, 1994.

25. NAACCR Registry Operations Committee. *Standards for Cancer Registries. vol 3: Standards for Completeness, Quality, Analysis, and Management of Data.* North American Association of Central Cancer Registries, 2000.

26. Seiffert, Jennifer, Susan Capron, and Jim Tebbel, (eds.), *Standards for Cancer Registries, vol. 4: Standard Data Edits.* Np: North American Association of Central Cancer Registries, 1996.

BIBLIOGRAPHY

The following represent the published standards for the standard setters identified in this chapter. Most are updated frequently, and registries should obtain current versions as they are published. Some of the earlier versions are also listed. The early versions are useful as historical documents and because they may still be applicable to data collected in the past. In addition to printed material, many of these organizations maintain Internet accessible services through which the publications can be ordered or downloaded.

American Cancer Society
Manual of Tumor Nomenclature and Coding. New York: American Cancer Society; 1951.

American Joint Committee on Cancer
Greene FL, Page DL, Fleming ID, et al, eds. *AJCC Cancer Staging Manual,* 6th ed.New York: Springer; 2002. See also editions 1 through 5.

College of American Pathologists
Cote RA editor. *Systematized Nomenclature of Medicine.* Skokie, Ill: College of American Pathologists; 1977.

College of American Pathologists. *Systemized Nomenclature of Human and Veterinary Medicine.* Northfield, Ill: SNOMED International; 1993.

Commission on Cancer of the American College of Surgeons
Data Acquisition Manual, rev. ed. Chicago, Ill: American College of Surgeons Commission on Cancer; 1994.

Fundamental Tumor Registry Operations Manual. Chicago, Ill: American College of Surgeons Commission on Cancer; 1992.

Cancer Program Standards, 2004. Chicago, Ill: American College of Surgeons; 2003.

Standards of the Commission on Cancer, vol. 11: Registry Operations and Data Standards. Chicago, Ill: American College of Surgeons; 1996.

Supplement to Standards of the Commission on Cancer, vol. 11: Registry Operations and Data Standards. Chicago, Ill: American College of Surgeons; 1998.

Facility Oncology Registry Data Standards, Chicago, Ill: American College of Surgeons; 2002.

Winchester DP, Brennan MF, Dodd GD, et al, eds. *Clinical Cancer Case: Selected Cases from the Tumor Board.* Philadelphia, Pa: Lippincott-Raven Publishers; 1995.

North American Association of Central Cancer Registries
Gordon B editor. *Standards for Cancer Registries, Version 5.0, vol. 1: Data Exchange Standards and Record Description.* Np: North American Association of Central Cancer Registries, 1996.

Menck H, Seiffert J, eds. *Standards for Cancer Registries. vol. 2: Data Standards and Data Dictionary,* 7th edition. Np: North American Association of Central Cancer Registries; 1995.

Hultstrom D, ed. *Standards for Cancer Registries. vol 2: Data Standards and Data Dictionary.* North American Association of Central Cancer Registries; 2002.

Seiffert J ed. *Standards for Cancer Registries, vol. 3: Standards for Completeness, Quality, Analysis, and Management of Data.* Np: North American Association of Central Cancer Registries, 1994.

NAACCR Registry Operations Committee. *Standards for Cancer Registries. vol 3: Standards for Completeness, Quality, Analysis, and Management of Data.* North American Association of Central Cancer Registries; 2000.

Seiffert J, Capron S, Tebbel J, eds. *Standards for Cancer Registries, vol. 4: Standard Data Edits.* Np: North American Association of Central Cancer Registries; 1996.

Surveillance, Epidemiology, and End Results Program

Comparative Staging Guide for Cancer, Major Cancer Sites, Version 1.1. Bethesda, Md: National Institutes of Health, National Cancer Institute; 1993.

SEER Extent of Disease—1988, Codes and Coding Instructions, 2nd ed. Bethesda, Md: National Institutes of Health, National Cancer Institute; 1992. NIH pub. no. 92-2313.

Summary Staging Guide. Bethesda, Md: National Institutes of Health; 1977 (Reprinted 2001). NIH pub no. 01-2313.

Young JL Jr, Roffers SD, Ries LAG, Fritz AG, Hurlbut AA, eds. *SEER Summary Staging Manual—2000: Codes and Coding Instructions.* Bethesda, Md: National Cancer Institute; 2001. NIH Pub. No. 01-4969

SEER *Program Code Manual,* rev. ed. Bethesda, Md: National Institutes of Health, National Cancer Institute; 1992. NIH pub. no. 92-1999.

World Health Organization

Fritz A, Percy C, Jack A et al, eds. *International Classification of Diseases for Oncology,* 3rd ed. Geneva, Switzerland: World Health organization; 2000.

International Statistical Classification of Diseases and Related Health Problems, 10th revision, vol. 1: Tabular List. Geneva, Switzerland: World Health Organization, 1992.

International Statistical Classification of Diseases and Related Health Problems, 10th revision, vol. 2: Instruction Manual. Geneva, Switzerland: World Health Organization; 1993.

International Statistical Classification of Diseases and Related Health Problems, 10th revision, diskette version. Geneva, Switzerland: World Health Organization; 1994.

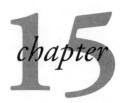

CODING OF NEOPLASMS

April Fritz
BA, RHIT, CTR

According to the dictionary, a code is a set of symbols arranged systematically for easy reference. The purpose of coding is to express a concept symbolically, allowing similar concepts to be grouped for the purposes of information retrieval. For example, take the concept of the color *red*. Red has many different names: rose, carmine, ruby, sanguine, cardinal, cherry, salmon, and vermillion—just to name a few. A data analyst who wanted to review cases that involved the concept of *red* would have to remember all the different synonyms in order to gather every case of *red*. However, if the original data collector had a system in which all of the different synonyms of red had the same code and such a code was assigned at the time of data collection, the data analyst could retrieve all cases that represented *red* in a straightforward manner by looking for a single code.

The act of coding is the process used to transpose text to codes. Most coding begins with a nomenclature, or a system of names. In the previous example, that nomenclature would have classified the major color groups for red, blue, yellow, and so forth, under which would be the lists of synonyms that represented the various color concepts. For cancer registries, the codes and disease nomenclature identify where the cancer started (topography) and what the tumor is (morphology).

HISTORY OF CODING NEOPLASMS

As early as 400 B.C., the Egyptians used codes. The Greeks, following Hippocrates' teachings, were the first to attempt to classify diseases into groups (the four humors).[1] In the seventeenth century, John Graunt of London recognized the need for classifying diseases,[2] and the first medical statistician, William Farr of the Registrar General's Office in England, labored for better, more uniform classification of diseases.[3]

In 1891, the International Statistical Institute formed a committee headed by Dr. Jacques Bertillon to prepare a classification for causes of death, and the first edition of the *International List of Causes of Death* was published in 1900.[4] Details of this early history and the beginning of the publication of the list are well documented in the introduction of the *International Classification of Diseases,* 1955 revision, published by the World Health Organization (WHO) in 1957.[5]

In the United States, a committee of the American Medical Association was convened to develop a nomenclature of diseases. This nomenclature was based on the one published by the Royal College of Physicians in 1869. In 1903, *The Bellevue Hospital Nomenclature of Diseases* was published. Between 1903 and 1933, eight other nomenclatures and coding books were developed in the United States. In 1933 came the first edition of the *Standard Nomenclature of Diseases,* and in 1942, the first edition of the *Standard Nomenclature of Operations* was published. These two nomenclatures became the *Standard Nomenclature of Diseases and Operations* (SNODO), 4th edition, published by the American Medical Association in 1952.[6]

SNODO's code structure consisted of a code for the topography (site), a hyphen, and a code for the etiology (cause). Although no one knew the etiology of cancer, the series of codes beginning with 8 was used for new growths, and various histologic types were filled in. The origin of the morphology section code numbers beginning with 8 developed from this.

By itself, coding did not provide access to data; it was coupled with indexing—a manual system of recording cases with similar codes in the same section of the index. For example, an index card was prepared for every code of major body sites. Medical records having the same site codes were indexed on the same card. The disease or procedure code was written in the column labeled with the first digit of the code. When beginning a study for a physician, one had to identify the appropriate code and go through all of the site cards for that code looking for entries for the specific disease or procedure. This was time-consuming, but it was the only system available at the time. The same coding and indexing system was used for cancer registries. The fifth edition of SNODO was the last edition ever published or used.[7]

After World War II, when the World Health Organization (WHO) was formed to deal with the health problems of the United Nations, it was given the responsibility for revising the *International Classification of Diseases* (ICD). Chapter 2 of ICD has always been assigned to neoplasms, including malignant neoplasms (cancers), benign neoplasms, in situ lesions, uncertain as to whether benign or malignant, and so forth.

Neoplasms are usually described first by their topographic site, the place in the body where the cancer originated (lung, breast, bone marrow, colon, etc.); next by their behavior, whether they are malignant, benign, insitu, or otherwise classifiable; and then by the cell type, also called the morphologic or histologic type, as determined by a pathologist using a microscope. The neoplasm chapter of the ICD is principally a topographic code that takes the behavior into account. Very few specific morphologic types are included: melanomas, lymphomas, leukemias, and multiple myeloma. Pathologists objected to this because they wanted to be able to identify, for example, whether a lung tumor was an adenocarcinoma, squamous cell carcinoma, small cell carcinoma, or some other histologic type. These tumors acted just as differently within the lung as various types of cancers acted in different parts of the body.

In 1951, the American Cancer Society assigned a committee principally composed of pathologists and statisticians to develop the *Manual of Tumor Nomenclature and Coding*.[8] This code book contained only a three-digit code: two digits for morphology and the third digit, preceded by a period, for the behavior. Tumor registries assigned as a topography code whatever was used in their hospital, either SNODO or ICD.

In the early 1960s, hospitals in the United States began using the *International Classification of Diseases* (ICD) for coding morbidity and mortality because it was easier to use and had more current terms; however, it was still not an ideal system. When the *International Classification of Diseases, 1965 revision* (ICD-8), was published,[9] users in the United States found that it did not meet the coding needs of hospital health records departments. Subsequently, two adaptations of ICD-8 were published in the United States. One was *International Classification of Diseases, Adapted for Use in the United States* (1967) (ICDA-8).[10] The other adaptation was developed and published by the Commission on Professional and Hospital Activities (CPHA) in Ann Arbor, Michigan. This book, *Hospital Adaption of International Classification of Diseases* (H-ICDA)[11] was used for coding by those hospitals who were members of CPHA, as well as others who preferred H-ICDA over ICD-8.

The College of American Pathologists decided in the early 1960s to develop a code for all pathologic terms, not just neoplasms. The culmination of their efforts was the *Systematized Nomenclature of Pathology* (SNOP), published in 1965.[12] It had been agreed upon ahead of time that when the book was finished, cancer data experts could use the neoplasm sections (sections 8 and 9) from this book and publish their own code book just for neoplasms. So in

1968, the American Cancer Society published the *Manual of Tumor Nomenclature and Coding*, 1968 edition (MOTNAC).[13] It consisted of a topography section based on the neoplasms chapter of ICDA-8 and a morphology section adapted from sections 8 and 9 of SNOP.

In the early 1970s, the World Health Organization started preparing for the ninth revision of ICD. During this revision, certain physicians expressed a desire to have a cancer supplement that included morphology. They looked around for a suitable morphology code and finally selected MOTNAC. After extensive field testing, a practice WHO had never tried before, the *International Classification of Diseases for Oncology* (ICD-O) was published in late 1976.[14] Naturally, the topography of ICD-O was based on the neoplasms chapter of ICD-9.

The ICD-O is a ten-digit code consisting of four digits for topography and four for morphology, followed by a slash (/) and a single digit behavior code indicating whether the tumor is malignant, benign, in situ, or otherwise classified (see Table 15-1). Most cancer registries collect only those tumors that are malignant (/3) or in situ (/2). Pathologists may use /6 (malignant, metastatic) or /9 (malignant, uncertain whether primary or metastatic). The registry, however, reports these neoplasms as C80.9, "unknown primary site," unless a primary has been determined through other diagnostic means. The sixth or last digit of the morphology code is for grading or differentiation and describes how much or how little a tumor resembles the normal tissue from which it arose. Acceptable sixth digits for solid tumors are 1, 2, 3, 4 and 9.

The ninth revision of the *International Classification of Diseases* (ICD-9) was published in 1977, with the morphology code numbers (M-codes) included in the alphabetic index and listed numerically in the back of volume 1, pages 667-90.[15]

ICD-9 encompasses two volumes: the tabular list (codes in sequential order) and the alphabetic index (alphabetic listing of terms and corresponding codes). ICD-9 was used by vital statistics offices for coding death certificates through 1998. However, it was not adequate for the multiplicity of other uses for coded data, such as healthcare review, reimbursement, and scientific studies. A clinical modification for the United States was published, the *International Classification of Diseases, 9th revision,*

Table 15-1
Example of ICD-O ten-digit code consisting of four digits for topography and four digits for morphology, followed by a slash (/) and a single digit behavior code indicating whether the tumor is malignant, benign, in situ, or otherwise classified.

Topography—Structure of Topography Code

C____ ____ . ____
(site)   (subsite)

Example: **C50.4**
Breast, upper-outer quadrant of breast

Morphology—Structure of a Morphology Code

M ____ ____ ____ ____ / ____ ____
(histology)   (behavior—grade)

Example: **M-8140 / 31   Well-differentiated adenocarcinoma**

M-8140	3	1
Tumor/cell type	Behavior	Differentiation

Adopted from Table 7. Structure of Topography Code, and Table 8. Structure of a Morphology Code. *International Classification of Diseases for Oncology,* 3rd ed., Geneva, Switzerland, World Health Organization; 2000:9.

Clinical Modification (ICD-9-CM), which added a third volume containing both a tabular list and an alphabetic index for operations and procedures.[16]

The ICD-9-CM is a numeric classification system. The tabular list is divided into 17 chapters; some are classified by condition and others by site. There are also two supplementary chapters with special classifications: V-codes (factors influencing health status and contact with health services) and E-codes (external causes of injury and poisoning).

Each chapter of the tabular list is further subdivided into sections, categories, subcategories, and subclassifications. Sections are groups of three-digit code numbers such as "Diseases of other endocrine glands" (250-259). A category within the section is one three-digit code number; for example, diabetes mellitus (250). At the four-digit level are subcategories of code numbers that further delineate the category, such as diabetes mellitus with ketoacidosis (250.1). A fifth digit is required in some categories within the tabular list. The five-digit code numbers are called subclassifications. Using the example of diabetes, the subclassification 250.10 is diabetes mellitus with ketoacidosis, adult onset,[17] as shown in Table 15-2.

The ICD-9-CM index is an alphabetic listing of diagnoses. These diagnoses are listed by main terms followed by modifiers and subterms, for example,

Diabetes, diabetic (mellitus) with ketosis, ketoacidosis 250.1[17]

To select the proper code in ICD-9-CM, the main word or term of the disease or procedure must be located in the alphabetic index. Usually only nouns are indexed. Modifiers and subterms must be reviewed carefully because they may affect the choice of the most appropriate code associated with the diagnosis. The most specific code must be selected, for example, 250.1 for diabetes with ketoacidosis, not simply 250. The code must be verified in the tabular list. Before the final code selection is made, all instructional notations, punctuation, symbols, and other coding conventions must be reviewed to determine the accuracy of the code selected.

Coding conventions used in ICD-9-CM include punctuation, symbols, typefaces, abbreviations, and other notations such as "includes" and "excludes" notes. Each of these tells the coder something about the code. These conventions must be followed to correctly code a diagnosis. Only one of the abbreviations, NOS (not otherwise specified), is used to code neoplasms in ICD-O. The tabular list of ICD-O contains no inclusions or exclusions to be reviewed that are not also printed in the index.

In ICD-9's alphabetic index under the term "neoplasm," anatomic sites are listed alphabetically. For each site, there are five columns indicating the behavior: malignant, benign, and so on. The coder selects the appropriate column based on the description in the medical record. In ICD-O, all primary cancers use the same anatomic site codes, and the behavior is indicated by adding a fifth digit to the morphology code after the slash.

Since its introduction, ICD-O has been used not only in cancer registries throughout the United States, but in the rest of the world as well. It has been translated into all the major languages of the world. The Surveillance, Epidemiology, and End Results (SEER) Program of the National Cancer Institute adopted ICD-O as its official code book for coding the site and histologic type of neoplasms,[18] and other standard setters in the United States, Canada and the rest of the world have designated ICD-O as the official reference for coding neoplasms.

In 1977, the College of American Pathologists published an extensive revision of SNOP, entitled the *Systematized Nomenclature of Medicine* (SNOMED).[19] It incorporated the neoplasm section as presented in the first edition of ICD-O. SNOMED has since been used for coding in many pathology laboratories all over the world.

Historically, there had usually been a ten-year interval between revisions of the ICD; however, the World Health Organization wanted the tenth revision to be a major one, so they extended the interval between revisions to 15 years. Oncologists were anxious to add new terminology and classifications to ICD-O, especially for lymphomas. A working party was formed by WHO to revise ICD-O. It was again decided to base the topography on the forthcoming tenth revision of ICD (ICD-10). There was a major

change in the codes, because WHO had decided it was necessary to go to an alphanumeric code in order to have sufficient room for expansion. Therefore, the topography section of ICD-O-2 contains C-codes. Many people thought this meant cancer, but it was purely coincidental. The first chapter of the *International Statistical Classification of Diseases and Related Health Problems, 10th revision,*[20] used the letters A and B for infectious and parasitic diseases, and because neoplasms were always coded in the second chapter, the next available letter of the alphabet was C.

The second edition of ICD-O was published in 1990.[21] Some "healthcare professionals" started using it immediately. Foreign countries had not used the first edition of ICD-O and were anxious to begin coding their data. The SEER Program implemented ICD-O-2 for their 1992 data after holding extensive training programs. Widespread use of ICD-O-2 by US cancer registries began in 1993.

The primary difference between ICD-O and ICD-O-2 is that the topography of ICD-O-2, which is based on ICD-10, has an alpha character C in front of the three digits, and the numeric digits range from 00.0 to 80.9. New morphologic terms were added and the lymphoma section was expanded to include terms used in the Working Formulation and some foreign classifications, such as the Kiel classification for lymphomas. The introduction and instructions at the beginning were expanded. The last few pages of the book list the new morphology code numbers, terms, and synonyms. The final page is very important because it lists the terms in the second edition that had been changed to malignant. Added to the grading or differentiation column in ICD-O-2 were codes for T- and B-cells when diagnosed for lymphomas and leukemias.

A new edition of SNOMED, now called the *Systematized Nomenclature of Human and Veterinary Medicine* (SNOMED International) was published in 1993.[22] This edition was published in four volumes by the College of American Pathologists. Volume 1 includes the morphology sections 8 and 9 of ICD-O-2. SNOMED International was the final printed version of this code scheme. Subsequent versions of the codes—SNOMED Reference Technology (RT)[23] and SNOMED Clinical Terms (CT)[24]—have been published in electronic format for use in computerized coding systems. Each new version of SNOMED has retained compatibility of the morphology sections 8 and 9 of ICD-O.

Table 15-2

Stylized Representation of Section of ICD-9-CM Tabular List

Division	Code	Meaning
Section	250-59	Diseases of other endocrine glands
Category	250	Diabetes mellitus
Subcategory	250.0	Diabetes mellitus without mention of complication
	250.1	Diabetes with ketoacidosis
Subclassification	250.10	Adult onset

The United States implemented ICD-10 for coding death certificates in 1999. However, with the availability of computers and other electronic mechanisms to assist with coding, it has become more complicated to change existing programs and hardware and to retrain coders. Studies have demonstrated that ICD-10 is not adequate to code morbidity in medical facilities, so a clinical modification of ICD-10 was necessary. The National Center for Health Statistics, which now operates under the Centers for Disease Control and Prevention (CDC), is involved in this modification, as well as the Centers for Medicare and Medicaid Services (formerly the Social Security Administration), because of their oversight of payments for hospitalization. Following comments on the initial draft, an updated draft of the clinical modification of ICD-10[25] was released in June 2003 for public viewing. As of early 2004, an implementation date has not been established for ICD-10-CM in the United States. Once the federal government has published a final notice to implement, medical facilities and other users of ICD-10-CM will have two years to comply. Final implementation is not anticipated until at least 2008.

Concurrent with the implementation of ICD-O-2 in North America, there were significant advances in the diagnosis of neoplasms, particularly the hematopoietic diseases (diseases arising in the lymphatic system and bone marrow). In particular, new cytogenetic techniques contributed considerably to the body of knowledge about lymphomas, leukemias, and other bone marrow conditions. As a result, the nomenclature for these diseases expanded and data collectors were unable to easily assign codes to the new terminology. In 1998, the World Health Organization again assembled a task force to assess whether new codes for the lymphomas and leukemias should simply be added to ICD-O-2 or whether a new edition was warranted. After receiving comments from many national registries, the decision was made to develop a new edition.

In addition to incorporating the WHO classification of hematopoietic and lymphoid neoplasms,[26] the editors of the new edition included the terminology of other WHO publications such as the *Histological Typing of Tumors*[27] series, known to pathologists as the "blue books" because of the cover color for the series' first edition. After a limited international field trial in 1999 and further refinements of the morphology codes, introduction, and index,

the third edition of the *International Classification of Disease for Oncology*[28] was published in late 2000 with implementation set by the North American Association of Central Cancer Registries (NAACCR) beginning with cases diagnosed on or after January 1, 2001.

There were no changes to the topography code structure between ICD-O-2 and ICD-O-3; ICD-O-3 continues to be based on ICD-10. However, some terms changed behavior code, affecting their reportability. Eleven terms changed from borderline (/1) to malignant (/3) and therefore reportable to all cancer registries. These include all of the refractory anemias, polycythemia vera, and several other hematopoietic diseases. Six neoplasms previously coded as malignant, the various cystadenomas of the ovary and pilocytic astrocytoma, where changed from malignant (/3) to borderline (/1), making them not reportable as of 2001 diagnoses. However, by agreement among North American standard setters, pilocytic astrocytoma will continue to be reported as a malignancy because if its significance as a childhood tumor and the effect that excluding those cases would have on incidence rates over time. The principal impact of the third edition was the inclusion of about 780 morphology terms and synonyms, roughly two-thirds in the first part of the list (M-8000—M-9580) and one-third in the lymphomas and leukemias section.

To reflect contemporary pathology practice and terminology, a number of acronyms were added to ICD-O-3 as synonyms of the terms they represent. For example, one of the primary morphology term for breast cancer is "ductal carcinoma in situ," but it is commonly reported as "DCIS." Both terms are coded to M-8500/2 in ICD-O-3. On the other hand, ICD-O serves as a reference manual for legacy data as well, so virtually all terms from older classifications have been retained. Terms that are truly archaic, such as *lymphosarcoma*, are marked with [obs] as an indication that use of the term is discouraged because better, more definitive, and descriptive terms are available. Another example in ICD-O-3 is the term *hepatoma*, which is marked with [obs] because the preferred terminology is now hepatocellular carcinoma, of which there are four distinct and separately coded subtypes.[29]

Another issue that arose from the inclusion of certain new codes was the correct coding of tumors that contain multiple histologic types, in particular the new combination codes 8523/3, infiltrating duct mixed with other types of carcinoma, and 8524/3, infiltrating lobular mixed with other types of carcinoma. These two codes are intended to describe a single lesion containing multiple histologic types. They should not be used to code multiple independent tumors of differing histologic types in the same primary site. This same principal applies to other combination codes in ICD-O-2 and ICD-O-3. The evolution of coding over three editions of ICD-O requires a solid understanding of the implications of adding new codes or combining old codes and how those changes and data conversions affect incidence reporting in population-based registries.

A number of side issues related to the implementation of ICD-O-3 were identified during the development process, all of which are related to the increasing reliance of cancer registries on electronic databases. These included timely revision of cancer registry software to accommodate ICD-O-3 codes, development of reference tables incorporating the new codes, storage of ICD-O-3 codes in cancer registry databases, and converting ICD-O-2 codes to ICD-O-3. Because of NAACCR's efforts to standardize data collection and data transfer, a task force was formed for the first time to prepare guidelines for implementing ICD-O-3. Conversion tables for ICD-O-2 to ICD-O-3 and vice versa, as well as conversion between ICD-O-3 and ICD-9 were developed, along with a new primary site/histology table listing the histology codes most commonly associated with each primary site. The guidelines published by the task force[30] included recommendations for implementation and storage of the codes, and recommendations for collecting or no longer collecting cases with codes that changed behavior, as well as alternatives for coding and storing cases when a registry's software installation might be delayed. The work of this task force set the standard for coordinated implementation of later changes in the cancer registry data set, such as Collaborative Staging and the 2003 treatment codes. As of the publication of this text, there are no plans to develop a fourth edition of ICD-O.

Figure 15-1, adapted from the introduction of the *International Classification of Diseases for Oncology,* Third edition (ICDO-3), shows all the code books used for neoplasms for the past seven decades.

Table 15-3 shows how the code structure for neoplasms has evolved from MOTNAC (1951) to ICD-O-3.

BASICS OF CODING NEOPLASMS

Just as the first edition of ICD-O had established, ICD-O-3 has a ten-digit code comprising a code number for topography (site), a code number for morphology (tumor type), a code for behavior, and a code for grade or differentiation. In ICD-O-3, the alphabetic index is used for coding both topography and morphology (the same as in ICD-O). The topographic terms begin with "C" and the morphologic terms with "M-," although recording these two characters and the punctuation (decimal point or slash separators) in a database is optional. Whereas in ICD-9 it is necessary to verify in the tabular list all code numbers found in the index in order to review any exclusions or other coding instructions, it is not necessary to do so in ICD-O because there are no special instructions in the numeric section that would alter the code number selected in the alphabetic section.

The coding guidelines for topography and morphology and the instructions for use at the beginning of ICD-O-3 are very detailed and should be reviewed carefully before coding is attempted. Refer to ICD-O-3 for the specific rules of topography and morphology coding. These parts of the book are often overlooked by users, especially those with computerized registries, because software vendors include both code numbers and terms in their systems. Most software programs allow an operator to key a number, after which the term appears on the screen, or to enter the term, after which the corresponding number appears. The simplicity of the computerized look-up system can result in coding errors. The coding rules at the beginning of ICD-O must be studied before beginning to code.

A related issue that bears comment is the importance of the "matrix principle." ICD-O is very flexible for coding the topography, morphology, and behavior of a particular neoplasm. When a data collector is dependent on a computerized system for assigning the code, some of that flexibility is lost. Therefore, it is important to remember that the purpose of the code is to describe what the pathologist

Figure 15-1
Historical Lineage of ICD-O

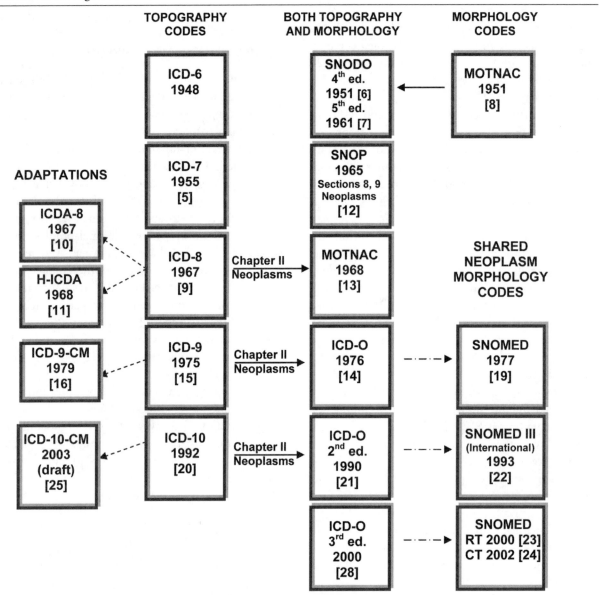

Note: Dates shown are publication dates, not implementation dates.

Adapted from Table 1. Coding of Neoplasms 1946-2000: Historical Lineage of ICD-O. *International Classification of Diseases for Oncology*, 3rd ed. Geneva, Switzerland: World Health Organization; 2000:2. Numbers in [brackets] refer to the publications cited in the reference section at the end of this chapter.

says about the tumor, including a different behavior if so stated by the pathologist. The "matrix principle" allows the data collector to change the behavior code from what is printed in the book or included in a reference table in a computerized cancer registry system in order to truly represent in coded form what the pathologist described.

SUMMARY

The quality of registry data depends on the care registrars take in reviewing available information and selecting the most accurate codes to represent the data they collect. To accurately code the primary site, histologic type, behavior, and grade or differentiation, a registrar must know every section in the cod-

Table 15-3
Evolution of Code Structure from MOTNAC and SNODO to ICD-O-3.

Diagnosis: poorly-differentiated infiltrating duct carcinoma of upper outer quadrant of right breast.

Pub. Year	Reference	Code	Meaning
1951	MOTNAC[8]	00.6	Infiltrating duct carcinoma
1961	SNDO 5th ed.[7]	190-8191F	Carcinoma of breast, infiltrating, differentiated
1965	SNOP[12]	0402 8503	Breast, right, infiltrating duct carcinoma
1967	ICD, 1965 ed.[9]	174	Malignant neoplasm of breast
1967	ICD-A[10]	174	Malignant neoplasm of breast
1968	H-ICDA[11]	174.0	Primary malignant neoplasm of breast
1968	MOTNAC 1968[12]	174.9 8503	Breast [NOS], duct carcinoma
1976	ICD-O[14]	174.4 M-8500/33	Breast, upper outer quadrant, infiltrating duct carcinoma, poorly differentiated
1978	ICD-9-CM[16]	174.4 M-8500/3*	Malignant neoplasm of breast, upper outer quadrant; *optional morphology code: infiltrating duct carcinoma
1976	SNOMED[19]	T-04004 M-8500/33	Breast, upper outer quadrant, NOS, infiltrating duct carcinoma, poorly differentiated
1992	ICD-10[20]	C50.4 M-8500/3*	Malignant neoplasm of breast, upper outer quadrant; *optional morphology code: infiltrating duct carcinoma
1990	ICD-O-2[21]	C50.4 M-8500/33	Breast, upper outer quadrant, infiltrating duct carcinoma, poorly differentiated
1993	SNOMED Int.[22]	T-04004 M-8500/3 G-F503*	Upper outer quadrant of breast [NOS], infiltrating duct carcinoma, *optional grade code: poorly-differentiated
1996	SNOMED RT[23]	T-04024 M-85003 G-F503*	Upper outer quadrant of right breast (body structure), infiltrating duct carcinoma (morphologic abnormality), *optional grade code: poorly-differentiated (grade)
2001	ICD-O-3[28]	C50.4 M-8500/33	Breast, upper outer quadrant, infiltrating duct carcinoma, poorly differentiated
2002	SNOMED CT[24]	T-04024 M-85003 F-02901*	Upper outer quadrant of right breast (body structure), infiltrating duct carcinoma (morphologic abnormality), *optional grade code: poorly-differentiated histological grade finding (finding)
2002	ICD-10-CM[25]	C50.41 M-8500/3*	Malignant neoplasm of right [female] breast, upper outer quadrant; *optional morphology code: infiltrating duct carcinoma

ing book. This is especially important for coding rules and conventions as detailed in the instructions for use at the beginning of ICD-O-3. Most studies conducted by researchers, physicians, and others require, at a minimum, one of these elements as a parameter for case selection. If the codes are incorrect, the results of the studies will be flawed and the credibility of the registry damaged. Accuracy must be the operational word for coding site and histology.

STUDY QUESTIONS

1. Name the current coding books used in the United States for (a) coding mortality and (b) coding neoplasms for cancer registries.
2. Describe at least two differences between ICD and ICD-O.
3. The complete code for a neoplasm contains ten characters. What are the principal parts of the code, and what do they represent?
4. What is the most important concern in coding neoplasms?
5. Name three organizations that have helped to develop the topography and morphology codes used to code neoplasms.

REFERENCES

1. Huffman EK. The standard nomenclature of diseases and operation. In: *Manual for Medical Record Librarians.* Berwyn, Il: Physician's Record Company; 1960: 207-44.
2. Greenwood M. *Medical Statistics from Graunt to Farr.* New York: Cambridge University Press; 1948: 28.
3. Registrar General of England and Wales. *Sixteenth Annual Report,* 1856; London: 1856; 75.
4. Bertillon J. Classification of the Causes of Death [abstract]. *Transactions of the 15th International Congress of Hygiene.* Demog. Washington, DC: 1912; 52-55.
5. World Health Organization. *Manual of the International Statistical Classification of Diseases, Injuries and Causes of Death,* 1955 revision vols. 1 and 2. Geneva, Switzerland: World Health Organization; 1957.
6. Plunkett RJ. Hayden AD, eds. *Standard Nomenclature of Diseases and Operations,* 4th ed. Philadelphia: The Blackiston Company; American Medical Association, 1952.

7. *Standard Nomenclature of Diseases and Operations,* 5th ed. New York: McGraw-Hill; American Medical Association, 1961.
8. *Manual of Tumor Nomenclature and Coding.* Atlanta, Ga: American Cancer Society; 1951.
9. World Health Organization. *International Classification of Diseases,* 1965 revision, vols. 1 and 2. Geneva, Switzerland: World Health Organization; 1967.
10. World Health Organization. *International Classification of Diseases, Adapted for Use in the United States,* vols. 1 and 2. Washington, DC: US Department of Health, Education, and Welfare; Public Health Service; National Center for Health Statistics; 1967. PHS publication no. 1693.
11. World Health Organization. *International Classification of Diseases, Adapted,* vols. 1 and 2. Ann Arbor, Mich: Commission on Professional and Hospital Activities (CPHA); 1968.
12. *Systematized Nomenclature of Pathology,* 1st ed. Skokie, Il: College of American Pathologists; 1965.
13. *Manual of Tumor Nomenclature and Coding,* 1968 ed. Atlanta, Ga: American Cancer Society; 1968.
14. World Health Organization. *International Classification of Diseases for Oncology.* Geneva, Switzerland: World Health Organization; 1976.
15. World Health Organization. *International Classification of Diseases,* 1975 revision, vols. I and 2. Geneva, Switzerland: World Health Organization; 1977.
16. *International Classification of Diseases, 9th revision: Clinical Modification,* vols. 1-3. Ann Arbor, Mich: Commission on Professional and Hospital Activities; 1978.
17. *International Classification of Diseases, 9th revision: Clinical Modification,* vols. 1-3. Ann Arbor, Mich: Commission on Professional and Hospital Activities; 1978: 159.
18. Young J, Percy CL, Asire AJ, eds. *Surveillance, Epidemiology, and End Results: Incidence and Mortality Data, 1973-1977.* National Cancer Institute monograph 57. Washington, DC: US Department of Health and Human Services, National Institutes of Health; 1981.
19. *Systematized Nomenclature of Medicine,* 1st ed., vols. 1 and 2. Skokie, Il: College of American Pathologists; 1976-1977.
20. World Health Organization. *International Statistical Classification of Diseases and Related Health Problems,* 10th revision, vols. 1-3. Geneva, Switzerland: World Health Organization; 1992.
21. Percy C, Van Holten V, Muir C, eds. *International Classification of Diseases for Oncology,* 2nd ed. Geneva, Switzerland: World Health Organization; 1990.

22. *The Systematized Nomenclature of Human and Veterinary Medicine,* vols. 1-4. Skokie, Il: College of American Pathologists; 1993.

23. Spackman KA, Campbell KE, Cote RA. *SNOMED RT: A Reference Terminology for Health Care.* Northfield, Il: College of American Pathologists; 2000.

24. SNOMED Clinical Terms (SNOMED CT). Northfield, Il: College of American Pathologists; 2002.

25. *International Classification of Diseases, Tenth Revision, Clinical Modification* (ICD-10-CM), US National Center for Health Statistics; June 2003. Available at: http://www.cdc.gov/nchs/about/otheract/icd9/icd10 cm.htm. Accessed January 29, 2004.

26. Jaffee ES, Harris NL, Stein H, Vardiman JW, eds. *World Health Organization Classification of Tumors. Pathology and Genetics of Tumors of Hematopoietic and Lymphoid Tissues.* Lyons, France: IARC Press; 2001.

27. World Health Organization. *International Histological Typing of Tumours,* 2nd ed. Geneva, Switzerland: World Health Organization; 1981-2000.

28. Fritz AG, Percy C, et al, eds. *International Classification of Diseases for Oncology,* 3rd ed. Geneva, Switzerland: World Health Organization; 2000.

29. Fritz A, Percy C. Introducing ICD-O-3: impact of the new edition. *Journal of Registry Management.* November 2000; 27(4):125-1320.

30. ICD-O-3 Implementation Guidelines. Springfield, IL: North American Association of Central Cancer Registries, November 27, 2000. Available at: http://www.facs.org/dept/cancer/coc/naaccr.html.

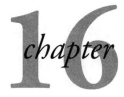

chapter 16

EXTENT OF DISEASE AND CANCER STAGING

Dianne Hultstrom
BS, RHIT, CTR

INTRODUCTION

The concept of describing disease by stage or extent of disease was introduced in 1929 by the League of Nations' World Health Organization. The first primary site so described was cancer of the cervix. Staging is a common language developed by medical professionals to communicate information about a disease to others.[1] The disease can be any acute or chronic disease such as cancer, diabetes, acquired immunodeficiency syndrome (AIDS), cardiovascular disease, or rheumatoid arthritis.

Staging for cancer has evolved over many years. Many groups have developed different staging systems. Some cover all cancer sites. Others are limited to particular ages, histologies, sites, study groups, or medical specialties. This chapter briefly discusses common staging schemes and classifications. The three most common staging systems used in hospital and central registries are reviewed in detail.

Staging is a shorthand method for describing disease. A coded format, such as a numerical system with increasing values meaning more involvement or severity, allows electronic analysis of cases with similar characteristics.

A short definition for staging is the grouping of cases into broad categories based on extent of disease. Extent of disease is a detailed description of how far the tumor has spread from the organ or site of origin (the primary site). Extent of disease is an anatomic categorization using descriptors to group individual cases in relation to the human body. Classification is the process of grouping cases based on specific criteria. Classification is an orderly arrangement showing relationships among groups.

Staging is coded shorthand or a notation describing disease in more general terms. By staging, characteristics about a case (precise extent of disease information) can be grouped into categories. Thus staging translates extent of disease classification about individual cancers into groups that can be studied or evaluated for prognostic significance.[1]

Elements to be considered in any staging system are the primary tumor site, tumor size, multiplicity (number of tumors), depth of invasion and extension to regional or distant tissues, involvement of regional lymph nodes, and distant metastases.

PURPOSES OF STAGING

There are several reasons for staging cancer cases. It is important for the medical practitioner to ade-

quately assess the extent of cancer in order to treat the disease in the most appropriate manner. Understanding the extent of disease assists the physician in determining the most appropriate treatment to cure the disease, decrease the tumor burden, or relieve symptoms.

Staging is also used to indicate prognosis. Data from historical sources can provide an estimate of the expected survival rate for a particular cancer with a corresponding extent of disease.[1] Histology, grade of the tumor, age, sex, race, and the efficacy of therapy play a part in determining the patient's prognosis and quality of survival.

Staging provides a means of comparing local institutional experience with national data. It can be used to compare treatment results based on common criteria for extent of disease. Staging expedites the exchange of data and assists in the continuing research on cancer. The health information record is the primary source of documentation for staging information.

STAGING SOURCES

Many sources in the health information record must be examined to determine the extent of disease. These sources are part of the diagnostic workup for the disease. These tests may be done on an outpatient basis or in a physician's office.

Physical Exam

For most cancers, the report of the physical examination should include the location of a tumor, including site and subsite, direct extension of the tumor to other organs or structures, and palpability and mobility of accessible lymph nodes. The probability of distant site involvement, such as organomegaly, pleural effusion, ascites, or neurological findings should be stated. In a breast cancer case, for example, the physical examination should describe the exact location of the tumor mass, clinical size of the tumor, and the condition of the skin surrounding the tumor, including changes in skin color and texture and attachment or fixation of the mass. The exam should include the entire axilla and regional nodal areas including the supraclavicular nodes.

Tumors of the head and neck area are evaluated with a general exam of the face and neck. The eyes, skin, ears, and nasal cavity should be examined in addition to mucosal surfaces of the nasopharynx, oral cavity, oropharynx, hypopharynx, and larynx. Digital and bimanual palpation of the oral cavity, oropharynx, and neck should be included in the physical exam.

Some organ sites are not easily examined clinically. A patient suspected of having a gastrointestinal tumor should have external palpation of the liver and abdomen. Females should have both a digital rectal exam and a pelvic exam. Males should have a digital rectal exam. Suspected lung cancer patients should have an assessment of cervical and supraclavicular nodal areas.

In all cases, other than lymphomas, nodes must be described by a clinician as "involved" in order to be considered to contain cancer. For example, if it is stated that nodes are enlarged, they are not considered to contain cancer until there is cytologic or pathologic confirmation. If there is matting or fixation, the medical practitioner may say that the nodes are involved with cancer.

Radiologic Procedures

X-rays, scans, and endoscopic procedures are useful for staging purposes. Radiologic reports should define the location of the cancer, the size of the tumor, involvement of adjacent structures, or existence of distant disease. They can help determine the resectability of the tumor. All radiologic reports should be reviewed to determine the extent of disease. According to the Commission on Cancer (CoC) of the American College of Surgeons, the following terms are to be interpreted as evidence of tumor involvement: *adherent, apparent, compatible with, consistent with, encroaching upon, fixation/fixed, induration, into, onto, out onto, probable, suspect, suspicious, and to.*[2] The following terms are to be interpreted as no tumor involvement: *approaching, equivocal, possible, questionable, suggests, and very close to.*[2]

X-Rays

The most common x-ray is the chest film, which is used for a variety of purposes. The posteroanterior and lateral chest x-rays are simple methods of detecting lung cancers or lesions metastatic to the lung from other primary cancer sites. The x-ray can show the tumor size, location, obstruction, pleural effusion, or invasion of adjacent structures such as the chest wall or mediastinum.

Mammography is an x-ray technique used to diagnose abnormalities in the breast. Usually, two views are taken of each breast, and the radiographs are examined for lesions or microcalcifications. The mammogram is useful in localizing suspicious non-palpable lesions. The area of concern is visualized while the breast is in the mammography unit. The radiologist injects dye or inserts a special hookwire needle into the suspicious area. The surgeon is then able to excise the abnormal area.

The most common x-ray used for the diagnosis of colon cancer is the barium enema. The large colon is filled with a barium solution and multiple x-ray films are taken. Polyps, as well as constricted and obstructed areas, can be seen. The upper GI series is useful in diagnosing lesions of the pharynx, esophagus, stomach, and small intestine.

One common radiologic exam used in the study of the urinary tract is the KUB, a frontal film of the abdomen used to examine the kidneys, ureters, and bladder. There are several other urinary tract x-ray exams that use a contrast medium (a radiopaque substance to delineate and define the contour of the structures). The intravenous pyelogram (IVP) follows the injection of the contrast media into a vein and displays the path of the media through the kidneys, ureters, and bladder. A retrograde urogram is carried out by inserting a cystoscope into the ureteral meatus, inserting a catheter through the cystoscope, and adding a contrast solution to study the renal pelvis and ureters. The location and size of tumors of the urinary tract can often be defined through these x-ray studies.

An angiogram is an x-ray study of the vascular system that is used to diagnose some cancers. A cerebral angiogram helps define the blood supply to brain lesions. Lymphangiograms are useful in the study of the vessels of the lymphatic system. They were widely used as a staging workup for lymphomas before the widespread availability of Computerized Tomography (CT) and Magnetic Resonance Imaging (MRI).

Scans

CT scanning is used for the examination of many parts of the body. The scan's images show cross-sectional "slices" of the body that are each a millimeter thick. A composite image is created by the computer and photocopied. The CT scan gives an accurate picture of the extent of disease and helps identify tumors at an early stage. CT scans are performed both with and without contrast media. CT scans can be taken of the head, chest, abdomen, pelvis, or the whole body. When a case is staged, the entire report should be reviewed for correct interpretation of the areas that are involved or not involved with tumor. Enlarged lymph nodes may also be seen on the CT scans.

Diagnostic nuclear medicine examinations or scans are used to identify abnormalities in the brain, salivary glands, thyroid, heart, lung, kidney, liver, spleen, and bone. The patient is given a radioisotope that emits gamma rays and permits the radiologist to see abnormal structures or functions. Bone scans can show metastatic lytic (destructive) lesions or blastic (overgrowth of bone) lesions of bone. For example, breast and prostate cancers are known to metastasize to the bone. Therefore, a bone scan may confirm or rule out the distant spread of disease. Liver and spleen scans can show the presence and size of a tumor. Brain scans can indicate the location or size of a tumor and associated vascular structures.

Endoscopy

An endoscopic exam involves using an instrument to examine internal passages or the inside of hollow organs or viscera. This can be effective in the nasopharynx, pharynx, larynx, esophagus, stomach, large bowel, bladder, and parts of the lungs. The common endoscopic procedures used in cancer diagnosis are listed in Table 16-1.[3]

A bronchoscopy is the examination of bronchi in the lungs. The scope can be inserted through the oral or nasal cavity. The pharynx, larynx, and trachea can be seen as the bronchoscope goes through to the bronchi. Using the flexible bronchoscope, the interior segmental and subsegmental bronchi can be visualized. The endoscopist looks for irregular bronchial folds, mucosal thickening, stenosis, friable tissue, and many other abnormalities such as a tumor mass. Normally, biopsies or bronchial washings are obtained during a bronchoscopic exam.

A proctoscopy is often done using a rigid scope. A sigmoidoscope is more flexible and can be used to observe the colon into the descending colon at greater than 30 cm. In the past, rigid sigmoidoscopes were often used, but they have been replaced with flexible sigmoidoscopes. Flexible scopes allow greater visualization of the sigmoid colon. A fiberoptic colonoscope is a flexible instrument that examines the colon to the cecum. Often, the physician will

Table 16-1
Common Endoscopic Examinations

Examination	Site Examined
bronchoscopy	bronchi
colonoscopy	colon and rectum
cystoscopy	urinary bladder
esophagoscopy	esophagus
gastroscopy	stomach
laryngoscopy	larynx
nasopharyngoscopy	nasopharynx, pharynx
ophthalmoscopy	interior of the eye
otoscopy	internal ear
panendoscopy	urinary bladder and urethra
proctoscopy	rectum
sigmoidoscopy	colon up to sigmoid flexure

Reprinted from Surveillance, Epidemiology, and End Results (SEER) Self-Instructional Manual for Tumor Registrars, book five. National Institutes of Health, National Cancer Institute.

photograph and biopsy any abnormalities or suspicious areas seen during colonoscopy.

A cystoscope is used to examine the interior of the bladder. It is inserted through the urethra, so the urethra can also be examined. Abnormalities can be surgically removed or electrocauterized during the cystoscopic procedure.

The entire endoscopic procedure report must be read to obtain pertinent information. Endoscopic reports define certain observations, tumor location, pertinent findings, diagnosis, or the impressions of cancer. For example, colonoscopy reports should state the distance of the abnormality from the anal verge. Esophagoscopy reports should state the distance of the abnormality from the incisors to help determine the exact location of the tumor. Any biopsies or washings sent for microscopic examination should be noted. It is important to locate copies of the pathology and cytology reports to confirm the diagnosis of cancer.

Some endoscopic procedures can be accomplished through natural openings in the body. Others must be performed through incisions into the body. For example, thoracoscopy is used to examine the pleural cavity. The instrument is inserted through an intercostal space. Mediastinoscopy is performed through an incision in the neck and allows visualization of the area between the lungs. The mediastinal lymph nodes that are examined for potential involvement by metastatic cancer can determine the unresectability of a lung cancer.

Laparoscopy, performed through an incision in the abdominal wall, allows the visualization of intra-abdominal structures. Laparoscopy is useful in gastrointestinal and gynecologic malignancies to diagnose both the primary organ and metastatic involvement. Needle biopsies of the liver are often done under the direct visualization of the laparoscope. Some surgeries can be completed as laparoscopic or laparoscope-aided procedures. A culdoscopy incision is made through the posterior vaginal wall and allows visualization of the cul-de-sac.

The endoscopic retrograde cholangiopancreatogram (ERCP) allows direct visualization and contrast x-rays of the ampulla of Vater and the duodenal mucosa. ERCP is helpful in diagnosing both pancreatic and bile duct cancers.

Tumor Markers

Cytologic tumor markers are tumor-specific substances in the blood serum or other tissues that can assist in determining the presence or absence of cancer.[4] They can help determine the initial tumor burden in both the primary site and distant sites. Tumor markers can be helpful in monitoring for recurrence. Care should be taken to seek tumor marker information to assist in determining stage.

The most common tumor markers used for prognosis in breast cancer are the estrogen receptor assay (ERA) and the progesterone receptor assay (PRA). Both are steroid hormone receptors. ERA and PRA are used to estimate the potential response to endocrine, or hormone, therapy. They help in the determination of prognosis and the management of breast cancer patients. Pieces of breast cancer tissue are analyzed in the laboratory to determine the ERA and PRA. The presence of estrogen and/or progesterone receptors denotes whether the cancer is growing in the presence of either or both naturally occurring hormones.

Cancer antigen 15-3 (CA-15-3), a tumor associated glycoprotein, is found in the serum. It can be useful in monitoring the presence of metastatic breast cancer and the patient's response to chemotherapy.

Prostate-specific antigen (PSA), a proteolytic enzyme, is used as a screening mechanism for prostate cancer. It can monitor the presence of metastatic disease in patients who have undergone a radical prostatectomy. PSA is not effective for mass screenings because elevated PSAs can also be found in aging patients and in association with benign prostatic hypertrophy (BPH) and prostatitis.

One oncofetal antigen, carcinoembryonic antigen (CEA), has been used for many years to monitor colon, lung, breast, and pancreatic cancers. Rising serum levels of CEA may indicate disease recurrence many months prior to clinical manifestations.

Cancer antigen 125 (CA-125) is a glycoprotein associated with ovarian carcinoma cells. Elevated levels appear in about 75% of ovarian cancer patients and may be associated with tumor burden and recurrence. CA-125 is used to monitor patients for residual or recurrent disease.

Alphafetoprotein (AFP) is an oncofetal antigen that is useful in monitoring patients with nonseminomatous testicular cancer and certain types of ovarian cancer. Human chorionic gonadotropin (hCG) is a hormone that can be detected to assess the prognosis and to monitor treatment response in patients with germ cell tumors, breast cancer, choriocarcinoma, and testicular carcinoma.

Flow cytometry has recently become an important clinical test to determine cellular DNA ploidy (the number of sets of chromosomes in a cell) and S-phase (the percentage of cells in active DNA synthesis). In flow cytometry, cells are stained with a special dye and then analyzed in a flow cytometer by using a laser beam to measure the fluorescence of cells. The results are charted in a histogram showing the distribution of DNA in the cells.[5] Results of flow cytometry are helpful to determine prognosis, monitor treatment response, and document tumor recurrence. Tumors demonstrating an abnormal number of chromosomes, such as tetraploidy, polyploidy, or aneuploidy, are more likely to be aggressive than tumors that are diploid (have the normal two sets of chromosomes).[6] Tumors with a low S-phase have a better prognosis.

Pathologic Exams

The most common and accurate methods of diagnosing cancer include microscopic examination of either tissues or cells. Cells examined are usually obtained from fluid around the suspected site of cancer. Tissues examined are usually removed from the primary or metastatic site of a cancer.

There are many kinds of biopsies to remove tissue for a cancer diagnosis. An aspiration biopsy is obtained by using a needle to suction fluid, cells, or tissue into a syringe. A bone marrow biopsy is the removal of bone marrow from one of the body's larger hollow bones.

Excisional biopsies attempt to remove the entire tumor. Incisional biopsies remove only a portion of the tissue. Often, the biopsy specimens are quickly frozen, thinly sliced, and examined to determine the presence or absence of cancer cells (frozen sections). Permanent sections are then made, and the diagnosis from the permanent sections should take precedence over frozen section reports.

Surgical resections involve removing more tissue from the body, including margins of normal tissue and/or regional lymph nodes. The pathologist can often determine staging by examining the primary tumor, surrounding tissue, and regional nodes when there is a "total" resection of the tumor. The information from a total resection takes precedence over biopsy reports and operative notes.

Quite often, there are several tissue samples, biopsies, or surgical resections for one cancer. When staging a cancer, it is important to review all pathology reports for the clinical diagnosis, gross description of the specimen, and postoperative diagnosis.

The gross description of the specimen should include the total size of the tumor. Both the gross and microscopic descriptions should state whether the surgical margins are involved by tumor. The pathology report should contain information about the primary site and the spread of disease in surrounding tissues. It is important to note all areas, organs, or structures involved with tumor.

The pathology report contains the histologic type of cancer and the grade of the tumor (how closely the cancer cells resemble normal tissue). Grade is normally expressed as Grade I through III or as well differentiated, moderately differentiated, and poorly differentiated, respectively. Tumors can also be described as anaplastic or undifferentiated (Grade IV).

The final diagnosis of the histologic type takes precedence over preliminary reports and frozen sections. The microscopic description takes precedence over the gross description. Occasionally, pathologic specimens are sent to other centers for consultation, and the final pathology report may not be signed until all consultations have been returned.

The most important information in a pathology report includes source of the specimen, primary site, tumor size, histologic type of cancer, grade of tumor, and the extent of disease within the organ of origin and beyond. The type, size, location, number of lymph nodes removed, and number of nodes containing tumor should be noted. This information is often required for accurate staging.

Pieces or chips of tumor should not be added together to determine tumor size. If the patient has received preoperative radiation therapy, the size of the tumor should be recorded as found in radiology reports prior to radiation therapy. *Multifocal* and *multicentric* are synonymous terms. The size of the largest of the multifocal tumors should be used for staging.

Autopsy reports are a type of pathology report that contain detailed information about organs and structures of the body. They are considered the most complete pathology reports. In summary, pathology reports, or reports of tissue, contain information about biopsies, frozen sections, tissue aspiration or biopsy of bone marrow, surgical specimens, and autopsies.

Cytology reports describe the microscopic examination of cells in body fluids such as sputum, bronchial washings and brushings, pleural fluid, peritoneal fluid, spinal fluid, aspirations from bone marrow, and cervical smears. The Papanicolaou (Pap) smear, used for detection of abnormal cervical cells, is probably the most widely known cytology specimen. Cells can also be obtained by fine-needle aspiration to diagnose cancers of the liver, pancreas, breast, and lung. The most common ways of obtaining cells include brushing the lining of an organ, puncturing a cavity and removing fluid, scraping the lining, or using a swab to obtain secretions.

Thoracentesis is a puncturing of the thoracic, or chest, cavity for the removal of fluid. Paracentesis is the puncture of the abdominal cavity for removal of fluid.

There may be multiple cytology reports. It is important to note the source of the specimen, the histologic description, and pertinent findings, along with interpretations.

Surgical Reports

All surgical procedures should be noted in a written operative report, either as a separate entry or as part of a progress note. Pertinent observations from operative procedures should be noted, including the location of the tumor and any direct extension, nodal involvement, or metastatic spread. Information from the operative or procedure report supplements the information noted in the pathology report. The operative report should state whether the procedure was considered curative or palliative. If a palliative procedure is done, any residual tumor remaining may be biopsied.

Non-cancer-directed surgeries such as cystotomy, gastrotomy, laparotomy, and thoracotomy may contribute information on involvement of organs, tissues, or lymph nodes that were not resected. Bypass surgery may be performed to create a passage around a tumor, often for palliation of symptoms. Bypass surgeries such as esophagogastrostomy, gastrostomy, and urethrostomy may provide information on the extent of tumor involvement.

To summarize, cancer-directed surgery reports should describe the removal and size of the tumor. Observations of regional lymph nodes, adjacent structures, and organs should be included. The pathology report will confirm the presence or absence of tumor in resected specimens.

Progress Notes and Discharge Summaries

Progress notes summarize diagnostic findings and patient status on a daily basis. The progress notes should be read to supplement and clarify information from laboratory tests, x-rays, scans, endoscopies, procedures, and histologic reports. The final progress note or the discharge summary should summarize all diagnostic, surgical, and pathologic findings. The stage of cancer should be stated.

THE DISEASE PROCESS OF CANCER

According to the theory of cancer growth or the natural history of cancer, cancer originates in a single cell. The cell continues to divide and grow in the organ of origin, spreads to adjacent tissue or regional lymph node drainage areas, and then spreads to distant organs or structures. Cancer can spread directly from the organ of origin through the bloodstream into distant organs without involving adjacent organs and regional lymph nodes.

Many cancers go through a matured course, advancing in tumor size or involvement to regional nodal involvement and eventually to distant metastasis. Small tumors can metastasize, with the first sign of the cancer being the metastatic disease.

STAGING SYSTEMS

Requirements for Staging

The Surveillance, Epidemiology, and End Results (SEER) Program of the National Cancer Institute (NCI) collects cancer data from designated population-based cancer registries in various areas of the country. There are two staging classifications developed by SEER: extent of disease and summary stage. Extent of disease (EOD) coding is required for all SEER programs funded by the NCI through 2003.

The Commission on Cancer (CoC) of the American College of Surgeons requires that the American Joint Committee on Cancer (AJCC) staging system be completed on all applicable sites and histologies.[2](p17) The CoC requires summary staging on the sites or histologies not included in AJCC staging.

Summary Staging

Summary staging is based on the theory of cancer growth previously described in this chapter under the heading Disease Process of Cancer. The SEER Summary Staging Manual 2000 includes a staging scheme for all sites and histologies including the reportable hematopoetic diseases.[7]

Intraepithelial, noninvasive, or noninfiltrating cancer is described as in situ. In situ tumors fulfill all microscopic criteria for malignancy except invasion of the basement membrane of the organ.

A *localized* tumor is confined to the organ of origin without extension beyond the primary organ. There can be no evidence of metastasis elsewhere in the body. Descriptive terms such as *perineural invasion, lymphatic invasion,* and *blood vessel invasion,* imply local involvement when applied to tissue from the organ of origin.

Regional extension of tumor can be by direct extension to adjacent organs or structures or by spread to regional lymph nodes. When assigning this stage, it is important to establish that the cancer has spread beyond the organ of origin. Distant spread must be ruled out based on all scans, physical exams, and clinical impressions available in the health information record.

Areas of tumor in lymph node drainage areas are considered regional nodes involved with cancer. For example, in colon cancer, metastatic nodules in the pericolic or perirectal fat or in adjacent mesentery (mesocolic fat) without evidence of residual lymph node tissue are considered regional lymph node metastasis if the nodule has the form and smooth contour of a lymph node.[8] In breast cancer, "cancerous nodules in the axillary fat adjacent to the breast, without histologic evidence of residual lymph node tissue, are classified as regional lymph node metastasis."[8](p 225) Nodes in a specimen of unknown original location are recorded on the abstract as regional nodes. Most often, discontinuous or non-contiguous growth is recorded on the abstract as being positive for evidence of distant disease. Discontinuous growth that is thought to be regional disease must be handled on a site- specific basis.

If the cancer has spread to parts of the body remote from the primary tumor, it is recorded on the abstract as *distant* disease. Common metastatic sites include bone, brain, liver, lungs, and distant lymph nodes. More difficult or controversial areas include some of the following examples: malignant cells in cytologic exams of fluid from a thoracentesis or paracentesis are indicative of regional or distant disease; liver involvement may be mentioned as both "regional" and "distant" for some sites such as the pancreas, transverse colon, or hepatic flexure. If there is direct or contiguous spread of tumor into the liver, the appropriate regional stage may be used. When involvement of the liver is discontinuous or there are multiple diffuse lesions, the distant staging may be the most descriptive.

There are several common routes of tumor spread, as seen in Figure 16-1. Direct extension

Figure 16-1
Interpretation of Spread of Disease

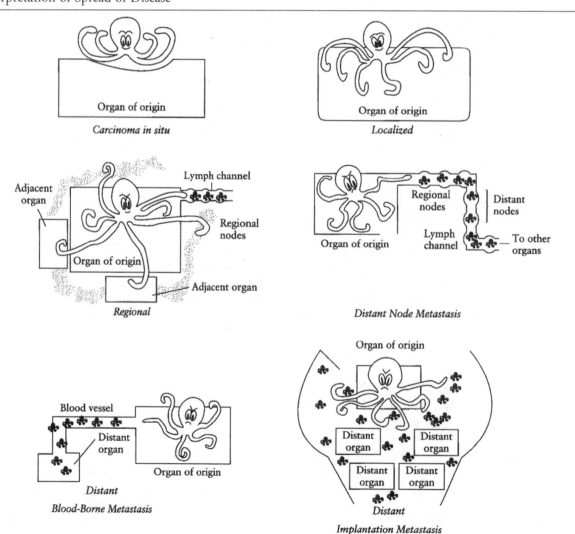

Reprinted with permission of the Surveillance, Epidemiology, and End Results Program, National Cancer Institute.

occurs when the cancer first invades the organ of origin, extends through the organ wall, invades adjacent connective tissue, and eventually extends to neighboring organs and structures. Tumor can also spread through the vascular and lymphatic systems because they transport fluids throughout the body. Malignant cells invade the lymph or blood vessels in the primary site and pass through the lymphatic or vascular system to other sites in the body. They can become entrapped in lymph nodes or enter blood vessels and implanted in adjoining organs or sites supplied by those blood vessels. Lung and liver are common sites of metastasis because blood flows directly through them.

Cancer cells can also spread by implantation that occurs when tumors perforate serosal surfaces and disseminate into body cavities. The cancer cells may implant on the lining of the thoracic or abdominal cavities. Sometimes there is insufficient information to assign a stage, such as in cases without diagnostic workups or cases in which there is ambiguous or contradictory information.

SEER Extent of Disease Coding

SEER extent of disease (EOD) coding has gone through several revisions and now includes schemes for all sites of cancer. The EOD coding scheme consists of a ten-digit code.[9] It incorporates three digits for the size and/or involvement of the primary tumor, two for the extension of the tumor, and one more as a general code for lymph node involvement. Four more digits are used after these six: two for the number of pathologically positive regional lymph nodes and two more for the number of regional lymph nodes that are pathologically examined. The code is based on clinical, operative, and pathologic diagnoses of the cancer. EOD coding incorporates all information available within two months following diagnosis. The size of tumor recorded is the size before radiation therapy. Examples of tumor extension codes for the colon are shown in Table 16-2.

As the depth of invasion increases in a site, the extension code increases. In order to ensure accuracy, it is important to review the extent of disease (EOD) codes and the coding instructions at the time of abstracting. Each site has a different scheme.

Regional lymph nodes are listed for each applicable site. Regional lymph nodes do not apply to sites such as the brain, lymphoma, and the hematopoietic system. These cancers include

Table 16-2

Extent of Disease Codes for Colon Cancer as Classified by the Surveillance, Epidemiology, and End Results (SEER) Program

Description of Tumor Extent	Codes
Noninvasive tumor	00
Polyp, noninvasive	05
Localized tumor in colon	10-30
Tumor invasive through bowel wall or adjacent structures	40-66
Tumor with distant involvement	70-85
Unknown extension	99

leukemia, multiple myeloma, and other hematopoietic and reticuloendothelial neoplasms. The lymphoma scheme reflects systemic symptoms at diagnosis. Positive and examined regional nodes are not applicable to lymphomas.

The EOD coding scheme provides a value, or code, for the lymph node field for all sites. Adjacent (regional) lymph nodes may be classified for size, laterality, number, and the distance of the nodes from the organ of origin. Lymph node involvement is also a hierarchical code.

When lymph nodes are described as fixed, matted, or mass, they are considered to be involved with tumor. Terms such as *palpable, enlarged,* or *lymphadenopathy* do not indicate involvement in solid tumors. A clinical or pathological statement must verify the presence of tumor.[9](p8) When staging lymphomas, however, any of these terms indicate involvement. Nodes that are part of a resected primary site specimen should be considered regional nodes.

The extent of disease coding scheme records the number of regional nodes found positive for cancer at pathologic examination. The number of regional lymph nodes pathologically examined must also be recorded.

The EOD coding system also includes a scheme for Kaposi's sarcoma. There is no staging system for this disease in the American Joint Committee on Cancer staging system.

American Joint Committee on Cancer (AJCC) Staging System

The concept of a classification scheme that would encompass all aspects of cancer distribution in terms of primary tumor (T), regional lymph nodes (N), and distant metastasis (M) was first introduced by the International Union Against Cancer, or Union Internationale Contre le Cancer (UICC), in 1958 for worldwide use.[10] The American Joint Committee for Cancer Staging and End Results Reporting (AJC) was established in 1959. The AJC changed its name to the American Joint Committee on Cancer (AJCC) in 1980. Staging schemes were developed to be consistent with the practice of medicine in America and used the basic premise of the TNM system: cancers of similar histology or site of origin share similar patterns of growth and extension.[8](p3) This group published a series of site-specific staging schemes from 1962 until 1974. The American Joint Committee on Cancer (AJCC) published the first edition of the Manual for Staging of Cancer in 1977. Every few years, a new edition is published with updates and new schemes for additional cancer sites.

The AJCC staging scheme is based on the evaluation of the T, N, and M components and the assignment of a stage grouping.[8](p3) The T element designates the size and invasiveness of the primary tumor. The numerical value increases with tumor size and extent of invasiveness.[8](p5) For example, a small lesion confined to the organ of origin would be coded as T1; larger tumor size or deeper extension into adjacent structures, tissues, capsules, or ligaments as T2; larger tumor size or extension beyond the organ of origin but confined to the region, T3; and a massive lesion or one that directly invades another organ or viscera, major nerves, arteries, or bone, T4.

The N component designates the presence or absence of tumor in the regional nodes. In some sites, there is an increasing numerical value based on size, fixation, or capsular invasion. In other sites, numerical value is based on multiple node involvement or number or location of the regional lymph nodes. The 6th edition of the AJCC Cancer Staging Manual has added identifiers to the breast cancer chapter to indicate the absence or presence of isolated tumor cells (ITC) or small cell clusters in regional lymph nodes detected only by immunohistochemical (IHC) or molecular methods.[8](p227) The M component identifies the presence or absence of distant metastases, including in lymph nodes that are not regional.

The stage group is assigned using the table listed in each chapter. Stage 0 reflects minimal involve-

ment, usually carcinoma in situ, whereas Stage IV indicates either greatest tumor involvement or distant metastasis.

The general rules for the AJCC staging system are defined in the AJCC *Manual for Staging of Cancer.* Further explanation can be found in the *UICC TNM Supplement 1993* and the *Workbook for Staging of Cancer,* a self-instructional book published by the National Cancer Registrars Association. Before staging a cancer, the appropriate site-specific staging system must be determined. Certain sites include only specific tumor histologic types. Some sites require microscopic confirmation to verify the histology.

The point of evaluation determines the staging basis. Clinical staging basis is assigned after the staging workup is completed, but before any definitive treatment has begun. Evaluation is based on information from the physical exam, imaging, endoscopy evaluations, and biopsy (biopsy information can only be used for T value if size is not a criteria for the T value). The clinical staging basis is defined for each site in the *AJCC Manual for Staging of Cancer.* Rules applicable to one site do not necessarily apply to another.[11]

The pathologic staging basis is assigned after the resection of the primary tumor and analysis of the surgical specimen. Most sites require the removal and examination of regional lymph nodes. Each site schema must be reviewed for the applicable rules.

Two other staging basis are less commonly used. An autopsy-staging basis is completed after the death and postmortem examination of a patient. Recurrent or retreatment staging is applied after a disease-free interval and when further treatment is planned. Biopsy confirmation is required.

Collaborative Staging

The American Joint Committee on Cancer in collaboration with the CoC, the NCI/SEER program, the CDC/NPCR program, NAACCR, and NCRA has developed a Collaborative Staging (CS) System for use beginning with cases diagnosed on or after January 1, 2004. The CS system was developed to assure the collection of a unified data set in all registries and to permit a translation or other method of conversion between the TNM staging system of the AJCC and the SEER Summary Staging System.[12]

CS resolves rules issues for timing and combines clinical and pathologic data for a best stage. CS is based upon a modified EOD system and includes all elements necessary for TNM and SS staging. Fifteen data items are used to accommodate CS; six of the data items include information on tumor size, EOD, regional lymph node involvement, and distant metastasis; six site-specific factors (formerly known as tumor markers) are also part of the CS data set. Three new fields have been added to assist in determining the staging basis for the size and extension of the primary tumor, regional lymph node and metastatic involvement. The CS System includes a computer algorithm to derive the AJCC T, AJCC N, AJCC M, AJCC Stage Group and AJCC T, AJCC N, AJCC M descriptor fields as well as Summary Stage 1977 or Summary Stage 2000.[13]

Other Common Staging Schemes

- *Colon and Rectum Staging*
  In 1929, Dukes described a staging classification for cancer of the rectum. Simpson and Mayo modified Dukes' scheme for colon cancer in 1939. Astler, Coller, and others made further modifications. The Dukes staging system and its modifications are still in use by many clinicians today. In 1988, the TNM system was modified to correspond with the Dukes system. A comparison of these staging systems is shown in Table 16-3.[14]

- *Prostate Staging*
  The American Urological Association (AUA) had its own staging scheme for prostate cancers.[15] With the publication of the AJCC *Manual for Staging of Cancer*, 4th edition, urologists are abandoning the AUA staging scheme and adopting the AJCC staging scheme. The two systems are comparable, as seen in Table 16-4.

- *Gynecologic Staging*
  The International Federation of Gynecology and Obstetrics (FIGO) adopted the first classification of clinical extent of disease for cervical cancer in 1961. The Union Internationale Contre le Cancer (UICC) has approved the use of FIGO classifications that correspond to the AJCC staging system.[8(p241)] Historically, endometrial staging was based on extent of disease; however, in 1971, the FIGO committee included the size of the uterine cavity, the involvement of the cervix, and histologic differentiation in the staging.[16] Size of the uterine cavity is no longer a factor in the assignment of the T value (FIGO/AJCC, 1992).

- *Melanoma Staging*
  Two classification schemes are often used for melanoma. Breslow's microstaging is a measurement of the depth of invasion from the basal lamina to the greatest depth of tumor penetration.[17] It is a more accurate indicator of prognosis because the thickness of the skin varies in different parts of the body.[17(pp1618-19)] Breslow's

Table 16-3

Comparison of Staging for Colon and Rectum Sites by Three Different Systems

Level of Bowel Involved	Dukes' Classification	Astler-Coller Classification	AJCC Staging
Mucosa		A	Tis
Submucosa	A	B1	T1
Muscularis propria (partial)	A	B1	T2
Muscularis propria (entire)	B	B2	T3
or colonic serosa			T4
or adjacent organs			T4
Positive nodes—any	C	C	
1-3 positive nodes			N1
4+ positive nodes			N2
Positive nodes along unnamed vascular trunk			N3
Distant metases		D	M1

Table 16-4
Comparison of Staging for Prostate Cancer by the American Urological Association (AUA) and American Joint Committee on Cancer (AJCC) Staging System, 4th ed.

Involvement	AUA	AJCC
No palpable lesion	A1	T1
Focal/less than 5%	A2	T1a
Diffuse/more than 5%		T1b
Identified by needle biopsy; elevated PSA		T1c
Confined to prostate		
Less than half a lobe		T2a
More than half a lobe		T2b
Both lobes		T2c
Small, discrete nodule	B1	
Large or multiple areas	B2	
Localized to periprostatic area		
Unilateral extracapsular	C1	T3a
Bilateral extracapsular	C1	T3b
Invades seminal vesicle(s)	C2	T3c
Metastatic disease		
Invades other structures		T4a
Fixed to pelvic wall		T4b
Pelvic lymph node metastases	D1	N1-3
Bone or distant metastases	D2	M1

Table 16-5
Clark's Level of Invasion Classification for Melanoma

Level	Level of Invasion
I	Confined to the epidermis
II	Invasion of papillary dermis
III	Invasion of papillary-reticular interface
IV	Invasion into reticular dermis
V	Invasion into subcutaneous tissue

Table 16-6
Breslow's Depth of Invasion Classification for Melanoma

Vertical Thickness Groupings
0.75 mm or less
0.76 mm to 1.50 mm
1.51 mm to 3.0 mm
More than 3.0 mm

depth of invasion is measured in millimeters of vertical thickness by the pathologist. Clark's level of invasion relates to involvement of specific layers of the skin and is used along with Breslow's depth of invasion to determine the T value in the AJCC staging scheme.[17](pp1618-19) The greater the thickness and invasion through the layers of skin, the higher the stage. Tables 16-5 and 16-6 depict these two classifications.

- *Lymphoma Staging Scheme*
The Ann Arbor staging classification is commonly used for the staging of lymphomas and is the scheme defined in the AJCC *Manual for Staging of Cancer.* Originally developed for Hodgkin disease, this staging scheme was later expanded to include Non-Hodgkin lymphoma. In addition to the schemes just described, there are many staging schemes for specialized sites and cancers in use throughout the world. It is important to be aware that they exist.

TIME FRAMES FOR INCLUDING EXTENT OF DISEASE IN STAGING

The Surveillance, Epidemiology, and End Results (SEER) extent of disease coding and summary staging are based on combined clinical and operative/pathologic assessment and should include all information available through the completion of surgery(ies) in the first course of treatment or within four months of diagnosis in the absence of disease progression, whichever is longer.[7](p10) The American Joint Committee on Cancer (AJCC) clinical staging is determined after the staging workup is completed and before any treatment has started. AJCC pathologic staging is completed after the completion of surgery(ies) in the first course of treatment or within four months of diagnosis in the absence of disease progression, whichever is longer.

GENERAL GUIDELINES

The following list includes general guidelines for staging for all schemes:

- Stage grouping can only be applied to cancers that are alike in site, histology, or both.
- Accurate and complete assessment of the cancer is necessary before staging.

- Rule out distant disease first. When metastatic disease is documented, there may be no need to look for information about the primary tumor and regional lymph node status.
- A few cases are unstageable. The "unstageable" category should be assigned only after all efforts to identify the extent of disease have been exhausted or the site or histology does not meet criteria for staging.
- It is mandatory to stage uniformly using the same staging classification in order to compare data or results.
- It is important to seek further information if staging information is unclear in order to ensure the quality of data.

The following list includes general guidelines for AJCC staging:

- Pathologic staging for AJCC is based on a combined clinical (including diagnostic tests and examinations) and operative or pathologic assessment.
- When there is doubt about assigning the correct stage, select the lower (lesser) category.
- Classifications are revised as medical science progresses. It is important to use the most current edition of a staging system. Changes to a new edition should be made at the beginning of a diagnosis year.
- It is important to verify physician staging. Request substantiation if a physician's staging does not correlate with the information in the health information record.
- Multiple ambiguous terms that classify tumor involvement or extension are listed in the ROADS by the CoC.
- Cases diagnosed after January 1, 1995 must have the T, N, M, and stage grouping documented in the health information record by the managing physician, according to the Commission on Cancer. In 2005, staging forms are required to be on the patient's chart and they are helpful in determining and documenting the stage.

COMMON CONCERNS WITH STAGING

- The stage of a cancer is sometimes confused with the grade of a tumor by new registrars. Terms such as *well differentiated* and *undifferentiated* are tumor grades.

- The rules for each staging scheme must be reviewed for each site and histology. The AJCC staging staging systems, EOD, and summary staging systems list the sites and histologies to which specific staging schemes apply.
- The term *microinvasion* implies invasion through the basement membrane (an anatomic landmark), indicating that the stage is invasive instead of *in situ*.

Some cases of cancer are difficult to stage appropriately. Problem situations include the following:

- Diagnostic tests done on an outpatient basis with results not documented in the hospital health information record
- Tests and biopsies done in a physician's office and sent to freestanding laboratories for assessment
- Conflicting information about the exact location, size, and involvement of the tumor

There are many resources available for staging cancers. The registry should have adequate access to appropriate references. Staging manuals for the most commonly used systems (collaborative stage, summary staging, AJCC staging, and SEER extent of disease) provide comprehensive guidelines. These should be routinely reviewed at the time of abstracting to verify the staging classification.

The CoC requires that staging be documented on the staging form and completed by the managing physician. This requirement does not negate the need for the registrar to understand staging. Verification is necessary at the registry level to ensure the accuracy and completeness of data. It is imperative that staging be correct when registry data are reported and analyzed.

The patient's treatment is based on the extent of disease. The prognosis of the disease can be estimated by the stage and other factors such as age, aggressiveness of tumor, and the presence or absence of other medical conditions. In certain stages of disease, quality of life issues may influence treatment decisions. The stage of disease is used in research studies and in the analysis of cancers.

STUDY QUESTIONS

1. Define staging.
2. List three uses of staging information.
3. Why do staging schemes change?

156

4. Describe two ways that cancer cells can metastasize to other parts of the body.

5. How do the clinical and pathologic staging bases differ in the American joint Committee on Cancer staging system?

6. What is the CS System and how what issues does it resolve?

REFERENCES

1. Fritz A and Hulstrom D. *Workbook for Staging of Cancer*, 2nd ed. Alexandria, Va: National Cancer Registrars Association; 1999.

2. Commission on Cancer. *Standards of the Commission on Cancer: Facility Oncology Registry Data Standards (FORDS).* Chicago, Ill: American College of Surgeons; 2002: 18.

3. Shambaugh EM, *Self Instructional Manual for Tumor Registrars*, Book Five, 2nd ed. Bethesda, Md: National institutes of Health, National Cancer Institute; 1993, 123. NIH publication no. 93-1263.

4. *A Guide to Recent Advances in Tumor Markers.* Abbott Laboratories, Diagnostics Educational Series 97-9366/R.; 1991:1-40.

5. Sklar J, Principles of molecular cell biology of cancer: molecular approaches to cancer diagnosis. In DeVita VT, Hellman S, Rosenberg SN, eds. *Cancer Principles and Practice of Oncology*, 4th ed. Philadelphia, Penn. J.B. Lippincott; 1989: 96.

6. Zackon I, Goosby C. A clinician's guide to flow cytometry. In *Contemporary Oncology.* Montvale, NJ: Medical Economics Publishing; 1994: 14-36.

7. Young J, Roffers SD, Ries LAG, Fritz AG (eds), SEER Summary Staging Manual—2000: Codes and Coding Instructions, National Cancer Institute, Bethesda, Md; 2001: 10 NIH Pub. No 01-4969.

8. Greene FL, et al. *American Joint Committee on Cancer Staging Manual,* 6th ed. Springer-Verlag; 2002: 3, 5, 115, 227.

9. Fritz AG, Ries LG. *SEER Extent of Disease, 1988.* Bethesda, Md: National Institutes of Health, National Cancer Institute; 1998, pp. 1-9. NIH publication no. 99-1999.

10. Seiffert J, Shambaugh EM, Weiss MA, et al. *Comparative Staging Guide for Cancer, Major Cancer Sites,* Version 1. 1. Bethesda, Md: National Institutes of Health, National Cancer Institute; 1993: p. 1-6. NIH publication no. 93-3460.

11. Sobin LH, Wittekind CH. *TNM Classification of Malignant Tumours,* 6th ed. New York, NY: Wiley-Liss; 2002: 15.

12. American Joint Committee on Cancer. *Collaborative Staging Manual and Coding Instructions,* Version 1.0. Collaborative Stage Task Force. Chicago, Ill: American Joint Committee on Cancer; 2002.

13. Douglas LL. Collaborative stage: an update. *Journal of Registry management.* 2001; 28:4.

14. Cohen A, Minsky B, Schilsky R. Colon cancer. In DeVita VT, Hellman S, Rosenberg SN, eds. *Cancer Principles and Practice of Oncology,* 4th ed. Philadelphia, Pa: J.B. Lippincott; 1989: p. 940.

15. Hanks G, Myers C, Scardina P. Cancer of the prostrate. In DeVita VT, Hellman S, Rosenberg SN, eds. *Cancer Principles and Practice of Oncology,* 4th ed. Philadelphia, Pa: J.B. Lippincott; 1989: 1087.

16. Holleb A, Fink D, Murphy G. *American Cancer Society Textbook: Clinical Oncology,* Atlanta, Ga: American Cancer Society; 1991: 486.

17. Sefel B. Cancers on the skin. In DeVita VT, Hellman S, Rosenberg SN, eds. *Cancer Principles and Practice of Oncology,* 4th ed. Philadelphia, Pa: J.B. Lippincott; 1989: 1618-19.

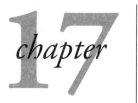

CANCER TREATMENT

Donna M. Gress
RHIT, CTR

INTRODUCTION

Cancer-directed treatment is defined in the *Standards of the Commission on Cancer, Volume II: Facility Oncology Registry Data Standards* (FORDS), as "treatment intended to modify or control the malignancy."[1] Currently, surgery, radiation therapy, and systemic therapy which includes chemotherapy, hormone therapy, immunotherapy, endocrine therapy and hematologic transplants, are the recognized and accepted methods of treating patients with cancer. The physician makes treatment decisions (a treatment plan) for each patient based on a number of disease- and patient-specific factors. The diagnostic and staging workup provides disease-specific information such as primary site, metastatic sites, histology, clinical stage, and tumor grade. The physician combines this information with patient-specific information including age, overall health status, mental status, and women's menopausal status to select the appropriate treatment or combination of treatments.

The first course of therapy is the treatment that is planned at the time of initial diagnosis.[1] Refer to Chapter 19, General Principles of Abstracting, for brief descriptions of rules for abstracting treatment. Most authorities agree that the first and second courses of treatment have the greatest chance of eliminating the cancer. Subsequent methods of treatment are usually "salvage" therapy given to prolong survival or to improve the quality of life.

Careful data collection by cancer registries has been essential in directly enhancing advancement in cancer diagnosis and treatment, as well as patient survival. Changes in breast cancer treatment are a dramatic example. The patient's quality of life improved when surgical treatment changed from radical mastectomy to modified radical mastectomy. This important change occurred because analysis of oncology data proved that survival time was not significantly affected in patients who had the less debilitating modified radical mastectomy. Analysis of recurrence data proved that most breast cancers recurred in distant sites. Up to that time, surgery and regional radiation therapy were used to treat patients with breast cancer who had positive nodes. Chemotherapy was added to the first course of treatment to destroy the systemic micrometastases (microscopic secondary tumors). The effectiveness of tumor markers, such as estrogen receptors and progesterone receptors to guide treatment choices, was proven by long-term data collection and outcome analysis. Physicians could use these tumor markers to predict whether the addition of hormones to the first course of therapy would prevent or delay disease recurrence. The addition of chemotherapy and hormone therapy to the first course of treatment for breast cancer patients has improved survival time and decreased the recurrence rate.

It is imperative that cancer registrars collect complete and accurate treatment data. This chapter defines the different methods of treatment and how the information should be collected.

SURGERY

Surgery is the oldest form of treatment for cancer and, until recently, was the only treatment modality that could cure patients with cancer.[2] Surgeons play a critical role in diagnosis, treatment, and rehabilitation of the cancer patient, and the prevention and palliation of cancer. The registrar records surgeries other than preventive as either non-cancer directed or cancer directed. Definitions of the codes for surgery are usually specific to each primary site.

Preventive Surgery

Preventive surgery is used for patients who have a congenital or genetic trait that creates a high risk of developing cancer. An example would be a patient with familial polyposis of the colon. Without a preventive colectomy, half of these patients would develop cancer of the colon by age 40, and virtually all would develop cancer of the colon by age 70.[3] The cancer registrar cannot collect information on preventive surgery using the current standard data sets.

Diagnostic Surgery

The surgeon uses diagnostic procedures to identify the histologic type of cancer and stage of disease. Aspiration biopsies, needle biopsies, and incisional biopsies remove enough tumor tissue to allow a cytologic or histologic examination of the specimen. Each of these types of biopsy leaves gross tumor in the body.

Biopsies of regional and distant tissue or organs are used to confirm the stage of disease. A staging laparotomy in Hodgkin disease, for example, is used to rule out occult abdominal disease, thus accurately determining the stage of disease. A suspicious lesion in the liver may be biopsied to prove or disprove the presence of distant metastasis. A biopsy that removes only a fragment or portion of the tumor, primary or metastatic, is recorded in the abstract as surgical diagnostic and staging procedures.

Surgical Treatment

Surgery is an important part of the treatment plan in patients with solid tumors and is often used to cure patients whose tumors are localized at the time of diagnosis. These surgical procedures remove all of the primary tumor, leaving gross margins free of tumor. The procedures may also partially or totally remove the organ of origin.

Most patients receive both surgery and adjuvant treatment because approximately 70% have micrometastases when they are diagnosed.[4] Adjuvant therapy is defined as chemotherapy given following surgery or radiation to localized disease. Localized disease is removed surgically, and appropriate adjuvant chemotherapy is used to destroy the micrometastases. As with localized tumors, surgery removes all of the primary tumor, leaving margins grossly free of tumor. The surgical procedures may also partially or totally remove the organ or tissue of origin.

When a patient is diagnosed with regional tumor extension, cytoreductive surgery is performed to remove as much gross disease as possible. Because distant micrometastases are often present in patients with regional disease, the first course of therapy usually combines surgery with the appropriate adjuvant chemotherapy. Cytoreductive surgery is beneficial only if adjuvant treatments can control or eliminate the residual disease. These surgical procedures usually remove the primary organ and affected regional tissue or organs. For some primaries such as ovarian cancer, surgery is used to reduce the bulk of tumor so that adjuvant therapy will be more effective. Debulking procedures may or may not totally remove the primary tumor or organ of origin.

Surgery is currently being used to remove solitary or limited metastases to the lung, liver, or brain. Surgical treatment of distant metastases is usually limited to patients with disease that is not highly responsive to adjuvant treatment and limited to one site of distant metastasis.

Each of the surgical procedures described above is recorded in the abstract as first course of treatment surgical procedures of primary site, scope of regional lymph node surgery or surgical procedures of other site.

RADIATION THERAPY

Radiation kills cells by damaging their deoxyribonucleic acid (DNA), thereby affecting the ability of the cell to divide. The decision to treat the tumor with radiation is based on the location of the primary tumor and whether the tumor cells are radiosensitive. Radiosensitive tumors respond by promptly showing regression after moderate doses of radiation.[5] Because radiation affects both normal and cancerous cells, radiation fields are very carefully planned to exclude uninvolved vital organs and tissues. Radiocurability means that the normal tissue tumor relationship is such that curative doses of radiation can be used without excessively damaging the normal tissue. Radiocurative tumors include carcinoma of the cervix, larynx, breast, and prostate. Radiocurative tumors other than carcinomas are Hodgkin disease and seminomas.[5] Radiation may be the only therapy necessary for radiocurative tumors.

Types of Radiation

Radiation is delivered as brachytherapy, teletherapy, or stereotactic radiosurgery or is added to a liquid base (iodine 131 [I-131] or strontium 90) and delivered through intravenous or intracavitary devices. With brachytherapy, the radioactive material is encased in rods or beads that are placed in direct contact with the tumor. Teletherapy refers to the standard method (external beam) of delivering radiation from a source at a distance from the body. Stereotactic radiosurgery involves focusing the radiation beam on a small area and delivering very high doses. Finally, radioactive particles can be attached to small molecules and given intravenously. For example, I-131 is used intravenously to treat thyroid cancer, and strontium 90 is used to treat bony metastases. Each of these types of radiation is recorded in the "radiation" field as first course of therapy.

New Types of Teletherapy

Teletherapy includes new methods of delivering the radiation which include three-dimensional conformal radiation therapy (3D-CRT) and intensity modulated radiation therapy (IMRT).

3D-CRT allows radiation to be delivered to tumor more accurately in higher doses. It uses computerized tomography (CT), positron emission tomography (PET) or magnetic resonance imaging (MRI) scanners to produce images of the tumor area. These images are transferred to a computer that measure the size and location of the tumor and nearby healthy tissue. The amount of radiation targeted at the tumor is determined. This is most beneficial for tumors that are irregular in shape or found in delicate areas such as the brain, or those surrounded by normal tissue that is highly sensitive to radiation. Parts of the body commonly treated with 3D-CRT are prostate, brain, lung, head, and neck.

IMRT is a new form of 3D-CRT. The difference is that IMRT treats the tumor with small beams of different strengths of radiation, whereas 3D-CRT uses beams of the same strength. IMRT is a technique in which higher doses of radiation are applied to certain parts of the tumor tissue. Since the tumor can vary in thickness, this minimizes areas of the tumor that would receive more radiation than other areas. It also supplies a more consistent dose of radiation aimed at the tumor while sparing healthy tissue.

Radiation and Surgery

Radiation is often used as adjuvant therapy to surgery because radiation failures usually occur in the center of the tumor. Surgery can effectively remove the gross tumor, but there may be a limit to the amount of adjacent tissue that can be removed without impairing function. Radiation therapy rarely falls in the periphery of tumors, where small numbers of well-vascularized tumor cells are found. Using surgery to remove gross tumor, followed by radiation to treat microscopic residual cells, can be very effective. An example of radiation surgery combination is the treatment of a Stage I breast cancer patient with lumpectomy and axillary dissection followed by radiation therapy to the intact breast and axilla.

Radiation may also be used preoperatively for unresectable tumors or tumors that may seed (disseminate cells) during surgery. If the tumor is unresectable, radiation is used to decrease tumor bulk to the point where resection is achievable. A patient with endometrial cancer may be treated with intrauterine radium implants prior to surgery to prevent seeding.

Radiation and Chemotherapy

Radiation therapy is sometimes combined with chemotherapy to improve patient outcome. Chemotherapy is added to the radiation regimen to control systemic micrometastases or to increase radiosensitivity.

SYSTEMIC THERAPY

Systemic therapy includes chemotherapy, hormone therapy, immunotherapy, endocrine therapy, and hematologic transplants.

CHEMOTHERAPY

Chemotherapy is a systemic method of cancer control. Cells divide by going through the cell cycle, in which the key events are the synthesis (S-phase) of DNA, mitosis (M-phase), and the actual division of the parent cell into two daughter cells (Figure 17-1).

Chemotherapy interferes primarily with DNA synthesis and mitosis (the S and M phases of the cell cycle). Most chemotherapy drugs can destroy only actively dividing cells, so they cannot kill all of the cancer cells in a single dose. The killing effect of chemotherapeutic agents has a definite selectivity for cancer cells over the normal host cells.[6] Although individual cancer cells do not divide faster than their normal tissue counterparts, the population of cancer cells generally have a higher growth fraction (the number of cells undergoing division at any one time).[6(p192)]

Chemotherapy is used as a definitive curative treatment for some diseases such as Hodgkin disease, leukemia, and testicular cancer. For other cancers, it is an adjuvant therapy used in combination with surgery or radiation therapy to control micrometastases or increase radiosensitivity. It is also used when a patient is initially diagnosed with metastatic disease or has recurrent disease after initial treatment with surgery or radiation therapy.

Figure 17-1
The Cell Cycle

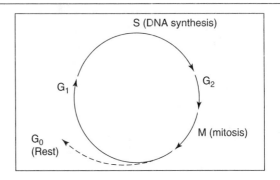

Chemotherapy is usually given in a combination regimen consisting of more than one chemotherapeutic drug. Combining drugs that work at different points in the cell cycle increases the killing effectiveness of chemotherapy. In addition, combinations of drugs can be selected to decrease cumulative side effects and the development of resistance.

Table 17-1 lists the more common chemotherapeutic agents used for cancer patients. The cell-cycle phase that is affected by each chemotherapeutic agent is shown, along with the method of administration.[7]

At times, a patient may not be able to tolerate a chemotherapeutic agent, and the physician may change the prescribed regimen by replacing that agent

Table 17-1

Common Chemotherapeutic Drugs by Cell-Cycle Phase Active and Type of Administration

Anti-Cancer Drug	Cell Cycle Phase Active	Administration
I. Alkalating agents		
A. Nitrogen mustards		
1. Mechlorethamine	NS	IV
2. Cyclophosphamide	NS	IV, IM, PO
3. Melphalan	NS	IV, PO
4. Chlorambucil	NS	PO
5. Ifosfamide	NS	IV
B. Allsyl sulfonates—busulfan	NS	PO
C. Nitrosourea		
1. Carmustine (BCNU)	NS	IV
2. Lomustine (CCNU)	NS	PO
3. Semustine	NS	PO
4. Streptozocin	NS	IV
D. Ethylenimines—thiotepa	NS	IV
E. Triazines—dacarbazine (DTIC)	NS	IV
II. Antimetabolites		
A. Folate antagonists		
1. Methotrexate	S	IV, IM, PO, IT
2. Trimetrexate	S	IV
B. Purine analogs		
1. Thioguanine (6-TG)	S	PO
2. Mercaptopurine (6-MP)	S	IV, PO
C. Pyrimidine analogues		
1. Cytosine arabinside	S	IV, IM, SQ, IT
2. Fluorouracial (5-FU)	NS	N, PO
III. Antibiotics		
A. Anthracyclines		
1. Doxorubicin	S	IV
2. Daunomycin	S	IV
3. Idarubicin	S	IV
B. Bleomycin	G_2, M	IV, IM
C. Mitomycin	P	IV
D. Dactinomycin	P	IV
E. Mithramycin	NS	IV

(continued)

Table 17-1
(continued)

Anti-Cancer Drug	Cell Cycle Phase Active	Administration
IV. Vinca alkaloids		
A. Vincristine	M (late S)	IV
B. Vinblastine	M (late S)	IV
C. Vindesine	M (late S)	IV, PO
V. Enzymes-L-asparaginase	S	IM, IV
VI. Miscellaneous		
A. Hydroxyurea	S	PO
B. Procarbazine	NS	PO
C. Carboplatin	NS	IV
D. Cisplatin	NS	IV, IP
E. Epipodophyllines		
1. Etoposide (VP-16)	G_2, S	IV
2. Teniposide (VM-26)	G_2, S	IV

Key:

Cell-Cycle Phase

S   DNA synthetic phase
M   mitosis
G1   growth phase
G2   growth phase
NS   nonspecific, kills during all phases of division and in G_0
P   kills proliferating cells, not G_0

Methods of Administration

IV   intravenous
IM   intramuscular
PO   oral, by mouth
SQ   subcutaneous
IP   intraperitoneal

with another better tolerated drug (for example, replacing cisplatin with carboplatin). If the replacement drug is in the same group (antimetabolite, alkylating, or natural product) as the original drug, it is still recorded in the abstract as initial treatment.

Classes of Chemotherapeutic Agents

• *Antimetabolites*
Antimetabolites replace natural substances as building blocks in DNA molecules, thereby altering the function of enzymes required for cell metabolism and protein synthesis. Their action is most pronounced during the S-phase of cell division. Antimetabolites have three classifications: folic acid analogues (such as methotrexate), pyrimidine analogues (such as 5-fluorouracil), and purine analogues (such as 6-mercaptopurine). Folinic acid (leucovorin) bypasses the enzymatic block produced by methotrexate and "rescues" normal cells from the effect of methotrexate. Cancer cells, however, which lack an active transport enzyme for leucovorin, are not "rescued."

- *Alkylating Agents*

  Alkylating agents cause cross-linking of DNA strands, abnormal base pairing, or DNA strand breaks, thus interfering with DNA replication.[8] Dividing cells are the most sensitive to alkylating agents, but resting cells are also affected. Alkylating agents include chlorambucil, cyclophosphamide, thiotepa, and busulfan. Because bone marrow and gastrointestinal tract cells have high growth fractions, alkylating agents commonly cause bone marrow suppression and gastrointestinal disturbances.

- *Natural Products*

  Antitumor antibiotics prevent nucleic acid synthesis and block DNA translation and ribonucleic acid (RNA) transcription. Although they act throughout the cell cycle, some are more effective during the S- and M-phases. Examples of antibiotics used in chemotherapy are actinomycin D, doxorubicin, and mitomycin.

  Plant alkaloids are derived from the periwinkle plant and interfere with cell division by inhibiting mitosis (the M-phase of the cell cycle). Plant alkaloids include vinblastine and vincristine.

  L-asparaginase is an enzyme that inhibits the growth of tumor cells unable to synthesize L-asparagine, an amino acid necessary for protein synthesis.

Methods of Administration

Chemotherapy drugs are given by one of several routes, depending on the drug (see Table 17-1). Some are given orally and absorbed through the gastrointestinal tract into the bloodstream. Others are given intravenously and carried throughout the body by the bloodstream. Although these two methods are the most often used, other methods are used to concentrate the drug dosage or to overcome barriers to drug absorption. These types of administration can include intrathecal, pleural, pericardial, intraperitoneal and hepatic artery injections.

Intrathecal administration (injection into cerebrospinal fluid surrounding the brain and spinal cord) is used when a drug does not cross the blood-brain barrier. Most intrathecal medications are given by spinal tap, which involves inserting a needle into the spinal fluid sac around the spinal cord in the lumbar region. An access device called an Omaya reservoir, which directly connects to the ventricular system, may be implanted and chemotherapeutic agents injected into the device. Intrathecal injections are used primarily for meningeal leukemia or lymphoma.

Injections directly into the pleural space are used to fuse the parietal and visceral pleura to control malignant pleural effusion. The medicine injected may be a chemotherapy drug or an irritant or sclerosing agent such as tetracycline. Injections can also be made into the pericardial space to control effusions.

Intraperitoneal infusion (injecting chemotherapy into the peritoneal cavity) is used to destroy tumor cells present in the peritoneal fluid. Ovarian cancer often spreads throughout the peritoneal cavity by seeding free tumor cells into the peritoneal fluid. Intraperitoneal infusion gives a concentrated chemotherapy dose to the peritoneal fluid and the visceral surface of the peritoneal organs but spares systemic side effects.

Hepatic artery infusion (inserting a catheter into the hepatic artery) is one of the methods used to deliver a concentrated chemotherapeutic dose to the liver.

HORMONE THERAPY

Hormones are natural substances produced by the body that control reproduction, growth, and metabolism in distant organs. Certain body tissues such as breast and prostate require hormones to develop. When cancer originates in these tissues, it is often hormonally responsive. This means that it responds to hormonal manipulation, which includes the administration of hormones or interference with hormone function.

Hormones are not usually given as a single agent to attempt to cure cancer. Hormones may be used to prevent or delay recurrence of cancer after other modalities of treatment have removed the gross primary tumor and chemotherapy or radiation has treated systemic and regional micrometastases. An example is a breast cancer patient who had the primary tumor and positive axillary nodes removed surgically, received systemic chemotherapy and regional radiation, and was placed on tamoxifen, a synthetic antiestrogen, to prevent or delay recurrence. Hormones may also be used to inhibit the growth or spread of hormonally responsive tumors. For example, low-stage prostate cancer can be treated with leuprolide (Lupron) injections.

Hormonal Administration

Hormones can be administered orally, intravenously, or intramuscularly.

- **Hormone Replacement Therapy**

  When cancer-directed therapy removes a gland that produces hormones that are necessary for bodily function, those hormones must be artificially replaced. Replacement hormones are not abstracted as cancer-directed therapy, with the exception of thyroid replacement. Thyroid hormone replacement inhibits the production of thyroid-stimulating hormone (TSH) by the pituitary. Because TSH can stimulate thyroid tumor growth, the thyroid replacement decreases TSH production and inhibits cancer growth. Therefore, thyroid replacement is recorded in the abstract as cancer-directed treatment in patients with thyroid cancer.

- **Steroids**

  Steroids are recorded as treatment in the same field as hormones. Steroids are cytotoxic to lymphoid malignancies and, therefore, are often part of combination chemotherapy regimens for these tumors. In other situations, steroids may alter the immune system response and the cancer cells' reaction to chemotherapy, thereby improving treatment response. Prednisone and dexamethasone are the steroids most commonly used as chemotherapy.

  If a steroid is given for supportive care, it is not recorded in the abstract as treatment. Examples are megestrol acetate given to improve appetite and dexamethasone given to reduce brain swelling and therefore decrease neurologic symptoms caused by brain tumors.

IMMUNOTHERAPY

Immunotherapy manipulates the interactions between the body's immune system and the tumor. Immunotherapy, or biological response modifier therapy, is usually administered after the bulk of tumor has been destroyed by surgery or chemotherapy. Interferon, interleukin, and Bacillus Calmette-Guerin (BCG) are some of the more commonly used immunotherapy drugs. Immunotherapy is the newest type of cancer-directed therapy and is still under intensive investigation.

ENDOCRINE THERAPY

Endocrine therapy is the suppression or withdrawal of hormones through the use of radiation or surgical procedures. These procedures prevent the naturally occurring hormonal activity from taking place and thereby altering the growth of hormone dependent tumors.

For example, a patient with prostate cancer may have an orchiectomy to prevent the production of testosterone. This surgical procedure is recorded in the abstract as a hematologic transplant and endocrine procedure because the surgery prevents hormone production rather than removes cancer tissue.

HEMATOLOGIC TRANSPLANTS

Bone marrow transplants and stem cell harvests are performed to restore the function after chemotherapy or radiation therapy has caused myelosuppression or bone marrow ablation. They are recorded in the abstract as hematologic transplant and endocrine procedures. These procedures are used in a variety of malignancies. Patients are treated with myeloablative doses (lethal to bone marrow cells) of chemotherapy and/or radiation therapy to kill remaining tumor cells, after which bone marrow or stem cells are given to restore marrow and immune system function.

OTHER THERAPY

Cancer treatment for the newly reportable hematopoietic diseases can be supportive care, observation, or any treatment that does not meet the usual definitions and cannot be assigned to the other specific treatment data items. These treatments may include phlebotomy, transfusions and aspirin. They are recorded as other treatment.

Other therapies include treatments whose action or efficacy has not been clearly defined. Examples include experimental therapies that have not been approved by the Food and Drug Administration (FDA), double blind studies in which the study is still in progress and the drug's mechanism of action is not known to investigators, and non-FDA-approved agents used outside of research settings. Laetrile and herbal remedies are in this class of treatments.

PALLIATIVE PROCEDURES

Palliative procedures relieve symptoms and include the procedures of surgery, radiation therapy, systemic therapy, and pain management therapy.

Palliative surgery is used to improve the patient's quality of life by reducing pain or correcting functional abnormalities. Bypass surgery for unresectable colon cancer is performed to correct a functional abnormality. Because this procedure does not modify or control the malignancy, it is recorded as palliative procedure. On the other hand, palliative surgery may involve the removal of a painful primary or metastatic tumor mass such as a solitary spinal metastasis. Because this procedure does remove cancer tissue, it is recorded as surgical procedure of primary or other site.

Palliative radiation is often used for pain control. Patients with painful bony metastasis are treated with radiation to alleviate or control the pain. Because the radiation makes no attempt to treat the primary tumor, it is recorded in the abstract as a palliative procedure.

Pain management therapy with no other palliative care is also recorded as a palliative procedure.

ANCILLARY DRUGS

Ancillary drugs are not directed at the malignancy but enhance the effects of the cancer therapy. Some ancillary drugs are folinic acid (Leucovorin) used in combination with 5-FU, allopurinol used to prevent uric acid formation, and growth-stimulating factors (G-CSF, GM-CSF) used to repopulate bone marrow.

CANCER ASSOCIATED WITH ACQUIRED IMMUNODEFICIENCY SYNDROME (AIDS)

Immunosuppressed patients are at an increased risk for malignancy. Acquired Immunodeficiency Syndrome (AIDS) was identified as a new disease in 1981 because of the occurrence of Kaposi's sarcoma and Pneumocystis pneumonia in homosexual men. Kaposi's sarcoma in the AIDS patient usually presents in a disseminated stage with lesions on the skin surface, visceral surfaces of internal organs, and gastrointestinal lesions. Only the treatments intended to reduce or modify the Kaposi's sarcoma, such as radiation therapy to the skin lesions, should be recorded as treatment.

SUMMARY

Treatment is a method to destroy, modify, or remove primary, regional, or metastatic cancer tissue. The approach can be a surgical procedure, radiation, the administration of medication, hematologic transplant or endocrine procedures. The treatment plan is determined by a physician and based on patient and disease characteristics. First course of therapy (planned at initial diagnosis) and second course of treatment (initiated due to additional disease) have the greatest opportunity to eliminate the cancer.

Treatment for cancer has changed dramatically over the years and has improved survival time and decreased the recurrence rate. Surgery, radiation therapy, and chemotherapy are the mainstay approaches, although the effectiveness of other therapies continues to be measured. The cancer registry abstract must contain complete and accurate treatment data to evaluate the outcome.

STUDY QUESTIONS

1. What is the purpose of a biopsy?
2. Why is chemotherapy combined with surgery?
3. Describe stereotactic radiosurgery.
4. What is the definition of cancer treatment?
5. Describe endocrine treatment and give an example.

REFERENCES

1. Commission on Cancer. *Standards of the Commission on Cancer, vol. II: Facility Oncology Registry Data Standards.* Chicago, Ill: American College of Surgeons; 2002.
2. Rosenberg SA. Principles of surgical oncology. In DeVita VI, Hellman S, Rosenberg SA, eds. *Cancer: Principles and Practice of Oncology,* 3rd ed. Philadelphia; J. B. Lippincott; 1989: 215, 220-21, 251, 262.
3. Mendelsohn MT. The growth fraction: A new concept applied to tumors. *Science.* 1960; 132: 1496.
4. Craig C, Stitzel P. *Modern Pharmacology.* New York, NY: Little, Brown & Company; 1982: 745-57.
5. Shambaugh EM, Nayfield SG, Swenson TM, Kruse MA, eds. *SEER Program Self Instructional Manual for*

Tumor Registrars, Book 8, 3rd ed. Bethesda, Md: National institutes of Health, National Cancer Institute; 1994. NIH Publication No. 94-2441.

6. Balis F, Holcenberg JS, Poplack DG. General principles of chemotherapy. In Pizzo AT, Poplack DG eds. *Principles and Practice of Pediatric Oncology.* Philadelphia, Pa: J. B. Lippincott; 1989: 192.

7. Hutchison C, Roffers, S, Fritz A, eds. *Cancer Registry Management Principles and Practice.* Dubuque, Iowa: Kendall/Hunt Publishing Company; 1997.

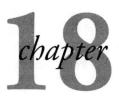

CLINICAL TRIALS

Karen I. Christie
MA, CTR, CCRA

INTRODUCTION

To collaborate in research efforts, hospitals and other institutions have formed regional, national, and international clinical trial groups. These groups formulate scientific studies involving specific medical conditions, diseases, or target populations in order to improve cancer prevention, diagnosis, treatment and outcomes. Clinical trials frequently have institutional (primary) members, and affiliate members. Each institutional member designates a principal investigator (PI) who is responsible for conducting the studies designed by the clinical trial group in his or her institution. Most clinical trial groups have full-member institutions that annually accrue large numbers of patients on studies. Affiliate members have a responsible investigator who, in a manner similar to the principal investigator, conducts studies in local institutions. Typically, a smaller number of patients is accrued each year by affiliate institutions. Their cases are reported to the full-member institution with which they are affiliated.

The terms *clinical study, clinical trial,* and *protocol* are often used interchangeably; however, each has a different meaning.[1] A clinical study is a scientific approach to evaluating disease prevention, diagnostic techniques, and treatments. A clinical trial is a subset of a clinical study that evaluates investigational (nonstandard) medications, treatments, diagnostic and preventive techniques or devices, or a combination of these elements. A protocol is the written document that provides the parameters for the clinical trial.

CLINICAL TRIAL PHASES

Clinical trials are usually completed in three phases. These phases are not always completed in the same order, but each phase must be completed for the trial to be considered scientifically valid. In addition, phase IV trials are often conducted by pharmaceutical companies with drugs they hope to have approved by the Food and Drug Administration (FDA). Phase IV studies provide additional details regarding a drug's safety and efficacy profile. Most national oncology trial groups, however, use only the first three clinical trial phases.[1](pxxiii)

Phase I clinical trials are designed to test the initial safety of new drugs, devices, treatment modalities, or combinations of these elements. They are designed to determine the estimated tolerable dosage range of the agent or the toxicities resulting from its use on human subjects. Phase I trials are often conducted on seriously ill volunteers who are no longer responsive to conventional treatments. The results of Phase I trials are considered preliminary.

Phase II clinical trials are sometimes divided into Phase IIa and Phase IIb trials by pharmaceutical companies. Phase IIa trials are pilot trials focusing on dose responses, frequency of drug dosage, or other areas of safety and efficacy. Phase IIb trials are well-controlled trials representing the most rigorous demonstration of efficacy. They are sometimes called pivotal trials.[1](pxxii) Most national clinical trial groups do not distinguish between Phase IIa and Phase IIb trials but refer to them simply as Phase II studies.

Phase III clinical trials compare the research drugs, methods, or devices being studied with standard treatment. These trials are sometimes separated into Phase IIIa and Phase IIIb. Phase IIIa includes trials conducted after efficacy has been established but before the submission of a New Drug Application (NDA) or other dossier to the FDA. Phase IIIb includes trials conducted after regulatory submission of an NDA or other dossier. Most trial groups refer to all these trials as Phase III. This is usually the final testing phase.

COOPERATIVE OR INTERGROUP CLINICAL TRIALS

Sometimes two or more clinical trial groups join forces to form an "intergroup" so that larger numbers of patients from a wider geographical area can participate in their studies. In this manner, specific diseases of a rare nature can be carefully studied in an expeditious manner, since patients are accrued more rapidly than if only one group conducted the study. Each cooperative group is held accountable to the National Institutes of Health (NIH) for the performance of its members.

THE INSTITUTIONAL REVIEW BOARD

Definition and Purpose

Before any clinical trial (Phase I, II, III, or IV) can be initiated in a hospital or clinical setting, federal law requires that it be approved by an institutional review board (IRB). The IRB is a committee whose membership, composition, purpose, and functions are specified by federal law.

The fundamental purpose of the IRB is to provide a complete and adequate oversight of research activities commonly conducted by the institution. The basic goal of the IRB is to protect the rights of all human subjects participating in such research.

History

Throughout history, there have been healers who have attempted to cure the illnesses prevalent in their societies. Until the twentieth century, however, little thought was given to the protection or the rights of the patients.

After World War II, the Nuremberg Code (printed in 1949) was developed in response to the horrors of the brutal human-subject research conducted on concentration camp prisoners by the Nazis. This code defined basic human rights, especially for research subjects. It placed the responsibility for the welfare of these subjects squarely on the shoulders of the investigator. Peer review was not yet advocated in this document nor in the Declaration of Helsinki (1964), which also gave the investigator sole responsibility for the welfare of the subjects.

The first contemporary document to address peer review of research programs and practices was issued with the opening of the National Institutes of Health (NIH) Clinical Center in 1953. This document set forth guidelines for use in intramural research conducted at the NIH Clinical Center. It also paved the way for the international acceptance of peer review within the medical research community. The guidelines said that written consent must be obtained from the subjects if the experiments were considered dangerous. The administrative procedures required the documentation of the doctor-patient relationship, an area where privacy had not previously been subject to invasion.[2,3]

The Drug Amendments Act of 1962 also had an impact on the regulation of human research. It was enacted in response to worldwide reaction to the tragic effects on unborn infants whose mothers had ingested a drug called thalidomide.[4] Previously, the FDA had allowed and even encouraged clinical investigators to use a high level of imagination and freedom in pursuing their research objectives. They were to be guided by their own professional judgment and controlled by their own ethical standards and those of their institutions.[2](p208), [3](p209)

The Drug Amendments Act authorized the secretary of Health, Education, and Welfare (now known as Health and Human Services) to regulate the testing of new drugs. It required the consent of subjects involved in these tests. In 1965, the National Advisory Health Council proposed the establishment of institutional review boards (IRBs) for clinical research and investigation involving human subjects.

Three purposes were given for establishing these IRBs:

- Protection of the rights and welfare of individuals involved in clinical research studies
- Guarantee of the appropriateness of the methods used to secure informed consent from research subjects
- Articulation of the risks and benefits potentially involved in the experiments[5]

In subsequent revisions of the Drug Amendments Act, the principle of prior peer review was extended to all institutions funded with grant monies by the U.S. Public Health Service. In addition, the principle of general assurance was set forth. As stated in a revision of the guidelines governing IRBs, dated May 1, 1967, this principle is as follows:

"The committee must be composed of sufficient members of varying backgrounds to assure complete and adequate review . . . [Furthermore,] the membership should possess not only broad scientific competence to comprehend the nature of the research, but other competencies as necessary in the judgment as to the acceptability of the research in terms of institutional regulations, relevant law, standards of professional practice, and community acceptance."[2](p208), [3](p210)

Since these guidelines were issued, more refinements in the requirements governing board members have been added. Many regulations have redefined the composition, purpose, and goals of the IRBs. Currently, IRBs provide a complete review of all research activities in their institutions. Their aim is to protect all human subjects involved in research from undue harm and to ensure the rights of all human subjects.

Federal Requirements

In order to be approved to perform research, each institution must comply with the regulations set forth by the Department of Health and Human Services (HHS). A written general assurance must be sent to the secretary of HHS covering the requirements listed in Table 18-1.[5](p6)

Table 18-1

Overview of Requirements for Institutions Conducting Research

1. Principles governing the institution must be defined.
2. Institutional responsibilities toward protecting the rights and welfare of human subjects must be defined.
3. An institutional review board must be established.
4. Adequate meeting space must be available for the institutional review board.
5. Provisions must be made for sufficient staff to support institutional review board review and record-keeping duties.
6. Written procedures for the institutional review board to follow when conducting research reviews must be defined.
7. A current list of members including name, profession, earned degrees, and other pertinent information must be maintained.
8. Records with reviews of research being conducted must be kept.
9. Unforeseen risks to subjects or others from research must be reported to the Department of Health and Human Services.

The Office for Protection from Research Risks (OPRR), a division of NIH, issues OPRR *Reports,* which present discussions of IRB functions, as well as updated IRB rules and regulations. There are certain minimal standards in the composition of IRB membership that must be met by each institution. Some of these are listed in Table 18-2.[5](p7) In addition, each IRB member must have certain specific qualities as listed in Table 18-3.

A member who has submitted a research proposal for review may be called upon by the IRB to furnish information on the proposal, but that member cannot participate in the review itself. Research studies can be reviewed only at convened IRB meetings when most members are present and eligible to participate. At least one nonscientific member must be present. There must be a majority consent by the participating members for the approval of studies. Any IRB member with a conflict of interest (for example, owning shares in a drug company whose drug will be used in the study) is not allowed to participate in the review of the study in question.

Detailed minutes of each IRB meeting must be recorded and must include all actions taken and a detailed analysis of each vote. Additionally, the minutes must include the basis for disapproval of projects. Summaries of controversial issues and the actions taken in regard to them must be documented. The IRB must keep copies of all reviewed research proposals, scientific evaluations, approved sample consent forms, progress reports, and reports of injuries or toxic exposure to study subjects.

Copies of all correspondence between the IRB and the investigators must be kept for a minimum of three years after the completion of the research. These records must be made accessible for inspection and copying by the HHS within a reasonable amount of time after they are requested.[5](p9)

The IRB has the right to suspend any study if NIH regulations are not followed, if the study is not conducted according to federal and institutional requirements, or if unexpected or serious harm occurs to subjects. Noncompliance with HHS rules by clinical trial investigators must be reported to the OPRR.[5](p7)

Approval of Clinical Trial Studies

IRBs usually provide application packets containing forms that must be completed by the investigator. These forms are reviewed by the IRB during the process of study approval. The answers to the questions on the forms ensure compliance with federal and IRB requirements by the investigator.

Before approving a research study, the IRB must decide whether several criteria have been met:

- The potential benefits to the subjects must be greater than the risks inherent in the study.
- Risks to subjects must be minimized by using procedures consistent with sound research design.
- Appropriate procedures completed for diagnostic or treatment purposes should be used for research purposes.

Table 18-2

Partial List of Institutional Review Board Membership Composition Requirements by the Office for Protection from Research Risks

1. Minimum of five members
2. Male and female members
3. More than one profession represented
4. Minimum of one nonscientific member (e.g., law, clergy, etc.)
5. Minimum of one member not affiliated with the institution and not part of any employer's immediate family

Table 18-3

Required Qualities of Institutional Review Board Membership

1. Expertise in matters relating to each member's particular field
2. General knowledge of clinical medicine and clinical research, with the exception of members in nonscientific professions
3. Knowledge of the institution's commitments and regulations, the laws applicable to it, and its expected standards of professional conduct
4. Concern for the welfare of vulnerable subjects
5. Sensitivity to, and knowledge of, community attitudes
6. Ad hoc consultants (nonvoting) with special skills and competencies

For example, a blood test that has diagnosed leukemia could be used as the required blood test for the study. This use of one test or procedure for two purposes is known as *piggybacking*.

When reviewing research study applications for approval, the IRB must consider only the risks and benefits that may immediately result from the research. Selection of subjects must be equitable; in order to determine equitability, the IRB must consider the purpose of the research and the setting in which it will be conducted. For example, a study on prostate cancer would be justified in accruing only males, whereas a lung study should have representation from both sexes. If subjects are vulnerable to influence or coercion (for example, persons with severe physical or mental illness, or economically or educationally disadvantaged individuals), appropriate safeguards must be taken to protect their rights and welfare.[5](p8)

Informed Consent

The approval of a research study depends primarily on the informed consent form. The description of the study and procedures must be written in non-technical language. The OPRR has set criteria for what must be included in an informed consent form.[5](p9) Many of these criteria are listed in Table 18-4. Measures must be taken to ensure that subjects understand the study before signing the consent form.

If the research involves more than minimal risk to the subject, a statement must be included about compensation or medical care available if injury occurs. If compensation is available, this must be explained to the subject, as well as where further information can be obtained. Other clauses may be included in the consent form at the behest of the IRB or the study group.

Consent must be informed and must be voluntary. The subject must be mentally competent to understand the information before making the decision to participate in a clinical trial. Other clauses pertaining to the protection of vulnerable subject populations, such as pregnant women, prisoners, fetuses, and children, can be included if applicable. The basic clauses must be addressed before a research study can gain IRB approval.

Table 18-4
Specific Requirements of an Informed Consent Form

1. Statement that the study involves research
2. Explanation of the research
3. Expected duration of the subject's participation
4. Description of the procedures
5. Identification of any experimental procedures
6. Description of any reasonably foreseeable risks or discomforts
7. Description of benefits to the subject or to others
8. Alternative procedures or treatment, if any, which may benefit the subject
9. A statement regarding the extent to which confidentiality of records identifying the subject will be maintained
10. Contact(s) for answers to pertinent questions about the research
11. Contact(s) in the event of a research-related injury
12. Statement of the subject's rights
13. Statement that participation is voluntary
14. Statement that refusal to participate will not result in loss of benefits or a penalty to the subject
15. Statement that the subject may discontinue participation in the study at any time without penalty or loss of benefits

Annual Renewal of the Institutional Review Board Approval

Once initial approval of a study has been granted, the IRB must renew its approval each year unless the renewal interval is otherwise noted. Forms for the renewal process are sent to the principal investigator by the IRB when the review is due. These forms must be submitted prior to the IRB review. Each institution may require additional documentation for the review process.

Approval of Clinical Trial Revisions

Study changes or revisions by the clinical trial group that can affect subjects must be reviewed by the IRB as they occur. Certain changes must be reflected in the consent form. All pertinent changes or revisions must be submitted to the IRB for approval before being used or enforced.[6] Administrative changes such as new phone numbers or minor changes in eligibility (e.g., lower blood values) are not necessarily required to be submitted to the IRB. Each IRB differs in its requirements for the submission of study revisions.

THE OFFICE OF SPONSORED RESEARCH

Purpose and Function

HHS requires each institution involved in research studies to maintain a liaison office, or clearinghouse, which is often called the Office of Sponsored Research or Grants Administration. This office serves as a liaison among the institutions, the Department of Health and Human Services, and other research groups, foundations, or individuals who grant funds to the principal investigators.

The Office of Sponsored Research submits the institution's general assurance to the appropriate federal and research groups. It controls and coordinates the funding of research for the institution. The staff may serve as nonvoting members of the IRB.

Filing of the HHS Form

Once the IRB has approved a study, the PI must submit a form to HHS to document the full IRB approval and date. Copies are distributed to the Office of Sponsored Research, the principal investigator, and the appropriate clinical trial group to facilitate the opening of the study. The clinical trial group will not allow the institution to accrue patients on the study without a copy of this form. The form must be completed and resubmitted each year after the IRB has reapproved the study. It demonstrates the institution's compliance with both IRB and HHS regulations.

ASPECTS OF THE CLINICAL TRIAL

Patient Eligibility

Patient populations are defined in detail in the study protocol. Records of prospective subjects must be reviewed to determine which are eligible for the study. If a patient meets the study eligibility criteria, the attending physician usually discusses the study with the patient or family members. Most studies specify a time frame for a patient's diagnosis date and specific diagnostic tests that must be completed before the patient is eligible for registration. Clinical criteria are defined and may include stage of disease, performance status, and specific values for many required diagnostic tests.

The consent form is presented to the patient after the study has been explained. The form must be written in language that a layperson can understand. It is read to or by the patient or guardian. All questions must be adequately answered. If the patient agrees to participate in the study, the consent form is signed by the patient or guardian, the principal investigator, and other witnesses.

Patient Registration

Patients must be registered for the study by the clinical trial group. This is usually done by telephone or facsimile. The various treatment arms or branches of the study are defined within the protocol, which should also include a schema of the treatment arms. The schema defines the treatment modalities and dosages for each arm.

In studies with more than one treatment arm, the patient is placed on a study arm by randomization, or chance, to eliminate statistical bias and ensure valid results. This is done by personnel at the trial group operations office, who key specific patient information into a computer programmed to choose an arm at random. To make certain that each arm of the study will accrue subjects with varying prognoses or expected outcomes, some studies further separate,

or stratify, certain factors (such as histology, stage of disease, age, and similar variables). The study arm chosen by the computer is then revealed and a case number assigned at the operations office. In blind studies, the study arm is not known to the patient and or the doctor (double-blind).

Data Collection

After patient registration has been completed, the treatment plan is arranged by the physician following the chosen study arm. Each study has a set of forms designed by the clinical trial group. Two basic types of initial data are required by the trial group: clinical data and films, and treatment plan information. These data must be collected in a timely fashion and submitted on approved forms.

The clinical trial groups rate the timeliness and accuracy of data submissions. These ratings and the number or percentage of patients accrued are part of the overall score, that institutions receive from trial groups. Some trial groups allocate grant monies based on this scoring system.

Drug Accountability

It is a federal requirement that all drugs used in clinical trials be stored securely at all times when they are not being dispensed or inventoried. Drug inventory and accountability are evaluated by the clinical trial group during site visits. This is another factor in determining the institutional scores previously mentioned.

Follow-Up Data

After a patient completes the initial treatment, a follow-up examination schedule is arranged according to the requirements of the study. Follow-up is typically conducted on a progressive scale (for example, starting at once a month, then going to once every three months, then every six months). After five years of survival, annual follow-up visits are usually recommended for the duration of the patient's disease free interval. The protocol specifies required follow-up intervals and tests to be performed. As with other aspects of the patient's care, the follow-up data are recorded on forms and submitted to the trial group according to the assigned schedule.

CLINICAL RESEARCH ASSOCIATES

Most major clinical trial groups have been in existence for decades. During most of that time, data managers processed studies for IRB approval, composed consent forms, and collected patient data for individual departments or institutions. These managers were often trained in related healthcare areas, most commonly in the field of nursing or radiation therapy. They were often expected to combine other job responsibilities with the data management of clinical trials.

With the ever-increasing number of large scale national clinical trials and groups, many institutions have dedicated full-time positions to the data management of clinical trials. The personnel hired for these positions were usually trained in related healthcare fields but not necessarily in nursing. These positions were often categorized as clerical, but the duties required highly skilled personnel with medical knowledge, including knowledge of specific diseases. These data managers came to realize a need for formalized recognition and standardization of their skills and knowledge.

In 1989, at the behest of the National Cancer Institute, a group of data managers began working together to form a professional organization. The position title of clinical research associate (CRA) was adopted because it describes the functions and responsibilities of these individuals. In October 1991, the CRAs formed an organization called the Society of Clinical Research Associates (SoCRA).

Since then, the status and contributions of CRAs have increased within most of the national clinical trial groups. Recently, CRAs have taken a more active role in the trial groups by serving on committees with physicians and other healthcare professionals. They now have significant input in the development and performance of new clinical trials. SoCRA has set worldwide professional standards for CRAS.

SoCRA set formal certification standards for CRAs in 1994. The first group of certified clinical research associates (CCRAs) meeting certification requirements was announced in the spring of 1995. In the summer of 1995, SoCRA held its first 10-day training course, a supplemental course for CRAS, at Duke University. The first certification examination was administered in September 1995, at SoCRA's annual meeting.

THE RESEARCH TEAM

The research team conducting clinical trials consists of the principal investigator (a physician), other physicians, one or more CRAS, nurses, technologists, pharmacists, and statisticians. The entire team is responsible for compliance with all institutional and federal regulations while conducting research trials.

INSTITUTIONAL SITE VISITS

The federal government requires principal investigators (Pls) and the institutions participating in clinical trials sponsored by the National Cancer Institute (NCI) to participate in audits (inspections), or site visits, at regular intervals. Clinical trial group personnel and peers of the PI conduct these site visits every three to five years. A representative from the NCI often accompanies the auditors to observe the audit and ensure that it is done in a procedurally and ethically correct manner.

There are specific requirements that the PI and other institutional staff must meet for an acceptable site visit rating. The purpose of the site visit is to verify the following:

- The information submitted on the data collection forms can be supported by the primary patient treatment records, health records, and films at the facility.
- Quality control procedures such as drug inventories for investigational agents meet the required federal standards.
- Policies for IRB review and patient consent are designed for the protection of human subjects.

The institution is normally notified 6 to 10 weeks in advance and given specific instructions to prepare for the site visit. Approximately two to four weeks before the visit, the clinical trial group sends the PI a list of specific studies and cases to be reviewed. Generally, this list consists of approximately 10% of the accrued cases from both the member and affiliate institutions. The cases are selected for review at random in the operations office of the clinical trial group.

Customarily, it is the CRAs that are designated to organize the site visit and assist the auditors in the review process. The PI must be available to explain any medical discrepancies that might be discovered.

At the conclusion of the site visit, the inspectors present an overview of the findings to the PI and other staff.

The PI receives a copy of the final written report several weeks after the visit. A formalized response must be sent to the clinical trial group by the PI within a designated period of time. Both documents must then be forwarded to the NIH by the clinical trial group.

CLINICAL TRIAL GROUP MEETINGS

Clinical trial groups usually host meetings twice each year to examine the ongoing results of each trial. Principal investigators and other members of the research team are invited to attend. Committees meet to discuss research procedures, and educational presentations are offered to the members. The quality assurance committee often meets to assess the overall scores of member and affiliate institutions.

Written reports on current findings for each open clinical trial are compiled and distributed to the attendees. These meetings offer members opportunities to network with their peers, design new studies, and improve the current studies.

REPORTING AND PUBLICATION OF CLINICAL TRIAL STUDY OUTCOMES

In recent years, the publication and distribution of information gleaned from clinical trials have had a significant impact on the practice of medicine. Results of clinical trials have led to improved outcomes in the prevention, diagnosis, and treatment of various diseases. Clinical trial groups and PIs publish their data in medical and scientific journals for medical professionals on a continuing basis. This reporting is vital for the expansion of knowledge and the prospect of cures. Statistics, written summaries, and explanations of treatment techniques are critical for the acceptance of these data by the medical and research community.

IN-HOUSE TRIALS

In-house clinical trials are studies designed by physicians or other staff at an institution and sometimes shared with affiliate members for study accrual. Generally, in-house studies are simpler in design than the studies generated by the national clinical trial groups. The accruals on these studies are usually not large, and the endpoints may be less complex than those of larger national studies. In-house studies must be approved by the institutional review board before activation. The success of an in-house study can lead the PI to design a more complex study based on the same premise. Studies such as this are sometimes modified by national clinical trial groups and made available for national accrual.

ETHICS

The issue of ethics is extremely important in clinical trials. *The Belmont Report,* published several years ago by the federal government, describes the ethical principles and guidelines established for the protection of research subjects. These include respect for persons, beneficence, and justice.[7]

All members of the research community are obligated to ensure the integrity of informed consent, the fair assessment of risks and benefits to the patient, and the just and equitable selection of subjects for research studies.[7](p18) Refer to Chapter 2 and Appendix I of this textbook for further information on ethics and legal issues.

SUMMARY

The membership of a clinical trial group consists of several institutions with investigators who design and administer research studies. A clinical study is the classification of scientific approaches to evaluate a disease and its prevention, diagnostic techniques, and treatments. A clinical trial is a subset of a clinical study that evaluates investigational medications, treatments, devices, or diagnostic or preventive techniques in three basic phases. A protocol is the written procedural guide for a clinical trial.

Three phases are used to categorize clinical trials. Phase I trials are preliminary trials that test toxicity of the investigational techniques and establish basic safe dosage levels of investigational drugs. Phase II trials determine safety and efficacy of investigational drugs or techniques. Phase III trials are the final testing phase for clinical trial groups. These trials provide additional information about the agents or techniques being investigated. Phase IV trials are used only by drug or device manufacturers to gain additional information about the product being tested.

Each clinical trial has a principal investigator who is responsible to the clinical trial group for conducting the research. Most national oncology clinical trial groups are funded through the National Cancer Institute of the National Institutes of Health. An institutional review board must review and approve a clinical trial and its informed consent form before patient accrual can begin.

The institutional review board (IRB) is governed by strict federal guidelines. It must review all new and ongoing research studies within its institution. The composition of the IRB committee is regulated by specific federal requirements. The committee must have both scientific and nonscientific members with various stated qualifications and backgrounds. The IRB's main function is to protect the rights of human subjects participating in research. The IRB has the right to terminate any research study if unexpected risks arise or if the study is not being conducted according to NIH guidelines for approved protocols.

The informed consent form is an important document containing information for the subjects who participate in research studies. Certain elements must be present in every informed consent form. Most of these elements relate to the protection of human subjects. This form must present the study information to the subject in nontechnical language. The subject must understand the information before signing the informed consent form. The principal investigator and witnesses must also sign the form.

Institutions participating in research must have a department or office to serve as a liaison between the institution, the Department of Health and Human Services, and various research foundations and clinical trial groups. This office is often called the Office of Sponsored Research or Grants Administration. It keeps records of specific studies in the institution that are compliant with HHS and IRB regulations and administers research funds and grants to the institution.

Clinical trial protocols outline trial procedures, patient eligibility criteria, registration procedures, treatment or techniques, and timelines for tests, follow-up, and other endpoints. Study-specific data collection forms are distributed by the clinical trial groups. The sponsoring groups also set and monitor data collection schedules for each study case.

The research team conducting clinical trials consists of physicians and other healthcare professionals, including clinical research associates, nurses, technicians, pharmacists, and statisticians. Each member of the team is responsible for ensuring that the trial is conducted in an ethically and procedurally correct manner.

In-house studies are clinical trials conducted within private institutions, with simpler designs and smaller accruals than national clinical trials. They also need IRB approval before patient accrual can begin. These studies are important and, if successful, can lead to larger, more complex trials by national groups.

Site visits are conducted to evaluate the compliance of member institutions with the regulations of the federal government and the involved national clinical trial group. These visits are conducted every three to five years according to strict standards. It is the auditor's responsibility to verify the data collected at the institution through an inspection of the primary patient records, films, and other sources. Institutional ratings are determined by the auditors for each site visit.

Clinical research associates are responsible for collecting and managing the data resulting from clinical trials. They are generally trained in healthcare-related areas and are knowledgeable in medical and research fields.

Advances in medicine are the ultimate result of clinical trial studies. It is important for clinical trial investigators to report their findings to the medical and research communities in order to advance longer survival periods and enhanced quality patient care.

STUDY QUESTIONS

1. Define a clinical trial. How does it differ from a clinical study and a protocol?
2. Define the term *institutional review board*. What is the main purpose of this group?
3. What is informed consent? Why is it important?
4. Describe one of the three phases of a clinical trial.
5. Why is *The Belmont Report* considered important to researchers? List the three principles stated in this report.

REFERENCES

1. Spilker, B. *Guide to Clinical Trials.* New York: Raven Press; 1991: xxi-xxiii.

2. Levine R. *Ethics and Regulations of Clinical Trials.* Baltimore/Munich: Urban Schwarzenberg; 1981: 208.

3. U.S. Department of Health, Education and Welfare. *Issues in Research with Human Subjects.* Bethesda, Md: National Institutes of Health; 1980: 136, 209-210.

4. Freund P, ed. *Experimentation with Human Subjects.* New York, NY: George Braziller; 1970: 410-11.

5. U.S. Department of Health and Human Services. *OPRR Reports: Code of Federal Regulations Title 45—Public Welfare, Part 46—Protection of Human Subjects.* Bethesda, Md: Public Health Service Act; 1991: 6-9, 137.

6. Radiation Therapy Oncology Group. Site Visit Facility Preparation Instructions. Philadelphia, Pa: The Group; 1991: 1.

7. The National Commission for the Protection of Human Subjects of Biomedical and Medical Research. *The Belmont Report: Ethical Principles and Guidelines for the Protection of Human Subjects in Research.* Washington, DC: Department of Health, Education and Welfare; 1985: 18. (Note: the OPRR now sponsors this report.)

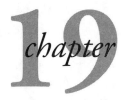
chapter 19

GENERAL PRINCIPLES OF ABSTRACTING AND CANCER REGISTRY FILES

Carol Hahn Johnson
BS, CTR

Carol L. Hutchison
CTR

INTRODUCTION

An abstract is an abbreviated record that identifies the patient, the disease, the cancer-directed treatment, and the disease process from the time of diagnosis until the patient's death. The registry may report to multiple agencies such as the Commission on Cancer (CoC) of the American College of Surgeons (ACoS); Surveillance, Epidemiology, and End Results (SEER) Program; or a regional or state registry. These agencies' case-inclusion and reporting requirements, as well as the institution's reportable list, should be used to decide which data items are collected on the abstract.

The abstract is usually divided into different sections, which are listed in Table 19-1. As molecular-biological studies have progressed, tumor markers have become more relevant in cancer diagnosis and treatment; therefore, some abstracts contain information about the tumor markers.

The abstract is the basis for the rest of the registry's functions. Without the summary data of a patient's cancer experience, no other registry function can take place. Data collection and abstract development should be based on the three major objectives of any cancer registry, which are listed in Table 19-2. For the most part, this chapter discusses the data set described by the CoC for approved hospital cancer programs.

DATA STANDARDS

Using standard data collecting rules and data definitions ensures uniform data. The primary value of data lies in the comparison of the institution's data with data from other databases. In order to compare data, collection of the items to be compared must be made in the same manner using the same rules. The CoC has published *Facility Oncology Registry Data Standards (FORDS),* a data-collection manual for CoC-approved cancer programs.[1] This manual must be the basis of the data collection efforts of all CoC-approved cancer programs. Use of the manual ensures that data collection is the same in all institutions and makes comparison of data more relevant. Detailed information regarding data standards can be found in another chapter of this textbook.

It should be recognized from the beginning that accuracy and consistency are of utmost importance. Methods of ensuring the accuracy of data should be established early. Quality control begins at the time of data collection or abstracting. The *FORDS* manual provides codes for data consistency, which must be used in CoC-approved cancer programs. Policies and procedures should cover special or difficult issues for consistency purposes, which is the most important rule in data collection. An error can be corrected more easily if the data item has been collected in a consistent manner. A simple global change to the database may be all that is needed.

Any changes in codes or staging schemes should be recorded in the procedure manual. If the registry software converts old codes into the new structure, the conversion date should be documented so that data can be easily identified if there are errors.

In addition to *FORDS,* other resources for CoC-approved cancer programs are necessary. At a minimum, the registry should have a medical terminology textbook, the *SEER Summary Staging Manual 2000,* and the most recent editions of the *American Joint Committee on Cancer Manual for Staging of Cancer,* and *International Classification of Diseases for Oncology.* The registry should also secure the latest information regarding regional or state registry requirements. Refer to other chapters of this textbook for further information regarding coding and staging.

Table 19-1
Common Sections in a Cancer Registry Abstract

- Patient identification
- Cancer identification
- Stage of disease at diagnosis
- First course of treatment
- Outcomes
- Case Administration

Table 19-2
Three Major Objectives of a Cancer Registry

1. Identify and access all cases meeting the criteria for inclusion in the registry in a manner that allows useful retrieval of the data.
2. Develop and implement a quality control program that will ensure data of unimpeachable quality.
3. Disseminate the data while maintaining the patients' confidentiality.

ABSTRACTING TIME FRAME AND SUSPENSE LISTING

Availability of information and intended use of the data are key factors in determining the abstracting time frame. The "customers" (the people who request data) must be considered when making this decision. It is important for the cancer committee, administration, or other healthcare professionals to have access to current statistics collected in the registry. As hospital environments change, analysis of cases diagnosed or treated in the facility has become increasingly important to hospital administrators. This type of information can be abstracted at the time of initial diagnosis.

SUSPENSE CASES

Most registry software systems allow the registrar to enter the information that is currently available and save the case as a "suspense" case, which is a reportable case awaiting completion. The registry software should be able to generate a listing of all suspense cases, which typically includes: patient name, patient identifier, date of diagnosis or date of first contact, and primary site.[2]

The suspense list may include cases that, on further inspection, do not fit the criteria for entry into the registry. Refer to Chapter 8, Cancer Registry Management, for information regarding the reportable list. Chapter 12 titled Case Ascertainment, provides further information on casefinding and determining whether the case should be included in the registry.

Information can be abstracted when a patient is discharged from the hospital, and the case should be placed in suspense until it is time to complete it. Some registrars find it more desirable to concurrently abstract cases as information becomes available, especially since more treatment is now done on an outpatient basis. Some treatment may be done in freestanding facilities, and the registrar may need to contact the physician to secure this information for case completeness.

If concurrent abstracting is being done, it is critical to establish a procedure for marking or labeling the abstract as incomplete until the first course of therapy and all data items have been abstracted. It is important to ensure data (especially patient treatment) are complete and accurate, and an established procedure will document the process. No analysis of

first course of therapy can be made until all data are collected and recorded.

In institutions approved by the CoC, abstracting must be completed within six months after the date of first contact.[2] Typically, the complete workup, cancer staging, and planned first course of treatment are usually complete within a six month period.[2] A procedure must be in place to assure the cancer registry abstract is complete within the required time frame.

CASE CLASSIFICATION AND THE DATA SET

The class of case (analytic or nonanalytic) categorizes cases for analysis purposes. The CoC and central registries can change the definition of analytic status. Manuals must be reviewed for analytic definition. The class of case is important and must be assigned correctly as it can affect the administrative reports, which are used for planning and evaluation of service areas.

The following is an overview of certain items included in cancer registry abstracts and where the information can be found in the health record. The actual definition of each data item can be found in the *FORDS* or other appropriate data manuals.

Patient Identification

The patient identification section consists of the following data items that identify the patient or descriptors: Accession number, sequence number, medical record number, social security number, patient's name, patient's address at diagnosis, place of birth, date of birth, race, Spanish origin, sex, primary payer at diagnosis, comorbidities, complications, and the physicians who were involved in the diagnosis and treatment of this cancer.

Most of the information to complete the patient identification data items is usually found on the registration form or the institution's cover sheet (face sheet) for a patient's health record. The eight-digit date of birth and social security number are helpful to the registrar in matching cases or avoiding duplicates and in matching deaths from state death listings.

Accession Number

The accession number is a unique eight-digit number assigned to the patient by the cancer registrar. It is usually generated by the computer software. The first four digits of the number indicate the year in which the patient was first seen for cancer in the reporting institution. The rest of the number is the sequential order in which the patient was identified by the registry or abstracted into the database. For example, if a patient had a positive biopsy in January of 2004 and was the first case identified in 2004, the accession number would be 20040001. It is important to assign accession numbers that include the year in which the patient was first seen in the institution. If, somehow, the patient was not identified for inclusion into the registry until 2005, the accession number should still begin with 2004. Because the accession number identifies the patient, the same number is used for all additional primaries that the patient may develop, regardless of the year in which subsequent reportable tumors occur.

Sequence Number

The sequence number identifies separate primaries for each patient. The sequence number allows the registry to identify patients who have multiple primaries. If the patient has only one primary cancer (malignancy), the sequence number is 00; if the patient has more than one primary cancer, 00 is changed to 01 to indicate that this is the first of several or more primaries. Each subsequent primary is labeled according to the sequence in which it occurred.

It is important to note that the sequence number indicates the number of primary cancers the patient has had in his or her lifetime, not just the number of primary cancers diagnosed or treated at the reporting facility. For example, if a patient is diagnosed or treated at the reporting institution for lung cancer and has a history of breast cancer diagnosed and treated elsewhere, the institution would assign the lung cancer a sequence number of 02 to reflect the fact that it is the second primary for the patient. Sequence numbering is defined in the *FORDS.* Reportable-by-agreement cases now have unique sequence numbers, which were first described with the release of the FORDS in 2002.

Physicians and Institutions Involved with the Case

The names of all physicians involved with the case (such as surgeons and referring, consulting, and following physicians) should be recorded. This information is useful in obtaining additional information

regarding complete first course of treatment and follow-up or patient status for outcome reporting. This information can also be used in administrative reports about physician activity or referrals.

Cancer Identification

The cancer identification section contains data items that describe the disease and contains additional administrative information: class of case, facility referred from, facility referred to, date of first contact, date of initial diagnosis, primary site, laterality, histology, behavior code, grade/differentiation, diagnostic confirmation, tumor size, regional lymph nodes examined, and regional lymph nodes positive. The data elements "hospital referred from" and "hospital referred to" establish patterns of referral, which can be used by administration to identify patient migration patterns. Categories of patients referred from certain areas can be further defined and analyzed by creating subgroups using age, ethnicity, primary payer at diagnosis, and so on. This information can be used in developing marketing strategies and in program planning.

The date of initial diagnosis is the first time a medical practitioner confirms the presence of cancer. Quite often, it is the date of a pathology report, but it may also be based on a laboratory value, radiology report, or physical examination of the patient prior to biopsy. Ambiguous terminology is defined in the *FORDS* to ensure consistency in establishing the date of diagnosis.

The admission history, physical examinations, radiology studies, and laboratory studies performed during the current admission and any earlier admissions are the sources of information used to determine the site, histology, and extent of disease. The admission history and physical may provide clues to where the workup was done prior to admission. The admitting diagnosis is used to determine whether the diagnosis of cancer has already been made and the patient is being admitted for confirmation or whether the diagnosis is currently unknown. For some sites, the physical examination may provide information about laterality. It is important to look for copies of, or reference to, outside studies in the patient's record.

Stage of Disease at Diagnosis

The section for stage of disease at diagnosis contains data items that identify the stage of disease and items that confirm and support the assigned stage. The staging information must include the assessment of three components: tumor (T), node (N), and metastasis (M), which have numerical subsets. In effect, the system is a shorthand notation for describing the clinical and/or pathologic anatomic extent of a particular malignant tumor at diagnosis. A clinical or pathological stage group is determined from these three components.[3] The staging categorization for the summary stage or collaborative stage must be recorded according to the current manuals.

The pathology report contains important information about histology and is helpful in assigning a stage. More information on staging and extent of disease can be found in Chapter 16 of this textbook. If the primary tumor has been completely excised, the pathology report should include the size of the primary tumor. If the primary tumor has not been excised, the next best determination of size is usually a radiographic study. Supporting staging information can be found in mammograms for breast, sonograms for prostate, and Computerized Tomography (CT) or Magnetic Resonance Imaging (MRI) scans may for other parts of the body.

First Course of Treatment

This section contains data items that describe the surgical procedures, radiation therapy, chemotherapy, hormonal therapy, immunotherapy, hematologic transplant, and endocrine procedures, as well as palliative procedures. All treatment fields should be recorded according to the definitions in the registry's data dictionary. Surgical procedures include biopsies of the primary tumor or of a metastatic site. Operative reports provide information on exactly whether the tumor was biopsied or excised. This information may affect the staging of the cancer.

Determining first course of treatment can be difficult. First course of therapy is the treatment that is either given or planned at the time of initial diagnosis. Some treatment regimens may take a year or more to complete. An example of an extended first course of treatment could be a patient diagnosed with inflammatory carcinoma of the breast. The patient is diagnosed by biopsy and treated with several cycles of chemotherapy (which may take five months or more). At that time, a mastectomy may be done. After the patient has recovered from the mastectomy, radiotherapy may be given. If all of this treatment was planned when the patient was initial-

ly diagnosed, it should be included in the first course of therapy.

The opposite situation can also happen. A patient may come in with a primary tumor of the colon. Diagnostic workup may include liver function studies and other tests that indicate no metastatic disease. Surgery would be a complete removal of the primary tumor. If, at the six-week postoperative checkup, liver function studies are abnormal and a scan shows hepatic metastases, the patient would be placed on chemotherapy. The chemotherapy was not planned at the time of initial diagnosis. The chemotherapy was given because of disease progression or recurrence. The second course of therapy is treatment initiated either because the disease did not respond to the first treatment, or because the disease progressed or recurred.

Outcomes

The outcomes section consists of the follow-up fields: date of first recurrence, type of first recurrence, date of last contact or death, vital status, cancer status, following registry, follow-up source, and next follow-up source.

The date of first recurrence has increased in importance as quality of survival is being studied more intensely. In some cases, the goal may be to delay recurrence rather than to prevent it. The date of first recurrence is determined by a physician and always follows a disease-free interval (the patient must be completely free of disease before a recurrence can be recorded).

If a date of first recurrence is reported, the type of first recurrence must also be recorded. This may be either local recurrence, which is recurrence of the primary tumor itself; regional recurrence, which is recurrence beyond the limits of the organ of origin; or distant recurrence, which is disseminated recurrence or recurrence that is remote from the original primary tumor.

Follow-up data include the name, address, telephone number, and relationship of a relative, friend, or neighbor who is most likely to know how to locate the patient. Multiple listings for contacts are common. The name of the spouse should be recorded for married adults and the next of kin for children. These data items can usually be found on the facility's registration form or cover sheet. These items are used to obtain follow-up information.

Follow-up information on the initial abstract includes the last date the patient was known to be alive or the date of death. The status of the cancer must be recorded. This information is updated at least annually according to CoC requirements. The facility's cancer committee may choose to require more frequent follow-up for some sites. More detailed information about follow-up can be found in Chapter 14 of this textbook.

Case Administration

The case administration section contains override flags and identifies coding systems used to abstract the case, the version of coding manual that was used to abstract the case, the reporting facility, and the abstractor who coded and abstracted the data.

PATIENT INDEX

The patient index[2] is an alphabetical list of patients in the registry's database since its reference date. The list must contain date of birth, date of diagnosis, date of last contact or death, histology, laterality, medical record number, patient name, primary site(s), sequence number, and sex. If registries serve multiple facilities, the patient index includes facility identifiers. The reporting system can generate a master patient index, but the list must be in natural language, not computer codes (in other words, the codes must be translated into English).

ACCESSION REGISTER

The accession register is an annual, sequential listing of all eligible cases included in the registry's database. It is sorted by accession year. The accession register includes, but is not limited to accession and sequence number, date of initial diagnosis, patient name, and primary site. If a registry serves multiple institutions, the register must include facility identifiers. The accession register is used to audit other registry files, monitor casefinding, assess the work load, plan cancer conferences, and select cases for quality review.[2] Reportable-by-agreement cases may also be included in the register.

Numerical gaps in accession numbers are allowed. If a case is deleted from the database for a legitimate reason, the accession number must not be reused for another case. This prevents any chance of two cases having the same accession number. If the case had been reported to a state, central, or nation-al registry before it was deleted and the number was used for another case, the collecting registry would have the original case identified with that accession number, which would create multiple problems. Many regional, state, and national registries use the hospital accession number as the patient identifier.

SUMMARY

The most valuable database is one that is complete with flawless information. The labor that goes into abstracting the data from the health record is offset by the usefulness of the data. It is important to remember that the data input must be accurate in order for the data output to be reliable. The ability to produce reports beneficial to physicians, researchers, administrators, and other healthcare professionals is of paramount importance to the future of the registry. Registry data and the outcomes can be used as internal or external benchmarks.

The content of the data set should be carefully considered before data analysis. Data standards and codes must be in place and meet the requirements of the governing body.

STUDY QUESTIONS

1. List common sections of the cancer registry abstract.
2. What diagnostic tests can be used to find the tumor size or staging information?
3. What determines the data set that will be collected by the cancer registry?
4. What is the significance of a sequence number?
5. Where would the registrar find most of the patient identification information?
6. How is the first course of treatment time period determined?
7. List two files commonly required for cancer registries?

REFERENCES

1. Commission on Cancer. *Facility Oncology Registry Data Standards.* Chicago, Ill: Commission on Cancer; 2002.
2. Commission on Cancer. *Cancer Program Standards 2004.* Chicago, Ill : *Commission on Cancer;* 2003.
3. Greene FL, Page DL, Fleming ID, et al. *AJCC Cancer Staging Manual,* 6th ed. New York, NY: Springer-Verlag; 2002.

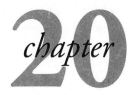

chapter 20

MONITORING PATIENT OUTCOME: FOLLOW-UP

Donna M. Gress
RHIT, CTR

INTRODUCTION

The primary purposes of follow-up are to ensure continued medical surveillance and to monitor the health status of the population under investigation. Follow-up information provides the documentation of residual disease or its spread, recurrences, or additional malignancies and vital status. Subsequent treatments must be included in the patient database.

Outcome and end-results data enable researchers, physicians, and others to assess clinical standards and quality of care. Follow-up information must be comprehensive. To produce survival data, successful follow-up must be maintained. These factors necessitate an organized system of long-term surveillance. The follow-up system can promote optimal patient care and provide a valuable record of patient outcomes.

CONFIDENTIALITY

The issues of confidentiality must be emphasized when obtaining patient data, especially follow-up information. Cancer registries must have policies and procedures approved by the cancer committee,[1,2] including a procedure for both written and verbal contacts.

It has been reported that, occasionally, follow-up information has been obtained by cancer registry staff pretending to be representatives of organizations other than the hospital. This method of obtaining follow-up information is both unethical and illegal; misrepresentation is not a lawful practice. Chapters 4–5 of this text provide detailed information about confidentiality and relevant laws that should be reviewed. The National Cancer Registrars Association's *Code of Ethics* (see Appendix I of this textbook) also addresses the issues of confidentiality and staff conduct.

HIPAA

In 1996, the Health Insurance Portability and Accountability Act (HIPAA) was passed. HIPAA requires that when changing insurance, pre-existing conditions cannot be denied (the portability part of the law); it calls for common sense privacy and security protection of the personal patient information (the accountability section); and mandates standardized health transactions and coding to decrease administrative overhead.[3] See Chapter 4 in this text-

book for a more complete discussion on HIPPA. Although clear-cut and universally acceptable interpretations of the possible effects HIPAA may have on follow-up are not yet available, some caution may be warranted. The Commission on Cancer of the American College of Surgeons has addressed this issue in their "Frequently Asked Questions Received by the CoC Related to *HIPAA*" in their *HIPAA Security Policies and Procedures,* revised July 10, 2003. Their opinion is that registrars can continue to obtain treatment and follow-up information from other hospitals and physicians, even those not on staff at the registrar's hospital. Under the HIPAA Final Privacy Rule, private practice physicians may disclose patient Protected Health Information (PHI) to hospitals for the purpose of treatment, payment, and healthcare operations. Quality assessment/improvement, treatment, and follow-up information are all considered healthcare operations.[4] NAACCR has provided an opinion: Private practice physicians and hospitals may continue to provide treatment and follow-up information to hospital cancer registries without patient authorization. Although private practice physicians and hospitals are health providers, and thus covered under the provisions of the HIPAA privacy regulations, they may continue to provide cancer patient follow-up and treatment information to hospital cancer registries without patient authorization when both the physician and the hospital have or previously had a relationship with the patient. Again, this information is considered part of the covered healthcare operations.[5]

REQUIREMENTS OF THE COMMISSION ON CANCER

The Commission on Cancer (CoC) of the American College of Surgeons requires approved cancer programs to maintain an 80% follow-up rate for all analytic reportable patients from the cancer registry reference date. A 90% follow-up rate is maintained for all analytic reportable patients diagnosed within the last five years, or from the cancer registry reference date, whichever is shorter.[1] The follow-up rate is calculated on all eligible reportable patients, both living and dead. The rate is also calculated based on patients, not on individual primaries. If a patient has multiple primaries in the registry, they are just counted once in the follow-up calculations.

The CoC considers a patient to be delinquent if no contact has been made with the patient within fifteen months after the date of last contact.[2] An institution may request its registry to follow certain patients with various tumor types, sites, or stages more frequently than annually.

Names of patients who are lost to follow-up (delinquent) should remain in the follow-up system until follow-up is obtained. The follow-up system must be audited periodically to determine that all patients lost to follow-up remain in the system and are continually pursued for current follow-up.

The CoC requests follow-up statistics at the time of an institution survey; the follow-up calculations are part of the survey application. Most registry software systems have a programmed report for calculating these statistics. The information used for CoC calculations is illustrated in Figure 20-1.

POLICIES AND PROCEDURES

The cancer committee is responsible for the supervision of the cancer registry.*[1] Follow-up rates should be monitored by this governing body. If the cancer registry experiences problems obtaining follow-up, the cancer committee should be informed. The cancer committee should be directly involved in finding solutions to problems that the registry encounters, including difficulties with follow-up.

Cases and Frequency

The cancer committee determines the types of cases to be followed. Though the cases listed in Table 20-1 are not included in the calculation rates for cancer programs approved by the CoC, individual institutions may choose to follow them.

The frequency of contact and procedures for initiation of follow-up are also established by the cancer committee. Follow-up letters are usually initiated at 12 months after the most recent date of contact in order to obtain information before the case is considered delinquent. Some registries send physician letters at 13 months to allow the patient the entire anniversary month to complete their annual follow-up visits.

Method

The cancer committee also determines the sequence of contacts or sources for follow-up. Permission must be given by the governing body or appropriate physician to contact patients. The method and system must be approved by proper authorities and documented in a policy and procedure format. Cancer registries may need to request permission from the physician before contacting patients.

Blanket permission may be granted by the medical staff at the request of the cancer committee. This request is usually channeled through the medical executive committee. If the request is denied, blanket permission to contact patients from individual physicians may be necessary. Letters granting permission should be kept on file in the registry.

Blanket permission is most frequently granted when the procedure is well described in the request. Sample letters or dialogue to be used in contacts should be provided to the person(s) from whom the permission is being requested. The medical staff may wish to impose some restrictions. For instance, the registry staff may be instructed not to mention the patient's diagnosis unless the patient does so first. This restriction has often been applied in the past and can help alleviate problems for the registry staff.

The cancer committee should decide if letters are to be signed by the registry staff or the cancer committee chairperson. A policy should be defined for the registry staff for initiating telephone calls to patients and contacts other than physician offices. Often, cancer registrars are required by the governing body to identify themselves by another title, such as *follow-up registrar,* rather than using the term *cancer registrar.*

Occasionally, a patient will contact the registry in response to a follow-up letter, requesting a referral to a new physician, an appointment, or general information. A policy should be established to manage such situations.

Data Set

The Commission on Cancer (CoC) of the American College of Surgeons core follow-up data items for approved cancer programs are listed in Table 20-2.[2]

Personnel Requirements and Resources

An adequate staff and budget must be provided to handle the follow-up volume. The staff must be trained and qualified to represent the institution in this process. The work area must be quiet during communication with patients and other contacts. Equipment needs will affect budgetary considerations.

The follow-up function of the registry can enhance the public relations of the institution. The person conducting follow-up must convey profes-

Figure 20-1
Follow-Up Calculations

	Exclusions	Total
Patients to Be Followed—Total Cases in Database Minus the Following:		XX
Less additional primaries for patients (patients are counted not each primary)	x	
Less patients prior to reference date	x	
Less benign and borderline patients prior to 1/1/04 (except juvenile astrocytoma which should be recorded as 9421/3)	x	
Less carcinoma in situ of cervix, CIN III, PIN III, VIN III, VAIN III, AIN III cases	x	
Less skin ca on or after 1/1/03, histology 8000-8110	x	
Less skin ca prior to 1/1/03, histology 8000-8110, AJCC stage group II, III, IV	x	
Less non-analytic patients (class of case 3, 4, 5, 6, 7, 8, 9)	x	
Less patients not yet completed	x	
Less residents of foreign countries (excludes US territories, Virgin Islands and Puerto Rico)	x	
Less patients reportable-by-agreement	x	
Less patients whose age exceeds 100 years and who are without contact for more than 12 months	x	
Final Subtotal of Patients to be Followed (to be used as "A" in calculations below for all patients since reference date)		XX
Less patients greater than 5 years since reference date if the database contains more than 5yrs of cases	x	
Final Subtotal of Patients to be Followed (to be used as "A" in calculations below for all patients within last 5 years of reference date)		XX

                                                                                                                        %

I.   Calculation of All Analytic Reportable Patients from Cancer Registry Reference Date

     A. Subtotal (reportable patients required to be followed)   100%

     B. Less number dead (vital status = 0)   %

     C. Subtotal of cases living (vital status = 1)   %

     D. Current follow-up (alive within last 15 months)*   %

     E. Lost to follow-up (delinquent, more than 15 months from date of last contact)   %

          *D should be >80% to be in compliance with standards

II. Calculation of All Analytic Reportable Patients Diagnosed Within the Last Five Years or from the Reference Date, Whichever Is Shorter

     A. Subtotal (reportable patients required to be followed with diagnose date less than or equal to last 5yrs of registry or from reference date, whichever is shorter)   100%

     B. Less number dead (vital status = 0)   %

     C. Subtotal of cases living (vital status = 1)   %

     D. Current follow-up (alive within last 15 months)*   %

     E. Lost to follow-up (delinquent, more than 15 months from date of last contact)   %

          *D should be ≥90% to be in compliance with standards

(continued)

Figure 20-1
(continued)

NOTE FOR FOLLOW-UP CALCULATIONS:
A-B=C
D+E=C
B+D+E=A (100%)
B+C=A (100%)
B+D= follow-up rate
E=lost to follow-up rate

Calculate percentages for D by dividing D by A x100.
Calculate percentages for E by dividing E by A x 100.

Table 20-1

Types of Reportable Cases Excluded from Calculations of CoC Follow-Up Rates for Approved Cancer Programs

- Residents of foreign countries
- Cases that are reportable-by-agreement
- Patient whose age exceeds 100 years and who are without contact for more than 12 months

Table 20-2

Required Data-Set Items, Follow-Up Data

- Date of first recurrence
- Type of first recurrence
- Date of last contact or death
- Vital status
- Cancer status
- Following registry
- Follow-up source
- Next follow-up source (method)

sionalism and be knowledgeable about available resources and general institutional information. This person must be comfortable talking about cancer with others, because this subject can potentially be disturbing to the contacts.

A telephone and telephone line are mandatory when managing follow-up procedures. The person conducting follow-up should have access to a computer with Internet access for working with the registry follow-up. Depending upon the facility's budgeting process, postage may need to be requested for the budget.

Telephone directories from cities in referral areas are helpful in obtaining addresses in addition to telephone numbers. City directories with street addresses are also helpful in locating correct mailing addresses, but using physician rosters can be more time-effective and accurate. The Internet can provide the telephone book resources on-line and can be searched using name, address and other criteria for both physicians and patients.

The Internet has become a very useful tool in identifying patients that have expired. It can provide specif-

ic dates and places of death on patients where information is vague. There are a number of websites based on the government's Social Security Death Index. Two sites are www.ssdi.genealogy.rootsweb.com and www.ancestry.com/search/rectype/vital/ssdi/main.html. Patients can be searched by name or social security number, and on some sites by last known residence or birth and/or death dates. Another option is the National Obituary Archive (NOA). This can be found on the website www.arrangeonline.com. Cases can be searched by name, last known residence, or a range of approximate dates of death.

The type of follow-up letter generated by the computer is a factor in deciding what stationery to use. The type of envelope used for mailing the letters also must be considered. For example, different software systems require either labels or window envelopes for follow-up letters. Most cancer registries provide a self-addressed, stamped envelope in which to return the reply.

Sources and Other Contacts

The follow-up process actually begins with the initial abstracting process. All information that may be useful for follow-up must be abstracted first. If a patient is transferred to another hospital for treatment, the registry or other department there should be listed as a follow-up contact. Other follow-up contacts can include home care, nursing homes, or hospices. It is helpful to document any unusual circumstances such as blindness, difficulties in hearing, or the fact that the patient does not speak English.

Other possible sources to consider are listed in Table 20-3; however, the cancer committee must authorize the registry staff to contact them. The method and dialogue of follow-up must be designated by the cancer committee. Most registries also review obituaries and compare them with their patient index files.

Table 20-3

Partial List of Sources Used for Obtaining Follow-Up Information

- Armed Forces locating services
- Bureaus of vital statistics
- County assessor offices
- County welfare departments
- Credit bureaus
- Death indexes or searches
- Departments of motor vehicles
- Embassies or consulates
- Employers or unions
- Halls of records (recorded marriages and births)
- Healthcare finance administrations
- Hospices
- Insurance companies
- Internet websites
- Local, county, or state records
- Other registries (for example, hospital, central, or state)
- Professional organization directories
- Public housing and public utilities
- Religious organizations
- Schools and alumni groups
- Social security administration
- State boards of certification and licensure
- Visiting nurse and home care agencies
- Voter registration

The National Cancer Registrars Association does not endorse any of the sources listed in Table 20-3. However, these sources have been reported by cancer registrars as effective tools.

When mailing follow-up letters to patients, families, or friends, stamping "Address Correction Requested" on the envelope is useful. The United States Postal Service will usually return the letter with a forwarding address within a certain time period.

Registrars have reported success when sending letters by certified mail, return receipt requested. When the patient signs the card, the United States Postal Service carrier dates it. The signature must be verified with the health information record. If the signatures match, the follow-up is reliable.

Follow-Up Letters

Follow-up letters should be developed for each type of contact. These letters represent the facility and must be approved by the appropriate hospital committees, the hospital administration, or the cancer committee. All letters should identify the hospital and registry, either by using hospital stationery or printing the information in the letter. The registry telephone number should also be included.

Letter content depends on the type of contact. Letters to nonmedical contacts must be written in a language that is easily understood. Hospital policy determines whether the word *cancer* is mentioned in the letter. Exercise caution in using this word, especially if in situ or benign cases are followed. A separate letter must be designed for these contacts that do not use the word *cancer*. Letters to physicians or other healthcare contacts can include technical or disease-specific information.

It is important to use direct phrasing in an understandable language in order to obtain a response. Contacts must understand what information is being requested and a clear message facilitates a quicker response than ambiguous terminology or wording. Samples of successful follow-up letters are shown in Figures 20-2, 20-3, 20-4, and 20-5.

THE FOLLOW-UP PROCESS

Initiation of Follow-Up

Follow-up should be generated each month. A control list of patients due for follow-up can be compiled and compared manually or electronically to

Figure 20-2
Sample Follow-Up Letter to Physicians

To: James Smith, M.D.   Date of letter: 11/17/04
          123 Any Street
          Anytown, XX 99999   Last follow-up date
                                      other hospital #

From: John Doe, M.D.   Re: Doe, Jane Mary
         Chair, Cancer Committee   Date of Birth: 1/1/40
                                        Diagnosis: breast CA
                                        TR#: 910123/00 (Accession and Sequence)

An annual follow-up of registered cancer cases seen at Anytown Medical Center is conducted by the Cancer Registry. We would appreciate receiving the latest information you have on the patient listed above. Please direct questions to the Cancer Registry at (999) 555-9999

Patient Status:

1. **Alive**—Date last seen or contacted: _____

    A. Status of Neoplasm   B. Quality of Survival

        No evidence of cancer _____   Normal activity   _____
        With evidence of cancer _____   Symptomatic and
                                         ambulatory   _____

        Cancer status *unknown* _____   Ambulatory more than
                                         50%, occasionally
                                         needs assistance   _____

        New areas of recurrence
        and/or metastasis   _____   Ambulatory less than
                                         50%, nursing care
        Site: _____   needed   _____

                                         Bedridden, may require
                                       hospitalization   _____

    C. Additional therapy within the last year
        Surgery: _____   Date: _____
        Radiation: site _____ rads: _____ Date: _____
        Chemotherapy: _____   Date: _____
        Hormone therapy: _____   Date: _____
        Other: _____   Date: _____

2. **Expired**—place: _____   Date: _____
    Cause of death: _____   Autopsy? _____Yes _____No

Patient referred to: _____

New patient address: _____

Comments: _____

Figure 20-3
Sample Follow-Up Letter That Can Be Sent to Nursing Home or Convalescent Hospital

---

Date of Letter: 11/17/04

Care Convalescent Home
1234 Any Street
Anytown, XX 99999

An annual follow-up of all patients treated at Anytown Medical Center with a diagnosis of cancer is conducted by the Cancer Registry. Our record show that the patient listed below was transferred to your facility. To complete our records, we would appreciate information regarding the patient. Any questions may be directed to the Cancer Registry at (999) 555-9999.

Sincerely,

John Doe, M.D.
Chair, Cancer Committee

Re: Doe, Jane Mary   Last Follow-Up Date:
Date of Birth: 1/1/40   Accession Number/Sequence:
Diagnosis: Breast CA

Patient Status:
1. **Alive**—Still in your facility: _____ Yes _____ No
   If answer is no—date transferred: _____
                    —where transferred: _____

   A. Status of Neoplasm   B. Quality of Survival

       No evidence of cancer   _____   Normal activity   _____
       With evidence of cancer _____   Symptomatic and
                                                  ambulatory   _____

       Cancer status *unknown* _____   Ambulatory more than
                                                  50%, occasionally
                                                  needs assistance   _____

       New areas of recurrence
       and/or metastasis   _____   Ambulatory less than
                                                  50%, nursing care
       Site: _____   needed   _____

                                              Bedridden, may require
                                              hospitalization   _____

2. **Expired**—place: _____   Date: _____

   Cause of death: _____   Autopsy? _____Yes _____No

Comments: _____

Patient's Attending Physician: _____

Address: _____

Figure 20-4
Sample Follow-Up Letter to Patient

Date: 11/17/04   Last F/U Date:
                                                  Accession number/Sequence Number

Jane Mary Doe
123 Patient Street
Anytown, XX 99999

Dear Jane Mary Doe,

The staff of Anytown Medical Center has a continuing interest in its patients and would appreciate receiving the information requested below concerning your condition since you were treated here. We recommend that you have a physical examination annually or more often if warranted by you or your physician.

What is the condition of your general health at the present time?

_____

Have you had any further medical or surgical treatment relating to the cancer since leaving this hospital? If so, please describe briefly:

_____

_____

Who is your physician now?   _____

Physician's address: _____

If your address given above is not correct, please provide present address:

_____

Telephone Number: _____

If you are unable to complete this questionnaire, it would be greatly appreciated if you could obtain the assistance of a friend or relative and supply as much information as possible.

Any further comments you may wish to make may be written on the reverse side of this letter. A stamped, return-addressed envelope is enclosed for your convenience. Thank you for taking the time to respond to our patient information letter. We at Anytown Medical Center are genuinely interested in your health and look forward to hearing from you soon. Any questions may be directed to the Cancer Registry at (999) 555-9999.

Sincerely yours,

John Doe, M.D.
Chair, Cancer Program

Figure 20-5
Sample Follow-Up Letter That Can Be Sent to Relative or Friend

Date of Letter: 11/17/04   Last Follow-Up Date:
                                                      Accession number/Sequence Number

Susan Doe
123 Friend Street
Anytown, XX 99999

Dear Susan Doe,

The staff of Anytown Medical Center has a continuing interest in its patients and has been unable to contact

       Jane Mary Doe

For purposes of follow-up, we are most anxious to communicate with a number of our former patients. If you have any knowledge of the whereabouts of this patient, we would appreciate it if you would record the information at the bottom of this page and return it to us in the enclosed return-addressed envelope. Any questions may be directed to the Cancer Registry at (999) 555-9999.

Thank you for your assistance.

Sincerely yours,

John Doe, M.D.
Chair, Cancer Program

Please provide:

Present whereabouts of JANE MARY DOE

Address: _____

City and State: _____

Telephone Number: _____

Present condition: Apparently well _____ Not well _____

hospital admission and outpatient records, if other methods do not exist to notify the registry of recent activity in patients' files. If the patient has returned to the facility, records are obtained and appropriate information extracted. Some health information management departments automatically route the record to the cancer registry if a diagnosis of cancer is coded (whether coded active, metastatic, or "history of") allowing the information to be updated on a more current routine basis. Some registries have identified in the hospital database all those patient names that are also in the registry database. All registry names must be entered into this hospital database just once, and new names added on a routine basis when cases are abstracted. This allows registries to automatically receive a listing each month of all of the names in their registry database that had returned to the facility that month. It eliminates the need to look up the same names year after year. This list can be used to update the follow-up information before the control list is compiled, eliminating many of those who would have been due for follow-up.

If the patient has not returned to the institution, follow-up letters are usually mailed to the managing or referring physician. Letters may be sent to other physicians involved in the care of the patient. If physicians have not seen the patient since the date of last contact, follow-up letters are then usually sent to the nursing home, patient, family members, or other contacts.

If a response has not been received, letters are mailed to new sources until all potential sources have been exhausted. Follow-up procedures vary with different software systems. Letters can be generated individually or in a group, depending on the software.

Attempts should be made periodically to contact all patients who do not have current follow-up. By doing so, the registry can reduce the number of patients that are lost to follow-up and improve the registry's follow-up rate. Even though a patient becomes lost after three months, fifteen months from date of last contact, that should not end the attempts for follow-up. Persistence is usually successful.

Follow-Up Responses

When follow-up letters are returned, the return address on the envelope should be verified against the current address shown in the registry. The date should be requested in the letter for the patient or contact to complete. If the date is blank, the date

stamped on the return envelope can be recorded as date of last contact. Do not record the date of last contact as the date the letter was received in the registry, as it may have been in the mail system for a few days. If a patient has multiple primary cancers, all records should be updated with the date of last contact. Because the status of each cancer can be different, each is coded independently.

FOLLOW-UP FILES

Computerized Registries

Registry software systems incorporate abstracted follow-up information into appropriate fields and files within the system. Computerized registries rely on the software to compute the follow-up due date. The concept is the same for computerized registries as previously described for manual registries.

A computerized registry is more efficient than a manual registry, and the Commission on Cancer of the American College of Surgeons now requires approved cancer programs to maintain computerized records.

Manual Registries

Though most registries are computerized, information is provided in this chapter for a manual follow-up system. Older registries may use a manual system until existing cases are computerized. This information can help other registries or new cancer registries begin follow-up procedures until software is in place. A registrar may be asked by another department, such as research or community outreach screening programs, for assistance in setting up a follow-up system.

Manual registries need a method to indicate which patients are due for follow-up. The most common method is the dual tickler file. A follow-up or "tickler" card is created at the time of abstracting. An index card is satisfactory. This card contains patient identifiers, contacts, and date of last contact. Only one card should be prepared for a patient, regardless of the number of primary cancers. All cancers or reportable diseases should be listed on the patient's follow-up card.

A dual tickler file contains two sets of monthly guides. One set is for the current year, the other for the following year. A follow-up card is filed alphabetically in the same month last seen but in the following year. For example, if a patient was last seen on December 22, 2002, the follow-up card would be filed alphabetically in the December 2003 section, or the second set of months.

The dual tickler file is for tracking living patients that are due for follow-up. At the beginning of each month, follow-up cards should be pulled from the current month to prepare and mail letters for patients due for follow-up. As follow-up is received, the information should be processed as described.

The date of last contact should be recorded on both the abstract and patient follow-up card. When patient follow-up information is obtained, the abstract is retrieved to add the date of last contact. The follow-up card is removed from its current position, the date of last contact is updated, and the card is filed appropriately in the month due for follow-up the next year.

A section at the beginning of the tickler file should be designated for the cases that are over one year delinquent and those monthly guides have had to be moved to the back for the second part of the dual tickler file. At the end of each month that is over one year old, the remaining cards should be alphabetized together and the section marked with the year. The monthly divider cards are placed in the back of the dual tickler file for cases to be followed during the next year. For example, when sending out letters due for follow-up in December 2002, and the second half of the ticker file contains the months for 2003, cards for patients last seen in December 2001 would need to be removed from that monthly card and grouped with cards from January through November 2001. The December monthly section card is now needed for those whose next date of follow-up will be December 2003.

Regular attempts should be made to obtain follow-up information. All cases (represented by cards) needing follow-up should be reviewed routinely and continued attempts should be made to obtain follow-up until current information is obtained. This includes all delinquent cases.

CANCER REGISTRY BROCHURES

Some registries inform patients they will be followed each year by a cancer registry and physicians. This is explained in a brochure that is usually given to the patient within the first few weeks after diagnosis.[6]

The brochure can be provided in a folder with other resource materials. If the patient is in the hospital, the brochure and other information can be taken to the patient by the registry staff. Some registries mail the brochure with the patient follow-up letter to further explain the follow-up process.

The brochure explains the purpose of follow-up and registry functions. Confidentiality issues are addressed in the brochure. The brochure explains that the patient's information is made available for research analysis and that aggregate data are made available to other research databases such as the National Cancer Data Base. It would also inform them of the laws in their state regarding cancer reporting and if follow-up information is part of that program. Various types of additional information can be included within the brochure, such as current American Cancer Society statistics, and cancer prevention and control reminders.

The patient may be given a wallet-size card containing the registry's phone number and address. Some registries give patients a self-addressed stamped postcard to report their new address in the event that they move.

SUMMARY

Follow-up ensures continued medical surveillance and monitors the health status of patients. The course of disease or new malignancies can be tracked and clinical standards, and outcomes can be assessed by researchers and others, with accurate and timely data. The Commission on Cancer (CoC) of the American College of Surgeons has a required follow-up data set for approved cancer programs.

Confidentiality is extremely important, especially when working with follow-up. Follow-up policies and procedures must be approved by the cancer committee.

The CoC standards require approved cancer programs to meet certain follow-up percentages annually. Certain cases are not required to be included in these types of calculations. Follow-up rates must be monitored by the cancer committee. The cancer registrar must consider the timeline to initiate follow-up in relationship to when a case becomes delinquent. All patients must remain in the system, even if they are considered lost-to-follow-up.

Adequate staffing, equipment, and work areas must be provided for the registry to manage follow-up operations. Follow-up can augment hospital public relations with the community.

The follow-up process begins with the initial abstracting process. There are many sources in the health information record that can be used for follow-up purposes. The cancer committee or governing body, depending on institution policy, must give the registry staff permission to contact a source before they can initiate the contact.

Follow-up letters must be prepared for each type of contact. All letters should identify the hospital and registry. The wording of the letters is important to encourage a response. The Cancer Committee must decide if the word *cancer* should be used. If benign cases are followed, the word *cancer* must not be included in follow-up letters or dialogue.

Follow-up letters should be generated each month. Attempts should be made routinely to contact patients or others for updates. If a patient has more than one primary, the vital status of each must be recorded on the patient record.

A follow-up system contributes to a worthwhile record of patient outcome. Accurate survival data are only possible if successful follow-up is maintained.

STUDY QUESTIONS

1. What is the primary purpose of follow-up?
2. What is the required rate (percentage) for follow-up in programs approved by the Commission on Cancer of the American College of Surgeons?
3. After what time period are cases considered delinquent if no contact has been made?
4. List three types of patients that are not required to be followed in programs approved by the Commission on Cancer of the American College of Surgeons.
5. Explain the benefit of providing patients with cancer registry brochures.

REFERENCES

1. Commission on Cancer. *Cancer Program Standards 2004.* Chicago, Ill: American College of Surgeons; 2003.
2. Commission on Cancer. *Facility Oncology Registry Data Standards.* Chicago, Ill: American College of Surgeons; 2002.
3. Health Insurance Portability And Accountability Act Of 1996 (HIPAA) Public Law 104-191, 104th Congress, August. 21, 1996.
4. American College of Surgeons Commission on Cancer. *HIPAA Security Policies and Procedures,* "Frequently Asked Questions Received by the CoC Related to HIPAA," revised July 10, 2003.
5. North American Association of Central Cancer Registries. "Frequently Asked Questions and Answers about Cancer Reporting and the HIPAA Privacy Rule," revised March 31, 2003.
6. Greene F, Andrews K. "Patient follow-up brochure provided by the cancer registry." *News from the Commission on Cancer of the American College of Surgeons.* 1993; 4(2): 6-7.

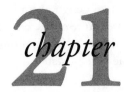

chapter 21

QUALITY CONTROL OF CANCER REGISTRY DATA

Frances Ross
BA, CTR

INTRODUCTION

Registries seek to identify and enumerate every instance of a reportable condition within a defined population. Hospital cancer registries strive to include every reportable malignancy diagnosed or treated within their patient populations. The registration process is rarely perfect and a variety of errors can occur: nonreportable cases can be erroneously included, reportable cases omitted, and cases misclassified. The function of registry quality control is to maximize correct reporting and to characterize the reporting process in measurable terms. This ultimately allows the registry to produce accurate and useful information about cancer incidence and cancer care within its population.

DEFINITIONS

Quality is usually defined as fitness for use.[1] If the overall features and characteristics of a product fulfill the needs of its users, it is of high quality. Quality characteristics must be operationally defined and quantifiable. An operational definition includes both the type of measurement and the limits of acceptability. Examples for a cancer registry could include "Ninety percent of all cases must be registered within 4 to 6 months from the date of diagnosis" or "One hundred percent of the computerized edit checks must be passed before the record is stored in the database."

Quality control involves a carefully planned set of activities by which database managers monitor current quality and take appropriate remedial action to positively affect future quality.

Careful planning requires a comprehensive review of every aspect of operations, including the scope of reporting, abstracting procedures, computer software, training, use of data, and so on.

Monitoring current activities includes the measurement of various aspects of operations. Examples include the calculation of the percentage of missed cases, the percentage of core data coded "unknown," or the lag time for production of an annual report. Communicating the current state of operations to everyone who is involved with or influential in the operation of the registry (registrars, programmers, administrators, physicians, and data users) is an important part of the process.

Taking appropriate remedial action involves not only correcting mistakes but also repairing flaws in system design, introducing new procedures to eliminate future errors, retraining personnel, and initiating activities to foster improvement in quality, even when the current state is within acceptable standards.

Positively affecting future quality ensures that the remedial action has the desired effect and no unforeseen negative side effects are introduced. Quality control requires a continuous loop of measurement, communication, and action.

BASIC METHODS

The basic methods of cancer registry quality control are acceptance sampling, process controls, and designed studies. Acceptance sampling is the inspection and subsequent acceptance or rejection of a product. Computerized edit checks are an example of acceptance sampling for registry data. Serious and frequent use of the registry data can also prove to signal potential errors and underscore quality.

Process controls represent a higher level of quality control sophistication. Statistical methods are used to measure the state of a process and trigger a review when the process exceeds established limits.

Some hospitals are focusing on organizational quality improvement programs that have been proven successful in business and industry for understanding customers' needs, analyzing business processes, and instituting proper measurement methods. One example is Six Sigma, which is a statistical measure of variation that reflects process capability. The sigma scale of measure is perfectly correlated to such characteristics as defects-per-unit, parts-per-million defective, and the probability of a failure error. The Six Sigma method complements and adds effectiveness to existing improvement methods.[2] Process controls such as this are often used to monitor timeliness of reporting in a cancer registry.

Designed studies are used to optimize a system by investigating the current level of quality through a formalized plan and analysis. Reabstracting studies are an example of designed studies.

REQUIREMENTS

Prerequisites for quality control of cancer registry data include a list of reportable malignant conditions, data definitions, coding guidelines, and training for data abstractors. A reportable list is necessary to outline the scope of the registry and to define the criteria for case inclusion.[3] Most errors in hospital cancer registries fall in the direction of underreporting (missed cases) but overreporting can also occur (by including benign or ineligible cases or duplicate cases).

A list of the data items to be collected, along with data definitions, valid codes, allowance of blanks, and "unknown" codes, is essential. These should be written, reviewed, and updated regularly in an abstractor's manual. The manual should also provide additional guidelines for interpreting and coding unusual situations, ambiguous documentation, or special requirements.

Training, both initial and ongoing, is necessary to ensure that data items are collected accurately and consistently across different registries and across time.

COMPONENTS

A distinction should be made between quality control of registry operations and quality control of data. Registry operations have a much broader scope, and include complete casefinding, timely reporting, policies and procedures manuals, and staff training. Quality control of data is limited to the specific characteristics of accuracy, completeness, and timeliness of the information reported. Accuracy can be described by such terms as *consistency, reliability, validity, reproducibility,* and *concordance.* Completeness of data is the comprehensiveness of the data set collected, the specification of code values (as opposed to blanks and "unknown" codes), and the avoidance of omissions (overlooking additional therapy or follow-up information). Timeliness is the degree to which various stages of the registration process occur on schedule. This has important implications for systems management, data accuracy, and utility.

STRATEGIES

Various strategies are available to ensure accuracy, completeness, and timeliness of data: visual review, edit checks, review of output reports, statistical analyses, physician supervision, reabstracting studies, and test case studies.

Visual Review

Every abstract tells a story. Registrars should visually review the paper abstract with English-language

descriptions of codes before data entry or a computer-generated abstract after data entry, for logical consistency among data elements. For example, if the behavior code[4] is 2 for in situ then the summary stage[5] should be 0, meaning in situ as well. Trends in errors, such as putting in the wrong year or skipping a required field, may be spotted easily and eliminated quickly. The value of this method may diminish as registrars become more experienced. Its effectiveness should be re-evaluated periodically.

Edit Checks

Along with visual review, data edit checks are another form of acceptance sampling. Nearly every registry uses some form of computerization with data edit checks. These provide a cost-effective method of quality review and check 100% of the cases. Types of data edit checks include range or allowable code checks, interitem checks, interrecord checks, and interdatabase checks (see Table 21-1).

Different systems have different edit checks and different loopholes. Repeated use of a particular computer software package will familiarize users with its processing routines and how errors can occur. Errors can often be identified by reviewing reports and data lists generated by the computer. For example, edit checks on the field "laterality" may issue warnings only, since skin of scalp and neck (C44.4), overlapping lesion of skin (C44.8), and

Table 21-1
Examples of Computerized Data Edit Checks

- Allowable range check
- Interitem check
- Interrecord check
- Interdatabase check
  —Value for sex must be one of the following codes: 1 = male, 2 = female, 3 = other (i.e., hermaphrodite), 4 = transsexual, 9 = unknown.
  —If sex = male, site cannot be cervix, endometrium, or other female genital organs.
  —If patient is marked dead on one primary cancer, patient cannot be marked alive on another primary cancer.
  —If patient has colon cancer in hospital cancer registry, then disease index and other hospital records (i.e., billing) should be consistent with colon primary diagnosis.

Table 21-2

Sample Report of Case Count by AJCC Group
for Larynx Cancers

AJCC Stage Group Larynx Cases	
0	3 cases
I	15 cases
II	10 cases
IIA	1 case
III	4 cases
IV	5 cases
99	8 cases
Blank	4 cases
Total:	*50*

skin NOS (C44.9), are not considered paired sites. If
a user overrides the warning message, assuming that
this case is an exception when it is a true error, then
the error would be entered into the database. A
report listing patient name, site of cancer, and laterality code sorted by site, could quickly identify errors
or records that merit review.

Statistical Analysis

Statistical reports are another useful tool for identifying unlikely, questionable, or erroneous codes.
Sometimes edit checks at data entry are insufficient
to prevent certain errors or inconsistencies, and statistical reports can make them obvious. A report
generated from a selected group of larynx cancer
cases, with a count of cases by AJCC stage group,[6] is
shown in Table 21-2. Since stage group IIA is invalid
according to the AJCC manual chapter for larynx,
the case coded IIA is certainly in error. The cases
coded as 99 or left blank might also be reviewed to
determine whether they could have been coded more
specifically.

Statistical reports can be especially useful in
evaluating data completeness. The frequency with

which data fields contain valid values, specific values,
or blanks can be measured for any data item. A comparison of reports on all cancer cases by sex is shown
in Table 21-3. Clearly Hospital C does not meet
high quality standards! This report quickly reveals
that the abstractor is failing to collect an important
piece of information that is most likely available in
source documents.

Physician Supervision

Physician supervision is critical to the integrity of
registry operations. In fact, the Commission on
Cancer (CoC) of the American College of Surgeons
states that "the cancer committee ensures the quality
of cancer registry data by establishing and implementing a quality control plan to monitor multiple
areas of cancer registry activity and accuracy and
completeness of cancer registry data."[7] Physician
involvement enables accuracy checking not only with
source documents but with the source of the healthcare information (practitioners). Communication
between the registrar and hospital physicians enables
each to gain a greater understanding of the other's
roles and constraints. It can lead to clarification of
documentation and underlying assumptions each
one makes during routine job performance. Regular
communication with practitioners can improve the
accuracy of data entered, as well as of reports generated on request. Hospital physicians should serve as
resources to the registry, answer questions, and develop policies and procedures. A random review of at
least 10% of all cases should be performed by the
physician advisor. The examples shown in Figures
21-1 and 21-2 may be helpful in documenting and
summarizing physician review of cases for quality
assurance by the cancer committee.[8]

Reabstracting Studies

Reabstracting studies are formal procedures conducted in order to check the accuracy of data in the

Table 21-3

Sample Report of Case Counts by Sex for Three Hospitals

Hospital A		Hospital B		Hospital C	
Male	223	Male	155	Male	78
Female	175	Female	301	Female	29
Other	2	Other	2	<blank>	315
Total:	400		458		422

Figure 21-1
Sample Form for Documentation of Physician Review of Registry Data

---

Hospital Cancer Data System
QUALITY ASSURANCE—PHYSICIAN REVIEW

Reviewed by: _____, MD   Date: _____

Charts abstracted: _____ (month/year)

Criteria:
1. The abstracting is completed within 6 months of discharge.
2. The histology and grade are coded correctly.
3. The primary site is coded correctly.
4. The class of case is correctly assigned.
5. The first course of treatment is coded correctly.
6. The staging information is coded correctly.

Directions:
1. If item audited is correct, record a (+) in the appropriate box.
2. If item is incorrect, record a (-) in the appropriate box.

Patient Identifier	Criteria Numbers						Comments
	1	2	3	4	5	6	

Action Taken:

Charts abstracted:_____   # Charts audited:_____   % Charts audited: _____

---

cancer registry against the original health record.[1] When reabstracting, the entire data set (or a specified set of core items) is completely recoded without reference to the original abstract. Preferably, the recoding is performed by someone other than the original abstractor. Typically, the objectives of a reabstracting study are as follows:

- To estimate rates of agreement between the registry data and the information in source documents
- To identify problems in the interpretation and coding of specific data

- To develop standard guidelines and rules for abstracting ambiguous situations

Reabstracting studies can be time-consuming and labor intensive and, therefore, are usually conducted on a small sample of cases. However, they can be particularly useful as an assessment and training exercise.

In order to carry out a reabstracting study, a written protocol should be formulated at the outset, stating the specific objectives of the study; sampling procedures; plans for analyzing the results; and the data items to be measured for accuracy, or agree-

Figure 21-2
Sample Form Documenting Count of Cancer Charts Reviewed for Quality Assurance

Hospital Cancer Data System
QUALITY ASSURANCE
Chart Review Summary-2004

Month	Total Abstracted	Percent Physician Review	Percent CTR Review	Percent Total Review
January				
February				
March				
April				
May				
June				
July				
August				
September				
October				
November				
December				

ment, rates. Major and minor disagreements are usually defined in order to assess the impact of errors on the results of research conducted using cancer registry data. Next, the charts to be reabstracted are identified, located, and recoded. Once the cases have been reabstracted, each case is then compared to its original abstract.

A workshop of cancer registrars participating in the reabstracting process provides a forum for discussing the differences in each case and reaching a consensus concerning the correct or accurate code for each item. Several important benefits may be gained by this process: individual cases in the registry database are corrected, model cases can be established for future reference, inadequate or ambiguous data definitions can be refined, and areas where additional training is needed can be identified.

The results of the reabstracting study should be summarized and reported to all concerned, and possibly included in the registry's annual report. Major and minor disagreement rates should be tabulated for each data item, as well as the reason for disagree-

ment, such as data entry errors or information from the chart was missed or miscoded. A formal presentation of results can lead to action such as targeted training to improve quality.

Test-Case Studies

Another strategy for measuring agreement among several abstractors is the use of test cases specially prepared for this purpose. Agreement rates are again measured based on how often or how closely different coders agree on each data item. The concept of reproducibility or reliability of data is based on the agreement among different coders using the same information. It is unlikely that a group of coders would have a high reproducibility rate on an inaccurate code. In formal test-case studies, the correct codes are determined by a panel of experts, often composed of data standards committees and medical advisors.

This approach was used by the Commission on Cancer of the American College of Surgeons in their 1999 patient care evaluation study on the quality of oncology data.[9] Seventeen case scenarios were assembled and edited from actual hospital patient records, which included melanoma, breast, colon, rectum, bladder, lung, and prostate cancers. The opportunity to participate was widely publicized among cancer registry professionals, including hospital-based registrars, central cancer registrars, and independent cancer abstractors. The results of this study indicated that the 971 participants had high rates of agreement with the preferred codes (>90%) for behavior code, morphology, tumor grade, laterality, and some elements of first course treatment. However, problems were identified in the areas where registrars must interpret, apply, and adhere to standard coding procedures. While some of these problems were related to the amount of training and experience each respondent possessed, others are inherent in the process of abstracting information according to multiple and complex sets of rules and guidelines. The results of this study were presented to the appropriate standard-setting organizations and to the National Cancer Registrars Association to initiate communication and educational efforts.

These two methods for measuring data accuracy—reabstracting and test-case studies—can be combined to provide direct descriptive information on the quality of the data and the reliability of the abstractors in the cancer registry studied. Reabstracting actual cases is beneficial because it reflects the true quality of the data currently in the registry, since the cases are chosen from those submitted under routine reporting conditions. The advantage of test cases is the relative simplicity and adaptability of the approach. Both strategies can be used as significant resources for training and modifying the work of individual coders, as well as for measuring and controlling the quality of data in a registry.

SYSTEMS TO MONITOR DATA QUALITY

The characteristics of data quality are accuracy, completeness, and timeliness. Monitoring is a critical aspect of quality control, and various methods can be employed to monitor these three components.

Accuracy

Edit rejection rates can be monitored by the computer and can be used to measure against a standard that is set for acceptable accuracy levels. When the

error-rate threshold is exceeded, a retraining program should be initiated. Reabstracting and test-case studies also provide information about data quality and can be helpful in targeting retraining efforts to the most needed areas.

Completeness

Data Completeness

Statistical reports are particularly useful in identifying problem areas. Errors of omission may be site-specific due to the nature of the disease or to the reporting process. Therapy information may be particularly difficult to obtain and special efforts may be required to identify where and how this kind of information can best be captured. Again, reabstracting studies can be helpful in identifying information that is systematically being missed. Additional action is necessary to improve data completeness in future abstracts.

Case Completeness

Routine monitoring of completeness of case ascertainment is an essential function of a cancer registry's operations. Accurate estimates of the incidence rates of cancer, as measured by population-based registries, depend on complete ascertainment of the new cases of cancer reportable to the registry.

A number of methods are used by registries to monitor completeness. Central registries use the NAACCR method, the historical data method, and casefinding audits to monitor completeness of reporting. Hospital-based registries use the historical data method and casefinding audits. Refer to Table 21-4 for ICD-9-CM codes, which are used to ascertain cancer cases from health information management department disease indices.

The NAACCR method was developed by the NAACCR Data Evaluation and Publication Committee, and is accepted as the standard for measuring completeness when evaluating a central registry for NAACCR Certification.[10] This method uses the rate ratios created when the five-year site- and sex-specific SEER incidence rates for the white population are divided by the five-year site- and sex-specific US mortality rates for the white population. When these rate ratios are multiplied by the five-year site- and sex-specific mortality rates for the population served by the registry being evaluated, they yield an expected incidence rate. The site- and sex-specific incidence rates are summed to create an overall can-

Table 21-4

Screening List of ICD-9-CM Codes For Casefinding

Certain ICD-9-CM* codes used by medical records departments for discharge diagnoses identify cases of neoplasms that are reportable to SEER. Casefinding procedures should include the review of medical records coded with the following numbers:

ICD-9-CM CODE

042.2	AIDS with specified malignant neoplasms
140.0-208.9	Malignant neoplasms (primary and secondary)
225.0-225.9	Benign neoplasm central nervous system
227.3	Benign neoplasm of pituitary, craniopharyngeal duct, craniobuccal pouch, hypophysis, Rathke's pouch, Sella turica
227.4	Benign neoplasm of pineal gland, pineal body
230.0-234.9	Carcinoma in situ
235.0-238.9	Neoplasms of uncertain behavior
237.0-237.9	Neoplasm of uncertain behavior pituitary gland, central nervous system, neurofibromatosis, von Recklinghausen disease
239.0-239.9	Neoplasms of unspecified nature
273.2	Heavy chain disease (alpha, Gamma and Franklin's disease)
273.3	Waldenstrom's macroglobulinemia
279.9	Unspecified disorder of immune mechanism
289.8	Acute myelofibrosis
748.1	Glioma,** astrocytoma, astroglioma, astroblastoma of nose
V07.3	Other prophylactic chemotherapy
V07.8	Other specified prophylactic measures
V10.0-V10.9	Personal history of malignant neoplasms
V58.0	Radiotherapy session
V58.1	Maintenance chemotherapy
V66.1	Convalescence following radiotherapy
V66.2	Convalescence following chemotherapy
V67.1	Follow-up exam following radiotherapy
V67.2	Follow-up exam following chemotherapy
V71.1	Observation for suspected malignant neoplasm
V76.0-V76.5	Special screening for malignant neoplasms

*International Classification of Disease, 9th Revision, Clinical Modification (4th ed., October 1991)
**Glioma of nose (SNOMED M-26160) is not reportable.

cer incidence rate. The completeness rate of a central cancer registry can be estimated by comparing the actual incidence rate calculated by the registry to the estimated expected incidence rate. The original model has been empirically tested and modified to account for variations in racial composition and in case fatality rates for different populations. In addition to determining the completeness of case ascertainment rate ratio, NAACCR has identified two other activities which, when carried out by central cancer registries, may significantly impact the number of incident cases included in the registry. These

activities are death certificate clearance and the rigorous review and elimination of duplicate cases.

The historical data method compares the expected number of cases (based on previous year experience) with the current period in question. This method is simple and effective. However, fluctuations in the numbers of cases across and between years may be the result of changes in the health care system in the population covered by the registry. For example, in a central registry, if a large military base closes and the result is a decrease in the population, there will likely be a reduced number of cases.

Hospital-based registries may experience site-specific fluctuations in the number of cases reported per year because of events such as changes in the hospital's medical staff (i.e., if the hospital brings on a prostate cancer specialist there will likely be more prostate cases in the registry than in prior years when the specialist was not on staff) and the hospital's cancer screening activities in the local community.

Casefinding audits typically involve the use of a statistically controlled study whereby casefinding sources were investigated and scrutinized for possible missed cases. Re-examination of source documents and planned casefinding audits provide the most direct estimate of completeness but are also the most expensive. NAACCR and the NCI SEER Program have been conducting these casefinding audits for many years now.

Timeliness

Two ways to monitor timely reporting are outlined here. In the first method, registrars calculate the number of cases abstracted to date for the current accession year as a percentage of the total number of cases expected for the current year. This is then compared to the amount of time that has elapsed to date in the current accession year, minus the allowable reporting time frame. For example, if the reporting time frame is six months, then by January 1, half of the cases for the previous year should have been abstracted and entered into the registry. Similarly, on January 1, if the number of cases abstracted so far is 50% or more of the total number expected for the previous year, the registry is within timeliness standards.

The CDC's National Program of Cancer Registries has as its timeliness goal, 90% of a year's expected cases be reported within 12 months of the close of the year of diagnosis, and 95% within 24 months of the close of the diagnosis year.

Another approach to monitoring timeliness is to have a computer program automatically calculate the lag time between the date of diagnosis and the date of data entry. Each case is then marked with a lag-time value, and the number of cases above and below a set threshold can easily be reviewed. When the percentage of cases beyond the acceptable time lag increases to a certain point, action must be taken to reduce this number to within acceptable timeliness standards. Data items needed to monitor timeliness include

Date of diagnosis, Date of admission or first contact, and Date record transmitted to central registry.

SUMMARY

Quality control involves a carefully planned set of activities for database managers to monitor current quality and take appropriate remedial action to positively affect future quality. The characteristics of data quality are accuracy, completeness, and timeliness. The basic method of cancer registry data quality control are acceptance sampling, process controls, and designed studies. Various strategies available to ensure data quality includes visual review, edit checks, output review, statistical reports, physician review, and reabstracting studies. Quality control involves a continuous loop of measurement, communication, and action, leading to continuous quality improvement.

STUDY QUESTIONS

1. Give two examples of acceptance sampling used for cancer registry data.
2. Describe three examples of computerized data edit checks.
3. Describe three methods of monitoring completeness.
4. Name three prerequisites for quality control of data in a cancer registry.
5. Describe two methods of monitoring timely cancer reporting.

REFERENCES

1. Hilsenbeck, SG, Glaefke GS, Feigl P, et al. *Quality Control for Cancer Registries.* Bethesda, Md: US Department of Health and Human Services, Public Health Service, National Institutes of Health; May 1985.
2. Harry M, Schroeder R. *Six Sigma, The Breakthrough Management Strategy Revolutionizing the World's Top Corporations.* New York, NY: Doubleday; 2000.
3. Young JL, Roffers SD, Ries LAG, et al, eds. *SEER Summary Staging Manual—2000:Codes and Coding Instructions.* National Cancer Institute; 2001. NIH Publication No. 01-4969.
4. Commission on Cancer. *Facility Oncology Registry Data Standards.* Chicago, Ill: American College of Surgeons; 2002.

5. Fritz A, Percy C, Jack A, et al, eds. *International Classification of Diseases for Oncology,* 3rd ed. Geneva, Switzerland: World Health organization; 2000.

6. Fleming ID, Cooper JS, Henson DE, et al, eds. *Manual for Staging of Cancer* 5th ed. Chicago, Ill: American Joint Committee on Cancer; 1997.

7. Commission on Cancer. *Commission on Cancer Cancer Program Standards, 2004.* Chicago, Ill: American College of Surgeons; 2003.

8. National Cancer Data Base and National Cancer Registrars Association, Inc. *Advanced Quality Improvement Workshop-Student Workbook.* Chicago, Ill: American College of Surgeons; 1992.

9. Malnar K, Phillips JL, Fritz A, et al. Quality of oncology data: findings from the Commission on Cancer PCE study. *Journal of Registry Management.* 2001; 28(1):24-34.

10. Tucker TC, Howe HL. Measuring the quality of population-based cancer registries: the NAACCR perspective. *Journal of Registry Management.* 2001; 28(1) 41-44.

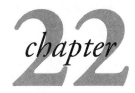

COMPUTER PRINCIPLES

Ted J. Williamson
MD, PhD, CTR

LeeAnn W. McKelvey
MAT

THE COMPUTERIZED REGISTRY

The computer has become a central part of almost every aspect of cancer registry work. It has automated the data collection, storage, use, and printout of registry information. In several short decades, registrars have become sophisticated computer users. The cancer registry was a relative latecomer among database applications. This is not necessarily a bad thing. Database software designers have been able to learn from the mistakes of the past and use that knowledge to improve modern cancer registry systems. There is no question that registry computerization can improve registry data utility. However, it is important to have realistic expectations of what an electronic database will and will not do for registry operations.

A computerized registry will *not* save much time in the abstracting process (Registrars will still have to locate the records and, within the records, search for needed information), prevent the need to track down the doctor in order to get him or her to complete the staging forms, resolve coding ambiguities (There will always be patients whose disease classification is unclear), make tracking hard-to-follow patients any easier, allow a hospital to replace a registrar with an untrained data entry clerk, or reduce a registrar's work load or stress level.

Computers free users from some of the tedious and repetitive chores often associated with the cancer registry. For consistency purposes, cancer registry standard-setting agencies, such as the North American Association of Central Cancer Registries and the Commission on Cancer (CoC) of the American College of Surgeons (ACoS), have expanded and standardized the *data sets* to be collected.

Computerized registries perform invaluable tasks for a registrar. For example, a computerized registry *will*

- offer opportunities for more efficient casefinding;
- digitize and store the abstracted and patient data;
- automate data editing;
- facilitate follow-up record keeping;
- provide lists and reports;
- perform statistical analysis (survival calculations);
- facilitate the cancer registry's real missions: *using collected patient data to monitor patient care and outcomes against continuously evolving standards and ensuring that patients receive the best and most current care;*
- eliminate tedious aspects, such as typing letters, counting and sorting file cards, and preparing lists manually;
- offer easier and more flexible adaptation as data coding standards change. It is far simpler to convert data to a new staging system electronically than to perform longitudinal studies on cases staged on three or four different systems;
- provide access to email;
- provide word processing and access to spreadsheet, presentation, and other management software;
- provide Internet access and other telecommunications facility;
- systematize registry operations.

Before computerization, the data in many, if not most, registries had been virtually inaccessible without tedious hours of sifting through paper abstract cards and files. A well-managed computer registry can be the key to accessing the information. A strong electronic edit checking system within the computerized registry can improve data quality and consistency, an achievement essential to useful outcome studies. Flexible and fast reporting functions can reduce days of manual labor to minutes of keyboard work.

Registry technology is enhanced when a hospital's cancer committee and the medical staff are committed to using the information as a tool to improve and reshape patient care within the community. Contributing data to the *National Cancer Data Base (NCDB)* and reporting to state central cancer registries are certainly important functions of a computerized registry. However, the real value becomes apparent when these new tools are used to identify and define areas where facilities can improve patient care.

SOFTWARE: REQUIRED ELEMENTS OF A CANCER REGISTRY

There are also components essential to a computer program for maintaining cancer registry data. These include a setup for data entry, a query system to search for cases, and a means of reporting results. Experienced vendors did not become seriously interested in registry software design until the early 1980s. Prior to that time, virtually all registry systems were developed locally for whatever *mainframe* computer happened to be available. In the absence of national standards, it was not uncommon to find certain critical elements missing from these systems. Even today, there are registry systems in place that have fine capabilities for data entry but very limited means for presenting the data in any useful form other than a printed abstract. This section briefly describes the key elements that should be present in any registry software design, whether commercial or from a local drafting board.

Data Entry

Data entry system design subtleties within a registry, especially the organization of data entry *fields and screens,* can have a significant impact on a registrar's efficiency. For purposes of definition, the *data entry field* is a point of entry for a single piece of data, often represented as a highlighted window on the data entry screen. The term *screen* is often used to represent a collection of data fields presented on one integral display. Several sequential screens are usually required for complete data entry of one abstract. Unfortunately, the medical record may not be organized in a fashion that is compatible with the sequential structure of data entry into the cancer registry software. The usual screen organization is to group fields into demographics, diagnostics, treatment, and follow-up. A program should allow a registrar to bypass fields that are irrelevant to a given patient; for example, fields for ERA and PRA in a patient with prostate cancer.

The registry system's ability to provide automatic coding (autocode) assistance in fields that use standardized coding, such as American Joint Committee on Cancer (AJCC) staging or International Classification of Diseases for Oncology (ICD-O) site and histology coding, also significantly reduces a registrar's work load. The computer registry system that can present site-specific AJCC staging onscreen at the press of a key can greatly assist registrars with coding.

The best modern registry systems utilize graphic interfaces that closely follow the conventions of Windows. Anyone familiar with Windows-based word processing systems should be able to easily perform data entry within these systems.

Data Edit Checking

Electronic data entry certainly has improved the life of the registrar and provided greater accessibility to data. However, the axiom "garbage in, garbage out" still prevails, and the value of registry data would have progressed little, were it not for the unique potential of the computerized registry system to *edit check* data as they are being entered. *Edit check* literally means to monitor the data input process, preventing the entry of obviously incorrect data and alerting the operator to potentially suspect data. For example, if "female" is entered in the field for sex, "prostate" should not be entered in the field for site. Mention the term *edit check* and most cancer data specialists immediately think of inter-field edits, but a strong edit-checking system actually functions at four levels: data coding and format edits, inter-field edits, inter-record edits, and completeness edits.

Data Coding and Format Edits

These are the front line of defense against bad data. The minimum qualification any registry software program should meet is the ability to prevent entry of data values that are not logical or not possible for a given field. In the past, most locally developed programs and many commercial systems were very weak in this area. As a simple example, consider a field for Summary Stage. There is a standard coding system for this field that dictates only eight valid codes, numbers from the list 0, 1, 2, 3, 4, 5, 7, and 9. Any computerized registry should reject an entry of 6 or 8 into this field. Yet, in many older registries, the Summary Stage field is still contaminated with the letters O and L. These were entered mistakenly by someone of an earlier generation who had learned to type on an economically designed manual typewriter, for which lowercase l ('el') and the number 1, and uppercase O ('oh') and the number 0 shared common keys. A second example comes from one analysis of an older commercial registry system. The registrar had to type a descriptive word into an open, 12 character, free-text field to record summary stage. A frequency table data analysis revealed 11 different spellings of *local,* 15 different spellings of *regional,* and a few fields with stray characters that had no relevance whatsoever. Using a free-text field for a codeable data item is one of the worst violations of quality data system design.

A data format edit ensures that the data entered meet standardized structural requirements. For example, the histology code and behavior code should be separated by a slash (/) (e.g., 8140/3). Similarly, for readability, telephone numbers should have hyphens between the area code and prefix and between the prefix and suffix.

Inter-Field Edits

An electronic *inter-field edit* is a feature of some software systems that makes a logical comparison between data entered in one field and data entered in another, testing for consistency between the two statements. In addition to the obvious case of the female patient with prostate cancer, another example involves the various dates entered into a registry. Dates should have a logical progression: birth date should precede date of diagnosis, which should precede date of treatment, which should precede date of follow-up. Date of last follow-up shouldn't be later than the current date.

    Some inter-field edits are absolute and inviolable, such as female/prostate or date order. Others should be less strictly enforced. For example, Surveillance, Epidemiology, and End Results (SEER) has published a table with thousands of entries defining allowable combinations of site and histology code. In general, anything not in this table should prompt an *edit check warning*. For example, there is no seminoma of the uvula on their allowed list of combinations. Sometimes, however, nature actually violates these rules. There is an age/histology edit that says Wilms tumor should not be seen in adults. Yet, occasionally, Wilms tumors do appear in older adults. This biological reality leads the SEER edit checks to allow for *overrides*. Currently there are 18 inter-field edits that have overrides, such that when an override is set, then the data edit check should be suppressed. Each override is itself a data field, as defined in the North American Association of Central Cancer Registries (NAACCR) data record. When that field contains the number 1, it is an indication that the registrar recognizes the edit check conflict but has been satisfied that it is in fact a valid combination. For the most current information on overrides, consult the latest edition of the NAACCR Standards for Cancer Registries.

Inter-Record Edits

Just as rules of consistency within a patient record are crucial, SEER has defined a set of rules for consistency between records for patients with multiple primary neoplasms. This is where *inter-record edits* come into play. As an obvious example, the patient

shouldn't be alive with one primary and dead with another. For these reasons, inter-record edits are of special interest to central registries.

Completeness Edits

It is certainly important that each data item entered use the proper coding and format and be consistent with other data entries. It is equally important to ensure that all data fields needed to meet the minimum reporting requirements of a registry have been filled. At the very least, this list would include the required elements defined by the Commission on Cancer (CoC) of the American College of Surgeons and/or state registry, if applicable. The electronic registry should have the ability to conduct *completeness edits,* which identify missing elements, not only at the time the data are being entered, but also on a batch basis, so that all of the records created in a given time period can be audited for completeness. The tools that accomplish this assume various forms. Ideally, the registrar should be able to identify any patient subgroup and, on demand, generate a list identifying the patient records with missing data elements, and what those elements are.

Standardizing Edits

Decades ago the SEER program of the National Cancer Institute (NCI) pioneered editing rules for registries with a standardized set of inter-field edits. For many years registry software vendors varied widely in the degree and manner to which they incorporated edits in their programs. Some early registry programs provided only named blank fields for typing text with no edit control at all. Needless to say, data quality with these systems was frequently very poor.

    With the move to centralized registry data collection, it became apparent that strong standards would be necessary if the data collected were to offer any value in studies of patterns of care and outcomes. This problem transcended cancer registries and affected a myriad of other registries of interest to public health (trauma, cardiac, etc.). To address these problems, the Centers for Disease Control undertook a project to develop a software tool that could be used by virtually any agency to enforce quality control on large blocks of data. The result is a public domain program known as "GenEdits." With this program anyone can write a set of edit rules (in a computer format known as a "metafile") for virtually any kind of data.

The responsibility for designing and maintaining cancer registry metafiles has been assumed by NAACCR in a cooperative effort with the CoC. Numerous metafiles have been created covering all manner of situations from central registry operations to edits hospital registries should satisfy before reporting cases to the state. Most registry software incorporates these edits in some fashion or other. It is also relatively easy for registrars to test files exported in the NAACCR or NCDB formats using the GenEdits program (it is a DOS program but it runs in the Windows environment). Some vendors, and some states, will provide ready-to-run packages of the GenEdits program and metafiles. The GenEdits program and metafiles can be downloaded from the NAACCR website (www.naaccr.org).

Operation of GenEdits is fairly intuitive. The user selects the metafile (edit rules) to be exercised, names the target file and the report file, and specifies several other operational characteristics. It runs quickly and generates a text file report that can be read with any word processor. Many organizations require data to be edited by GenEdits before data submission.

Query System

A query system is a software feature that allows the user to identify a specific subgroup of patients for reporting or analysis. Until recently, query systems were non-standardized. Some systems offered a simple but very restricted design in which only predefined criteria could be chosen from a list; others had great flexibility but required extensive knowledge of mathematics and/or programming. Structured query language (SQL), which is discussed later in this chapter, seems bound to emerge as the standard for database queries.

There are a few standard qualities that every registry query system should have. Foremost among these is the ability to allow the registrar to make queries without assistance from the IT Department. Equally important is the ability to construct a query from any combination of data fields. The query system should be self-documenting; it should be capable of printing and preserving the query instructions for later verification that the intended query was successfully run. Finally, the system should allow the registrar to reuse the query instructions. The latter issue is particularly important as registrars enter the era of relational databases, with their verbose and sometimes tedious query instructions.

REPORTING

Lists, Letters, and Abstracts

Many registries have adopted nearly standardized formats for their reporting tasks. Accession register listings, follow-up letters, and comprehensive abstracts tend to take the same form from one registry system to the next. Certainly, any cancer registry software should be able to provide a variety of these reports on demand. Similarly, the registry should be able to sort the patient files for listings in virtually any order. There is a strong need for flexibility in reporting, since physicians and hospital administrators recognize the value and availability of registry data. An effective cancer registry should also have some means for generating ad hoc reports incorporating data from any field. It is very important for cancer registry staff to review commercial cancer registry software systems when selecting a registry computer system. Cancer registrars can "shop" for cancer registry software systems at the National Cancer Registrars Association annual conferences in the exhibitor area. Most cancer registry software companies have displays available at these conferences for staff to view the newest version. Oftentimes, software companies will provide demonstrations on-site where IT staff, administrators, and others interested in the software can evaluate systems. An evaluation tool of various functions and capabilities can be developed for comparison purposes.

Statistics

Computerized registries rarely need to include a comprehensive statistical package, particularly if the registry provides a means for ad hoc exporting of data into electronic formats that can be read by one of the many powerful third-party statistics software packages on the market. However, reliance on these packages also forces the registrar to learn a much broader software base, and sometimes imposes expectations of unreasonable statistical sophistication. Therefore, registry systems should provide a certain minimum set of statistical functions. For example, registry software should be able to generate frequency tables on any reasonable data field, such as age or status at last follow-up.

Another essential element for statistical reporting is survival analysis. Even though survival analysis can be found in commercial statistical packages, it is seldom structured in a manner that suits the special needs of the cancer registry. At the minimum, a registry system should support analysis of survival from diagnosis to date of last follow-up. However, often there should be more alternatives. For example, medical oncologists tend to be more interested in survival from the date of initiation of treatment to the date of first recurrence, and quality assurance staff might be interested in the elapsed time between date of diagnosis and date of first treatment.

Survival calculations are always approximations of real life, wherein the survival of a group is estimated at fixed intervals, typically three months or one year. These intervals are certainly adequate for diseases where patients have a long natural life expectancy, such as prostate cancer. It may be useful for some cancers to be analyzed at intervals of one to four weeks.

Advanced Capabilities

An active registry needs to perform a number of computer-based tasks that may not be supported by vendor-developed registry software. An example is the need to provide graphic summaries of data for reports and presentations to cancer conferences and public forums. Audiences have become accustomed to high-resolution, full-color, presentation quality graphics. Fortunately, the marketplace includes products that meet this need. Usually registry data management software is required only to export data summaries in any one of a number of standard formats. Once these files have been exported, however, the registrar needs to be familiar with the use and capabilities of the graphics software package.

Database Adaptability

When it comes to data set definition, the cancer registrar must respond to many agencies, including the special requirements of the state registry, the CoC, the NAACCR, the American Joint Committee on Cancer (AJCC), the Joint Commission on Accreditation of Healthcare Organizations (JCAHO), the World Health Organization (WHO), and others. These agencies work closely together to improve the cancer registry data set. Due to new technology and information, organizations such as the AJCC, ICD-O, and CoC have redefined their systems and

data set. The data set and its coding rules inevitably are going to change. A cancer registry data system must be able to add new data fields from time to time. It also should allow for revision of the coding rules for data fields. When the coding rules for a field change, the system should support updating all historical cases to the new system.

PUTTING IT ALL TOGETHER

A computer workstation is created by putting all the pieces together (motherboard with CPU, disk drives, console, operating system, and peripheral devices such as printers). Aptly termed, this is where most registrars spend most of their hours entering and editing patient information, gathering data for studies, maintaining current follow-up, and organizing various functions such as the cancer committees, cancer conferences, etc. If a facility's cancer registry department has more than one registrar, more than one workstation may be needed.

Networking Concepts

Each active member of a cancer registry staff should have a workstation with a computer, email, and Internet access. A network configuration should be considered for access to data and work productivity.

The basic network concept is quite straightforward. It is to put all of the data in a central location, usually on a microcomputer with a large reservoir of memory. This computer is called a *server*. Attach several workstations to the server and let them access those data simultaneously. In other words, each person working in the registry can access a computer at the same time, using the registry software or another software. Like all community functions, though, the network must maintain rules of operation or the registry will experience a kind of byte anarchy. The most important of these rules for cancer registry is also the most obvious; two people cannot try to edit the same patient data at the same time. A patient's cancer registry data are usually organized in one or more "records," each containing a fixed number of data elements in a given order. A typical cancer registry database might, for each patient, have one demographic record and, for each primary site, a diagnostic record, a treatment record, and one or more follow-up records.

Record locking prevents two cancer registrars from accessing the same record at the same time, which is important so the most current information is available to each registrar editing patient information. The cancer registry software must, however, allow other registrars to access a patient's record when another registrar is editing it for viewing or reporting purposes.

The networking system just described is said to have *file server architecture*. In such systems, the server's primary responsibility is to allow files or pieces of files to move back and forth to workstation PCs. Generally speaking, the workstation is responsible for data integrity. A newer type of networking is called *client/server architecture*. The principal difference between client/server and file server architecture is the role the server computer takes in data management. In the client/server system it takes a much more active role in management of the data than in the file server system. For example, the server of a client/server system has the programs that determine whether or not a registrar should even have access to the data. Once the data are released to the workstation, the server ensures that appropriate record locking takes place. Then, upon the data's return, the server ensures that their quality is acceptable enough to be placed back into the main data file. The server in the client/server system also reassembles the database in the event of a power failure or other system failure during a critical operation. The server keeps continuous backup copies of data and can return the registrar to the point in his or her work just prior to system failure. This continuous backup, however, should never replace manual backups; rather, it should supplement them.

Finally, with the emergence of client/server architecture, standards have emerged for communication between databases that allow for hospital-wide data sharing, which includes the cancer registry. Currently, some cancer registry software programs interface with the hospital medical record and other department-specific software (e.g., Pathology, Radiology, Admissions, etc.). Relevant information from the patient's record can be automatically downloaded into the registry software in a standardized format.

The accepted data format and transmission standard known as Health Level 7 (HL7) is similar to the modern food-product industry's standards for packaging and labeling. The government has endorsed HL7 for increased medical and hospital use as a data format and transmission standard. Some hospital and central registries are starting to use HL7 as a data standard. Traditionally, registries have used flat ASCII file format and transmission standards. HL7 is an alternative format and data transmission standard, which provides an unlimited, structured patient record. Registry staff should acquaint themselves with the basics of HL7 technology.

Remote Operation

With today's telecommunication ability, including modems, the Internet, and common remote operation, many registrars are able to access their cancer registry software from home or other off-site locations. Additionally, some cancer registry software programs provide Internet-based operation. Remote operation requires data encryption and firewall protection. Internet technology will continue to evolve and improve in many ways that will enhance cancer registry operation. For example, new technology provides wireless, DSL, and cable Internet access.

Necessary Skills

The first registrars to use microcomputer software systems were often forced to become conversant in the challenging and sometimes unfriendly details of DOS in order to keep their system alive. In some institutions, the Information Technology (IT) Department has assumed the hardware and baseline software maintenance tasks, while cancer registrars work with the vendor for software support. Depending upon the institution, registrars may not be permitted to install software updates. In most cases, either the IT staff or the software vendor will provide support to the cancer registry.

Because of technical progress, the registrar should not only be knowledgeable in cancer registry rules, but also should be knowledgeable in statistics, graphics, and technical writing. A registrar is well advised to become conversant in the use of word processors, spreadsheets, and presentation software.

What about Structured Query Language (SQL)?

SQL is a standardized query language for requesting information from a database. Historically, SQL has been the favorite query language for database management systems running minicomputers, but increasingly SQL is being supported by PC database systems because it supports distributed databases

(databases that are spread out over several computer systems). SQL enables several users on a local area network (LAN) to access the same database simultaneously. There are different dialects of SQL; however it is the closest thing to a standard query language that currently exists.

MANAGING A COMPUTERIZED REGISTRY

The Data Set

The development of data standards has progressed to the point where cancer data coding in North America has converged to a common format and through data pooling projects such as the National Cancer Data Base, the registrars' efforts are beginning to have an impact on patient care.

Abstracting: To Paper or On-Line?

A *paperless registry* is permissible, although it can be difficult for cancer registrars when most cancer information comes from multiple sources such as the hospital record, oncology office or area, radiation oncology setting, etc. Furthermore, these sources of information are never organized by the flow and sequence of data entry screens rigidly controlled by most registry systems. Few facilities providing oncology care are so vertically organized as to concentrate all of the data of interest to a registrar in a single record. Some cancer registrars working in a *paperless registry* with *on-line abstracting* have two monitors side-by-side, one for the cancer registry software and the other to access medical information systems, or they use a split screen on a single monitor. The electronic registry faces perils from several sources including hardware failure, badly written software, harmful viruses, and poor backup management.

Backup

Many registrars, when discussing their backup and virus protection policies, will state, "The IT Department takes care of nightly backup."

No matter what reassurances a registry may receive from its IT department, the registrars are ultimately responsible for the data's safety and integrity. Registry data are expensive, about $75-$100 per abstract, if not more. If a registry loses all of the data for a 10,000-case paperless registry, sev-

eral hundred thousand dollars worth of effort (about 20-30 registrar years) have also been lost. This section offers some simple guidelines to help prevent backup nightmares.

Establishing Backup Responsibilities and Policies

Every registry should have a written and readily accessible policy manual, including a policy for registry backup. In that policy, the registrar should define precisely who is responsible for backup, the backup schedule, and procedures for making sure that backup has accomplished its goal, providing a current source for completely restoring a registry in the event of a computer hardware catastrophe. Assigning the responsibility for backup should be relatively simple; deciding how and how often to do backup is a bit more problematic. The registrar must work with the IT department to assure a safe backup is operational.

The interval between backups should be no longer than the amount of time a registrar is willing to spend re-entering data in the event of a system failure, as all data added to the system after the backup would have to be re-entered. A small registry accessioning one or two hundred patients a year might find it sufficient to back up once a week. For busy registries, a system that backs up at least daily could be a sound investment.

Large registries on networks should be equipped with hardware capable of *disk duplexing,* also known as disk mirroring. On these systems, every transaction is written to two identical hard drives simultaneously, and backup is continuous. The theory behind duplexing or mirroring is that data are lost only in the very unlikely event of both hard drives failing at the same moment. Many hospitals have now implemented so-called "RAID" systems in which the data is spread over multiple hard drives in a manner that allows any one of them to fail without interrupting system operations or losing data.

Disk duplexing and disk mirroring are *never* a substitute for periodic backup to a separate device.

Backup Methods

Backup systems must meet three fundamental criteria. They must be relatively inexpensive, readily available, and easy to use. At the present time, there are several types of systems that can meet all of these criteria.

Floppy disk: This was one of the first methods available and may still be satisfactory in many registry environments. Floppy disks certainly meet the three criteria above, but they suffer from an inconvenience factor. A 3.5-inch disk holds only 1.44 megabytes of data; most registries contain many megabytes of data. Therefore, special programs are required that distribute the data over multiple floppy disks, and human attention is necessary to feed the floppy disks into the system one at a time. The time investment in regular floppy disk backup can be quite substantial. Some utilization for backup purposes has been made of Zip and Jazz drives, which extend the capability provided by floppies.

Tape backup: Cassette-style magnetic tape actually preceded the floppy diskette as a medium for storing data on microcomputers. However, the early cassettes had very limited capacity. Tape backup systems have evolved rapidly in terms of capacity and reliability, although they are still relatively slow because of the mechanical practicalities of physically moving tape from one spool to the other. To compensate for this, most tape systems now come with software that allows the user to schedule tape backup to activate at night or at some other time when the computer system is not in use.

One disadvantage of tape systems is that the integrity of the backup can't be tested until the entire backup is restored from tape to a hard drive. More than one microcomputer operator has dutifully made tape backups only to find in a moment of crisis that the tapes were not readable. The solution to this is to test the tape system periodically, restoring the entire backup to an available hard drive. This should occur at an interval shorter than the longest interval of tape backups. For example, if tape backups are run on a three-month cycle, check tape integrity at least every two months. While this is the ideal situation, in reality it is rather rarely done.

A final comment on tape backup: The cost of a tape cassette, usually in the range of $25, is really quite insignificant compared to the value of the data, yet it is not uncommon to find cancer registrars equipped with only two or three backup tapes. This is a very false economy. A sufficient number of tapes would be the number needed for a minimum of six complete backups, using one set of three for rotating nightly backups and another set of three for rotating monthly backups. With this plan, even in a worst-case scenario, a registrar can go back as far as two to three months to obtain an intact copy of the data. Also, magnetic tape does age and wear; tapes should be completely replaced every year or two.

Backup to a hard drive: This is probably one of the most under-utilized yet time- and cost-efficient backup options. A few years ago, it would have been virtually unthinkable to rely on backup to a hard drive because of hard drive costs. Today, however, the costs can be more than offset by the time saved by a registrar. The concept is simple: in a single-user environment, a computer is equipped with two independent hard drives. In a multi-user environment, two or more workstations with hard drives are available, each with sufficient space to back up an entire registry. For nightly backups, a registrar simply copies the entire registry from its home hard drive to a designated directory on another.

In general, backup to another hard drive has several advantages over backup to a floppy disk or tape. It is many times faster than the two other backup alternatives, and, most importantly, a registrar can test the integrity of the backup very easily. All that must be done is to run the registry software from the backup directory with an operation that would access data over the entire registry, such as calculating percent lost-to-follow-up. *Remember:* Backing up to another hard drive is the fastest, most reliable choice to ensure data integrity. Removable hard drives, that can be easily pulled out of the host computer and taken to a remote storage location, are available today for less than $100.

CD-ROM: Plummeting prices have made the CD-ROM a very attractive back-up alternative. For a few pennies one can easily make a resilient and reliable backup of even the largest registry to a medium that is compact and can be stored indefinitely.

DVD-ROM: Another type of reliable backup for the registry is the DVD-ROM, a type of optical disk technology similar to the CD-ROM. The DVD specification supports disks with capacities of from 4.7GB to 17GB and access rates of 600KBps to 1.3 MBps. One of the best features of DVD drives is that they are backward-compatible with CD-ROMs, meaning they can play old CD-ROMs, CD-I disks, and video CDs, as well as new DVD-ROMs.

A Health Maintenance Program for a Registry Computer System

It is relatively easy, requiring more discipline than effort, to ensure that a registry system is healthy and well protected. Backup policies must always be tailored to the local registry environment, the intensity of activity on the registry, and, of course, the available equipment. Most registry specialists strongly encourage conducting backups to at least two different media, for example, floppy disk and tape or hard drive and tape. An alternative schedule might have IT back up nightly to tape and registrars back up monthly to floppy or hard drive.

Figure 22-1 is an example of a well-planned backup schedule for a fictional hospital. The system is equipped with a competent tape backup system and enough tapes for a three-tape backup cycle. In addition, the hospital invested in a second hard drive large enough to accommodate three complete backups of the registry system (all data files and programs). The hard drive is set up with three directories to receive the backup copies, which we'll call A, B, and C. At the end of each working day, the registry is copied from its home drive to one of the directories on the backup drive. The first day it is copied to directory A, the second day to directory B, the third day to directory C, and on the fourth working day, the cycle closes itself and the new copy is made back to directory A after the old contents of directory A have been deleted. This cyclic approach, with multiple backup directories, helps avoid the problems encountered if only one backup directory is utilized and the primary registry system fails in the middle of a backup, leaving both the primary and the backup copies damaged. Because the tape system requires more operator interaction and computer time, it is used less frequently. This situation calls for a monthly cycle with three tapes, the most recent tape being stored off-site after the backup is made. This type of backup plan should be implemented in addition to the system backups that MIS may be making on the network.

Testing the tape backup system is more complicated than testing a backup to a hard drive. Use the "restore" option of the tape backup software, return the registry data to a hard drive other than the parent hard drive (the hard drive where work normally occurs), and then try to run it. Be careful. Tape backup software tends to remember where the data came from and will want to restore the new data to that location unless it is told otherwise. The tape software might restore the registry to its state of several weeks ago, resulting in the loss of all subsequent work; therefore, restoring data from tape must be done with care. Since tapes are used relatively infrequently in this example, it would be sufficient to test them at intervals of about three months.

Although this backup schedule might look a bit complex at first, it will consume far less time than would be spent re-abstracting and entering two or three months of data. As an undisputable rule, the time it takes to complete these backup methods is always well invested. There is no cost to a registrar greater than that of lost information.

Viruses

One reason to adopt a regular backup program is to protect a registry against *viruses*. Computer viruses have the potential to damage or delete an entire data set. Any hospital or registry operation is at risk from computer viruses, even large medical organizations such as national health agencies. While all hospitals maintain virus protection systems, it is virtually impossible to keep these systems absolutely current and closed to outside assault.

A virus is a computer program designed with certain special characteristics that enable it to damage or destroy the contents of a computer hard drive or floppy disk. One of these characteristics is a virus's ability to make copies of itself. In fact, the world's

Figure 22-1

Example of a healthy computer maintenance program

Backup Method	\multicolumn{14}{c}{Working Days}
	1	2	3	4	5	6	7	8	9	10	11...	20	21	41	61
Hard Drive Backup	A	B	C	A	B	C	A	B	C	A	B...	B	C	41	61
Hard Drive Backup Test	A												B	C	A
Tape Backup	A												B	C	A
Tape Restore Test	A														B
Clean Tape Drive	X												--	--	X
Virus Monitoring	X	X	X	X	X	X	X	X	X	X	X...	X	X	X	X

first documented computer virus did just that and nothing else, but it made so many copies that it quickly filled up the hard drive on a mainframe computer system and caused the system to crash. Modern viruses are more insidious. They can insert their copies into critical locations such as other programs or the *boot sector* of a diskette or hard drive, the first portion of a disk or drive read when a computer starts up. Then when the infected program is run or the system booted, the virus resumes its replication/infection cycle. The real threat of viruses, however, comes from their ability to damage data by erasing files, corrupting the file allocation table, or doing any number of other nasty things to a registry.

With reasonable precautions, a registry should be well protected. Although most IT departments have precautions in place, below are a few guidelines:

- A meticulous backup program is a must, including maintaining backup copies that are held for at least two or three months.
- Purchase, install, use, and regularly update one of the quality virus protection software packages. Be sure it is updated regularly with the latest *virus signatures.*
- Minimize the contact your computer system has with files from outside the registry. Never allow staff to bring diskettes from home with the latest games, downloads from on-line services, or other software. When a system must be updated by floppy diskette, the diskettes should be tested with virus-checking software before being used.
- For a hospital-wide network, verify that the IT department has a regular program of virus prevention.
- Never, ever *boot* a system with a floppy diskette in place in the floppy drive. One of the most common sources of viral contamination of a hard drive is from the boot sector of a floppy diskette inadvertently left in the disk drive when rebooting.

WHERE THE MONEY GOES: THE COST OF COMPUTERIZATION

Paying for a computerized cancer registry may be difficult for many hospital financial directors.

Abstracting information and providing annual follow-up can cost approximately $100-$200 per cancer patient. Most of this cost is personnel. But beyond personnel, money should be allocated for computer hardware and software.

The least significant of all expenses in a registry should be the computer *hardware.* Consider some simple arithmetic. A complete and high-quality computer workstation can be outfitted for less than 5% of a typical registrar's annual salary, and can be expected to function adequately for at least four or five years.

Software, on the other hand, can be a fairly significant part of the budget. The registry seeking new software should make a very careful analysis of the many commercial options. Costs of purchase or lease, installation, training, and support should be amortized over five to ten years. A registrar must balance the ability of the software to meet the institution's needs. The match of software and registry may never be perfect, but it will be much better if it is preceded by a thoughtful layout of registry goals and financial priorities.

SUMMARY

The microcomputer is a tool that brings great potential to hospital cancer registry operations. Over the years, it has rewritten the registrar's job description, requiring new skills and introducing new responsibilities. To take full advantage of a computerized registry, the registrar must have a basic understanding of computer operations, agility with DOS and Windows, and familiarity with software tools that support registry operations. Added responsibilities include the discipline to take full advantage of the software's data quality assurance capabilities, and to establish and maintain a comprehensive backup and system maintenance program.

With a solid foundation of registry skill, uniform and reasonable coding standards, and quality software, the computerized cancer registry can become what it was intended to be: a system to monitor patient treatment and outcomes, ensuring that patients receive the best and most current care.

CHAPTER GLOSSARY AND BASIC CONCEPTS

ACoS: American College of Surgeons

Address: an identification, such as a name, label, or number for a register or location in a computer's storage.

ASCII: American Standard Code for Information Interchange: codes developed to translate keystrokes into electronic bits of information, and vice versa. These codes are transmittable over telephone lines or translatable by a computer's processor.

Backup: the process of safeguarding data by copying or duplicating files onto computer media separate from the original location of the file, such as floppy disks, magnetic tape, or a hard drive.

Bit: most basic and smallest unit of data storage or memory housed in an electronic, microscopic bipolar (on/off) switch.

Bits and Bytes: The term bit comes from *b*inary dig*it*. A bit is represented by either 0 or 1, the two numbers used in binary notation. The bit of data is maintained in an electronic microscopic device much like a kind of bipolar switch (a switch that can be on or off). Any computer has hundreds of millions of these bit-sized switches embedded in little black squares or rectangles called microchips.

The first big computers were developed before the invention of the transistor. In those days, one bit of information was stored in a tiny doughnut-shaped electromagnet whose north-south polarity could be switched by changing the electrical current in wires that wrapped around it. The center of an electromagnet is called its core, and computer memory was therefore called core memory. Magnetic cores have long since disappeared from computers, but some books refer to a computer's memory as "core memory."

The information one bit stores can be interpreted in several ways: as an answer to a question (yes or no), as the status of a device (on or off), or, most commonly, as a simple "binary" number (0 or 1).

Although a computer has many uses for information stored at the bit level, it usually works with bits collected together in groups of eight, a unit called a *byte*. With a byte, a computer can keep track of numbers from 0 to 255. To represent numbers much bigger than 255, groups of bytes can be assem-

bled together. Programmers call a group of two bytes a *word* (16 bits). For most purposes, a byte is similar to a letter or digit.

Microcomputers make use of very large numbers of bytes. Terminology had to be developed to express these numbers. For this purpose, the early programmers turned to *kilo* (thousand), *mega* (million), and *giga* (billion). But they did it with a twist because of binary number sequencing. Whereas a kilogram is exactly 1,000 grams, a *kilobyte* (kb) is actually 1,024 bytes, and a *megabyte* (Mb) is 1,048,576 bytes. These numbers happen to be more natural to computers that work with bits, because each bit can express two values and 1,024 is the tenth power of two $(2x2x2x2x2x2x2x2x2x2)$. In bit notation, 1,024 can be expressed more tidily than 1,000: 1,024 is expressed as 10000000000; 1,000 is expressed as 01111101000.

Boolean logic: the mathematics of logical relationships between objects; for example, "greater than," "less than," and "equal to."

Boot: to load a program or application into a computer; when a computer loads or starts its operating system.

Boot sector: the portion of a floppy or hard disk allocated for the special programs required to start a computer.

Byte: a group of eight bits.

CD-ROM: Optical disks (CD-ROM) are the newest mass storage media and are rapidly replacing floppy disks for distribution of software and backup. Instead of magnetic fields, they rely on microscopic pits in a reflecting surface to represent bits. Like hard drives and flexible diskettes, the pits are arranged in concentric circles. As the disk spins, light from a tiny laser beam is scattered by the pits and sensed by an optical detector to create the electronic signals needed by the CPU. Their large capacity (typically 650–700 megabytes) and very low cost (much less than a dollar per disk) makes them a very practical disposable backup medium. For confidentiality purposes, discs must be appropriately stored and disposed of.

Character Set: The early computer engineers borrowed technology from the now-antiquated teletype machines. The teletype was to the telegraph what the fax has become to the teletype. To send a message, a teletype operator used a typewriter-like keyboard.

Each keystroke was converted to a code in the form of electronic bits of information (in groups of seven rather than eight) that were then sent over telephone lines to a receiving typewriter that converted the codes back to a keystroke. The codes were eventually standardized according to rules known as the American Standard Code for Information Interchange, or ASCII (pronounced AS-kee).

The teletype machines used only seven bits for their codes because seven bits can be used to represent numbers from 0 to 127 and 128 numbers were more than enough to represent all of the characters on a typewriter keyboard. IBM extended the coding to eight bits (0–255) and used the extra 128 numbers to represent special graphic characters for a variety of purposes including writing mathematical equations with Greek characters and building lines, boxes, and tables. Several versions of ASCII coding are used regularly, but they differ primarily in the use of the extended character set. For example, many printer manufacturers use the extended character values for special character sets such as italics. The use of eight bits also expands the options for defining the codes that control the CPU (character set). Figure 22-2 illustrates one version of the ASCII standard that is known as the *IBM Extended Graphics Coding* list. It gave DOS programmers the ability to build frames and boxes on the screen.

This information demonstrates that computer engineers must convert the characters with which we communicate to the only form in which a computer can communicate numbers. If a programmer wants to put the greeting "Hello!" with a smiley face next to it on the monitor screen, his or her program must first contain a sequence of numbers that the computer will interpret as CPU instructions, translate what follows as text, and then send it to the video display. Imbedded in this list of instructions are the numbers to be converted to text or other characters. The numbers in Figure 22-3 represent the programmer's friendly message using the IBM Extended Graphics coding system.

Computers can only deal with numbers that are represented by the "on" or "off" state of groups of microelectronic switches. The computer can interpret these numbers as literal numbers, instructions to the CPU, or keyboard and graphics characters. Users communicate with computers by typing on a keyboard, which translates keystrokes into byte-sized numbers. Computers communicate with people

through the video display, which translates the numbers from the CPU into meaningful characters. Even the mouse must communicate with numbers. When you move the mouse across the pad, it is sending the CPU a stream of numbers representing its relative change in position.

Client/server architecture: a computer networking system in which the server allows and facilitates files or pieces of files to move between the server and workstations, or between workstations themselves, and takes an active role in data management. In this system, the server determines who has access to data, takes care of record locking, ensures data integrity when it is placed from the workstation back into the server's data file, and maintains continuous data backups.

Cluster: a group of one or more sectors of storage that is the basic unit in which DOS allocates disk space. The number of sectors in a cluster varies by disk type and operating system.

CoC: *Commission on Cancer of the American College of Surgeons.*

Code: a generic term for the text of computer programs.

Compiler: a computer program that translates second- and higher-generation pseudo-english language into machine language instructions that the computer can understand and process.

Completeness edit: monitoring data input to ensure that all data fields needed to meet minimum reporting requirements are filled, and to identify missing or empty fields.

Computer data pathway: There are three key components to a working computer: the CPU, its memory, and the program. How do these components mesh together to make the computer a functioning and useful machine? Figure 22-4 presents a schematic illustration. Usually, the CPU chip and the memory chips reside on a surface called the motherboard. They are connected through a set of electrical pathways called a *data bus*. The CPU has the ability to retrieve a byte from anywhere in memory. A typical modern microcomputer will have anywhere from 64 to 512 megabytes (MB) of memory (512MB= 4,294,967,296 bits). The cancer registry software does not use all of this, as the computer "operating system" takes a large portion and the rest is shared

Figure 22-2
IBM Extended Graphics Coding List

0	32	64 @	96 `	128 Ç	160 á	192 └	224 α
1 ☺	33 !	65 A	97 a	129 ü	161 í	193 ┴	225 ß
2 ●	34 "	66 B	98 b	130 é	162 ó	194 ┬	226 Γ
3 ♥	35 #	67 C	99 c	131 â	163 ú	195 ├	227 π
4 ♦	36 $	68 D	100 ■	132 ä	164 ñ	196 ─	228 Σ
5 ♣	37 %	69 E	101 e	133 à	165 Ñ	197 ┼	229 σ
6 ♠	38 &	70 F	102 f	134 å	166 ª	198 ╞	230 μ
7 ●	39 '	71 G	103 g	135 ç	167 º	199 ╟	231 τ
8 ◘	40 (	72 H	104 h	136 ê	168 ¿	200 ╚	232 Φ
9 ○	41)	73 I	105 i	137 ë	169 ⌐	201 ╔	233 Θ
10 ◙	42 *	74 J	106 j	138 è	170 ¬	202 ╩	234 Ω
11 ♂	43 +	75 K	107 k	139 ï	171 ½	203 ╦	235 δ
12 ♀	44 ,	76 L	108 l	140 î	172 ¼	204 ╠	236 ∞
13 ♪	45 -	77 M	109 m	141 ì	173 ¡	205 ═	237 φ
14 ♫	46 .	78 N	110 n	142 Ä	174 «	206 ╬	238 ε
15 ☼	47 /	79 O	111 o	143 Å	175 »	207 ╧	239 ∩
16 ►	48 0	80 P	112 p	144 É	176 ░	208 ╨	240 ≡
17 ◄	49 1	81 Q	113 q	145 æ	177 ▒	209 ╤	241 ±
18 ↕	50 2	82 R	114 r	146 Æ	178 ▓	210 ╥	242 ≥
19 ‼	51 3	83 S	115 s	147 ô	179 │	211 ╙	243 ≤
20 ¶	52 4	84 T	116 t	148 ö	180 ┤	212 ╘	244 ⌠
21 §	53 5	85 U	117 u	149 ò	181 ╡	213 ╒	245 ⌡
22 ▬	54 6	86 V	118 v	150 û	182 ╢	214 ╓	246 ÷
23 ↨	55 7	87 W	119 w	151 ù	183 ╖	215 ╫	247 ≈
24 ↑	56 8	88 X	120 x	152 ÿ	184 ╕	216 ╪	248 °
25 ↓	57 9	89 Y	121 y	153 Ö	185 ╣	217 ┘	249 ·
26 →	58 :	90 Z	122 z	154 Ü	186 ║	218 ┌	250 ·
27 ←	59 ;	91 [	123 {	155 ¢	187 ╗	219 █	251 √
28 ∟	60 <	92 \	124		156 £	188 ╝	220 ▄	252 ⁿ
29 ↔	61 =	93]	125 }	157 ¥	189 ╜	221 ▌	253 ²
30 ▲	62 >	94 ^	126 ~	158 ₧	190 ╛	222 ▐	254 ■
31 ▼	63 ?	95 _	127 ⌂	159 ƒ	191 ┐	223 ▀	255

Figure 22-3
IBM Extended Graphics Coding System

```
(72) (101) (108) (108) (111) (33) (1)
 H    e    l    l    o    !   ☺
```

Figure 22-4
Some Computer Data Pathways

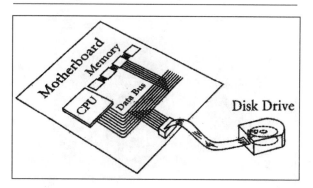

with other programs. Complete information on the memory type can be found by right clicking "My Computer" (usually located on the Desktop), then clicking on properties and then the "general" tab.

Console (Keyboard, Monitor):

Keyboard: Users talk to their computers through the *console* by typing at a keyboard, moving a mouse, or touching the monitor screen. The computer responds with recognizable images or readable characters on the monitor screen.

The computer keyboard is a flat, rectangular piece of plastic covered by keys for data entry. Most computers come with a keyboard called the enhanced 101-key keyboard, which has 101 basic keys (there may be additional manufacturer-specific keys as well), many of which are special to computer use and go beyond the basic alphanumeric keys.

Each keyboard has four main sets of keys that serve very different purposes: the typewriter keys, function keys, cursor-control keys, and the numeric keypad. Most of the time, a registrar will use the "typewriter keys": alphanumeric keys laid out like a standard QWERTY keyboard, and a few special computer keys such as Ctrl and Alt. The function keys, labeled F1 through F12, provide shortcuts to a variety of tasks, depending on the program or application running. The cursor keys (also called the arrow keys) move the cursor (the little flashing rectangle) on the screen. These keys are usually used when editing text, but like the function keys, they depend on the application in use. Finally, the numeric keypad, laid out in traditional 10-key form, serves for fast numeric entry and also as a backup cursor keypad. Despite these commonalities, not every computer keypad is the same as the next. Keys such as the escape "esc" and the back slash "\" may be placed in any of a number of sites on the keyboard.

Monitors: Regardless of the kind of monitor, it is important to understand a bit about the inner workings of this piece of equipment. Monitor systems are

actually made up of two parts: the screen and the *graphics adapter* hidden in the depths of the computer. Basically, what the graphics adapter does is provide the electronic circuitry that controls the monitor and converts bit and byte-sized numbers into the characters and color patterns that appear on the monitor screen.

The console may not seem very complicated at first glance; simply touch the letter or number keys on the keyboard, and the keyboard tells the computer to put those letters on the monitor screen. Touch an arrow key and the computer knows to move the cursor on the monitor screen up, down, left, or right. Move the mouse and the little arrow (cursor) moves. Refer back to the section on programming. A computer is able to read a list of numbers (the program) and, from that list, is able to solve problems or complete tasks. This is also how a monitor works with the computer.

CPU: *central processing unit:* the computer's microprocessor chip; often inappropriately referred to as the computer's "brain." As illustrated in Figure 22-5, the computerized registry depends on two CPUs working together (the computer and the registrar's brain); each one as important as the other. In fact, the computer's CPU merely takes over some of the more mundane aspects of the job so the registrar can focus on issues of judgment and patient care. Keeping sight of this relationship is essential: a computer can save the user time, but it cannot decide how best to take care of patients.

Data bus: electronic pathways on the motherboard that connect the CPU chip, memory chips, and peripheral devices.

Figure 22-5
Cancer Registry Computers Require Two Central Processing Units

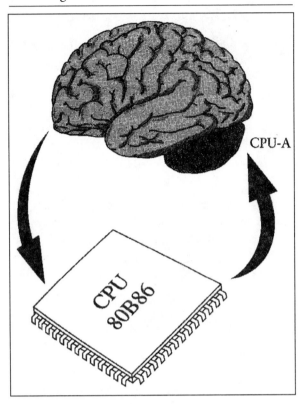

Data coding edit: a tool for monitoring data input to prevent entry of data values not logical or not possible for a given data field.

Data entry field: the point or place on the monitor screen where a single data item is entered into a computer.

Data field: the place where a particular category of data is stored in the database.

Data format edit: monitoring data input to ensure that data entered meet standardized structural requirements.

Data set: the list of items collected in a database.

Device: a piece of equipment; hardware.

Direct access: synonym for random access.

Direct/random access: the ability to read any portion of a data file from a data storage device without having to examine all preceding data in the file. This is done with the assistance of a table of contents, or file allocation table (FAT), which tells the computer exactly where to find information on the magnetic

surface. Floppy disks are direct/random access devices. Tapes are sequential or serial access devices.

Disk Drives: For several reasons, computers have used devices separate from the CPU for long-term data storage. It is not physically practical to equip a motherboard with enough memory to store all of the programs a user might want to run or all of the data a registrar might want to collect. Second, on-board memory is roughly 100 times more expensive than so-called *magnetic media* (tapes and disks). Finally, most computer memory is *volatile.* When a computer's power is removed the contents of the memory are lost.

Early computers relied heavily on reels of magnetic tape, which defined a bit by the direction of the magnetic field on a patch of tape it occupied. Magnetic tape is relatively inexpensive, but it has an enormous disadvantage in that it is a *serial access* device. This means that data and programs are laid out serially (end to end) from the beginning of the tape. To get to a particular piece of information on the tape, the computer must start at the beginning and examine all of the information that comes before the "target" piece of information.

By contrast, memory on a *hard disk* is a direct or *random access* device. With random access devices, each byte has an *address,* which is simply its relative position in the memory organization. A program simply has to supply the address to the CPU to get the contents directly (with help from the operating system). Note that the computer's on-board memory has the same basic properties. Random access memory is usually called RAM for short.

Floppy disks and hard drives are both direct/random access devices. They store bits and bytes of information in concentric rings on a magnetic surface. Information on a disk is organized in a linear fashion (starting from the innermost ring and working out), just as on magnetic tapes. However, a table of contents at the beginning of floppy disks and hard drives tells the computer where to find programs and data files. On computers with Microsoft operating systems (the usual case in registries), this table of contents is called the file allocation table, or FAT. Whereas the CPU can obtain data about 1,000 times faster than data on a hard drive can retrieve data in RAM, data on a hard drive can be retrieved as much as 10,000 times faster than data on tape. When hard drives first became available, their cost per byte stored was much greater than tape. In recent years, the cost of hard drives has decreased. In 1980, hard drives could cost over $500 per megabyte. In

1997, a hard drive cost 25 cents per megabyte and in 2002, a very large hard drive could be purchased for 15 cents per megabyte. And, like jet engines in airliners, hard drives have become much more reliable.

Disk duplexing: maintaining two hard drives with exactly the same information; often used as a form of backup.

DOS: *disk operating system:* a collection of programs that allows the PC and its user to manage information and the hardware resources on a computer.

Disk optimizing: the process of reorganizing the files stored on a hard drive to make sure each data file consists of contiguous clusters of information and to maximize disk operating speed.

DOS prompt: the set of characters DOS employs to tell the computer operator the computer is ready for input or information; the letter in the prompt tells the computer operator which disk drive is currently in use or is currently logged to; also called the "command prompt" (example: C:>).

DVD-ROM: A type of optical disk technology similar to the CD-ROM. The DVD specification supports disks with capacities of from 4.7GB to 17GB and access rates of 600KBps to 1.3 MBps. One of the best features of DVD drives is that they are backward-compatible with CD-ROMs, meaning they can play old CD-ROMs, CD-I disks, and video CDs, as well as new DVD-ROMs.

Edit check: to monitor the data input process, preventing input of erroneous data and alerting the user to potentially problematic data. *See also:* data coding edit, data format edit, inter-field edit, inter-record edit, and completeness edit.

FAT: *file allocation table:* table of contents held near the inner edge of a disk that tells the computer where to find programs or data files.

File server architecture: a computer network in which the server's primary responsibility is allowing and facilitating files or pieces of files to move between the server and workstations, or between workstations themselves. Within this system, the workstations are responsible for maintaining data integrity.

Floppy disk: a disk made of a flexible, magnetic substance used to store and access information. These disks are housed inside a rigid or semirigid plastic protective jacket and can be 5.25 or 3.5 inches in diameter. Also called diskettes or flexible disks.

Graphics adaptor: the electronic circuitry inside the computer that plugs into and controls the monitor.

GUI: *graphical user interface:* a computer operating system or program that allows the user to manipulate symbols or pictures on the monitor screen instead of entering discrete commands when accessing applications, procedures, or files.

Hard drive: a rigid magnetic disk used for storing and retrieving mass quantities of data. Unlike floppy disks, hard drives usually cannot be removed from the controlling hardware or housing within the computer. Also referred to as a hard disk or fixed disk.

Hardware: the physical components that make up a microcomputer, such as the printer, monitor, keyboard, and CPU.

HL7: *Health Level 7:* a voluntary standard developed to facilitate exchange of data between components of hospital and other medical information systems.

IBM extended graphics coding: a standard defining the use of the numbers 128 to 255 to represent screen and printer characters. This set of graphics uses numbers 176 to 223 to represent graphic characters for creating boxes and tables.

Instruction: a synonym for code (i.e., a line of program code)

Inter-field edit: monitoring and testing for consistency between data entered in one field and data entered in another field within a patient record with a single primary neoplasm.

Inter-record edit: to monitor and test for consistency between data entered in the same fields between two or more records for a patient with multiple primary neoplasms.

Kilobyte (KB): one thousand and twenty-four (1,024) bytes.

Machine language programming: an early and basic form of computer programming in which the programmer or engineer assembled a series of binary numbers that, when read into the computer's CPU, could be interpreted as program instructions.

Magnetic media: forms of memory storage, such as floppy disks or magnetic tapes, on which bits are stored on a magnetic surface.

Mainframe: a term applied to a class of computers characterized by their large size, expense, and data-processing capabilities; network microcomputers are gradually replacing mainframe systems.

Megabyte (MB): 1,048,576 (approximately one million) bytes; also called a "Meg."

Memory: short-term storage within the computer that the CPU uses to manipulate and work on information. CPUs can only work on information in memory; long-term storage requires saving information on disk.

Microchip: an electronic device, typically smaller than one square inch, housing microscopic electronic circuitry, used for memory storage inside the computer.

Minimum data set: the minimum required data fields a cancer registry system must maintain, as outlined by the Commission on Cancer of the American College of Surgeons and NAACCR.

Modem: *modulator/demodulator:* a device that converts electrical signals from a computer into an audio form transmittable over telephone lines and converts audio signals back to electrical signals to be received by a computer.

Motherboard: the main circuit board in a computer that houses microchips, such as the CPU chip and memory chips, as well as expansion slots for plugging in extensions. Also called planar, back plane, or system board.

Network: a system in which a number of independent computers are linked together to send files back and forth as well as share data and peripherals such as hard disks and printers.

On-line: abstracting, recording, or entering information from patient files directly into the computer database without completing a paper abstract first; a central part of a paperless registry operation.

Operating Systems: The operating system is the program that controls the computer, all other programs, and any software or hardware that saves information to, or loads information from, a disk. One of the first operating systems for microcomputers was simply called "DOS" (an acronym for "disk operating system"). "Windows" is the trade name for an operating system with a graphic interface to the user. Operating systems include programs that can link peripheral devices such as hard drives and printers to the CPU and memory through the data bus, or the pathway data take to travel to and from the CPU. They also must control interactions with the operator, taking input from the keyboard, mouse, and other devices, and responding with sounds and screen displays. When a registrar types a command at the keyboard, or clicks on a screen icon to start the cancer registry program, the operating system takes charge. It puts the program in memory, tells the CPU to go to the beginning of the program, gets the first byte (instruction), and then goes to work.

Over-ride: the ability to suppress a data edit and enter patient information generally not accepted in a particular field.

Paperless registry: a cancer registry that has eliminated the intermediary process of handwriting information from patient files onto abstract forms before entering it into the computer database. This type of registry is characterized by its lack of paper records and the need for file cabinets to store patient files.

Peripheral device: any device attached to the outside of a computer such as monitor, keyboard, modem, or printer.

Printer: There are many brands of printers on the market. Like monitors, printers come in a few basic forms: laser, ink jet, and dot matrix. In the past, dot matrix printers, like monochrome monitors, served most computer users' needs, producing text from word processing and database applications. Laser printers were usually too expensive to warrant purchasing except under special circumstances. However, as is the case with color monitors, high quality laser and ink jet printers are now readily available at very reasonable prices. Laser printers remain the best choice when large volumes of text must be printed. The registry budget will most likely determine the type of printer that is selected, whether it is an ink jet vs. laser printer for color graphics, etc.

Each printer requires specific software, a printer driver, installed on the computer. Most hospitals have Information Technology (IT) support staff to assist with printer hardware and software issues.

Program: set of electronic instructions or steps telling the computer how to manipulate its bits and bytes to solve a problem or approach a task; also called an "application."

Programmability: Computers can do as their name aptly suggests, "compute" (calculate, reckon, or manipulate), and store meaningful information. A CPU needs guidance to manipulate its bits and bytes. Electronic instructions, commonly called a program, provide this guidance. Conceptually, these instructions are relatively simple. They can tell the CPU to move numbers from one location to another, add or subtract the contents of two bytes, and do a few other basic operations. It is the combination of simple operations that creates complex ones (for example, the multiplication of 3x4 gives the same answer as the addition 4+4+4).

How does the CPU receive instructions to save or process information? As a first step, a computer programmer designs a list of byte-sized numbers, each representing a coded instruction for a particular operation the CPU should perform. This list, the program, is placed in the computer's memory, where the CPU can access it. Then the CPU extracts the program's first instruction from memory, interprets it, performs the action, and moves on to the next one. In general, each instruction code does just one tiny part of a program's work. A simple operation such as addition may require dozens of instructions; a comprehensive cancer registry program may employ several million instructions. Fortunately, modern microcomputers can process millions of instructions per second, so a complex task such as completing a patient abstract can be done in a reasonable amount of time.

Early programmers had to create each program instruction separately, often by punching columns of holes in paper cards or tape. Each hole position represented a bit of information; in bit notation a hole equaled 0 and no hole equaled 1 (or vice versa). The cards or tape were fed through electromechanical devices that converted the holes (or lack thereof) into numbers and then stored them in the computer's memory. Programming in this fashion was called *machine language programming.*

Engineers soon developed alternatives to this tedious process: *second-generation languages* (2GL) referred to by acronyms such as FORTRAN, COBOL, BASIC, and C. Some registry systems now use third-generation languages such as dbase. Fourth-generation tools have also evolved and become common computer languages for cancer registrars to use. Each generation has removed the programmers even further from inserting *instruction code* byte by byte, while at the same time delivering more powerful features, such as Windows compatibility.

There are many computer languages. Most languages have been optimized for specific purposes. FORTRAN (FORmula TRANslation), one of the first (circa 1954), has primarily scientific applications such as computer-aided drafting and statistical computation, so the code looks a lot like ordinary algebra. COBOL is a wordy language, popular for business applications such as financial management and banking. BASIC was designed for simplicity; a language for the common person. It borrowed heavily from FORTRAN. The designers of C (which followed developmental languages called A and B) were looking for a blend of power and flexibility; C is used commonly for graphics and databases. At one time or another, all of these languages have been used to develop cancer registry programs.

With any of these languages, engineers can design programs at a standard keyboard by typing in words or expressions in forms resembling common English or algebra, as shown in the example in Figure 22-6. However, when the CPU receives its instructions from a program, they are actually noth-

Figure 22-6

A Simple Edit Check as It Might Appear in FORTRAN

```
IF (HISTO EQ. '9800' AND. AGE LT. 30 AND.
        DEATHCAUSE EQ. '204.0') THEN
    WRITE (*,'(" SEER 1F43: Verify diagnosis ")')
    PAUSE ' '
END IF
```

This piece of code will alert the operator with a message on the monitor screen when the patient is less than 30 years old with a diagnosis of 'Leukemia, NOS' (98 00) and a recorded ICD-9 cause of death of 204.0, acute lymphatic leukemia. This is one of the standard SEER edit checks required of all registry programs.

ing like what is seen in Figure 22-6. Instead, the programmer must first feed his or her efforts through the computer using yet another program, called a *compiler,* which translates the scripted code into byte-sized machine language instructions that the CPU can understand. The compiler simply saves the programmers a lot of tedious and repetitive work because the engineer no longer has to enter information one byte at a time. The first compilers were written the old-fashioned way, in machine language.

Query: in computer registry terms, a question guiding a search for cases, usually focused on assessing common qualities or characteristics of a specific group or subgroup of patients.

Query system: a software feature that allows the user to identify a specific group or subgroup of patients for reporting or analysis.

RAM: *random access memory:* all memory accessible by the microprocessor at any given point in time; the main type of working memory in a PC.

Random access: a method of accessing data wherein the CPU can go directly to exact location of the source of information requested without having to examine all locations preceding the desired one; also called *direct access.*

Record locking: a data protection system that allows only one user at a time access to a specific record for editing. This prevents users from overwriting each other's data and entering erroneous or altering correct information. Some record-locking systems allow other users to access data (for viewing purposes only) when another user is making changes to the data.

Remote access: the ability to link two computers kept in separate locations, usually two work stations, via a modem.

Screen: The computer monitor's image. In abstracting a collection of data entry fields presented simultaneously on one screen; an abstract is typically comprised of several screens.

Second-generation languages: (2GL) computer programming languages that simplified the programming process by allowing the engineers to write program code in a language that closely resembled the mathematical notation to which they were accustomed.

Sector: a section of a disk or hard drive; most sectors hold 512 bytes of information.

Serial access: a method of accessing data, wherein the CPU starts the search for the desired information at the beginning of the data source. All information preceding the desired information on the source must be examined before the "target" is located. Magnetic tapes are serial or sequential access devices.

Server: a computer dedicated to managing a network, storing common programs and data used by many people on the network, and directing data transfer via dedicated lines outside the local network. Server computers usually maintain large amounts of memory and several large disks for storage.

Software: a series of instructions (program) loaded into a computer that tells it how to accomplish a task or solve a problem.

SQL: *structured query language:* a standardized system for designing questions, with which a user or engineer can access information stored in a database.

Tape backup: a method of backing up data stored in a computer to magnetic tape.

Virus: bits of program code designed to inhibit or destroy computer or software function.

Virus signature: program code fragments, much like human fingerprints or DNA virus code, that signify the presence of a virus in a computer system.

Volatile: in computer memory, devices that lose all stored data the moment the power source is interrupted or shut off.

Windows™: a computer graphical user interface (GUI) program developed by the Microsoft Corporation that allows the computer user to access applications, procedures, and files by manipulating pictures on the monitor screen.

Word: a group of 16 bits, or 2 bytes.

Workstation: a user's entire computer system including motherboard and CPU, disk drives, console, disk operating system, and peripheral devices.

STUDY QUESTIONS

1. What is a bit? What is the difference between a bit, a byte, and a word?
2. A workstation and a server are both types of computers. How are they used? How are they

similar to one another? Different from one another?

3. What is the purpose of backups? Discuss the methods and relative benefits and drawbacks of each type of backup presented in this chapter.

4. What are computer viruses? How can a registrar protect against them?

REFERENCES

1. Phillips JL, Menck HR. Computerization. In: Menck H, Smart C, eds. *Central Cancer Registries: Design, Management and Use.* Chur, Switzerland: Harwood Academic Publishers; 1994.

2. Coleman MP, Bieber CA. CANREG: Cancer registration software for microcomputers. In: Jensen OM, Parkin DM, MacLennan R, Muir CS, Skeet RG, eds. *Cancer Registration Principles and Methods.* Lyons, France: 1991. IARC Scientific Publication No. 95.

3. Williamson TJ, McKelvey LW. Computer principles. In: *Cancer Registry Management Principles & Practice.* Dubuque, Iowa: Kendall/Hunt Publishing Company; 1997.

4. Skeet RG. Manual and computerized cancer registries. In: *Cancer Registration Principles and Methods.* Jensen OM, Parkin DM, MacLennan R, Muir CS, Skeet RG, eds. Lyons, France: IARC; 1991. IARC Scientific Publication No. 95.

5. Menck HR, Parkin DM. *Directory of Computer Systems Used in Cancer Registries.* Lyons, France: IARC; 1986.

6. Menck HR. Selection of cancer registry software. *Oncology Issues.* 2002; 17: 32–34.

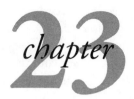

chapter 23

DATABASE MANAGEMENT SYSTEMS

Carol L. Kosary
MA

AN INTRODUCTION TO DATABASES

Data Storage BC (Before Computers)

Since the beginning of human civilization, we have been involved in the collection, organization, and retrieval of information. For a very long time information was stored in the wisdom and stories of tribal elders with human memory as the main method of storage. As civilization progressed, the amount of information increased beyond the point where it was practical to trust to the fallibilities of the memory of a few. The technology of writing was invented, and with it, information came to be stored on media such as clay tablets, and later, with the invention of parchment and paper, on scrolls and finally in voluminous repositories called books. The first person ever to record numbers in a storage medium (clay tablets) was probably a Sumerian accountant somewhere in the lower Mesopotamian river valley about 3200 BC.

With the invention of moveable type, the number of books increased. Soon large collections of books were gathered in libraries, the first real databases. Since the usefulness of any library (or any other database for that matter) is only as good as its data storage and retrieval efficiencies, early librarians defined and developed standardized filing and retrieval protocols. In time, many library collections expanded to include millions of volumes, each comprising hundreds or even thousands of pages, and storage technology grew to include filing cabinets, colored tabs, and three-ring binders. By the time computers burst upon the scene, information was accumulating at such an alarming rate that it seemed certain that it would eventually bury all of civilization under mountains of paper.

The Evolution of the Modern Database

A database is an organized collection of information. Databases excel in managing and manipulating structured information. Consider the phone book. A phone book contains several pieces of information—names, addresses, and telephone numbers—for each subscriber in an area. With the introduction of computers, they were quickly applied to the problems of information storage and retrieval. The first solutions follow the same paradigms and metaphors currently in use in paper-based systems. The first computer databases were "flat file" systems, based on discrete files in a virtual library. Files of archived data were called *tables* because they looked like the tables used in traditional file keeping. The rows of the table were called *records* and the columns *fields*. See Table 23-1 for a sample phone book in a flat file system.

Flat files proved to be very inefficient. In order to find a record, the computer would have to read through the entire file. With hundreds, thousands, or even millions of records, this soon proved to be very time consuming. The solution to this problem was the invention of the database as a computerized record keeping system. The characteristics of a database are that they are compact, fast, easy to use, current, accurate, support an easy sharing of data between multiple users, and are secure.

Database Models

A database model provides a description of both the storage structure of the data in a database and the methodology used to store and retrieve that data. Database models are abstractions but are useful. The analysis and design of these models has been the cornerstone in the evolution of databases. As the models advanced, so did database efficiency.

The databases in cancer registries, in all likelihood, will be one of two types, hierarchical or relational.

Hierarchical Models

A hierarchical model employs two concepts to structure data, *records* and *parent-child relationships* (PCR). While in a flat-file, *record* is used to define a row in a table. In a hierarchical model, *record* defines a collection of data that provide information on an

Table 23-1
Sample Flat File System

Name	Address	Telephone Number
John Adams	77 W. Strayer Ave.	555-4578
Jane Bellows	1278 Georges St.	555-2596
Herb Carlson	35 E. 5th St.	555-4658
David Danes	159 South St.	555-9245
Mary Erlan	8819 Granger Dr.	555-7435

Figure 23-1

An Example of a Hierarchical Model for Some Fictitious Cancer Registry Data

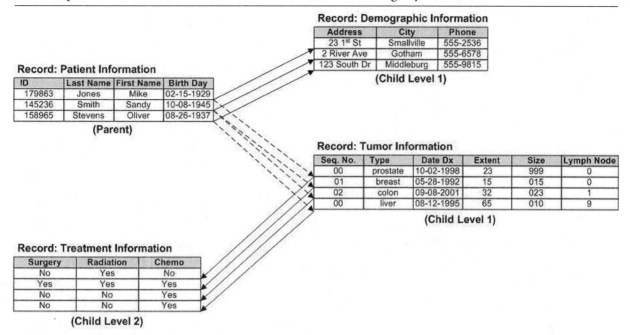

entity (such as patient information). The PCR defines the relationship between a parent record and one or more child records. An example of a hierarchical model for some fictitious cancer registry data is illustrated in Figure 23-1.

In this example the parent record is a group of variables defining patient information. It relates to two child records, defining demographic information and tumor information. Note that in the case of the tumor information record that more than one tumor may exist for a patient. The child record defined by tumor information further relates to a lower level child record that defines treatment information for each tumor.

The hierarchical model can be more efficient than a flat file. For instance, in the above example, a change in address would only require a change in the demographic information table. However, in order to retrieve, insert, update, or delete from the database, an understanding of how the data was structured is required.

Relational Models

Chances are very good that a cancer registry's database will follow a relational model. A relational database model consists of a series of *tables*. In each table,

different types of information are stored, such as a table containing patient demographic information. Each table is made up of horizontal rows called *records,* or *tuples,* that contains data entries for a single entity, such as information for a single patient, or a single cancer, and vertical columns called *fields* that consist of individual data items or *attributes.* All tables in a database are referred to as a *domain.* Each table is identified by a unique name that can be used by the database to find the table. A user only needs to know the table name in order to use the data. An example of a relational model for some fictitious cancer registry data is illustrated Tables 23-2, 23-3, and 23-4.

This example is of a relational database with three tables, Patient Information, Tumor Information, and Treatment Information. The more darkly shaded columns in both tables are the *primary-key* fields. A primary key uniquely identifies a record in a table.

Relational databases are very common. Microsoft Access or Oracle are both very common relational databases. SQL, or Structured Query Language, is a computer language for both accessing and creating relational databases. The advantages of the relational model are discussed below.

Table 23-2
Patient Information

ID	Last Name	First Name	Birth Date	Address	City	Phone
179863	Jones	Mike	02-15-1929	23 1st St.	Smallville	555-2536
145236	Smith	Sandy	10-08-1945	2 River Ave.	Gotham	555-6578
158965	Stevens	Oliver	08-26-1937	123 South Dr.	Middleburg	555-9815

Table 23-3
Tumor Information

ID	Seq. No.	Type	Date Dx	Extent	Size	Lymph Nodes
179863	00	prostate	10-02-1998	23	999	0
145236	01	breast	05-28-1992	15	015	0
145236	02	colon	09-08-2001	32	023	1
158965	00	liver	08-12-1995	65	010	9

Table 23-4
Treatment Information

ID	Seq. No.	Surgery	Radiation	Chemo
179863	00	No	Yes	No
145236	01	Yes	Yes	Yes
145236	02	Yes	No	Yes
158965	00	No	No	Yes

DATABASE MANAGEMENT SYSTEMS

Cancer registrars deal not merely with a database on a computer but rather what can be referred to as a database management system (DBMS). A DBMS is a software system, made up of *hardware* and *software,* used to control the storage, retrieval, and management of large data sets. In order to optimize data retrieval and provide fast access to data, it is essential to have a detailed knowledge of the computer's operating system and file management organization. With a DBMS, the need for the user to possess such knowledge is eliminated. The DBMS shields the physical implementation of the data files form the user and provides an operating-system independent interface, making storage, retrieval, and data management easier.

Possible Computing Environments

The information system architecture, that is the hardware upon which the Registry's DBMS is operating, will depend on when the registry DBMS software was developed. Regardless of what architecture is in place, however, all consist of similar elements. They will have a user interface, some method of data management utilizing some type of database, and a means of computation management.

The user interface, sometimes called a front end, generally consists of a keyboard, a video display, and possibly a mouse. The most common in use today are the dumb terminal and the personal computer, or PC. The databases could consist of flat files, hierarchical of relational databases. Computation is supported through programs written in a number of computer languages.

The very oldest DBMS's, those that were developed before the mid to late 1980s, may still be operating on computers configured in a *mainframe architecture,* utilizing what is now referred to as late third generation mainframe or minicomputers. Under this configuration, all data management and computational tasks are conducted within the central host computer. Users interact through a dumb terminal that captures keystrokes and transfers the information of the host. Computer programs for supporting the data management and computational tasks will generally be written in older programming languages, such as COBOL or Fortran, which may cause various limitations in processing speed or access. A further limitation is the lack of easy support of graphical user interfaces, or GUI's, or access to multiple databases. Typical mainframe architecture is pictured in Figure 23-2.

Those DBMS's that were developed during the early years of the next (fourth) generation microprocessors may be operating utilizing a *file-sharing architecture.* This configuration was common with the original PC networks. Under this configuration, the network server downloads files from a shared location to desktop PC's. The requested user job was then run on the desktop computer. Databases were generally flat files and software was generally programmed in such languages as BASIC or C. This configuration worked if the shared usage was low,

the need for updating was low, and the volume of data to be transferred was low. Due to these limitations, this was never a very satisfactory configuration. Typical file-sharing architecture is pictured in Figure 23-3.

Due to the limitations of the file-sharing architecture, the *client/server architecture* emerged. This approach introduced a database server to replace the file server, allowing user queries to be answered directly, reducing network traffic by providing a query response rather than a file transfer. It also improved multi-user updating through a GUI front end. The databases are usually relational and software is programmed using such modern languages as C++.

Client/server architectures can be *two-tier* or *three-tier.* See Figure 23-4. In a two-tier arrangement, the user system interface is located in the user's desktop, and the database management services are in a server that is a more powerful machine that services many clients. Processing management is split between the user system interface and the database server. A two-tier arrangement is a good solution when the number of users is small. When the number of users increases, performance will deteriorate. Three-tier architecture emerged to overcome these limitations. In three-tier architecture, a middle tier is added between the user system interface and the database server. This middle tier can perform a variety of functions, from queuing, application execution, or database staging.

Figure 23-2
Typical Mainframe Architecture

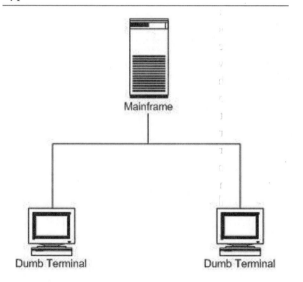

Figure 23-3
Typical File-Sharing Architecture

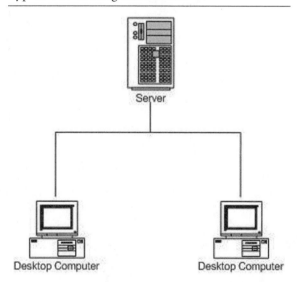

Figure 23-4

Typical Two-Tier and Three-Tier Client/Server Architectures

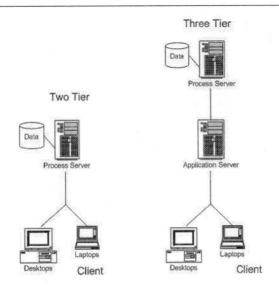

Characteristics of Any Database Management System

All DBMS's share a number of characteristics. At their core, all are involved in taking care of database storage, modification, and retrieval operations. All will have some method of checking that data integrity and consistency rules are upheld. All will have a means of insuring that access is limited to only those users who are authorized. All will control concurrency by way of not allowing multi-user access to the same record at the same time, and all will have some manner of transaction logging as a means of data protection.

Before a DBMS can be used to store and retrieve data, a database must be created, the data to be stored must be defined, and the relationships between the data and their constraints must be given. Database design is the process of deciding how to organize this data into record types and how the record types will relate to each other. The DBMS should mirror the organization's data structure and process transactions efficiently.

Database administrators will perform the job of creating and implementing the detailed database design. Users, however, may find themselves involved with the database administrator in determining the design of the database since they are the ones with the detailed information on the required

data, the relationship between the data, and any and all data constraints.

If a cancer registrar is involved in the design of a database, the systems analyst and database administrator may use something called a *conceptual data model.* This is a method for getting at the various properties of the data in the computer. For example, to identify a patient, a cancer registrar may need to store the properties name, patient number, address, etc. Groups of data that have similar properties are called entities. For instance, patient, cancer occurrence, and treatment are data entities. Data entities are often interrelated; a patient is related to an occurrence of cancer that is related to a treatment. These relationships can be described in an *entity relation diagram.* Graphical tools that assist the user in defining the conceptual model are available. An example is given in Figure 23-5.

Data consistency and integrity will be insured and maintained through effective edits. Again, a cancer registrar may be required to work with the systems analyst and database administrator assigned to the DBMS in order to insure that each data item within the database is associated with the appropriate edits. These edits may include *field edits,* which insure that only the valid values associated with a

Figure 23-5

Entity Relation Diagram

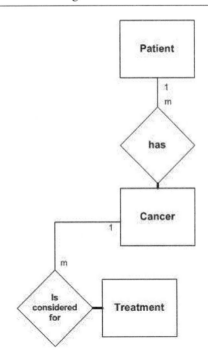

particular data item are allowed; *within record edits*, which would check for impossible conditions between two or more data items with a record, such as a female only cancer entered for a patient who is identified as male; and *between record edits*, which would identify such situations as a new address for a patient who has been diagnosed with an additional cancer.

The systems analyst or database administrator will be responsible for data security. This is generally controlled through the use of passwords, which may go so far as to limit a given user's ability to view and update either the entire database or subsets of the database. For example, only certain persons within the cancer registry may be allowed to update data elements based on the results of edits. Or only certain persons are allowed access to the most confidential data elements, such as patient name and social security number. A cancer registrar may have responsibilities for helping to develop registry security procedures, such as determining the formats passwords must adhere to, how often passwords must be changed, and who has access to what data.

The systems analyst or database administrator will also be responsible for insuring the integrity of the database by insuring that the DBMS has been designed in such a way as to prohibit more than one user from updating the same record at the same time. If a cancer registrar becomes aware that this is not happening with the DBMS, it should be brought to the attention of the appropriate computer professions immediately.

Database Management System Support of Consolidation

Many of the cancer registry functions which would be handled by a registry DBMS, such as case selection, abstracting, editing, and report generation have been previously discussed in other chapters. With the possible exception of editing, particularly complex edits involving checks between patient records or edits involving complicated conditions, record consolidation is the most highly dependent on registry computerization.

Within a cancer registry, various pieces of information are received related to a given cancer case. In a perfect world, all information pertaining to an occurrence of cancer in a patient would be received and entered into a registry's database only once and

in complete form. Cancer registration, like life, is almost never perfect. A hospital cancer registry may receive various pieces of information regarding a patient from numerous sources within the hospital, such as separate reports from the departments of medicine, surgery, and pathology, all of which contain parts of the total information required. It may not be practical to wait for all of these pieces to be fully assembled within a patient's medical record.

Data collection at a central cancer registry dealing with cancer diagnosed within a state or region will be further complicated by information arriving from multiple sources. Many patients are diagnosed by one facility; receive surgery from a second; and radiation, chemotherapy, or other forms of treatment from a third facility. A large hospital-based registry or a central registry can have tens if not hundreds of thousands of cancer records on their databases. With this magnitude of data, it is impossible to deal with data management without the aid of the computer.

Record Linkage

Consolidation requires the use of special software designed to match records. Records can be matched by comparing personal identifying data items from each record in an attempt to determine whether two or more records pertain to the same person. Common data items may include name (last name, first name, initial of first name), social security number (or parts of social security numbers, such as the first "so many" digits), sex, and such name variations as *Soundex*. Matches can be made *deterministically* or *probabilistically*. A deterministic match is one that had been made (or determined) with 100% certainty. Depending on how the DBMS software has been designed, a deterministic match may require no human intervention, with the computer making all necessary updates and corrections to the database.

In probabilistic matching, the computer assigns a score to a potential match indicating a probability that the identified match is in fact correct. Probabilistic matching may identify anywhere from one to many potential matches, requiring a hand-on determination by a cancer registrar as to whether any of the potential matches are in fact correct.

Matching may be conducted by comparing one record against the entire database. This would be the type of matching done in those instances where a new potential record is being entered. One-to-many matching and consolidation can be illustrated by the following example.

Suppose the cancer case for patient Jane Smith shown in Figure 23-6 has been found through a pathology report from the Oak Street Pathology Lab.

Some time later an abstract is received from St. Mary's Hospital. When it enters the database, a match is indicated to an existing record, patient Jane Smith's breast cancer found through the pathology report from Oak Street Pathology Laboratory.

Further, additional information, such as Jane Smith's middle initial, along with further treatment information has come in with the abstract. This additional information can be consolidated into the original record for Jane Smith, now known as Jane B. Smith. (See Figure 23-7.)

To illustrate a many-to-many match, consider the following case. When all of the records in the registry database are matched against each other, two separate records are found: one for Jane B. Smith diagnosed with breast cancer and the other for J. Belle Smith, diagnosed with colon cancer. (See Figure 23-8.)

When these records are compared, the cancer registrar determines that Jane B. Smith and J. Belle

Smith are in fact the same person. The two records are consolidated into one record for Jane Belle Smith containing information on two separate cancers, the breast and colon primaries.

Future Directions of Cancer Registry Database Management Systems

Utilizing DBMSs designed around late third generation or fourth generation hardware will increasingly concern casefinding. This is already taking place today in some cancer registries utilizing electronic copies of pathology reports. The text of these reports is *parsed* and searched against lists of terms in order to retain only those report records that may be cancer. By having the computer perform this task, the cancer registrar will no longer have to perform the tedious task of manually screening what could be thousands of pathology reports in order to find the cancer cases. Also, since the computer has a much lower error rate than the manual procedure, electronic pathology reporting should result in fewer missed cases, while freeing valuable registrar time form more complex, less repetitive tasks.

It should be obvious that electronic pathology reports are just one of several casefinding sources which can be utilized in the future. A future direc-

Figure 23-6
An Example of a Patient Record

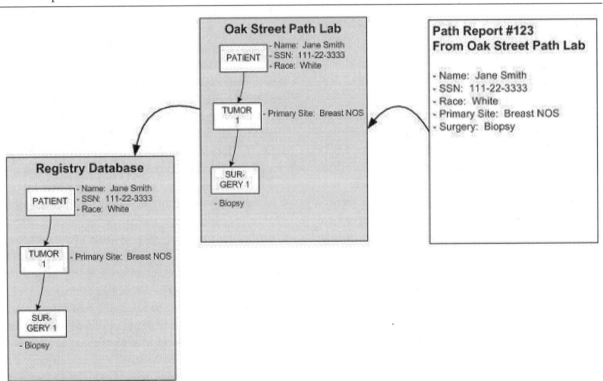

Figure 23-7

An Example of Probabilistic Matching Involving One Cancer

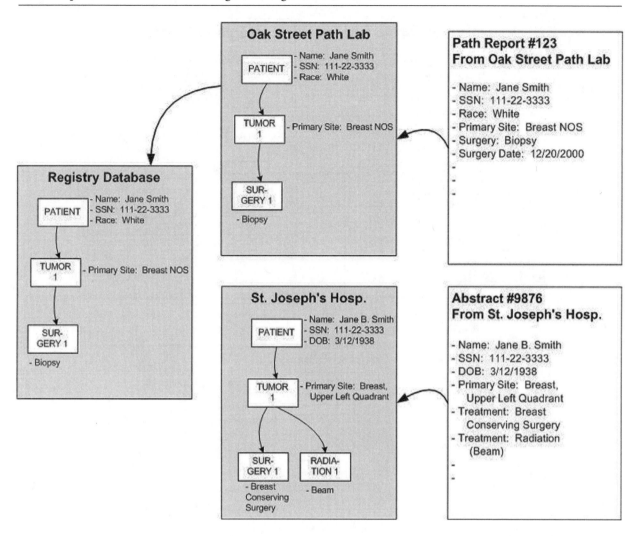

tion of cancer registry DBMSs will be identifying and realizing opportunities for harnessing the increasing power, size, and complexity of fourth and fifth generation computing hardware. This will create systems which fully take advantage of the capabilities of modern hardware and software, ultimately leaving the most complex functions and tasks to the skill and knowledge of the cancer registrar.

Beyond the task of casefinding, future systems have the potential to take advantage of upcoming advances in database design, which will permit the use of multiple databases possibly physically located on distant servers. With the increased ability to combine many different types of information, from data and text, to voice and pictures, future systems may incorporate the text of patient's electronic med-

ical records along with the voice recordings of physician notes and the digital images produced by various diagnostic devices, such as XRay and MRI.

The most exciting possibility, however, will come with the realization of the potential of the upcoming fifth generation of computers. As more data sources, such as electronic medical records, become available, the potential for future registry DBMSs to take advantage of advances in *Expert* or *Knowledge-based systems* or even artificial intelligence increase. Although it may sound the stuff of bad science fiction, even today the first attempts at autocoding cancer registry data obtained from electronic sources is taking place. It has only been 60 years from the development of the ENIAC to today's powerful desktop and workstation computers, and less

Figure 23-8
An Example of Probabilistic Matching Involving Multiple Cancers

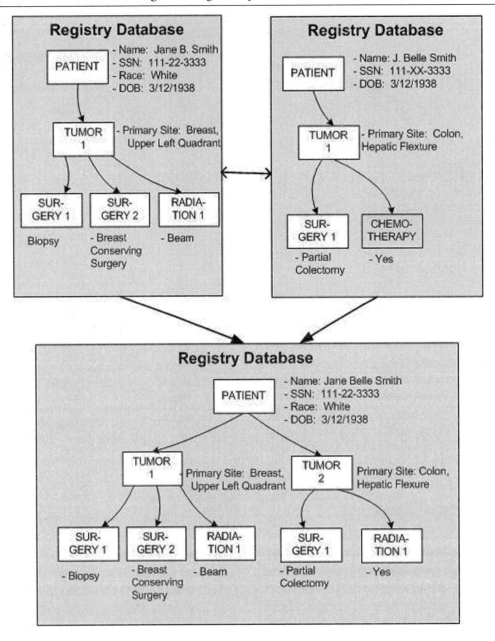

than 30 years from the introduction of the first microprocessor-based machines. There will be enormous changes in IT technology over the next several decades, and the impact it will make on registry DBMSs will be enormous.

STUDY QUESTIONS

1. What distinguishes two-tier from three-tier client server architecture? Which would be more appropriate in a cancer registry setting?

2. What is the purpose of consolidation? How is consolidation assisted by a registry's data management system?

CHAPTER GLOSSARY

Architecture: The framework or the concepts from which a system is developed.

Artificial Intelligence: Often referred to as AI; a subfield of computer science concerned with the derivation of new facts from known facts and inference rules, a procedure that combines known facts to get new facts. AI can be seen as an attempt to model aspects of human thought on computers.

Attribute: A column of a table in a relational database.

Client: A computer system or process that requests a service of another computer system or process (a "server") using some kind of protocol and accepts the server's responses. A client is part of a client-server software architecture.

Data: Representation of observations or concepts suitable for communication, interpretation, and processing by humans or machines. Interpreted data from information.

Data Management: The organizing, cataloging, locating, storing, retrieving, and maintaining data.

Database: A structured set of logically related data together with software to define the structure of the data and to obtain access to the data.

Database Management System: Software that handles all operations on data in a database.

Entity: An object having meaning in a particular context.

Entity Relation Diagram: Method to describe a data structure by entities that are important for the user and their relationships with other entities.

Expert system: Older term for a knowledge-based system.

Field: Part of a record containing one piece of data.

File: A data-storage entity that has a name and that is divided into logical records.

Graphical User Interface: Commonly referred to as GUI, a user interface containing windows, command buttons, and icons that the user can point at to issue a command, usually through a mouse.

Hardware: Physical equipment.

Information: Meaningful and useful facts extracted from data, or interpreted data.

Key: Part of a record that identifies that record.

Knowledge-Based System: a system consisting of an organized collection of knowledge and an inference mechanism stored in a computer to make decisions of solve problems.

Network: A system of interconnected computers and terminals, e.g., LAN or World Wide Web (www).

Operating System: The low-level software that handles the interface to peripheral hardware, schedules tasks, allocates storage, and presents a default interface to the user when no application program is running.

Program: Set of instructions or statements that let the computer perform a certain tasks.

Programming Language: A formal language for the representation of a computer program, also referred to as a computer language.

Protocol: A set of formal rules describing how to transmit data, especially across a network.

Record: The smallest logical unit in a file or database.

Relational Database: Database organization consisting of a series of tables, in which the rows are fixed-length records and the columns represent fields. Corresponding records in different tables are identified by means of keys.

Server: A computer system or process that provides some service to other (client) computer systems or processes. The connection between client and server is normally by means of message passing, often over a network.

Software: Computer programs and their documentation.

System: A combination of the people, procedures, programs, and machines used to perform a task.

Table: Part of a relational database, consisting of records with identical structures.

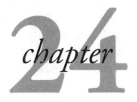
chapter 24

SNOMED CLINICAL TERMS®: MODERN TERMINOLOGY FOR USE IN CANCER REGISTRIES

Mary F. Kennedy
MPH

Patrick L. Fitzgibbons
MD

INTRODUCTION

It is estimated that the number of new cancer cases will rise from the 10 million per year reported globally in 2000 to 15 million per year globally by 2020.[1] Prevention of cancer, improved cancer detection, and effective treatment will become increasingly critical factors in decades to come. Shared care involving a wide range of clinicians in the acute, ambulatory, and home care settings is becoming commonplace. Because of the need to improve our capabilities in prevention, detection, and treatment, a systematic and comprehensive approach to cancer reporting has become an important global strategy for the war on cancer.

Cancer registries are vital for documenting, collecting, and reporting cancer cases, and constitute an essential resource for cancer researchers, public health communities, local practitioners, government programs, and the public. To effectively collect cancer data in a timely, efficient, comprehensive, and error-free manner, a terminology with detailed content is required. This standardized terminology content must include concepts of practical value to registrars and clinicians, yet allow flexibility of expression unique to institutions and individual cases. The terminology must also be able to assemble into complex statements at a highly granular or specific level and it must be compatible with legacy data from older terminology versions for unencumbered data collection. Shared access and more importantly, shared understanding of information across medical specialties, sites of care, and disparate computer systems are also important.

SNOMED Clinical Terms (SNOMED CT®) is a comprehensive clinical terminology used to code, retrieve, and analyze clinical data to meet the challenges of data collection, exchange, and analysis.[2] With the introduction of SNOMED CT, a new generation of global healthcare terminology is available for the cancer team to consistently document care and for cancer registrars to aggregate and retrieve cancer data. SNOMED CT encompasses the entire medical record, providing links to clinical knowledge bases for the sharing and exchange of cancer data.

SNOMED CT is a complete clinical terminology. It is a concept-based terminology that uniquely identifies each medical concept and its multiple descriptions and synonyms. This chapter presents a synopsis of many aspects of SNOMED CT. It is important to understand some of the basic components of SNOMED CT and how these components interact to create a tool that can be readily used in cancer registries.

BACKGROUND

SNOMED® International is a division of the College of American Pathologists (CAP), a not-for-profit organization, which advocates the advancement of excellence of patient care. The CAP is the world's largest association composed exclusively of pathologists, currently serving over 16,000 members. SNOMED International was established as a separate operating unit within the College in 1998 and oversees the strategic direction, scientific maintenance, and global distribution of SNOMED CT.

SNOMED International is committed to excellence of patient care through the development of a scientifically validated reference terminology that enables clinicians, cancer registrars, researchers, and patients to share common concepts worldwide. It embraces the following set of core values:

- Clinicians should determine content.
- Broad, inclusive involvement of diverse clinical groups and medical informatics is necessary.
- Minimal barriers to adoption and use must be maintained.
- Not-for-profit yet self-sufficient division.
- Quality focused on all levels.
- Quality improvement process open to public scrutiny and vendor input.

SNOMED International will maintain the scientific validity of SNOMED CT as it keeps pace with current healthcare discoveries, concepts, and technology. SNOMED CT is a registered HL7 vocabulary. It is compatible with all major messaging standards including HL7 and DICOM.

On July 1, 2003, the College of American Pathologists (CAP) announced the signing of a five-year sole source contract with the National Library of Medicine (NLM) to license English and Spanish language editions of SNOMED CT. This license will allow cancer registries to obtain the core content of SNOMED CT without charge. The NLM license agreement covers all states, US territories, and the District of Columbia; any US government facility wherever located that includes access to a system by

US government employees, designated representatives, and contractors for government purposes; and any public, non-profit, and for-profit entity wholly located in or incorporated in the US.

NEEDS OF THE CANCER REGISTRY

Electronic advances in an ever-shrinking world have brought the work of cancer registries to the forefront of global cancer detection and prevention. The World Health Organization (WHO) recently reported that in many parts of the world cancer registries are the only providers of available information on local cancer incidence. The WHO states that the "comparative value of the statistics which cancer registries produce depends upon the use of common methods, and definitions, so that international collaboration in this area has a very important role."[3]

From the time reporting facilities and medical personnel identify a reportable cancer case until the time the data is available for analysis and research, there are multiple steps involved to ensure that the data are accurate and complete. The potential for error is present at each step in the process, especially if any information is missing or there are discrepancies in the reports. Follow-up letters to physicians or facility medical record department review can involve a large amount of time and personnel. Multiple code sets, improper codes, or no codes at all require the expertise and time of a cancer registrar to assemble all patient information into a complete report.

SNOMED CT can capture the pathologic and other data elements that cancer registrars need to report. In the chart below, examples of reportable data elements are listed. These reportable elements, as well as other data elements, are captured in SNOMED CT, thus eliminating the need to access multiple code sets. See Table 24-1.

Table 24-1
Examples of Reportable Rate Elements Captured by SNOMED CT

Reportable Data Element	Examples of Data Element	Code in SNOMED CT?
Morphology	Islet cell carcinoma	☑
Grade	Gleason grade score 3 out of 10	☑
Primary site	Structure of head of pancreas	☑
Gender	Female	☑
Procedure	Laparoscopic biopsy of liver	☑
Laterality	Left lower quadrant	☑
Ethnicity	French	☑
Histologic type	Adenocarcinoma in situ	☑
Cause of Death	Viral pneumonia	☑
Cancer Treatment	Rituximab 500mg infusion concentrate	☑

Complete pathology reporting can be achieved using a standardized cancer case reporting protocol. Standardized cancer protocols and checklists will be discussed later in this chapter. Incorporating SNOMED CT into the checklists provides mappings, if needed, to report using either ICD-O-3 and/or ICD-9-CM.

SNOMED CT benefits cancer registrars in multiple ways. SNOMED CT represents relationships between concepts so data need only be entered once for each new case. SNOMED CT provides a standard for clinical information by providing a common reference point for data analysis within a software application. The structure of SNOMED CT allows for the linking of a cancer case to other clinical knowledge bases for data aggregation, information retrieval, and analysis of statistics. As a universal numeric terminology, SNOMED CT reduces barriers to communication within institutions, across diverse and often incompatible computer systems, between departments and registries, and even across language barriers.

THE ROAD TO SNOMED CT

The CAP developed its first nomenclature in 1965 to serve as a comprehensive tool for pathologists to code and retrieve their histology cases. This first work was known as SNOP, the Systematized Nomenclature of Pathology. The funds committed by the CAP Board of Governors were used to maintain SNOP and to cooperate with the Council of International Organization of Medical Science (CIOMS) to gain acceptance of this terminology worldwide.[4]

The positive response to SNOP led the CAP to consider expanding the coding work into other disciplines and healthcare professions. In 1974, 250 sites throughout the world field tested a new nomenclature version. This was followed by the introduction of an expanded 44,000-term vocabulary known as SNOMED II in 1979.

With the third edition of SNOMED in 1993, known as SNOMED International, SNOMED had expanded to more than 144,000 terms. SNOMED version 3.5, released in August 1998, contained 156,965 terms and codes. This was the last version in this edition.

In 2000, SNOMED Reference Terminology® (SNOMED RT®) was developed to be an integral foundation for the electronic medical record (EMR) and revolutionized the storage, retrieval, and aggregation of clinical information through its unique structure. Its distinctive design allowed for the integration of medical information in the EMR into a single data structure, facilitating interoperability and data analysis between a wide variety of systems and clinical records. SNOMED RT is a clinical terminology with interface and hierarchical referenced properties. "The terminology model used for data analysis, now called reference terminology, supports aggregation and analysis of clinical data. Aggregation is pooling data from multiple observers for multiple patients, and analysis is correctly answering queries based on data."[2] Interface properties are those features that focus on data collection at the user interface level and include such functions as navigating to find terms, data entry, natural language processing, and non-English translations. Reference properties are those features that focus on data retrieval, aggregation, and analysis.

Alpha development of SNOMED RT was done over a five-year period in collaboration with physicians and nurses in the Kaiser Permanente Convergent Medical Technology Project. Beta testing was carried out by over 40 developers and healthcare enterprises. This new edition of SNOMED was fully compatible with previous editions of SNOMED and included all the content from previous editions to ensure backward compatibility of coded historical data. It was initially released in November 2000 with over 121,000 concepts; 190,000 synonyms; and more than 340,000 relationships.

As SNOMED RT was being developed and refined, the College of American Pathologists and the United Kingdom's Minister of Health, on behalf of the National Health Service (NHS), formed a strategic alliance to create a convergence of SNOMED RT and the UK's Clinical Terms Version 3 (CTV3). Formerly known as the Read Codes, CTV3 brought highly granular primary care content to SNOMED RT. Together, the two merged works are known as SNOMED Clinical Terms® (SNOMED CT®). The result of these two works is a comprehensive and precise clinical reference terminology that provides clinical content and expressivities for clinical documentation and reporting.

SNOMED CT was first launched in January 2002. This terminology is an international, multilingual resource that can represent concepts and terms needed to encode the entire medical record including cancer diagnoses, procedures, treatments, and outcomes. As of the January 2004 release, SNOMED CT contains over 357,000 concepts; 944,000 descriptions relating to these concepts; and approximately 1.3 million relationships between concepts. Figure 24-1 depicts the size and scope of SNOMED CT relative to ICD-9 and ICD-O-3.[5]

SNOMED CT benefits cancer registries by allowing more descriptive capture of clinical data by a single terminology. SNOMED CT usage is made possible in the cancer registry (whether hospital, free-standing, central, or regional) through its unique design and compatibility via the registry's software application. SNOMED CT is *not* software, but rather a set of unique lookup tables in a data format. The data tables can be delivered in a number of different ways to adapt to the integration of different software applications. Users gain access to continual updates that are sent every six months. Since healthcare is continually changing and evolving, hardcover volumes of SNOMED CT are no longer available.

In the past, with each release of SNOMED, previous editions of SNOMED were no longer technically supported or updated. In keeping with this decision and to ensure that all users remain current, after the release of SNOMED CT, no additional updates will be made to any previous editions of SNOMED.

SNOMED CT AND ICD-O-3

The CAP has a long-standing relationship with the World Health Organization (WHO) and its

Figure 24-1
SNOMED CT Concepts and Terms, Size and Shape

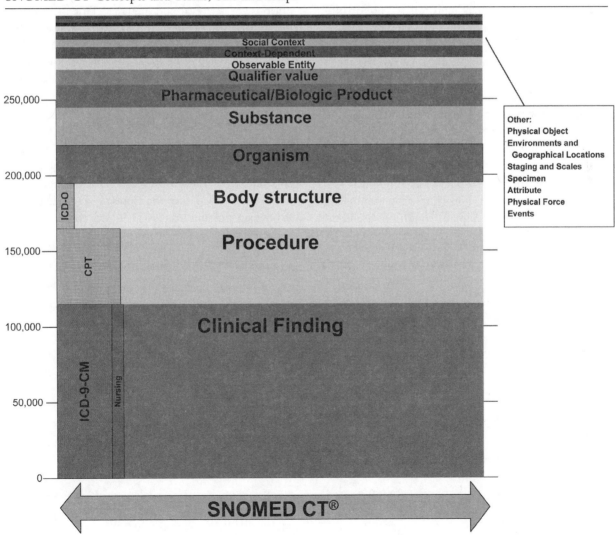

International Classification of Diseases for Oncology (ICD-O). At the time of the earliest edition of SNOP, the American Cancer Society (ACS) published a coding manual for cancer registrars. SNOP included two sections for neoplasms (sections 8 and 9) and an extensive topography section, which was much more complete and highly detailed than what was needed by the American Cancer Society at the time. An agreement was reached that allowed the ACS to use the SNOP neoplasm morphology sections 8 and 9 for their manual. This became the basis for the WHO's first ICD-O coding manual. Then in 1976, the CAP incorporated the morphology section of ICD-O as developed by WHO for its version of SNOMED II.

The codes for all morphology terms in subsequent editions of SNOMED continue to be identical to those that have a match in ICD-O. The topography concepts in SNOMED are more specific and are "mapped" to their appropriate concept in ICD-O. This allows cancer registrars the opportunity to continue to report in ICD-O codes if necessary.

Since the release of SNOMED RT, a link to the appropriate ICD-O morphology codes has been developed by the CAP. The history tables of SNOMED RT and now SNOMED CT will always contain all alphanumeric morphology codes found in ICD-O-3 (and any subsequent ICD-O versions) and any old or retired codes in ICD-O will continue to be connected to an appropriate code in SNOMED CT. In addition, in the ICD-O-3 edition, SNOMED CT morphology terms for non-neoplastic tumor-like lesions and some pre-malignant conditions are listed by a "M" followed by seven dashes and the phrase "(see SNOMED)" following the term. This is done to help the user differentiate benign neoplasms from malignant neoplasms.[6]

Another important difference between SNOMED and ICD-O is in the "many to one" terms in the topography section. Table 24-2 illustrates this difference. In ICD-O-3, "Heart" and the concepts below it all have the same code. In SNOMED CT, each one of these concepts has a separate unique code. This allows for greater specificity in coding the topographic site of a specimen.

Therefore, unlike the morphology codes, SNOMED CT must "map" to the appropriate topography codes of ICD-O-3. Historically, the SNOMED topography codes were denoted by a "T" code while the ICD-O-3 topography codes continue to begin with the letter "C."

While SNOMED CT and ICD-O-3 serve somewhat similar purposes, SNOMED CT is a more granular clinical terminology providing more options for retrieval and analyses. This is an intentional variation between the structure of SNOMED and ICD-O-3. Additionally, SNOMED CT is designed to work in modern computer systems using concepts that are related hierarchically.

SNOMED CT AND ICD-9-CM

SNOMED CT also contains a "mapping" table to ICD-9-CM. This table consists of single concept correlations of the Finding and Disease hierarchies of SNOMED CT and the closest ICD-9-CM term. Whenever possible, the ICD-9-CM codes with the highest level of specificity are selected.

Table 24-2
An Example of SNOMED CT Specificity

SNOMED CT Concept	SNOMED CT Code	ICD-O-3 Term	ICD-O-3 Code
Heart	T-32000	Heart	C38.0
Endocardium	T-32060	Endocardium	C38.0
Epicardium	T-39010	Epicardium	C38.0
Myocardium	T-32020	Myocardium	C38.0
Pericardium	T-39000	Pericardium	C38.0
Cardiac ventricle	T-32400	Cardiac ventricle	C38.0
Cardia atrium	T-32100	Cardia atrium	C38.0

Four categories of mapping exist between SNOMED CT and ICD-9-CM. They are:

- One to One SNOMED CT to ICD-9-CM map. The correlates currently are identical or synonymous approximately 12% of the time. An example of this is: "primary malignant neoplasm of central portion of female breast (ICD 174.1)."
- Narrow to Broad SNOMED CT to ICD-9-CM map. The SNOMED CT source code currently is more specific than the ICD-9-CM target code approximately 82% of the time. An example of this is: "malignant neoplasm of upper eyelid (ICD 173.1)."
- Broad to Narrow SNOMED CT to ICD-9-CM map. The SNOMED CT code is less specific than the ICD-9-CM target code. Additional patient information and rules are necessary to select an appropriate mapping. This currently occurs approximately 1% of the time. An example of this would be: "secondary malignant neoplasm of urinary system (ICD 198.1)."
- Partial overlap between SNOMED CT and ICD-9-CM map. Overlaps exist between correlates and additional patient information and rules are necessary to select an appropriate mapping. This currently occurs approximately 5% of the time.

SNOMED CT will continue to update its mapping tables to reflect the most recent updates to ICD-9-CM or any future versions.

OTHER CROSS MAPPINGS

SNOMED provides other mapping resources that allow cross-walks from SNOMED CT codes to matching codes in other systems. Based on the philosophy of "code once, use many times," these mapping resources help to minimize the re-entry of data. Current mappings besides ICD-O-3 and ICD-9-CM include:

- ICD-10
- Laboratory LOINC (integration)
- OPCS-4
- Nursing terminologies (e.g., NIC, Omaha System, etc.)
- CTV3 (integration)
- SNOMED RT (integration)

STRUCTURE OF SNOMED CT[7]

SNOMED CT is a comprehensive clinical terminology that is used to code, retrieve, and analyze clinical data. Its scope encompasses the entire medical record. The terminology is comprised of concepts, terms, and concept-defining relationships necessary to precisely represent clinical information across the scope of healthcare. All concepts are organized into 18 top-level groupings, called hierarchies which also contain numerous sub-hierarchies. Below are the 18 top-level hierarchies followed by an example for each (shown in parentheses):

Table 24-3
SNOMED CT Top-Level Hierarchies

• Clinical finding (*Hiccoughs*) This hierarchy also contains the sub-hierarchy of Disease (*Diverticulitis*)	• Physical force (*Friction*)
• Physical object (*Suture needle*)	• Procedure (*Biopsy of lung*)
• Observable entity (*Tumor stage*)	• Events (*Flash flood*)
• Body structure (*Parathyroid structure*) This hierarchy also contains the sub-hierarchy of Morphologically abnormal structure (*Medullary carcinoma*)	• Environments/ geographical locations (*Intensive care unit*)
	• Social context (*Organ donor*)
	• Context-dependent categories (*No nausea*)
	• Staging and scales (*Dukes staging system*)
	• Attribute (*Causative agent*)
• Organism (*Human papillomavirus*)	• Qualifier value (*Bilateral*)
• Substance (*Cerebrospinal fluid*)	• Special Concept (*Navigational concept*)
• Specimen (*Lymph node sample*)	• Pharmaceutical/ biologic product (*Tamoxifen*)

Of these top-level hierarchies, "Clinical Finding" and "Procedure" are known as **Main Hierarchies** and the other 16 are known as **Supporting Hierarchies.** In SNOMED CT, cancer registrars would be most familiar with the morphology and topography terms and codes used for reporting a primary cancer case. The "Body structure" supporting hierarchy includes topography codes but also contains the sub-hierarchy which incorporates the morphology codes. The "Body Structure" hierarchy is mentioned here so that a cancer registrar has a reference point in SNOMED CT when different elements of the hierarchy structure are explained later in this chapter. Additional examples of the content of each hierarchy will be given when these hierarchies are discussed further.

Hierarchies represent one of the ***basic elements*** of SNOMED CT. There are seven basic elements needed in the structure of SNOMED CT. The other basic elements are shown in the box below. An explanation of each of these basic elements and some components associated with them follows.

Table 24-4
The Basic Elements of SNOMED CT

I.	Concepts
II.	Descriptions
III.	Hierarchies
IV.	Attributes
V.	Relationships
VI.	Concept definitions
VII.	Relational tables

I. Concepts

A concept is a unique thought. Concepts are the most basic components in SNOMED CT and form its foundation. They are the key reference property from which data is compared. In SNOMED CT, concepts are abstract entities. Each concept has a unique numerical "Concept Identifier." Concepts can have multiple levels of "granularity"(specific or particular) and are organized into hierarchies. Everything in the SNOMED CT hierarchical tree is a concept.

The concept identifiers are meaningless numbers and imply no hierarchical information. This is intentional so that a concept may be organized into more than one hierarchy. For example, the morphology concept *Hairy cell leukemia* has the concept identifier *54087003*. All terms associated with this concept, including the preferred term, synonyms, other dialects, etc. can be retrieved through the Concept Identifier.

Concept *granularity* means "specificity" or "more refined" and refers to a particular level of detail. Concepts in SNOMED CT can represent one of many levels of granularity. This allows the

cancer registrar to code cancer cases at the desired level of detail. The hierarchical structure of SNOMED CT allows information to be recorded at very detailed levels and aggregated at either the same detail or a more general level. In addition, the information can also be retrieved along any concept defining characteristics.

The example below illustrates three levels of granularity:

- A broad concept level would be: *Neoplasm (morphologic abnormality)*
- A more granular level of the above would be: *Neoplasm, benign (morphologic abnormality)*
- A highly granular level of the above would be: *Intraductal papilloma (morphologic abnormality)*

II. Descriptions

Concept descriptions are the terms or names that are assigned to specific SNOMED CT concepts. (In SNOMED RT and previous versions of SNOMED these concept descriptions were referred to as "terms.")

For example, the SNOMED CT concept *25370001* contains, among others, the description *Hepatocellular carcinoma*. Each concept has one unique description called its "Fully Specified Name" (FSN) and one description called its "Preferred term." The FSN uniquely identifies every concept in a human-readable way. A concept can also have one or many other descriptions called "Synonyms." The FSN, the preferred term, and the synonyms each have unique numeric identifiers, called "Description IDs." The Description ID uniquely identifies each term in a machine-readable way and the Concept ID ties descriptions together that have the same meaning. By doing so, any preferred term or synonym can be used to express an idea and code a case.

Using the example in the above paragraph, the SNOMED Concept Identifier, the Fully Specified Name, the Preferred term, and its synonyms are related as follows:

CONCEPT ID: *25370001*

- Fully specified name: *Hepatocellular* carcinoma *(morphologic abnormality)*
  - Description ID: *755679015*
- Preferred term: *Hepatocellular carcinoma*
  - Description ID: *42540010*
- Synonym: *Hepatocarcinoma*
  - Description ID: *42543012*

- Synonym: *Hepatoma*
  - Description ID: *42546016*
- Synonym: *Hepatoma, malignant (UK edition)*
  - Description ID: *42544018*
- Synonym: *Liver cell carcinoma*
  - Description ID: 42542019
- ICD-O code: *M-81703* (referred to as SNOMED legacy code. This code is also the SNOMED ID.)

III. Hierarchies

As was previously mentioned, all concepts are organized into one of 18 top-level hierarchies. Each top-level hierarchy can in turn have numerous sub-hierarchies within them. SNOMED CT can be visualized as a tree with the 18 top-level hierarchies serving as the main branches off the trunk and the numerous sub-hierarchies representing the many smaller branches stemming from the main branches. The top-level hierarchies can be seen in Table 24-5.

Table 24-5
SNOMED CT Upper Level Hierarchies

- Clinical Finding
- Physical object
- Procedure
- Observable entity
- Body structure
- Organism
- Substance
- Pharmaceutical/ biologic product
- Specimen
- Physical force
- Events
- Environments/ geographical locations
- Social context
- Context-dependent categories
- Staging and scales
- Attribute
- Qualifier value
- Special concept

At each level further down a hierarchy, the concepts become more granular or specific. The example below shows the concept *infiltrating duct carcinoma* as it relates to the *Body Structure* hierarchy.

Figure 24-2
An Example of SNOMED CT Hierarchical Granularity

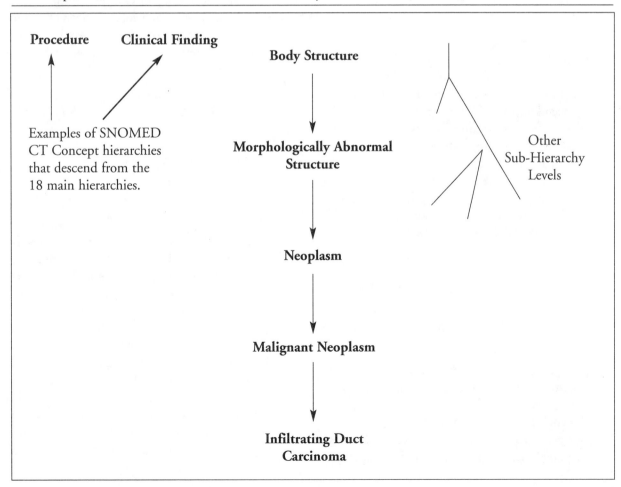

The Fully Specified Name, *infiltrating duct carcinoma (Morphologic abnormality)* would be found in the Body Structure hierarchy. If starting at the most granular level to its most top level, the sequence would be as follows:

Infiltrating duct carcinoma **IS A**
  Malignant neoplasm, primary which **IS A**
    Malignant neoplasm of primary, secondary, or uncertain origin which **IS A**
      Neoplasm which **IS A**
        Mass which **IS A**
          Morphologically abnormal structure which **IS A**
          Body structure, altered from its original anatomical structure which **IS A**
            Body structure which **IS A**
              SNOMED CT Concept ("root concept")

(More about the **IS A** relationships of concepts to each other will be described further when attributes are discussed.)

It is not always intuitive to understand the breadth of each of the top-level hierarchies by their name alone. The best way to understand what is included is to define and give examples from each of these top-level hierarchies.

1. **Clinical Finding**

   This hierarchy now contains the Finding and Disease (disorder) hierarchies, which were separate hierarchies in releases before January 2004. Concepts in this hierarchy represent the result of a clinical observation, assessment or judgment. These concepts are important for documenting clinical disorders and examination findings.

   Within the Clinical Finding hierarchy is the sub-hierarchy of Disease. Concepts that are descendants of Disease are always and necessarily abnormal.

   Examples: —*Diabetes mellitus (disorder)*
   —*Yolk sac tumor (disorder)*
   —*Cramp (finding)*
   —*Cold hands (finding)*

2. **Procedure**

   Procedures are concepts that are purposeful activities performed in providing healthcare. This hierarchy includes a broad range of activities including invasive procedures, administration of medicines, administrative procedures (e.g., medical record transfer), and contains the full range of activities in diagnosing and treating cancer.

   Examples: —*Endoscopic procedure*
   —*Prescription of drug*
   —*Fine needle biopsy of breast*
   —*Outpatient procedure*
   —*Sending of medical records to health authority*
   —*Insertion of radioactive isotope*
   —*Speech therapy*

3. **Observable Entity**

   Observable entities are concepts that when combined with a result, represent potential Findings, or "things you can ask questions about." A Finding could be thought of as composed of an Observable entity that is given a qualitative interpretation or a numerical value. For instance, *Visual acuity* is an *Observable entity*. However, *Reduced visual acuity* is a *Finding* since it is qualified by the interpretation *Reduced*.

   One use for Observable entities for the cancer registrar would be in coding headers on a template. For example, Gender (an observable entity) could be used to code a section of a form titled "Gender" where the user would choose male or female. The chosen gender then becomes a Finding.

   Examples: —*Distance of tumor from closest margin*
   —*Number of regional lymph nodes involved*
   —*Mitotic count score*
   —*Hepatitis C status*
   —*Visual acuity*

4. **Body Structure**

   These are concepts that include normal and abnormal anatomical structures used to specify the locations of diseases and procedures. Key concepts in the pathology report of a cancer patient are derived from this hierarchy. The topography codes ("C" codes of ICD-O-3) are found in this hierarchy. Body structure also includes abnormal body structures such as *Morphologic abnormality* concepts (the so-called "M" codes). Morphologic abnormality is included under Body Structure hierarchy and not the Disease hierarchy because *structural* changes on a cellular level in disease and abnormal development are being described in relation to its body structure. Since pathology reports are based on histologic characteristics and changes on the cellular level, the *Neoplasm* concepts, which are morphologic, are included in this hierarchy.

Examples: —*Iliac vein structure (body structure)*
—*Structure of mesentery of descending colon (body structure)*
—*Appendix structure (body structure)*
—*Fibrinous inflammation (morphologic abnormality)*
—*Lobular carcinoma (morphologic abnormality)*
—*Dystrophy (morphologic abnormality)*

5. Organism

This hierarchy contains organisms of etiologic significance in both human and animal disease including micro-organisms, infectious agents, fungi, and plants. The bacteria, viruses, and other infectious organisms that can affect immunosuppressed patients are also found in this hierarchy.

Examples: —*Cryptococcus neoformans*
—*Helicobacter pseudomonas*
—*Non-A, non-B hepatitis virus*
—*Perennial plant*

6. Substance

The substance hierarchy contains numerous sub-hierarchies such as: biologic substances, body substances, diagnostic substances, dietary substances, drug and medicament substances, toxic substances, abused, and substances. Ingredients used in pharmaceutical preparations are also included in sub-hierarchies. Physician and nursing orders are also included in this hierarchy.

Examples: —*Soy protein (substance)*
—*Cerumen (substance)*
—*Formalin fumes (substance)*
—*Contrast media (substance)*
—*Insulin (substance)*

7. Pharmaceutical/Biologic Product

In order to resolve ambiguity, clinical drugs were separated from raw ingredients of drug products found in the Substance hierarchy. The products in this hierarchy distinguish drug properties (products) from the chemical constituents of drug properties (found in the sub-

stance hierarchy). This hierarchy includes drugs, biological agents, blood products, and other manufactured products. Proprietary "branded" products are in a separate category called a Drug Extension since these items vary by country.

Examples: —*Capecitabine*
—*Antineoplastic agent*
—*Antidotes for pesticides*
—*Activated charcoal powder*
—*Vitamin D preparation*
—*Penicillin V 250mg tablet*

8. Specimen

This hierarchy contains the concepts that represent samples obtained for examination or analysis. Although these samples usually come from a patient, there are other concepts that do not have a human origin.

Examples: —*Tissue specimen from lung*
—*Knee joint synovial fluid*
—*Water specimen*
—*Cervical cone biopsy sample*

9. Physical Object

The Physical Objects hierarchy contains natural and man-made objects. Concepts in this hierarchy are of medical interest, especially in injuries.

Examples: —*Core biopsy needle*
—*Patient chart*
—*Tourniquet cuff*
—*Vena cava filter*

10. Physical Force

This hierarchy includes such characteristics as motion, friction, gravity, electricity, magnetism, sound, radiation, thermal forces (both heat and cold), humidity, and other categories mainly directed at categorizing mechanisms of injury.

Examples: —*Magnetic field*
—*Sonar*
—*Heat*
—*Fire*

11. Events

Included in the Events hierarchy are concepts that represent occurrences resulting in illness or injury such as accidents, falls, and others.

Examples: —*Environmental pollution*
—*Surgery performed on wrong patient*

—*Patient death or serious disability associated with medication error*

12. Environment and Geographic Location

This hierarchy includes different types of environmental locations such as treatment rooms, as well as geographical locations such as countries, states, and others.

Examples: —*Clinical oncology department*
—*Operating theatre*
—*Cancer hospital*
—*Hawaii*
—*Radioactive environment*
—*Health maintenance organization*

13. Social Context

Social conditions and circumstances contained in this hierarchy include such things as family status, ethnic and religious heritage, life-style, occupations, and others. These concepts may be used in developing a family tree to trace the genetic history of a cancer patient, to do current patient risk factors or factors that influence therapy decisions.

Examples: —*Cancer registrar*
—*Economic status*
—*Quaker religion*
—*Australian aborigines*

14. Context-Dependent Category

This hierarchy contains concepts that carry context embedded within the meaning and is used to attach additional information to a concept.

Examples: —*Family history of mental disorder*
—*Excellent response to treatment*
—*Biopsy planned*
—*Cancer confirmed*

15. Staging and Scales

The names of various staging schemes and assessment values reside in this hierarchy. The tumor, nodes, metastasis (TNM) grading system is included in this hierarchy.

Examples: —*WHO CNS tumor grading system*
—*FIGO staging system for cervical carcinoma*

16. Attributes

This hierarchy contains the concepts necessary to link two different concepts to each other. Attributes are also known as "roles" and attribute relationships are also known as "role relationships." Attributes are the bridges between the top-level hierarchies such as Disease and Procedure and Body Structure and Staging and Scales that connect concepts together to build the relationships in SNOMED CT. These attributes are useful for data retrieval and analysis.

Examples: —*Finding site*
—*Causative agent*
—*Severity*

17. Qualifier Value

Qualifiers make it possible for users to add further detail to a concept. Even though the attribute may be the same as a qualifier value, attributes are part of a unique concept in SNOMED CT that consists of one code (pre-coordination) while qualifiers are used to form relationships between concepts by connecting more than one concept (post-coordination).

Examples: —*Right*
—*Lateral approach*
—*Yellow*
—*Present*
—*In remission*

18. Special Concept

This hierarchy contains three sub-hierarchies of concepts in SNOMED CT. The *Non-current concept* sub-hierarchy includes concepts retired because they are outdated, found to be ambiguous, or other reasons. In order to maintain backward compatibility and access legacy data, these terms and codes are not deleted from SNOMED CT but retained and marked as retired (or inactive). The *Navigational concept* sub-hierarchy consists of concepts used to structure the display of hierarchies. The third sub-hierarchy is *Namespace concepts*. This is an internal sub-hierarchy that lists the organizations authorized to create new concepts.

Examples: —*Other lymphoid leukemia, NOS (Non-current)*
—*Clostridium species Q-Z (Navigational)*
—*Type of drugs H-M (Navigational)*
—*Poisoning/injury (Navigational)*

IV. Attributes

Attributes are the properties or characteristics that are used to characterize and define concepts. They

Figure 24-3
An Example of an Attribute Value Pair

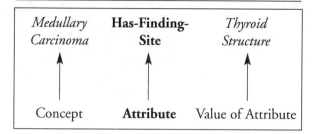

connect concepts together and build the relationships. An example of an attribute is "Finding site." The "Attribute-Value" pairs are the defining characteristics of SNOMED CT. For example, part of the definition of the concept *Medullary carcinoma* is the anatomic site affected. See Figure 24-3.

V. Relationships

These are the connections between the concepts in SNOMED CT. Every SNOMED CT concept has at least one relationship to another concept. These relationships are what characterize the concepts and give them their meaning. There are two types of relationships: *IS-A* relationships and *Attribute* relationships (see Hierarchies and Attributes sections above).

The **IS-A** relationship is also known as a "supertype-subtype" relationship or a "parent-child" relationship. SNOMED CT's hierarchies consist entirely of these IS-A relationships with some concepts having more than one **IS-A** relationship. The IS-A relationships connect concepts within a single hierarchy.

The relationships provide a consistent and computer readable means to consistently and completely retrieve all cases based on one or more selection criteria. For example,

Anaplastic Astrocytoma of Brain (Disorder) **IS A**
  Malignant glioma of brain which **IS A**
    Intracranial glioma which **IS A**
      Intracranial tumor which **IS A**
        Neoplasm of the Central Nervous System which **IS A**
          Neoplasm of Nervous System which **IS A**
            Neoplasm by body site which **IS A**
              Neoplastic disease which **IS A**
                Disease which **IS A**
                  SNOMED CT Root Concept

Therefore, one can retrieve a case of *anaplastic astromcytoma* for a cancer research project by retrieving all cases of:

- malignant glioma of the brain or any of the higher levels in the hierarchy
- primary malignant neoplasms of the brain
- diseases with a finding site equal to brain tissue structure
- morphology of anaplastic astrocytoma of brain

The attribute relationships for this concept characterize the concepts and give meaning to them as well as connect concepts in different hierarchies. The attribute relationships for the above example include:

Anaplastic astrocytoma **Has Finding Site** *Brain tissue structure*
Anaplastic astrocytoma **Has Associated-Morphology** *Astrocytoma, anaplastic*

The attribute relationships above connect the concept *Anaplastic astrocytoma* to the *Body Structure* hierarchy.

Both IS-A and Attribute relationships give concepts their meanings. IS-A relationships and attribute relationships are known as the "defining characteristics" of SNOMED CT concepts. They are essential properties of SNOMED CT concepts—defining characteristics—because they define what concepts mean and how they relate to each other.

VI. Concept Definitions

These are the formal concept definitions consisting of attributes and their parent concepts. All concepts in SNOMED CT have definitions that give explicit or precise meaning to each concept. A concept's definition consists of all of its relationships to other concepts—both **IS-A** relationships and *attribute* relationships. These formal definitions make all SNOMED CT concepts relational and hierarchical.

Relationships are the reference properties that allow the concept meaning to be processed by a computer. This is critical if information and data recorded in various ways is to be retrieved, interpreted, and shared. It is because of these formal definitions that sophisticated information retrieval queries can be done on data coded with SNOMED CT.

VII. Relational Tables

SNOMED CT is distributed to users as a collection of flat files that can be uploaded into relational tables. The technical structure is designed so that SNOMED CT is easy to install for use in many types of software applications and reference files. The structure fully supports the concepts, descriptions, relationships, and maps described in this chapter. The relationships between SNOMED CT concepts, and the linage of Descriptions to Concepts are all recorded in these tables. (A description of these relationships is beyond the scope of this chapter.)

SNOMED AND THE CAP CANCER PROTOCOLS

Surgical pathology reports contain vital information for the management of oncology patients. Physicians and healthcare providers have come to realize that the value of this information largely depends on how it is communicated.[8] Standardized reporting of surgical pathology cancer specimens ensures that all essential patient information is available to the oncologist, radiologist or any other physician involved in patient care. In 1992, Zarbo demonstrated that the use of a standard report form was 'the one practice significantly associated with increased likelihood of providing complete oncologic pathology information.[9]

In 1998, the College of American Pathologists published the first edition of the manual *Reporting on Cancer Specimens—Protocols and Case Summaries*.[10] The protocols in this guide are procedures designed to assist pathologists in providing clinically useful, relevant information and uniformity in reporting the results of their examinations of malignant tumor specimens. The protocols are continually reviewed and updated to insure that the latest relevant developments and changes are represented in a timely manner.

The protocols were originally published by the CAP Cancer Committee with input from the CAP Cytopathology, Surgical Pathology, Cell Markers, Neuropathology, and Hematology Committees as well as specialists from clinically related disciplines. This included surgical oncologists, radiologists, radiation oncologists, and medical oncologists. This multidisciplinary approach insures that the protocols specify all the information necessary to the referring physician to select primary or adjuvant treatments, estimate prognosis, and analyze outcomes. The uniform reporting format design provides cancer registrars and others in the collection of tumor data with the all the essential elements needed for the reporting of cancer cases.

The protocols are divided according to specimen site and procedural type. Although cytopathology procedures were originally included in the protocols, the most recent versions of the protocols have eliminated all cytopathology checklists, since these specimens generally do not allow for definitive tumor staging and histologic classification.

Each protocol is divided into two main sections. The long format contains detailed information and explanatory notes followed by specifically cited references and a bibliography. This section contains such items as details about the handling of specimens, tumor classification, grading, staging, pathologic prognostic factors, and other important pathology assessments. In general, the protocols endorse the use of internationally recognized standards such as the World Health Organization (WHO) classification of tumor types and the new American Joint Committee on Cancer, *AJCC Cancer Staging Manual, Sixth Edition* (2002) for tumor staging.

The short format section contains the cancer case summary. This summary has been put into a checklist format that includes important gross and microscopic features. The macroscopic section contains such things as specimen type, tumor site and size. The microscopic section includes items such as histologic type and grade, extent of invasion, margins, lymph node involvement, and distant metastasis. The CAP Cancer Committee has identified those elements in the case summary portion of the protocols that are considered essential elements of the pathology report. All checklists are regularly reviewed by the CAP Cancer Committee to insure consensus on which reporting elements are essential to the pathology report and which items may be clinically important, but not yet fully validated or regularly used in patient management. These essential elements have been deemed crucial by the CAP in order to provide patients and clinicians with appropriate data for staging, prognosis, and treatment.

Case summaries contain data elements in a synoptic ("checklist") format that supports electronic standardized case reporting. Each data element in the checklists contains the appropriate SNOMED CT code. Encoding the checklists using SNOMED CT, funded in part by the CDC, facilitates intra- and inter-institutional data capture and analysis across similar or disparate systems.

An example taken from the breast cancer checklist is shown on the following pages with corresponding SNOMED CT codes. The checklist data element is shown first, followed by the SNOMED CT code and wording.

(Note: The TNM Staging System for carcinoma of the breast of the American Joint Committee on

Cancer (AJCC) and the International Union Against Cancer (UICC) is recommended. The symbol "p" is used to refer to the pathologic classification of the TNM, as opposed to the clinical classification, and is based on gross and microscopic examination. pT entails a resection of the primary tumor or biopsy adequate to evaluate the highest pT category, pN entails removal of nodes adequate to validate lymph node metastasis, and pM implies microscopic examination of distant lesions. Clinical classification (cTNM) is usually carried out by the referring physician before treatment during initial evaluation of the patient or when pathologic classification is not possible.)

Table 24-6
Example Using the CAP Cancer Case Summary for Breast

Checklist Item	*SNOMED CT ID*	*SNOMED CT Fully Specified Name*
SPECIMEN TYPE		
Mastectomy	G-833A	Mastectomy sample (specimen)
LYMPH NODE SAMPLING		
Sentinel lymph node(s) only	R-003AF	Lymph node from sentinel lymph node dissection (specimen)
LATERALITY		
Right	T-04020	Right breast structure (body structure)
TUMOR SITE		
Upper outer quadrant	T-04004	Structure of upper outer quadrant of breast (body structure)
MICROSCOPIC/SIZE OF INVASIVE COMPONENT		
Greatest dimension: ___ cm (e.g., 1.2 cm)	R-00418	Tumor size, invasive component, greatest dimension (observable entity)
HISTOLOGIC TYPE		
Invasive ductal carcinoma	M-85003	Infiltrating duct carcinoma (morphologic abnormality)
Ductal carcinoma in situ	M-85002	Intraductal carcinoma, noninfiltrating, no ICD-O subtype (morphologic abnormality)
HISTOLOGIC GRADE/NOTTINGHAM HISTOLOGIC SCORE: TUBULE FORMATION		
Minimal: less than 10% (score = 3)	G-F60C	Breast tubule formation: Minimal <10% (score = 3) (finding)
HISTOLOGIC GRADE/NOTTINGHAM HISTOLOGIC SCORE: NUCLEAR PLEOMORPHISM		
Moderate increase in size, etc. (score = 2)	F-02B9E	Nuclear pleomorphism, moderate increase in size, etc. (score = 2) (finding)
HISTOLOGIC GRADE/NOTTINGHAM HISTOLOGIC SCORE: MITOTIC COUNT		
Less than 10 mitoses per 10 HPF (score = 1)	G-F610	Less than 10 mitoses per 10 HPF (score =1) (finding)

(continued)

Table 24-6
(continued)

Checklist Item	SNOMED CT ID	SNOMED CT Fully Specified Name
HISTOLOGIC GRADE/NOTTINGHAM HISTOLOGIC SCORE: TOTAL NOTTINGHAM SCORE		
Grade II: 6-7 points	G-F617	Nottingham Combined Grade II: 6–7 points (finding)
PRIMARY TUMOR (pT)		
pT1c: Tumor more than 1.0 cm but not more than 2.0 cm in greatest dimension	R-003C2	PT1c: Tumor more than 1.0 cm but not more than 2.0 cm in greatest dimension (breast) (finding)
REGIONAL LYMPH NODES (pN)		
pN1a: Metastasis in 1 to 3 axillary lymph nodes	R-003D3	Metastasis in 1 to 3 axillary lymph nodes (at least 1 tumor deposit greater than 2.0 mm) (breast) (finding)
SPECIFY: NUMBER EXAMINED		
Number examined (e.g., 1)	R-002AA	Number of regional lymph nodes examined (observable entity)
DISTANT METASTASIS (M)		
pMX: Cannot be assessed	G-F205	pMX stage (finding)
MARGINS		
Margin(s) uninvolved by invasive carcinoma	R-00423	Surgical margin uninvolved by malignant neoplasm (finding)
Distance from closest margin: _____ (e.g., 6 mm)	R-00481	Distance of malignant neoplasm from closest margin (observable entity)
Margin(s) involved by DCIS	R-00422	Surgical margin involved by ductal carcinoma in situ (finding)
EXTENT OF MARGIN INVOLVEMENT FOR DCIS		
Unifocal	R-00428	Surgical margin involved by ductal carcinoma in situ, unifocal (finding)
VENOUS/LYMPHATIC (LARGE/SMALL VESSEL) INVASION (V/L)		
Absent	F-02BAF	Venous (large vessel)/lymphatic (small vessel) invasion by tumor absent (finding)
MICROCALCIFICATIONS		
Present in invasive carcinoma	R-003B4	Microcalcification present in specimen (breast)(finding)

SNOMED CT has coded the elements in the checklists, including all TNM findings. This allows greater flexibility and specificity for cancer registrars because only one terminology is needed to report cancer cases.

As of January 1, 2004, the American College of Surgeons, Commission on Cancer (CoC) requires the use of the essential macroscopic and microscopic elements of quality pathological assessment as defined by the CAP cancer protocols as part of its Cancer Program Standards for Approved Cancer Programs. The CoC has endorsed the concept of the CAP cancer protocols specific for the tumor sites. Approval will require that at least 90% of surgical pathology reports contain all essential data elements identified in the CAP Cancer Protocols.

To view the most current version of the protocols, visit the CAP website at www.cap.org.

REQUEST SUBMISSION

Any terminology that is not continuously managed and modernized will quickly become outdated and unusable. Even though stability is important, the advancement of healthcare inherently mandates that new concepts will evolve over time and older concepts may actually change or be retired. SNOMED CT recognizes and supports this evolution proactively. SNOMED CT has an active update process in conjunction with licensees, clinical partners, and other stakeholders and welcomes comments and new concepts to review for possible inclusion into the SNOMED CT database.

SUMMARY

SNOMED CT, by its unique structure and comprehensive clinical terminology, is an ideal terminology for cancer registries to use to meet their reporting challenges. When using SNOMED CT, data is automatically integrated into numerous hierarchies for use in seemingly endless queries, with retrieval possible on multiple levels of granularity.

To learn more about SNOMED CT, please visit the SNOMED International website at: www. snomed.org.

STUDY QUESTIONS

1. What are the two types of relationships found between SNOMED CT concepts?
2. What is a concept in SNOMED CT?
3. Why are the morphologic terms such as malignant neoplasms contained in the Body Structure hierarchy and not in the Clinical Finding hierarchy?
4. What will the agreement between the CAP and the NLM mean for cancer registries in terms of SNOMED CT use?

REFERENCES

1. *Executive Summary. National Cancer Control Programmes: Policies and Managerial Guidelines,* 2nd ed. Geneva, Switzerland: World Health Organization; 2002: vii.
2. Spackman KA, Campbell KE, Cote RA. *SNOMED RT: A Reference Terminology for Health Care.* Proceedings of the 1997 AMIA Fall Symposium. Philadelphia: Hanley & Belfus; 1997: 640–644.
3. International Agency for Research on Cancer. *Biennial Report 2000–2001.* Lyons, France: World Health Organization; 2001: 2.
4. Wagner L, ed. *In Pursuit of Excellence: The College of American Pathologists, 1946–1996.* Northfield, Il: College of American Pathologists; 1997: 38.
5. Spackman, KA. *Presentation to the National Committee on Vital and Health Statistics, Subcommittee on Standards and Security Hearings.* Washington, DC; August 2002.
6. Fritz, A, et al., eds. *International Classification of Diseases for Oncology,* 3rd ed. Geneva, Switzerland: World Health Organization; 2002: 4.
7. *SNOMED Clinical Terms (SNOMED CT) Users Guide, January 2004 Release.* Northfield, Il: College of American Pathologists; 3–60.
8. Spackman KA, Hammond MA. Pathology standards in cancer informatics. In: Silva JA, et al., eds. *Cancer Informatics—Essential Technologies for Clinical Trials.* New York: Springer-Verlag; 2002: 166.
9. Zarbo RJ. Interinstitutional assessment of colorectal carcinoma surgical pathology report accuracy: a College of American Pathologists Q-Probes study of practice patterns from 532 laboratories and 15,940 reports. *Archives of Pathology and Laboratory Medicine.* 1992; 116:1113–1119.

10. Compton, C, et al., eds. *Reporting on Cancer Specimens: Protocols and Case Summaries, 1998.1.* Northfield, Il: College of American Pathologists; 1998.

BIBLIOGRAPHY

Aschman D. "SNOMED Clinical Terms—A Clinical Terminology for the Pharmaceutical and Biotechnology Industries," *Business Briefing: Pharmatech; 2002:* 1–4.

Bates PH. Breaking the ice jam: SNOMED upgrades cancer concepts. *For the Record.* May 2002; 9.

Bidgood W, Bray B, Brown N, et al. Image-acquisition context: procedure-description attributes for clinically-relevant indexing and selective retrieval of biomedical images. *J Am Med Inform Assoc.* 1999; 6:61–75.

Kudla K, Rallins M, SNOMED: a controlled vocabulary for computer-based patient records. *J Am Med Inform Assoc.* 1998; 69:40–44.

Landro L. Electronic medical records call for common language by doctors. *Wall Street Journal.* Thursday, August 15, 2002.

Skjei E. A giant leap for medical terminology. *CAP Today.* Northfield, Il: College of American Pathologists; January 1999: 2–5.

Southwick K. CDC taps SNOMED for cancer surveillance. *CAP Today.* Northfield, Il: College of American Pathologists; December 1999: 1–3.

Southwick K. Merging terminologies for a new mother tongue. *CAP Today.* Northfield, Il: College of American Pathologists; April 2002: 5–8.

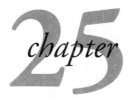

chapter 25

STATISTICS AND EPIDEMIOLOGY

Tim Aldrich
MPH, PhD, CTR

STATISTICS

Basic Concepts and Terminology

Fundamental to the concept of statistics is the recognition that the objective of statistics is to make a representation about a population. This linkage to the population is one reason for the close tie with epidemiology and its intrinsic study of disease in human populations. In order to calculate a specific numeric value for a population, a subset of subjects is selected to represent the *population*. This subset, or *sample* is then studied to derive the estimate of the numeric value of interest. The numeric value for the population [e.g., the true value] is called a parameter; the sample-based estimate of the value is called a statistic. As Figure 25-1 shows, the sample's relationship is to the population what the statistic's is to the parameter. This relationship is crucial to an understanding of how an analysis that is not based on all available data is believed to provide information about the entire population.

Statistical data is, by definition, meant to represent the population from which the sample was taken. To achieve this, there are many varieties of sampling schemes: simple ones, random, convenient, stratified, etc.[1] When a sample is drawn, the data from that sample may be used in several ways: (1) for comparison (i.e. with another sample, or with another population), (2) for description (i.e. simply to explain the characteristics of the population, (i.e. the survival time for lung cancer), or (3) for estimation (i.e. the response rate for adjuvant radiation therapy for Stage I breast cancer). When data is collected, it is not always of the same type; therefore the means of its analysis can vary.

Figure 25-1

Relationship of Statistics (from a Sample) to Statements about Data (Parameters) for the Population

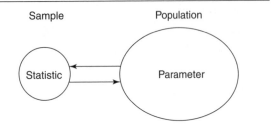

Types of Data

There are four types of data. Two of these data are regarded as qualitative (or also designated as categorical data), or simply classifications into related groups. That is to say, the numbers we may assign to these classifications in medical databases have no measurement value, per se. The other two forms of data are quantitative, i.e. the numbers are actual values or measures.

The first type of qualitative data is *nominal*, literally "naming" data. Nominal data is like race, or gender. We may assign the number 1 for women and the number 2 for men. But the number has no meaning, and the designations are for names we give to these classifications of people. The other sort of qualitative data is called *ordinal*. These categories are placed into an order, or ranking, but the numbers we assign to the classes do not really represent measures. Stage of disease is a fine example of ordinal data. Stage II is greater than Stage I, yet it may not truly be twice as much disease. We simply mean to show that Stage IV is an extreme value "away" from Stage 0, in an order or rank for the extent of disease that afflicts a patient. With both of these types of data (nominal and ordinal), there are particular methods of data descriptions used, and specific techniques for analysis.

The other type of data is quantitative, and in practice, the two types are not generally distinguished too closely from one another. First, there are *interval* data; these data are real measures or amounts based on a starting point that is arbitrary. Two examples of interval data from medicine are body temperature and survival. With body temperature, zero on the Fahrenheit scale is at one point, while the same value (zero) on the Celsius scale is at another point. In neither scale is the zero value truly devoid of temperature; "zero" value is simply the staring point for that scale.

With survival data, patients live for periods of time following a diagnosis, so each has a first year, second year, etc., in one-year increments. However, the first [calendar] years for all patients may represent different dates. One patient's first year of survival may transpire from May 31, 1990 to May 30, 1991, while another patient's first survival year is January 15, 1993 to January 14, 1994. Both live one-year after their diagnosis, but the starting point (zero date) is arbitrary. By contrast, *ratio* data may be the simplest of all measures. It represents measures or amounts based on a scale where zero means there is none. Some straightforward examples include size of a tumor mass, a person's height, or age. Next, we will examine ways to present data.

Frequency Distributions

When data is collected, there is always merit in depicting the specific observations visually. One speaks of the manner in which data are observed to vary as the "distribution" of the data. A long string of numbers is difficult to assimilate or interpret. And, without interpretation, data cannot become information. Therefore, we briefly touch on four simple diagrams for presenting the frequency distributions of sample data.

First, the simple *proportion* is easily recognized. The proportion is the part of the whole. Some view proportions as percentages. Two examples of data presented as proportions are shown in Figure 25-2. On the left is the familiar pie chart. The sizes of the pie's slices are the proportion of the whole represented by each stage group. On the right is a popular format, the stacked bar. The entire height of the bar is the complete sample of patient data; the segments are shaded in proportion to the fraction that each stage group represents. These diagrams are especially useful for nominal and ordinal data.

When one is dealing with counting categories, there is a well-established diagram, the *bar chart*. The bar chart is constructed so that one of its axis, here it is the *abscissa (or x-axis)* is labeled for categories (nominal or ordinal variables). The *ordinate (y-axis)*, is the actual count (interval or ratio variables). The bars of the chart do not touch to signify that they have no quantitative relationship. The height of the bars represents the amount in each category.

Next, there are means to present data from two variables taken from the interval or ratio scales. These are the more intricate presentation forms and likely the most crucial to grasp. These formats are usually referred to as *distributions*, although any representation of the content of a data set is rightly regarded as a distribution of the data. It is with these later representations, that certain, specific terms must also be applied for describing them. First however, let us examine the construction of these figures.

A *histogram* is comprised of bars. The bars on one axis are the intervals for a variable of interest. This variable may be discrete (e.g. whole number counts, as often used with age) or increments of a continuous measure (e.g., as with the size of a tumor mass). In either case, the data is often grouped into ranges, as 10 to 19 years, 20 to 29 years, 1.5 to 2.4 cm, 2.5 to 3.4 cm. Please note that the categories are mutually exclusive, and that they are contiguous (side-by-side). This adjacency of the bars is crucial to the nature of the data. Note that the bars of the histogram touch each other unlike the bar chart in Figure 25-3. In Figure 25-4, tumor size is the abscissa and the number of cases with tumor masses of that size is represented on the ordinate.

When one presents a histogram, there is always some consideration for how many bars to have, i.e. how many categories to use for grouping the data. As a general rule, seven to ten categories are preferred. Less than five categories can be "blocky," and over a dozen is "too busy" to be easily distinguished. When many figures are to be included in a report, or when

Figure 25-2
Two Examples of Data Presented as Proportions: Pie Chart and Stacked Bar

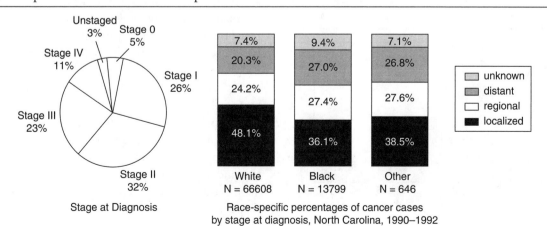

Figure 25-3
Bar Chart of the Number of Cancer Patients in a Series, by Anatomic Site

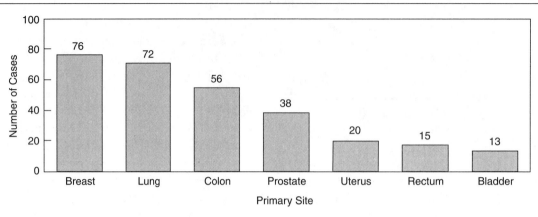

it is desirable to include data for more than one group on the same axis, the histogram is often replaced by a *frequency polygon* (Figure 25-5). This figure is simply composed of a line connecting the midpoints of the tops of each of the bars from the histogram. However, the visual effect permits multiple lines (representing different groups) to be superimposed onto one coordinate grid. A frequency polygon may also be called a line chart or an *ogive*. *One crucial consideration with the frequency polygon is to recognize that the area under the curve represents the same information as the histogram. That is, the area under the curve describes the proportion of the total data described by a specific value.*

When one seeks to analyze data, the distribution of the data is a pivotal consideration. Most often, the term "distribution" refers to the pattern formed by the histogram, or frequency polygon, over the *range*

Figure 25-4
Frequency Histogram of Tumors by Size of the Tissue Mass

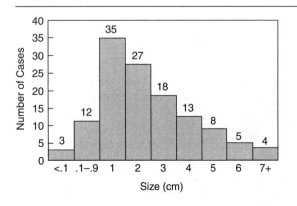

of values for the variable. The range of a variable is simply the difference between the highest value and the lowest. For example, in a group of persons, their weights may vary from 90 lbs. to 240 lbs. That represents a range of weights of 150 lbs (e.g. 240 - 90 = 150). The pattern of the weights, whether more at the lower end of the range, more at the higher end, or evenly spread out over the range is what is usually referred to as the "distribution."

Describing Distributions

When discussing statistics, it is important to use precise terms for describing the distribution of data over a range. Methods for such descriptions follow in the section after measures of central tendency. However, first let us examine the terms one uses to characterize the visual image represented by a histogram, or frequency polygon.

Figure 25-6 shows frequency polygons of three data sets. The three curves are all *symmetric*, that is the diagram is shaped the same above, as it is below, a certain point. However, the three curves differ in the manner by which they vary over the range of values. This aspect of the spread, or dispersal in the data is termed *kurtosis*. The shorter, flatter of the three diagrams is termed *platykurtotic*. As a means to visualize this term, one may think of a platypus. The highest diagram is called *leptokertotic*. One may envision two "leaping" kangaroos facing one another, with their long tails trailing out. However, it is the remaining diagram that is the most familiar in statistics and most important to describe. This middle distribution is *mesokurtotic* and is usually called bell-shaped. It is also referred to as the normal distribu-

Figure 25-5
Frequency Polygon of Number of Cases by Age

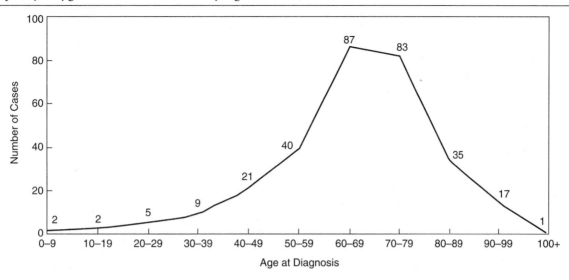

Figure 25-6
Representation of Three Distributions about a Common Point, with Differing Kurtosis

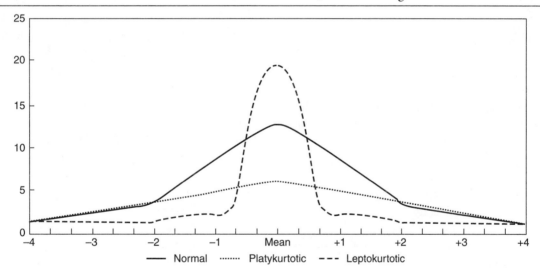

tion, as it occurs most frequently when one is studying biologic data in nature, or living systems.

Not all distributions are symmetric. On a two dimensional axis, there are only two ways that a diagram representing quantitative data may be dispersed. One direction is to the right; the other way the data may disperse is to the left. In Figure 25-7 are found representations of distributions that are *skewed*, that is, are drawn out in an extreme direction. When one describes skewing, one names the pattern in terms of the long tail. When a diagram trails off to the left, it is called *left skewed*, or *nega-*

tively skewed. This latter term is based on the idea that the tail is pointed back to the lower values of the range, or to the end of the axis that would eventually become negative values if they extended below the zero score. The alternative is a *positively skewed* distribution, or one that points to the right side of the figure.

When one inspects distributions of data, there is one consideration that is immediately apparent. The diagram is composed of many values, and the pattern can be described visually (with the terms from this section); but how does one describe the distribution

Figure 25-7
Representation of Skewed Distributions

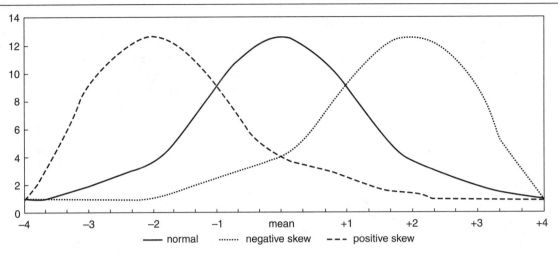

quantitatively? The aim is to identify one, or a few numbers, that will describe the distribution (or dispersal, or variation) of many observations.[2] The next section provides a way to meet the challenge of using a few numbers in place of many.

Measures of Central Tendency

This section will describe some of the most important terms in the entire field of statistics. The objective of this section will be to replace the distributions elaborated in the previous section with values—single numbers that will provide the description of the distribution of a sample data set without a diagram. The first aim then is to assign the location of the distribution along a number line. As shown in Figure 25-6, symmetric distributions are aligned about a central point. Further, the kurtosis describes the tendency of the observations to aggregate them about this central point. Logically then, the goal is to define a measure of this tendency toward the center, that is to say, a quantity for this central tendency.

Using the sample data from Appendix I, one may list the ages for the twelve children with Acute Lymphocytic Leukemia. In Table 25-1, these data are shown in the order from Appendix I, then they are re-ordered from lowest to highest ages. For the purposes of determining the three measures of central tendency, the values of the sample to be described must be in order (preferably ascending).

The simplest measure of central tendency is the "most frequently occurring value." In this sample,

that is age six years. This measure of central tendency, the age value of six, then is the *mode.* The next simplest measure of central tendency is the middle value, or *median.* This distribution is composed of an even number of observations, so that there is no middle value. The median may be a derived quantity, however. One takes the two middle values and finds their arithmetic average (i.e. add them together and divide by two; e.g. 5 + 4 = 9; 9/2 = 4.5); therefore the median is 4.5. One-half of the values will be found above this quantity, while one-half of the values will be less. If there are an odd number of observations, the exact middle value (even is it is repeated in the sample) is the median.

However, the most meaningful of the measures of central tendency is always derived, that is to say, it is usually not a value that is observed in the sample. Many know the formula for this measure as the arithmetic average, more properly called the *mean.* The mean has a specific symbol (an X with a bar over it). The X is used to denote a generic value, and the subscript refers to the order of the value (e.g., the second value would be represented by X_2. The total number of observations that comprise a sample is represented by the value of "n." So that X_n is the last value in a range. Below the data in Table 25-1 is shown the formula for the mean. This formula is read, "The sum (shown as the upper case of the Greek symbol Sigma) of observations, beginning from Number 1 and going to Number 12, is divided by the total number of observations."

Table 25-1

Childhood Acute Lymphocytic Leukemia Data From Appendix I, Measures of Central Tendency, and the Formula for the Mean

Ordered Observation	Age	Ordered Age		
X_1	7	1		
X_2	6	2		
X_3	5	3	Median = 4.5	
X_4	3	3		
X_5	6	4		
X_6	2	4	Mode = 6.0	
X_7	6	5		
X_8	4	5		
X_9	1	6	MEAN = $\overline{X} = \dfrac{\sum_{i=1}^{n} X_i}{n} = \dfrac{52}{12} = 4.33$	
X_{10}	3	6		
X_{11}	5	6		
X_{12}	4	7		
Total		52		

Now we have a measure of central tendency that is exactly quantitative (the mean), another that is positional (the median), and one that is simply the highest point on the curve (the mode). It is important to recognize that in all normal distributions (no matter what their kurtosis) there is only one mode. However, in nature, sometimes we are given distributions with more than one most common value. When there are two most common values, that distribution is termed a *bi-modal* distribution. Also, when a distribution is skewed, the effect is greatest on the mean. In a diagram of a skewed distribution showing the three measures of central tendency, the mean will be the one shown closest to the tail; pulled there by the skewed values.

Now there is the matter of dispersion about the measure of central tendency. The conventional term for this dispersal or variation for observations is the *variance*. The symbol for variance is the lower case Greek symbol sigma, if a printer cannot provide this Greek character, a lower case 's' may be used. Because variance is a squared quantity, the value of variance can often not be interpreted, e.g., years of age (...what is a year squared??). So to interpret the variation about the mean, the units must be the same as for the mean. This requires taking the square root of the variance, termed the *standard deviation*. In Table 25-2, the value of the standard deviation for

the children with Acute Myelocytic Leukemia has been calculated.

The calculation of variance introduces the term, *degrees of freedom*. Degrees of freedom are represented by the value n-1 in the denominator of the variance formula. The reason for this subtraction of one is based on the individual values that are free to vary once the sum and the number of observations is specified. *That is, if you know that eight numbers sum to 70, can you say what the value of the first number will be? No! Knowing that the age observed for the first child with acute myelocytic leukemia was seven, so that you know that the value of the next seven observations sums to 63, can you specify the value of the next observation? No! So this process continues until you have the ages of the first seven children known. With a summation of 70 to preserve, the age of the last child in this series must be 10, so that unlike the preceding age, it is "not free to vary."* As we are dealing with the variation of observations about the mean, if an observation cannot vary, the number of subjects that contribute variability to the calculation is reduced one. In other formula, in other calculations, the methods for determining the degrees of freedom is different, but it is always the number of observations that can vary and not change the sum of the observations.

Now, we have achieved our objective of being able to use a few numbers in the place of many. That

Table 25-2
Calculation of Variance and Standard Deviation

Observation	Age	Mean	$X_i - X$	$(X_i - X)^2$
X_1	7	8.75	-1.75	3.06
X_2	5	8.75	-3.75	14.06
X_3	6	8.75	-2.75	7.56
X_4	11	8.75	2.25	5.06
X_5	14	8.75	5.25	27.56
X_6	9	8.75	0.25	0.06
X_7	8	8.75	-0.75	0.56
X_8	10	8.75	1.25	1.56
Total	70		0.00	59.48

$$\sigma^2 = \frac{\sum_{i=1}^{n}(X_i - \overline{X})^2}{n-1} = \frac{59.48}{7} = 8.497$$

$$\text{Standard Deviation} = \sigma = \sqrt{\sigma^2} = \sqrt{8.497} = 2.915$$

is, two numbers that will describe a distribution. With the mean and standard deviation, one can define the quantitative central tendency point of a distribution and the extent of variation about it. One of the great merits of statistics is that the dispersion of observations about a mean value, in a normal or bell-shaped curve, is highly consistent. In Figure 25-8, the proportion of the distribution of observations that are represented under a normal curve is shown.

Within the values from the mean to one standard deviation will be contained about 34% of the total observations in a normal distribution. So that within the bounds of ± (plus and minus) one standard deviation value from the mean, there will be about 68% of all of the observations. Likewise, from the first standard deviation to the second two standard deviation value, the area under the normal curve is 13.5%, i.e. 13.5% of the observed values. Therefore, for the area from the mean to two standard deviation units, there are 47.5% of the total observations in the sample. Consequently, in the area ± two standard deviation unit from the mean, there is 95% of the observations in the sample. These relationships can be found in Table 25-3 as well. The tabled values for the areas under a normal

curve permit much finer determinations of the areas for smaller fractions of standard deviation units.

This process of recognizing areas under the curve is crucial to the process of statistical reasoning. The area under the curve is the proportion of observations from the sample that are distributed in those values. This fraction, proportion of the observations, can be viewed as a probability. For now, review Figure 25-8 and Table 25-3 with the perspective that about 34% of the observations lie within one standard deviation unit of the mean. Now, consider that the probability of a particular value lying between the mean and one standard deviation is about 34%.

Notice that Table 25-3 is arranged so that the area described is the proportion of the data between the mean and the value selected in units of the standard deviation. To clarify this, perform this simple exercise. We said that the area under normal distribution, between the mean and one standard deviation value was 34%. In Table 25-3, we see that it is exactly 34.13%. It is important to recognize the tabled values as decimal fractions and to be able to express those as percentages. Likewise, it is important to be able to express these areas. In order to find the area that is between the first and second values of a standard deviation, one must be able to visualize

Figure 25-8
Diagram of the Area under a Normal Curve

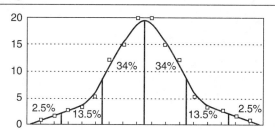

the areas. Notice that the area to the second standard deviation is 47.72%. Subtracting the area to the first standard deviation unit (47.72 - 34.13) gives 13.59; earlier in the narrative we referred to this area as about 13.5%. With the statistical table, much greater precision is possible than is often used. Notice that the exact point where 95% of the distri-

bution area is contained (47.5% on each side of the mean) is actually 1.96 standard deviation units. However, it is very common to see this value referred to as "two standard deviation units." Exercise care about when exact precision is needed and rounding is acceptable.

The next section of this text aims to clarify the concept of the area under the curve as a probability statement. This perspective (area as probability) is the basis to evaluate the likelihood of an individual observation belonging to a particular sample, to test data as belonging to a specific distribution, and for comparing the data from two different samples.

Tests of Significance

Understanding the perspective that standard deviation units may be used to describe proportions of a distribution is most vital to understanding the following

Table 25-3
Areas under the Normal Curve, Also Called a Z Table

%	.00	.01	.02	.03	.04	.05	.06	.07	.08	0.09
0.0	.0000	.0040	.0080	.0120	.0160	.0199	.0239	.0279	.0319	.0359
0.1	.0398	.0438	.0478	.0517	.0557	.0596	.0636	.0675	.0714	.0753
0.2	.0793	.0832	.0871	.0910	.0948	.0987	.1026	.1064	.1103	.1141
0.3	.1179	.1217	.1255	.1293	.1331	.1368	.1406	.1443	.1480	.1517
0.4	.1554	.1591	.1628	.1664	.1700	.1736	.1772	.1808	.1844	.1879
0.5	.1915	.1950	.1985	.2019	.2054	.2088	.2123	.2157	.2190	.2224
0.6	.2257	.2291	.2324	.2357	.2389	.2422	.2454	.2486	.2517	.2549
0.7	.2580	.2611	.2642	.2673	.2704	.2734	.2764	.2794	.2823	.2852
0.8	.2881	.2910	.2939	.2967	.2995	.3023	.3051	.3078	.3106	.3133
0.9	.3159	.3186	.3212	.3238	.3264	.3289	.3315	.3340	.3365	.3389
1.0	.3413	.3438	.3461	.3485	.3508	.3531	.3554	.3577	.3599	.3621
1.1	.3634	.3665	.3686	.3708	.3729	.3749	.3770	.3790	.3810	.3830
1.2	.3849	.3869	.3888	.3907	.3925	.3944	.3962	.3980	.3997	.4015
1.3	.4032	.4049	.4066	.4082	.4099	.4115	.4313	.4147	.4162	.4177
1.4	.4192	.4207	.4222	.4236	.4251	.4265	.4279	.4292	.4306	.4319
1.5	.4332	.4345	.4357	.4370	.4382	.4394	.4306	.4418	.4429	.4441
1.6	.4452	.4463	.4474	.4484	.4495	.4505	.4515	.4525	.4535	.4545
1.7	.4554	.4564	.4573	.4582	.4591	.4599	.4808	.4616	.4625	.4633
1.8	.4641	.4649	.4656	.4664	.4671	.4687	.4686	.4693	.4699	.4706
1.9	.4713	.4719	.4726	.4732	.4738	.4744	.4750	.4756	.4761	.4767
2.0	.4772	.4778	.4738	.4788	.4793	.4798	.4803	.4808	.4812	.4817
2.1	.4821	.4826	.4830	.4834	.4838	.4842	.4846	.4850	.4854	.4857
2.2	.4861	.4864	.4868	.4871	.4875	.4878	.4881	.4884	.4887	.4890
2.3	.4893	.4896	.4898	.4901	.4904	.4906	.4909	.4911	.4913	.4916
2.4	.4918	.4920	.4922	.4925	.4927	.4929	.4931	.4932	.4934	.4936

Table 25-4
Review of Frequency Distribution Using the Acute Lymphocytic Leukemia Data

Observation	Ordered Age	Absolute Age	Frequency	Relative Frequency	Cumulative Frequency
X_1	7	1	1	8.33	8.3
X_2	6	2	1	8.33	16.66
X_3	5	3	2	16.67	33.33
X_4	3	3			
X_5	6	4	2	16.67	50.00
X_6	2	4			
X_7	6	5	2	16.67	66.67
X_8	4	5			
X_9	1	6	3	25.00	91.67
X_{10}	3	6			
X_{11}	5	6			
X_{12}	4	7	1	8.33	100.00

concepts in this narrative on statistics. We will use the same information found in Table 25-1 to review this crucial concept. In Table 25-4, columns have been added to represent the area of the distribution (or probability for) represented by a specific observation. The statistical term for the number of occurrences of these values is their frequency. One speaks of the absolute frequency of the observations (how many observations have this value), the relative frequency (the proportion, or percentage, that have that value), and the cumulative frequency (the percentage of observations with this value or below). Another way to view the cumulative distribution is to consider the relative frequencies as "accumulating."

Take time to familiarize yourself with these values (frequencies). Notice how the three frequency columns relate to one another. Observe that the seven-year-old child represents an 8.33 proportion in distribution, and the probability for observing children younger than age seven in this sample is 91.67%. Now you are ready to explore the application of one of the most familiar of statistical tests. This method aims to evaluate the likelihood (or probability) of a specific observation being found in the sample for which it is observed.

The Z-Test

All of our lives, we are impacted by the use of the Z-test. The Z-test is the means most used by teachers for assigning grades in a manner termed "grading on the curve." Z-values are used for assigning persons to tax brackets, salary ranges, and even insurance rates. The Z-test is a familiar means of assigning a probability to a particular observation. That is the exercise shown in Figure 25-9 for the 14-year-old youth with Acute Myelocytic Leukemia. The questions being answered is, "What is the probability of observing a child 14 years of age or older with Acute Myelocytic Leukemia (AML), based on this sample data?" The resulting Z-score (1.80) can be located in the areas under the normal distributions (Table 25-3).

Enter Table 25-3 for the 1.8 value, then move across to the .00 column. This location on the table is equivalent to the distance from the mean to 1.80 standard deviation units (the heading for the column provides the third decimal place for a standard deviation value of interest). This tabled value shows that the area under the curve from the mean value to this observations is 0.4641 (recall that this is 46.41%).

In this sample of children with acute lymphocytic leukemia, the 14-year old is 5.25 years older than the mean value of 8.75 years. The standard

Figure 25-9
Calculation of the Z-test Using the Acute Myelocytic Leukemia Data

$$Z = \frac{X_1 - \overline{X}}{\sigma} = \frac{14 - 8.75}{2.915} = 1.80$$

deviation for this sample is 2.915 (this value was not shown in the earlier tables, you may calculate it for yourself if you choose). Examine the formula in Figure 25-9: by dividing the difference between the observation of interest (14 years old) from the mean (8.75 years), by the standard deviation value (2.915), one finds that there are 1.80 standard deviation units in the difference between the 14-year-old and the mean. The area under the curve from the mean to this point (1.80 standard deviation units) is 46.41%. Remember that this particular table shows the area for only one side of the overall distribution (e.g., the area from the mean out to the selected value of standard deviation). With the other half of the area under the curve below the mean representing 50%, the cumulative probability for observing children less than 14 years old is 96.41% (e.g., 46.41 + 50.00). The probability of observing children with AML who are 14 years of age or older, based on the distribution of this sample's data, would be 3.59% (100% - 96.41%).

Hypothesis Testing

Before we move on to the two statistical tests that this text will present, there is the matter of understanding the reasoning behind why one performs a statistical test. First, there is a hypothesis implied for the process. This hypothesis is called the *null hypothesis* (represented in notation as H_0). When one performs a statistical test, the objective is to determine the probability that the resulting statistic represents the finding that the null hypothesis is true. *It is conventional form to state the null hypothesis as "there is no difference" between the two measurements being compared.* Therefore, in research, the aim is to reject the null hypothesis that the two groups are not different, in favor of accepting an *alternative hypothesis* (H_a) that there is a "real" difference between the two groups (e.g. as the result of a different treatment, or some meaningful characteristic).

The process of statistical hypothesis testing is quite intricate. There are two ways that a "true" result can follow from a statistical test. One way is for the null hypothesis to be true, and the statistical test finds that it is true. The other "true" result is when the null hypothesis is false and the statistical test finds that it is false, e.g., the two groups are truly different. Consequently, with two ways to be right, there are two ways to be wrong. These errors are called *type I and II errors.*

Type I error occurs when the null hypothesis is true and the statistical test finds that it is false. This is also called the *alpha error,* it is the one most feared for medicine owing to the charge of the Hippocratic oath for physicians to "do no harm." It is for this reason that the driving force in most medical research is to have the chances of committing a type I error to be less than 5%, i.e., less than 0.05.

Most medical tests in years gone by were directed to finding new medications or better treatments. The possibility that there would be harm done to patients from erroneously accepting one treatment as better than another (when in fact it was not) led physicians to search for an acceptable probability level for this undesirable event. They sought out an august statistician, Dr. Karl Pearson, to advise them. Dr. Pearson indicated that he did not follow an exact probability himself with such decisions, rather he weighed the probability as a relative value. However, he observed that when the chances were less than one-in-twenty (i.e., five-in-100) he felt generally comfortable accepting that result. That is to say, that was the point to reject the null hypothesis and accept the alternative one. This advice has passed into the form of legend and has become an icon in medical research.

Type II error occurs when the null hypothesis is false, but it is accepted as true. This error was deemed more acceptable for medical applications, as it would result in no change from the current practice, and would lead to no potential harm for the patient. Over the years, public health researchers have come to place much emphasis on the option associated with not making the Type II, or *Beta error* when the null hypothesis is false. This is the circumstance when there is a true difference between the groups and it is found; such a result (measured as 1 – Beta) is called Power. One may then speak to the "power" of a study to find a difference between groups, when it truly exists.

In stating the result of a statistical test, one provides the *p-value*, where the "p" stands for the "probability," that this statistic is the result of a random observation. That is to say, one provides for the reader of the statistical test result, the probability that this observation (whatever the null hypothesis states) could have been obtained as a result of chance. The notation for presenting the p-value is usually to show an amount that the p-value is below. For example, the classic decision point (less than a 5% chance [0.05] of this observation) is shown as p < 0.05. The usual values assigned to the other measures mentioned in this section are as follows: for the Type II, or Beta error, use twice the value of the Type I or alpha error, that is often 0.10. This leads to the value for power (1 - Beta) conventionally being assigned at about 90%. Now, let us move on to learning about two statistical tests: one for quantitative data, the other for qualitative data.

Comparing Two Means

One of the most straightforward of all statistical tests is comparing two samples to see if they represent the same population. Another form is to ask whether a particular sample belongs to a particular population (e.g., compare the sample mean to the population mean). The null hypothesis for these tests states that the two means are from the same population, and that their difference is "due to chance." The alternative hypothesis asserts that their difference is beyond "chance," and the researcher may then offer an explanation why the two are different.

The t-Test

The t-test was developed originally for comparing the quality of beer samples. The inventor wanted to be able to make his determination about samples with fewer than 100 testings (the convention at that time). He developed the t-test as a special case of the Z-test with adjustments to the distribution for the statistic when smaller numbers of observations were used. When one compares the distribution of the t-statistic (Table 25-5) and the areas under the normal curve, they begin to draw relatively close after about 30 degrees of freedom. So, generally speaking, the t-distribution is favored when the sample sizes are less than 30 observations.

The t-test is designed to compare two means in order to determine whether they are statistically significantly different from one another. In that respect, it is much like the Z-test, where the p-value indicated the probability that one observation was statistically significantly different from the sample distribution of interest (suggesting that it may

Table 25-5
Critical Values for the t-Distribution

df	$t^{.20}$	$t^{.10}$	$t^{.05}$	$t^{.02}$	$t^{.01}$
1	3.078	6.314	12.706	31.821	63.657
2	1.886	2.920	4.303	6.965	9.925
3	1.638	2.344	3.183	4.541	5.841
4	1.533	2.132	2.776	3.365	4.032
5	1.476	2.011	2.571	3.247	4.604
6	1.440	1.943	2.447	3.143	3.707
7	1.415	1.895	2.365	2.998	3.499
8	1.397	1.860	2.306	2.896	3.355
9	1.383	1.833	2.262	2.821	3.249
10	1.372	1.812	2.228	2.764	3.169
15	1.341	1.753	2.131	2.602	2.947
18	1.330	1.734	2.101	2.552	2.878
19	1.328	1.729	2.093	2.539	2.861
20	1.325	1.725	2.086	2.528	2.845
30	1.310	1.697	2.042	2.457	2.750
40	1.303	1.684	2.021	2.432	2.704
120	1.289	1.658	1.980	2.358	2.617
160	1.287	1.650	1.975	2.350	2.607
200	1.286	1.653	1.972	2.345	2.600
Infinity	1.282	1.645	1.960	2.328	2.576

belong to another distribution). The t-test aims to test one distribution compared to another to determine whether they represent two different distributions or population. In the original setting, testing beer samples, the aim was to assure the quality of each batch before selling it. In that setting and with many others, it is usual to regard one of the distributions being tested as a surrogate for the population, being comprised of data that is "usual" or "standard."

With the t-test, a new measure of dispersion is used to evaluate the difference between the two means (much the way one evaluated the difference between an observation and the sample mean with the z-test). This new measure of variability however is referenced to the "population" and so is often called the *Standard Error of the Mean,* referring to the population mean (see Figure 25-10). Please give particular attention to the formula; it is very simple. It is the sample's standard deviation, divided by the square root of the sample size. Recall how variation is a squared quantity, hence the taking of the square root again, just as with the formula for standard deviation. The use of the sample size, *n,* for taking this square root means that greater precision is achieved with a large sample size, and lesser precision (or greater variation) will be associated with a smaller sample size.

Consider for a minute the interpretation of the SEM (Standard Error of the Mean). The description of the SEM is, "If 100 samples of the size N were repeated again and again, the true population mean would lie between plus and minus two [actually 1.96] of the SEMs from the sample mean, 95% of the time." One begins to see the logic that prompted the choosing of a smaller sample size. One hundred beer samples, however tasty, can be very daunting. This is especially true if the 100 samples were thought to need repeating 100 times—hence, the t-test, which uses only one sample and fewer observations. See Figure 25-11. This diagram shows how successive samples of the same size will have a

variety of means (due to natural variation). However, the successive confidence limits of these sample means will tend to encompass the true (population) mean. Some of the sample means provide closer estimation. In some instances, the population mean is nearer the boundary of the sample confidence limits, but nonetheless, most of the sample confidence limits based on the SEM (e.g., 95%) will contain the population mean. It is this tendency of the means toward the true population mean that is at the heart of statistical reasoning in fact, there is a theorem in statistics, based on using the means from repeated samples as a distribution themselves. The theorem, named the *Central Limit Theorem* may be stated: the bounds of the sample of means, would encompass the true, population mean, 95% of the time.

The matter of comparing a sample mean (or you may prefer to say distribution) to the population mean indicates that one has information from many other observations. This is exactly the instance with the beer testing; from years of testing and based upon the selected quality factors the company desired, the beer testers had a "standard" or "population" against which to compare each new batch of beer that they produced. This situation may be likened to a medical example, where one has long documented the response of patients to a particular treatment, so that one is then able to compare a new treatment to that large, earlier treatment experience in order to evaluate whether the new option represents an improvement.

Conversely, other considerations besides the treatment may have changed over time. Researchers will often prefer to compare the means of two samples,

Figure 25-11
Variability of Sample Means to Encompass the Population Mean (Illustration of the Principles of the *t*-test

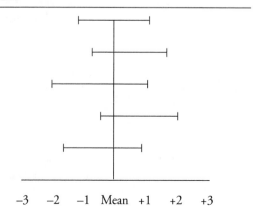

Figure 25-10
Formula for the Standard Error of the [Population] Mean

$$\text{Standard Error of the Mean} = \text{SEM} = \frac{\sigma}{\sqrt{N}}$$

i.e., persons treated with one options versus persons treated with the other, but during the same time period. *In either case, the t-test is the statistical method to use.* The actual mechanics of calculating the t-value however will vary slightly between these two options. Likewise, they will also vary somewhat if the two samples are matched, say for age at diagnosis. For a more thorough discussion of these differences in the ways of calculating the t-test, please consult other texts.[1,2,3,4] For this discussion, we will simply focus on our sample data set and compare the age distributions between the childhood myelocytic and lymphocytic leukemia cases.

With the t-test, one has a variety of expectations about the two samples; you may prefer to call these *assumptions* about the data. One expectation is that the means are not in some way related to one another. This consideration is often referred to as *independence of the means,* that is to say, they vary on their own without some dependence on one another. Another assumption is that the variation of the two samples are approximately equal. Often this equality of variance is not present, so the variation from the two samples must be pooled (added together in the relative proportions of the two samples). This is yet another way to calculate the t-test. This is the approach we will use here as we know these two samples have different variances.

For the sake of this text, computational formulae are not crucial. Rather the student should strive to grasp an understanding of the calculation process and the meaning of the resulting statistic.

All applications of the t-tests follow the same form: they seek to answer the question, "Is one mean close enough to the other, so that simple, random variation could have explained the difference observed between the two means?" If this question is answered, "yes," then one concludes that the variation between the two means is random and then accepts that the two samples are from one, or the same, population. For the beer application, such a result would mean that the new batch of beer may then be sold with confidence that it was the same quality of the other batches produced by this company. In a medical setting described before with two treatments, when the question is answered, "yes," the null hypothesis will lead the researcher to accept that the two treatments produce the same level of effect. However, if the t-test result shows that "no, the two means are too far apart to have resulted by chance, alone;" that means that the two groups are different from one another is a sub-

stantive manner. That difference may be regarded as the effect of the two treatments.

For our example, we will evaluate whether the two groups of children (those with lymphocytic leukemia versus those with myelocytic leukemia) have difference average [mean] ages. If the two means are not found to have significant statistical differences, then the difference between the means will be attributed to a random choice of which children had which leukemia, older or younger. However, if the mean ages are found to be different, one may infer that the two disease processes are different from one another, and that the difference in ages of the children affected may be one manifestation of this biologic difference.

Let us move on to the t-test calculation (Figure 25-11). As a first step, we see that the two means (4.33 and 8.75) are 4.42 years apart. The next step is to calculate the standard error for the two samples combined (the denominator of the first equation), as they have different variances (3.333 and 8.497 respectively). One successive calculation is nested within another calculation: the pooled variation of the two samples. This quantity is used for the estimate of the SEM.

Next, looking for this value for "t" in the t-distribution (Table 25-5), one enters the table for 18 degrees of freedom. Moving along the line, one sees that the value 11.947 is far greater than any of the tabled values for 18 degrees of freedom. Therefore, one declares that the probability of two samples (of these sizes) with mean ages that are this far apart (4.42 years) are not separated by random chance, rather the difference is "real" and open to interpretation. That is to say, this statistical relationship is represented as [p < 0.01]. We can describe this probability for these two samples actually representing the same [population] mean value, and this difference between them being random or chance (so that we would interpret the hypothesis wrongly, i.e. commit a type I error) is less that one in one hundred.

For the users of this textbook, there is no expectation that you must memorize the t-test formula. There is no need to be able to do the t-test calculation per se, although working through the sample solution shown in Figure 25-12 will help with understanding the process. What is crucial to readers is to recognize the use of the t-test with quantitative data (i.e. interval and ratio data) and for the purpose of determining whether the means of two samples represent the same population. Alternatively, the t-

Figure 25-12
Calculation of the t-Test Statistic Using the Sample Data for Lymphocytic and Myelocytic Data.

$$t = \frac{\overline{X}_1 - \overline{X}_2}{\sigma_{(\overline{X}_1 - \overline{X}_2)}} = \frac{4.33 - 8.75}{\sigma_{(\overline{X}_1 - \overline{X}_2)}}$$

$$= \frac{(3.33 + 8.497)}{(12 - 1) + (8 - 1)} \quad \sigma_p^2 = \frac{\sigma_1^2 + \sigma_2^2}{df_1 + df_2}$$

$$= \frac{11.83}{18} = 0.657$$

$$\sigma_{\overline{X}_1 - \overline{X}_2} = \sqrt{\frac{\sigma_p^2(N_1 + N_2)}{N_1 x N_2}}$$

$$t = \frac{(4.33 - 8.75)}{\sqrt{\frac{0.657(20)}{(12 x 8)}}} = \frac{4.42}{0.370} = 11.947$$

Please note how throughout these formulae, the sample sizes are closely involved.

test can also be used with the population mean, as mentioned above, in which case the objective is to determine whether the sample belongs to the population of interest.

Tests with Qualitative Data

Now then, how does one test such hypotheses with qualitative data? Not with the t-test! However, much of the actual process is the same (i.e., obtaining a test statistic, looking it up in a table, assigning a probability for that statistic having been reached by a random sampling process). The principal difference with this manner of analysis (qualitative data) is that it uses counts of observations within some category. As such, the test becomes one to evaluate whether the *observed* count is what was *expected*. As will be discussed later in the section on epidemiology, this evaluation of the observed versus the expected value makes this statistical test quite valuable for analyses of epidemiological data.

The Chi-Squared Test

A test that may be used with qualitative data (either nominal or ordinal) is called chi-squared, written in notation as X^2. The English "X" is the same form as the Greek letter "chi." Examine the formula for chi-squared (Figure 25-13) to see how the aspect of the value being squared is represented. Recall that this test is dealing with variability about an expected value. Just as variation was a squared quantity, so too is chi-squared.

The most familiar use of the chi-squared test involves tabular data. For this sample calculation, consider the gender distribution for the childhood leukemia cases, 16 males and 4 females. If one were to compare this observation to what might be expected with a random sample of 20 children, one could have the data shown in Figure 25-14.

The process for obtaining the expected values is to take the margin values (row total or column total)

Figure 25-13
Formula for the Chi-Squared Test Statistic

$$X^2 = \sum \frac{[(Observed) - (Expected)]^2}{Expected} = \sum \frac{[O - E]^2}{E}$$

Figure 25-14
Sample Data for Chi-Squared Calculation

	OBSERVATION		EXPECTATION		Chi-squared values for each cell	
	Male	Female	Male	Female		
Leukemia	16	4	13	7	0.69	1.28
Random Sample	10	10	13	7	0.69	1.28

for each of the four cells in sequence, multiply the appropriate two and divide by the total of the table. This resulting number is the expected value for the respective cell. For example, the expected number for the 16 male leukemia cases is obtained by multiplying 20 x 26 / 40; i.e. (16 + 4) x (16 + 10)/ (16 + 4 + 10 + 10). Once one of the values is obtained, it is easy to derive the other, because the margin values must remain "fixed." So if the first cell value is determined to be 16, then for the two margins containing this value of 16 to remain as 20 and 26 respectively, the expected values for the other two cells involved must be 4 and 10, respectively.

This constraint whereby the margin values and the total value for the data table are regarded as "fixed" is crucial to the chi-squared calculation. This same relationship (fixed margins and total) influences how one calculates the degrees of freedom for the chi-squared test. The degrees of freedom for chi-squared is the number of rows minus one (Rows - 1) multiplied by the number of columns minus one (Columns - 1). For the two-by-two table in Figure 25-13, that would be (2-1) x (2-1) = (1)(1) = 1 degree of freedom.

Solving the chi-squared formula then finds:

$$X^2 = \sum \frac{(O-E)^2}{E}$$

$$\chi^2 = \frac{(16-13)^2}{13} + \frac{(4-7)^2}{7} + \frac{(10-13)^2}{13}$$

$$+ \frac{(10-7)^2}{7} = 3.94$$

When one enters the chi-squared table (Table 25-6), with one degree of freedom, the value of 3.94 falls between the tabled values for 0.05 and 0.025. The manner in which this probability is shown then, with the chi-squared statistic, is: $X^2 = 3.94$, 1 df,

Table 25-6
Percentiles of the Chi-Square Distribution

df	0.1	0.05	0.025	0.01	0.005
1	2.706	3.841	5.024	6.635	7.879
2	4.605	5.991	7.378	9.210	10.597
3	6.251	7.815	9.348	11.345	12.838
4	7.779	9.488	11.143	13.277	14.860
5	9.236	11.070	12.832	15.086	16.750

$0.025 < p < 0.05$. This is read, "the probability of a chi-squared value of 3.94, with one degree of freedom is less than 5% but greater than 2.5%."

A Comment on Interpreting Statistical Results

When one has completed a statistical test, the p-value is obtained and interpretation can begin. Such a process can be very controversial, especially when the p-value is close to the decision point, say 0.055. In medical research, this eventuality is occasionally addressed with what is called a test for a "one-sided hypothesis." As you recall, the process of statistical testing is based on the concept of the null hypothesis. In conventional statistical testing, the null hypothesis is that the two data points being compared (e.g., sample means, observed and expected values) are not different. If they are found to be different from one another by the statistical test, that either one is greater or less than the other, or there are, two options. This greater or less possibility is a "two-sided hypothesis." This is "two-sided" perspective may be readily grasped when one considers the image of the bell-shaped distribution (Figure 25-8). The remaining probability of 0.05 is divided into 0.025 in each side of the distribution, for either a higher or lower observation.

However, if one wishes to optimize their analysis, there is a solution called the one-tail (one sided) hypothesis. Especially when the sample size for a study is small or the test in question will be difficult to repeat (e.g., an evaluation of a chemotherapy agent), one may shift the pattern of the significance area all on one side. To do this, one states the null hypothesis as "the mean of the standard treatment group will be equal to or less than the mean of the new treatment group." This makes the alternative hypothesis, the "treatment group will be greater than the standard care." Instead of a usual decision threshold of 0.025 (visualize a Z-value of 1.96), now a decision of statistical significance can be made at 0.05 (on one tail only). This is a Z-value of 1.64. Such maneuvering makes finding a difference between the groups somewhat easier. Whenever such a one-sided statement of the hypotheses is to be made, it should always be described in advance of the analysis, so that manipulation is not suspected.

Maneuvers such as one-side hypotheses are familiar aspects of medical research. However, such subtle manipulations pose a notable reason that statistical analyses should be conducted with the guidance of a professional statistician. This narrative has referred the reader to other texts for more in-depth information on statistical principles. Likewise, completing a formal course in statistics is encouraged. This recommendation that statistical tests be conducted with the consultation of a statistician is a similar precaution for working in this intricate subject area.

Other Tests, Non-Parametric Statistics

There are many other statistical tests that may be used from time-to-time with medical data analyses. Among the more familiar of these is Analysis of Variance (sometimes referred to as ANoVA, or the F-test). This method may be thought of as a comparison of the means from multiple samples, simultaneously. Consider the t-test as it might be used to evaluate the difference between mean survival for cancer patients on two different medications, two different histological types of cancers, or males versus females. With the F-test, one may evaluate each of these effects, simultaneously, one at a time, and test for interaction of the effects, e.g. female patients of one histological type on a particular medication. Analysis of variation is a wonderful, if daunting statistical method. If one wishes to use this sophisticated approach, consultation with a statistician is encouraged.

Multi-variable regression is another intricate statistical method that maybe encountered in medical research. Regression will provide t-test statistics as the results for comparisons between two subgroups in a multiple-group evaluation. A special form of this technique (logistic regression) is often used in epidemiological studies; the product statistic is the Beta coefficient. Again, use of regression analyses is recommended to be performed with statistical guidance.

One technique that is sometimes mistaken for regression is *correlation*. Correlation is used to analyze the variation between two variables that is related to their dependence on one another; a *rho* statistic is the product. Rho may have a value from + 1.0 (values for both variables rise and fall together) to - 1.0 (values for one variable rise when the value for the other declines). A zero value for rho means the two values are not dependant, or "correlated" with one another. It is interesting to note that one form of correlation (Pearson's) uses the actual values of the two variables, when another form (Spearman's) uses the order of the two variables when they have been ranked. This use of a rank value rather than the actual value is especially useful for skewed distributions. An adjustment of this type (using ranks [ordinal data] in place of

actual values [interval/ratio data]) is one form of non-parametric analysis.

Non-parametric statistics are widely used with medical research, usually because of small numbers of subjects or severely skewed distributions. This text will not explore these diverse methods to any degree, but several excellent texts provide a thorough treatment of them.[3,4] Among these non-parametric methods are the Mann-Whitney test, which is somewhat like a rank-order analysis of variance, and the Kruscal-Wallace test, for examining differences between two groups. When small samples are used to do analyses for nominal or ordinal variables, Fisher's Exact Test may be applied in place of the usual chi-squared test. Also, when small numbers of subjects are studied for survival effects, the Wilcoxon Signed Rank Test may replace the familiar survival methods discussed in the next section. Once again, it is strongly recommended that statistical guidance be sought with use of any of these non-parametric techniques.

Survival Analyses

Analyses of patient survival are central to the study of medical treatment. Survival is generally thought of as the interval from diagnosis until death; however, any time interval to a "failure" can be studied with survival techniques, for example the disease-free interval, the duration of symptom relief, etc. Survival analyses are based on what are called, "life tables." *Life tables* are used to calculate the *survivorship function* for any sort of failure-based outcome. A graph of the results from a life table is called a *survival curve*. In industry, survival curves are used to evaluate the time until mechanical parts wear out. In epidemiological studies, survival curves are used for analyses of cohorts of subjects whose disease risk is studied over time. In this text we aim to learn the simple approach for the techniques to do survival analyses; computer programs more easily address all of the complex modifications. It is crucial to understand the process for obtaining the survival function and interpreting the results.

With survival analyses, one begins by defining the time intervals of interest (See Table 25-7). In most medical applications, this is in whole years; however, some event may occur so rapidly that quarters, months, or even weeks may be used. The *number of subjects that begin the interval* must be determined. This number will decline with each successive interval as each line of the life table is completed. In the life table, one defines the *number of*

Table 25-7
Life Tables for Lymphocytic and Myelocytic Leukemia Data (Appendix 1)

Acute Lymphocytic Leukemia Data

Interval Years	Alive	Dead	Lost	Withdrawn	Effective # Exposed	Percent Dying	Percent Surviving	Cumulative Survival
0 - 1	12	1	0	0	12	0.083	0.917	0.917
1 - 2	11	1	1	0	10.5	0.095	0.905	0.803
2 - 3	9	2	1	0	8.5	0.235	0.765	0.635

Acute Myelocytic Leukemia Data

Interval Years	Alive	Dead	Lost	Withdrawn	Effective # Exposed	Percent Dying	Percent Surviving	Cumulative Survival
0 - 1	8	4	0	0	8	0.500	0.500	0.500
1 - 2	4	3	0	0	4	0.750	0.250	0.125
2 - 3	1	0	0	0	1	0.000	1.000	0.125

subjects that died (failed) during that interval. Next, comes one of the more subtle considerations with survival analyses, *censoring*. A censored observation involves a subject that began the time interval in consideration, but did not complete it. Death during the interval is a straightforward case for censoring. However, two other means of being censored are usually considered: these are subjects who are *lost-to-follow-up during the interval,* and ones who are *withdrawn alive.* In both of these latter cases, the subject began the interval, was eligible (alive) at the start of the time period. However, they did not complete the interval, and they did not die (fail). So they contribute their survival time to the interval, until they are censored (removed from the life table).

The inclusion of subjects who are censored other than by death (failure) is a fairly recent advance in survival analysis. Prior to this innovation, the *Direct Method of Survival Analysis* was used; this required that all subjects must have been available for survival throughout the complete interval of interest. With an analysis of five-year survival from cancer, only patients diagnosed at least five years earlier could be included in the analysis. For smaller facilities, this often meant that longer than five years might be required to accrue enough patients to do a survival analysis. The technique being presented here that uses the data censored other than from death is called the *Actuarial or Cohort Method of Survival Analysis.* Some people may refer to it as the "Kaplan-Meier" method after the authors of an early statistical paper on this technique.[5] In any case, the use of these data that are censored other-than-due-to-death has per-

mitted survival analyses to be performed in settings where the direct method would have led to protracted delays in order for enough subjects to be eligible for all of the time interval. The actuarial method takes the data for the time that a subject has survived, and uses it for the analysis as long as possible.

Subjects that are *lost-to-follow-up* are straightforward to understand [and were encountered with the direct method as well]. These are subjects for whom there is data to a certain date, then no more information is available. One removes "lost" subjects from contributing to the survival analysis on the date that a survival status was last known. The *withdrawn alive* category is handled in exactly the same way. If a subject was diagnosed a year-and-a-half before, they have survived the first full year, and one-half of the second year. Treating the subjects just as if they were "lost" permits that one-and-one-half of survival data to be included for the first two years of the analysis, where it would have been excluded with the direct method.

In practice, as many patients tend to be lost in January as in December, in March as in September—that is, as many in the first half of the year as in the second half. This pattern has led to the general routine of simply adding the number of these two censored categories together and halving them. That is to say, averaging them all together, each of the "censored" subjects will have contributed about one-half a year of survival. This amount of censored time (one-half of the lost and withdrawn categories) is removed from the available time period; this leads to the *effective number exposed.* To clarify this aspect of the analysis, consider the term "cohort" as used earlier to describe this method. When each person begins the interval, they are eligible to provide one-full interval (e.g., a year) of survival. Such an interval is conventionally termed a person-year; that is the individual/time unit composite. When we reduce by one-half the completed interval for those persons censored, we must remove that amount from the available survival in that line of the life table. In some situations, with some computer programs, the uncomplicated process of halving the number is not done in favor of the exact time that the persons contributed to the interval before censoring. Such rigor is often seen with clinical trials, but here we will consider the easier (halving the time units) procedure.

This *effective number exposed* is used for the denominator, and the number dying is the numerator, to obtain the *percent dying*. This is a simple form of the death (or mortality) rate for that interval. Perhaps it is easily seen, but nonetheless the difference from the percent dying and the whole is termed the *percent surviving*. One may simply subtract the percent dying from 100%, that is, 1.0 in decimal form (the preferred form for presenting life table data).

Now one has nearly completed the calculation of the survival function. The remaining step is the accumulation of the survival over successive time periods. When a person survives a later time interval, logically they will have survived the earlier ones as well. This dependency of the later time periods on the earlier survival rates is termed *cumulative survival*. At the close of the calculation for each line of the life table, the cumulative survival is obtained by multiplying the survival rate for the time-period-of-interest, by

each of the preceding survival rates (percent surviving). This value is the one that is drawn onto a line graph as the *survival curve* (Figure 25-15).

It is important to recognize that when depicting the *survival function* (drawing the survival curve) the starting point is always 100% or 1.0 (the complete population who began the study of interest). Often with life tables, a standard error will be provided. The calculation of such a measure was discussed before and will not be elaborated here. However, suffice it to say that a statistical test of the divergence of two survival curves takes the form of the t-test. One may also see graphs drawn that will have the 95% confidence limits (1.96 times the standard error) depicted as bounds or brackets on the survival curves. Thus, if the confidence bounds that are shown for one survival curve do not overlap those bounds shown for the other curve, then the two survival curves may be viewed as being statistically significantly different from one another (e.g., p < 0.05).

Survival analysis is the most advanced form of statistical procedure that we will examine in this text. Several, more comprehensive, texts have been referenced in this chapter. Completing of a basic course in statistics, for whatever application (business, agriculture, etc.) will help one grasp some of the subtle concepts involved with analyzing and interpreting statistical data. Methods for survival analyses will not usually be included with a standard statistical course. Usually, survival analysis is taught as a specialized course; in a business class it may be called failure analysis. Also, survival analysis content may be found in a course on clinical trails or even a course in epidemiological methods.

One of the foremost purposes for performing statistical analyses in medical settings is for studying the patterns of disease in human populations. This leads us logically to the next section of this text, the methods and techniques of epidemiology.

EPIDEMIOLOGY

Epidemiology is the basic science of public health. As such, it is concerned with studying the patterns of disease and health in human populations or groups of subjects. For a definition, consider epidemiology as *the study of the distribution and determinants of disease occurrence in human populations*. By *distribution*, generally one refers to the rates with which disease occur in groups of people, for example in terms of the places that they live. Epidemiologists may also

Figure 25-15
Survival Curves for Sample Data

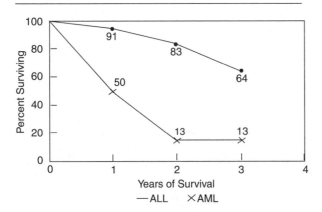

study disease in individuals, but even here that study is often described in terms of the characteristics of the person (e.g., age, race). Likewise, epidemiologists may study disease occurrence over time periods. These three attributes: *person, place,* and *time* are the basic aspects considered in evaluating the distribution of disease in human populations.

When an epidemiologist examines the disease patterns in human populations, these characteristics of the distribution of the disease may be likened to the newspaper accounts of "who, what, where, and when" an event occurs. A basic hypothesis of disease is that it should be a random event. When one group is seen to have higher rates, or the rates vary between locations or differ over time periods, this leads to questions of the "why" or "how" variety. Factors that explain the why or how are called determinants. They are not truly the cause of disease, but they represent attributes or actions that influence the risk for the disease to occur.

Epidemiologists regard three elements as crucial for the occurrence of disease (Figure 25-16). The "disease triad" is comprised of the *agent* (the actual biologic cause of the disease process, e.g., a bacterium); the *host* (a person is at risk for, or susceptible to contract the disease) and the *environment* (the place where the agent and the host encounter one another). Each of these three components of the disease process must be available for disease to occur. As public health is associated with the prevention of disease, it stands to reason that epidemiology is likewise directed to the same aim.

A basic tenant of epidemiology is that eliminating any one of the triad of disease can prevent disease. A few simple examples involve infectious diseases where vaccinations act to prevent disease risk by modifying the susceptibility of the *host,* purifying drinking water eliminates the *environment* when some disease risk can arise. With cancer risk, the disease process often seems much more complicated

than the triad concept implies. Nonetheless, one can identify examples of prevention actions based on eliminating exposure to a suspected carcinogen (e.g., stopping smoking) as a form of changing the *environment.* Prevention has many aspects, depending on what one is aiming to prevent (Figure 25-17).

Primary prevention is directed to preventing the occurrence of disease. For cancer, primary prevention is subdivided on the basis of interventions directed to the "host" versus the "environment." Host interventions include dietary changes and recognizing risky behaviors. Environmental, primary prevention actions, involve avoiding air pollution and reducing hazardous contamination. *Secondary prevention* is the level at which conventional medicine is practiced. At this level, the disease has occurred, and the objective is to prevent its threatening the life of the person or incapacitating them. Early detection and effective treatment are prominent components of this level of prevention. At *tertiary prevention,* the disease has occurred and the person's life has been impacted. This is the level of prevention where hospice operates. The usual aims for tertiary prevention are to reduce suffering and to prevent untimely death. Rehabilitation to recover productivity is also an example of tertiary prevention.

Epidemiological Reasoning

As an epidemiologist reasons over disease patterns in human populations, there is a specific, three-step sequence involved:

1 determination of a statistical association between an exposure and an endpoint;
2 formulation of a biologic inference (i.e., a hypothesis) about that relationship; and then
3 the hypothesis is tested.

In this *process of epidemiological reasoning,* measures of disease frequency are calculated for different person, place, and time characteristics (also often called an *exposure*). The process of deciding that a pattern of disease occurrence is statistically associated with a characteristic is evidence of the close reliance of epidemiology on statistical methods. The next section addresses the measures of disease frequency that are calculated for evaluating the pattern of occurrence between place, time, and persons. Following will be a section on the means for testing hypotheses based on these epidemiological observations.

Figure 25-16
Triad of Disease Occurrence

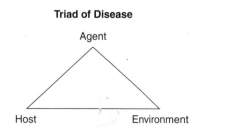

Triad of Disease

Agent

Host   Environment

Figure 25-17

Levels of Prevention

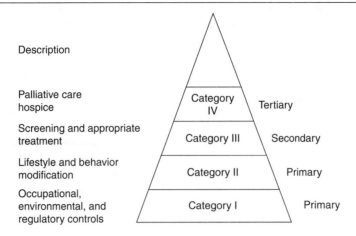

Epidemiological Measures

Epidemiology has been called an observational science because it studies what occurs in human populations without designing the pattern (as one might do with an experiment). The subtle distinctions of the various forms of epidemiology that are practiced today can be reviewed elsewhere.[6,7,8,9] Suffice it to say that when epidemiology studies are performed, there are measures of disease in the human populations; these measures take two forms: measures of frequency and measures of risk.

Disease Frequency

Disease occurs in human populations at different frequencies. Epidemiologists observe these different frequencies to describe the distribution of disease in human populations. Because disease is a spectrum (progressing from the pre-clinical state, to detectable pathology, advanced disease, and sequale or death) there are more than one measure of disease frequencies in human populations. First, there is *incidence,* a measure of the "force" of morbidity or mortality in a population. This quantity is always expressed with a time period that it references. Two examples might be the "incidence rate for colon cancer in Nebraska, in 1988," or the "the mortality rate for melanoma among white men in 1990." Notice that each example specifies the population at risk (Nebraska residents and white men, respectively) and the time period over which the cases or deaths occurred in that population and the time period of their occurrence.

$$Incidence = \frac{New\ cases\ of\ disease\ occurring\ \textit{over}\ a\ period\ of\ time}{Population\text{-}at\text{-}risk}$$

Incidence (new cases of disease) and mortality (death) rates are usually expressed in the form of occurring per some large round number. With few exceptions, this is 100,000. So if there were 93 new cases of cancer in 1995 for the town Smallville (population 25,791); the reported incidence rate would be (93/25,791) x 100,000 or 360.6/100,000. The Smallville cancer incidence rate would be reported as "360.6 per one hundred thousand population, in 1995." Please note the three crucial elements: number of new events (numerator), population at risk (denominator), and the time period of reference.

These characteristics are crucial for distinguishing the two prominent measures of disease frequency used by epidemiology to observe disease patterns in human populations. Because disease persists in populations, one often wishes to know how many cases there are present at a point in time. That measure is called *prevalence;* the formula follows.

$$Prevalence = \frac{Active\ cases\ of\ disease\ [new\ and\ existing]\ present\ \textit{at\ a\ point\ in\ time}}{Population\text{-}at\text{-}risk}$$

Using these measures, epidemiologist make comparisons between these frequencies in places (counties), between groups of people (e.g., men versus women), and over time to discern factors that indicate one (place, group, or time) is experiencing a higher rate of disease than another. Reasoning over these differences leads to hypotheses about why these differences exit, and tests to verify those hypotheses.

Measures of Risk

The preceding measures of disease frequency are *proportions.* That is the numerators are contained within the denominators. That means that the highest value they can attain is 1.0. Risk measures on the other hand are *ratio* measures. Ratios are fractions formed of two independent measures and can therefore exceed 1.0. The general form of all risk measures is shown below.

$$Risk = \frac{Observed\ disease\ frequency}{Expected\ disease\ frequency}$$

The measure of disease frequency may be an incidence measure, mortality, or prevalence. In any case, there is a comparison made. The caparison may be between two places, two population groups, or even two time periods. In any case, one of the measures is identified as the "expected" in order to provide a point of reference for the "observed" to be compared. When the observed and expected are the same, the resulting risk value is 1.0; this is the value for "no risk." As the risk of disease is greater for the "exposed" or "observed" group, the risk ratio rises.

There are also incidence ratios (sometimes called "relative risk") and mortality ratios. In general, these measures are referred to as rate ratios, abbreviated as "RR." Epidemiologists study the ratios as a means to quantify the risk associated with a certain factor. Consider the risk for lung cancer for asbestos exposure, often regarded as about 1.5. This means that one has about a 50% greater risk of contracting lung cancer if one has had asbestos exposure than if one has not. Contrast this to the risk for lung cancer among heavy smokers, often cited as 9.0. This is stated as "heavy smokers have nine *times* the risk of contracting lung cancer as non-smokers." It is important to recognize that risk, as a measure based on division, is multiplicative in its scale.

The risk for lung cancer among smokers is much greater than asbestos; thus the recognition of the magnitude of risk aids with identifying priorities for prevention. There is much more that can be said about measures of disease risk, notably that there are

measures for the impact of a factor in terms of the population risk. Such impact measures permit one to discern the portion of disease occurrence that can be attributed to a factor, or reduced by its prevention. However, before public health actions are taken, there is conventionally a testing of the relationship observed. Familiarity with the form of this "testing" or of these studies is an integral portion of understanding the discipline of epidemiology.

Epidemiological Study Designs

There are two basic research designs used with the study of epidemiology. One approach involves the identification of persons with a disease followed by characterization of those persons and comparing them to persons without the disease, for the same attributes (e.g., age, sex, race, etc.). Then an attempt is made to establish a causal linkage between exposure and effect. This approach may be termed "retrospective," as it looks back to the exposure history AFTER the disease or injury has occurred. The other approach involves the identification of an exposure or factor for which people are (e.g., population who are exposed verses non-exposed) with a search for a likely disease or injury endpoint. This approach is termed "prospective" as it looks FORWARD, from the exposure to the later occurrence of disease or injury.

Epidemiology studies always feature a study group and a comparison group. There are a variety of names given to each epidemiological study design listed here. The title of the design is not important, rather it is important to simply understand the means of organizing or collecting data to permit the analysis (comparison of population groups) that is desired for the hypothesis being evaluated.

Retrospective (Case-Control) Study Designs

Epidemiological studies are designed to find associations between exposures (cause) and disease (effect), and are based on the principle that exposure must occur before disease. However, as is apparent with the retrospective designs, the exposure-disease relationship does not always have to be measured in exactly that sequence.

These epidemiological designs may be called "case-control" studies. They are retrospective since both the exposure and the endpoint have already occurred at the time of the study analysis. This study design is also useful for studies of rare health events, i.e., cancer, birth defects, etc.

A casefinding system is needed for identifying all eligible cases; a similar system is also needed to select comparison subjects (e.g., sampling). Other cases of the same disease (e.g., a different type of cancer) may be used for this comparison purpose or health events of a different type entirely.[10,11,12] Restrictions are usually used with the selection of control subjects (e.g., age, race, and residence) to insure that the comparison group represents the population of interest.

The exploratory design is often chosen for generating hypotheses because of its rapid completion time and its relatively low cost. Exploratory case-control studies conducted within disease registries identified many of the geographic, demographic, and occupational risks that are known or suspected today for cancer.

The analytic version of the retrospective study design is characterized by the collection of very detailed exposure data, usually by interview.[13] Refined statistical techniques are available for studying the influence of confounding factors, but it is important that the necessary data be collected for the analyses to be performed. Larger numbers of cases and comparison subjects will be needed with this design as compared to the exploratory approach described just before. With so many levels of exposure, specialized statistical methods are used.[14,15] Statistical consultation is recommended with these more advanced methods of analysis.

The statistical analyses used with the case-control design are familiar (e.g., x^2). The usual risk measure that is calculated is the odd's ratio. In the following example calculations are from a community study where exposure to hazardous waste is suspected, Table 25-8.

The odd's ratio is a special estimation of the relative risk.[6,7,13] The calculation uses the cross-products of the two-by-two table (see Table 25-8). It is interpreted like other risk measures as the increase risk associated for the disease due to a history of the exposure.

Many pitfalls are common to this design, and most are beyond investigator control (e.g., the reliability of data from cancer abstracts or death certificates). The weakest link of a case-comparison study is usually the representativeness of the comparison group for the population of interest. One approach to improve the representativeness of the cases (i.e., persons with the disease of interest) is to exclude those cases that occurred in the past but are still alive at the time of the study (e.g., prevalent cases). To do this, only new cases of the disease may be made eligible for the study, e.g., as with cases identified from a population-based cancer registry.

Prospective Study Designs

These designs are often called "cohort" studies because they follow a group of persons (the cohort) through time. With this design, the long periods of follow-up can make them difficult to complete for chronic disease.[15] In the prospective or cohort design, exposure rather than disease is the initial classification for the start of the study. The analysis of data from a cohort study provides the measure of risk, called *relative risk*. See Table 25-9.

Clinical trails are a form of cohort study. The study "exposure" involves a difference in case management, but the follow-up to determine the outcome is still the usual form as with studies in the community. Community-based disease registries are the most common examples of follow-up (surveillance) of a group of exposed and non-exposed persons[16]; however, with this approach all persons in the population are studied and exposure status is

Table 25-8

Calculation of the Odds Ratio in a Case-Control Study

	Exposed Areas	Other Areas	Total
Cancer	24	12	36
Comparison subjects	29	43	72

Odds ratio = (24 x 43) / (29 x 12) = 2.97

Table 25-9

Calculation of Relative Risk

Relative Risk	Exposed Community	Rest of County
Cases of cancer	8	80
Population	3,600	720,000

Relative risk = (8/3,600) / (80/72,000) = 2.0.

determined after disease has occurred.[17] There are also surveillance efforts in progress based expressly on exposure, so-called *exposure registries* where more traditional follow-up of subjects is involved.[18] Unfortunately, characterizing exposures can be very difficult because humans live and work in many environments, and are exposed to complex mixtures at home, at work, and in the ambient environment.

There are also study designs referred to as *hybrid* because they are a departure from traditional methods. In the case of the "historical cohort," both the exposure and disease have occurred in the past, yet they are still studied in chronological sequence using historical data. Using available records (e.g., census, employment, medical, military) to define a population and characterize exposure history, the epidemiologist follows the [historical] cohort forward [to the present] to ascertain disease incidence. The key to this design is being able to identify some previously existing group with a well-documented exposure history, and to be able to obtain necessary information about the health outcomes of interest. An example of the historical cohort design is the study by the Centers for Disease Control of military personnel exposed to Agent Orange in the Viet Nam War.[19]

Another common form of analysis of data from cohort studies is the standardized incidence of mortality ratio (SIR or SMR). When small numbers of a health event of interest, e.g., cancers, confidence intervals may be placed upon the SMR with the Poisson distribution (rather than the normal one). The number of cases observed influences the precision of the SIR/SMR calculation; more subjects make for a more accurate study. One advantage of the cohort design if the use of person-years for analysis rather than numbers of individuals; see the following example for clarification.

Standardized Incidence or Mortality Ratio (SIR or SMR):

4,897 people studied for 12 years provides a study population of 58,764 person-years. Number of persons x number of years = person-years. In a community with a suspected hazardous exposure, there were:

Observed cases of cancer: 142
Expected cases of cancer: 126

$$SIR = 142 \setminus 126 = 1.12$$

In this method, the expected number of cases was obtained by multiplying the disease rates for the entire state by the population in the community to be studied. This method (using another population's data to obtain an expected value) involves the process of *standardization* or adjustment. Often the rates of disease must be adjusted for age, race, or sex differences between the two populations. These are subtle processes, but are crucial to avoid misinterpretation of the study results. Factors such as these (age differences in the two populations to be compared) produce bias in epidemiological studies. The next section discusses bias and means to control its effect.

Biases

All epidemiological research struggles against systematic errors - bias.[20] The principal sources of bias are: misclassification, selection, and confounding.

- **Misclassification bias** occur when subjects are assigned to the wrong groups, e.g., exposed or not exposed. These influences may be controlled as a part of the design of the research study, i.e., use of specific case definitions. In interview studies, subjects may try to please the researcher by reporting what they believe the study is seeking, or questions may be emphasized to "fish" for particular answers. Often too, cancer patients may recall earlier exposures in more detail exposures due to contemplations of their disease. For these instances, the subjects or even interviewers may be "blinded" to the study hypothesis, or to which "group" they are in, so they will not exaggerate effects, etc. When classification systems are changed (e.g., International Classification of Disease revisions), then cancer cases may be wrongly assigned (e.g. to leukemia instead of myeloma.) This is another form of misclassification bias.

- **Selection bias** occurs when all of the subjects in a population do not have the same opportunity to be included in a study. One of the classic examples of selection bias involves hospital cases. This particular bias, termed *Berkson's bias* for its first observer, occurs because persons in the hospitals do not represent the general population, e.g., they are generally ill. This means they may be more likely to be smokers, be overweight, etc. Other selection forces occur when only large hospital's data is used, only people with telephones are able to be contacted for recruitment, persons of low literacy or who are not English speaking cannot respond, etc. These biases are often addressed in epidemiological studies by the use of sampling strategies, or restricting study subjects to particular case and control groups.

- **Confounding** (mixing-up the effects from several risk factors) is best controlled at the time of analysis. Control for confounding involves the collection of information on all potential risk factors; then the influence of these traits can be segregated through careful analyses.

Screening

Screening is a large portion of the practice of epidemiology in a public health or disease control setting. Screening is a special form of what is sometimes called a cross-sectional study. The objective of the study is to evaluate the prevalence of a condition in the population. As the approach takes a "slice" of the disease frequency at a point in time, the description of a cross-section comes to mind. In any case, a screening study involves the prevalence of a disease state; in principle, this is undetected disease and the screening program represents a search for occult or (hopefully) "early" disease.

The evaluation of a screening process is based on the premise that the truth about the person's disease status is known. This contrast of the screening result and absolute "true" disease status is the basis for assessing the utility of a screening procedure (Figure 25-18). Screening may be best viewed as the search for diseased persons (a measure called *sensitivity*) and well persons (termed *specificity*).

Both sensitivity and specificity are described as percentages. In both cases, it is the percent of *truly* ill and *truly* well that the screening test is able to identify.

$$Sensitivity = \frac{A}{A + C} \qquad Specificity = \frac{D}{B + D}$$

An excellent screening test should have sensitivity and specificity greater than 90%. However, as only one test result may be used for determining disease status, the rise in sensitivity is usually compensated for by a drop in specificity, and vice versa. In clinical settings then, multiple tests are usually used to improve the accurate prediction of disease status. Putting several tests into a battery, where a person must fail all or a crucial number in order to be classified as "ill" is termed testing in *series*. Another screening option is to use a sequence of tests such that only persons identified as ill on the first test will receive the second test, etc. The persons classified as ill then are those found to be ill on all of the tests, this is called testing in *parallel*.

In today's setting of healthcare concerns, another consideration is the cost of confirmatory tests. Also, in circumstances where some risk is associated with follow-up of a positive test, the *positive predictive value* is a measure to be considered. Simply, this is the percentage of all persons tested as having the disease who will actually be found to have the disease (e.g., for whom the cost and risk of follow-up studies would have been justified).

$$Positive\ Predictive\ Value = \frac{A}{A + B}$$

Figure 25-18
Diagram of Screening Results

	Truly with Disease	Truly Well
Test As Diseased	A (Sensitivity)	B
Test As Well	C	D (Specificity)

As an object lesson in the implications of the positive predictive value, and the subtlety of prevalence data, consider a setting where there were 1000 cases of a disease that truly exist in a community where 100,000 persons are to be tested. With a sensitivity of 90% and a specificity of 90%, the test would correctly identify 900 of the cases; but erroneously classify 9,900 truly well persons as being ill. This would mean that 10,800 persons would have follow-up tests for the disease. However, for only 8.3% (900/10,800) would these studies be justified. In a tense healthcare climate, such ineffectiveness for cost would be unbelievable. For the persons bearing the costs or risks of follow-up studies, not to mention the emotions of being told they had a particular disease, this low positive predictive value could be unacceptable as well.

This concludes the overview of epidemiological principles. As the audience of this text is persons in the cancer registry field, a brief narrative on cancer epidemiology follows. First, some basic cancer biology is presented.

Primer of Cancer Epidemiology in the United States

Carcinogenesis is literally "the start of cancer." Cancer is an ancient term arising from the visual impression of a surgeon that a tumor appeared like a crab with legs extending into the surrounding tissue. The more appropriate term for the diseases we collectively refer to as "cancer" is malignant neoplasm. A neoplasm is a new growth. It is the malignancy of cancer that is the salient characteristic to define the disease. *Malignancy* refers to a tumor's ability to spread throughout the body from the site of origin. This process of spreading is termed *metastasis.*

It has long been recognized that the process of carcinogenesis occurred at a cellular level. A two-step process has been proposed for carcinogenesis, and coined the terms "initiation" and "promotion." *Initiation* means the transformation of a cell to one that has the potential for malignant growth. A later event causes a cell to grow rapidly, to metastasize as a result of uncontrolled growth; the latter distinct event is termed *promotion.* Initiation and promotion may be too simplistic for actual carcinogenesis.

Recent discoveries of oncogenes and a better knowledge of the process of cellular growth regulation have enhanced the general understanding of carcinogenesis. Likely, carcinogenesis requires a series of cellular-level events to transpire, some of which may require a specific sequence to be effective. Often, nutritional factors interact with these genetic events to provide a favorable potential for growth. Cells have many means to repair genetic damage. However, these repair capabilities vary in human populations. Also varying between people is the ability to detoxify chemicals that enter the body. These individual differences represent forms of personal susceptibility.

For the purpose of cancer epidemiology studies, it is necessary to recognize the genetic-level nature of carcinogenesis and to appreciate the interplay of multiple forces in order to achieve carcinogenesis. Some carcinogens are considered "sufficient" causes of cancer, meaning they can produce carcinogenesis without interaction with other agents (e.g., ionizing radiation). Some agents are necessary carcinogens, meaning that a particular cancer cannot occur without this agent being present (e.g., Epstein-Barr virus in Hodgkin Disease).

Understanding carcinogenesis is incredibly complex. But if we take as a "given," there is still much to understand about the disease, for all cancers are not the same. A common adage is that cancer is over 100 diseases. This perspective arises from the 40 or so anatomic sites where cancer strikes and the various cell types that are present at many of these sites.

Cancer is a historic disease, having been observed in ancient Egypt and Greece. Even dinosaur skeletons have been discovered with cancers. However, cancer "emerged" as a major public health concern in the middle of this century. The emergence of cancer as a leading cause of death is closely linked to the eradication of infectious diseases as major causes of death and the extension of life expectancy (see Table 17-10). Heart disease, cancer, and stroke are all diseases of aging, and as life expectancy rose, these causes of death rose as well, by attrition of the acute causes of death.

Cancer rates have varied, by gender, over the century (Figures 25-19 and 20). By the year 2010, cancer is expected to become the leading cause of death in the United States and the dominant basis for hospital admission. The most telling time trends are the precipitous rise in lung cancer death rates and the declines of uterine, liver, and stomach cancer mortality.[21] A discussion of cancer epidemiology must necessarily include the "big" cancers and the "bad" cancers. From Figures 25-18 and 19, one notes only 10 cancer sites, but over 40 types of can-

Table 25-10
Changing Order of Leading Causes of Death During the Twentieth Century

1910 **Influenza**	1950 **Heart Disease**	1990 **Heart Disease**
Tuberculosis	Cancer	Cancer
Diarrhea/Enteritis	Stroke	Stroke
Heart Disease	Accidents	Accidents
Stroke	Disease of Infancy	Influenza
Nephritis	Influenza	Diabetes
Accidents	Gen'l Arteriosclerosis	Cirrhosis
Cancer	Diabetes	Gen'l Arteriosclerosis
Disease of Infancy	Birth Defects	Suicide
Diphtheria	Cirrhosis	Disease of Infancy

Figure 25-19 and 20
Age-Adjusted Cancer Death Rates in the United States among Men and Women, 1930–1992

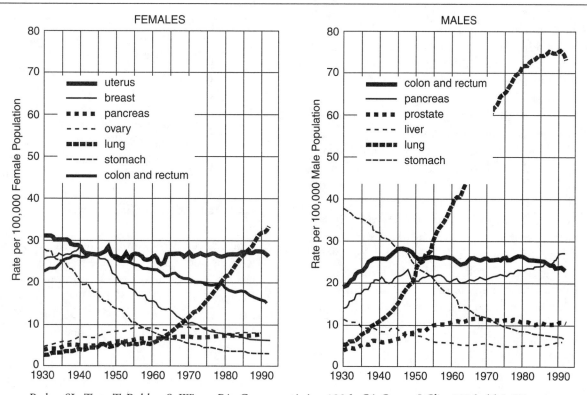

Source: Parker SL, Tong T, Bolden S, Wingo PA. Cancer statistics, 1996. *CA Cancer J Clin.* 1996; 46:5–27.

cer were spoken of before. The remaining 30 anatomic sites of cancer are less common than these, so they would crowd up along the bottom of the graph if they were included. Among the cancers shown in Figures 25-18 and 19, after 1960 there are only four "big" cancers: lung, breast, colorectal, and prostate.

It is instructive to note that these data offer a perspective of cancer in the world, as well. The pattern of cancer for 1930 to 1935 is much like that of the Third World today, i.e., stomach and uterine cancer predominate. As countries become more urbanized . . . industrialized . . . westernized, their cancer pattern shifts to be more like that toward the latter years of Figure 25-19. These changes, as well as studies of cancer patterns among migrants, are some of the strongest evidence for the assertion that "most cancers arise from environmental sources." However, the "environment" that statement refers to includes diet and lifestyle, both important considerations.

When one speaks of the "big" cancers, this refers to the common cancers. Lung cancer is the "biggest" cancer in terms of lives taken. However, one does not only think in terms of mortality; one must consider incidence, as well. Prostate cancer is the most common cancer among men, but lung cancer takes many more lives. A similar relationship exists for breast cancer and lung cancer in women.

Because of therapeutic advances, earlier detection, and greater access to state-of-the art care, more cancer patients today survive their cancer than die from it. This raises the issue of the "bad" cancers. Bad cancers are those for which the five-year survival rates are less than 50%. Among the "big" cancers (defined from Figures 25-18 and 19, after 1960), only lung cancer is "bad" by this definition. Stomach and liver cancer are quite rare in the western world and declining in frequency, yet they are leading causes of cancer death in Third World countries. The impact of lung cancer, as both big and bad, has led to a practice with some publications describing lung cancer patterns separate from all others. Some other cancers shown in Figures 25-18 and 19 are "bad" cancers, e.g., liver, stomach, pancreas, leukemia; yet these are mercifully rare.

The shifting patterns of cancer rates over the last three decades and the patterns from around the world have led to considerable debate of whether over-all cancer rates are rising. With the rising industrialization of many countries, the potential contri-

bution for environmental factors with cancer is central to this controversy. To better follow discussions of cancer, let us now review the general epidemiology of several cancers.

- Lung Cancer: This is the leading cause of cancer death in men and women. Increased risk is strongly associated with cigarette smoking - either direct or passive exposure. Occupational exposures include arsenic, organic chemicals, asbestos and ionizing radiation exposures, e.g., radon gas. These occupational risks are increased for smokers. Vitamin A deficiency is also a suspected risk factor.
- Prostate Cancer: Highest occurrence among blacks, primarily a disease of older age (> 65 years). Familial association and risk from dietary fat are suspected. Cadmium is a potential occupational risk.
- Breast Cancer: Most common cancer in women, primarily a disease of post-menopause (e.g., > age 50). Increased risk is associated with family history and no childbearing prior to age 30. A role for dietary fat is suspected.
- Colo-Rectal Cancer: Third leading cause of cancer death in both men and women. Associated with low fiber and/or high fat diet, history of polyps and inflammatory bowel disease.
- Uterine Cancer: Cervical cancer is a disease of young women, associated with early intercourse, multiple partners, and cigarette smoking. Endometrial cancer is a disease of older women; associated with infertility, estrogen therapy, and obesity.
- Oral Cancer: More common in men. Associated with cigarette, cigar, and pipe smoking; smokeless tobacco use; and alcohol consumption.
- Bladder Cancer: More common in whites and men. Smoking is a recognized risk factor. Workers in dye, leather, and rubber occupations are at risk.
- Pancreatic Cancer: Higher rates for blacks, males, and persons over age 65. Smoking is a recognized risk factor; dietary fat, chronic infections, diabetes, and cirrhosis are suspected risks.
- Skin Cancer: Common skin cancers occur in half of all people; however, a 98% survival rate has led to these cancers being excluded from most statistical reports. Melanoma is the most common lethal form of skin cancer. Fair complexion is a strong risk factor, as is excessive sun-

light exposure. Coal tar, pitch, creosote, arsenic, and radium are occupational risks.

- Leukemia: A disease of children and older adults; both sexes, all races. Certain genetic risks are known (e.g., Down Syndrome), as are viral agents (HTLV-1). Occupational risks are ionizing radiation and benzene.
- Ovarian Cancer: A disease of older women (> 60 years), and those women who have never borne children. Risk is increased by a history of breast, colo-rectal, and endometrial cancer.
- Brain Cancer: Increasing occurrence in recent years, suspected risks with job-related aromatic hydrocarbon exposures and non-ionizing radiation.
- Lymphoma: Increasing occurrence in recent years. A mixed group of diseases with many suspected risk factors including agricultural chemicals, viruses, and childhood exposures.
- Stomach Cancer: A leading cancer in developing countries, associated with nitrates in food.
- Liver Cancer: A leading cancer in developing countries, associated with Hepatitis B infection; cirrhosis; and occupational, aromatic hydrocarbon exposures.

For the purposes of cancer studies there are many considerations. Cancer is certainly difficult to study, especially from a population-based perspective; numbers of cases are small and the exposure issues are so complex. In addition there is the time scale of cancer. The interval from the induction of disease until it is clinically detected is termed *latency*. For most cancers, latency is believed to be 10 to 20 years.

An old adage says that "common things happen commonly and rare things happen rarely." From Table 25-11, one sees that lifestyle is the most common risk factor for cancer.[22] Lifestyle includes diet, tobacco use, alcohol consumption, and personal sexual history. As these are the common risk factors, it is not surprising then that the cancers associated with these common factors are likewise the more frequently occurring ones. This recognition of the "rare" cancers as ones that may represent environmental risks leads to the concept of so called "sentinel events." These are circumstances where the recognition of an unusual pattern in even a few, rare cancers can be informative.[23]

We have now given a quick orientation to cancer and its general epidemiological perspective.

Table 25-11

Percentage of Cancer Deaths Attributable to Different Factors

Factor	Range of Estimates	Best Estimate
Lifestyle:		
Tobacco	25-40	30
Diet	10-70	35
Infection	1-?	10
Reproduction and Sexual Behavior	1-13	7
Alcohol	2-4	3
TOTAL	39-100	85
Societal:		
Occupation	2-8	4
Industrial Products	<1-2	<1
Food Additives	?-2	<1
Medicines and medicinal procedures	0.5-3	1
TOTAL	4-15	6
Environmental:		
Pollution	<1-5	2
Geophysical Factors	2-4	3
TOTAL	3-9	5
Cumulative Attributable Risks	46-100	96

Finally, let us examine some of the considerations for conducting research.

Research Protocols

The performance of exploratory studies of cancer is an important consideration for advancing the "war" on cancer. Nationally, there is an effort to escalate the coverage of the United States population with cancer registries so that more information about cancer incidence will be available, more rapidly.[24] However, there is still much that can be done with local data bases and hospital-based resources.

When one identifies a hypothesis to be studied, one should develop a *research protocol*.[25] This is simply a detailed description of the study questions, the plan for conducting the study, and assurances about the process. In the description of the study questions, one may have a review of recent literature that relates to the topic, as well as preliminary data that may be the basis of the proposal. In the plan for conducting the study, there should be a detailed design for collecting the data that will be used for the analysis. Likewise the statistical methods intended for the analysis should be described. There should be a distinct section about the number of subjects to be studied and the adequacy for addressing the study questions. Consultation with a statistician may assist with the determination of these sample size needs.

In any study, there are assurances that must be made. Two of the more prominent of these are routinely addressed by Institutional Review Boards (IRBs). These topics are the assurance of confidentiality of the patient data and the protection of the subject's prerogative to decline to take part in the study. Unless the study will involve patient contact, no consent to take part in the study is usually required. However, common assurances for privacy include using numeric identifiers and destroying relevant data after the close of the study. A study proposal should close with a description of the significance of the research and its relevance to more global cancer research issues.[25]

Surveillance

Population-based cancer registries represent a form of public health surveillance.[26] *Surveillance* may be defined as a state of continual watchfulness. In the context of central cancer registries, that would be for a search for non-random patterns of increased occurrence of disease. The objective for such surveillance is to detect increases in disease risk, so that interventions may be applied. Also, surveillance maybe applied to evaluate such intervention activities. These methods are often involved with two other applications that will be touched upon briefly here, for completeness of the topic content.

First, a cluster analysis is exploratory surveillance. When evidence of disease clustering is strong, a case-comparison study may be used to test hypotheses suggested from the cluster evaluation. The case-comparison strategy is more analytic in its nature than is a cluster analysis. Next, within a surveillance system (e.g., a cancer registry), there is the potential for monitoring the course of rare cancers to continue, that is to be sustained over several years as an attempt to identify clusters as they are accruing. Such active surveillance may involve a process specified as "sentinel health event" [SHE] surveillance.[27]

Sentinel Health Events (SHEs)

In situations of cancer cluster investigations, often the public has difficulty understanding that one case of disease is not important, or significant. An analysis strategy using the principle that some disease cases **mean** more than others is called *sentinel event* reasoning. Simply stated, for some events their biologic meaningfulness is greater because of recognized characteristics that are known or suspected about the disease *etiology* [i.e., the causal mechanisms]. Selective surveillance for these health events can be very productive; and because by definition, these events are rare, there is reason to hope that their causation may also be more simple to study.

SHE surveillance strategy is borrowed from occupational medicine where it is applied to identify circumstances where safety or industrial hygiene interventions may be warranted from the occurrence of one or a very few specific health events.[27] Miller notes that "virtually every known carcinogen and teratogen has first been recognized by an alert clinician."[28] The *alert clinician* in each case was knowledgeable about disease occurrence in their own experience, so that when an unusual set of cases occurred, they took notice of it. From the original intent of sentinel event reasoning, the objective was to know enough about suspect exposures to anticipate what events might be expected as a sequela from them, so that the first case of one of those sentinel diseases would signal action.[29] Thus, rare diseases, or occurrences in unusual population groups, may represent sentinel health events.

Cancer Clusters

A troublesome aspect of cancer surveillance is evaluating cancer clusters. Assessing disease clustering is quite complicated. Two considerations are: the likelihood of simply finding a non-uniformity of the population (i.e., a densely populated residential area), rather than a meaningful cluster; and recognizing complex time trends (e.g., *secular trends* [in the general population]), before analysis. The strategy implicit with all of these methods is to detect clustering of cases, and that goal is not always the same as a detecting a generalized increase in disease rates. Consultation with persons experienced with these cancer cluster study methods is highly recommended for use of these controversial statistical methods.[30]

Geographic Methods

At the beginning of the twenty-first century, there is new technology to assist with geographic analyses of central cancer registry data. The advent of *Geographic Information System* (GIS) technology has been a boon to many large and small geographic area research applications. Address matching can be performed using specialized software.[31] Spatial analyses are in wide-spread use by centralized disease registries; it will facilitate cluster investigations and makes studies for small geographic subgroups (e.g., communities) very feasible.

The capacity that this technology has to: a) redefine population boundaries, b) assess disease distribution over irregular areas, and c) explore distance relationships, serves to make it an incredible tool for public health research and especially environmental epidemiology. Geographic Information Systems are especially useful for overlaying the distribution of cancer cases with other features of interest. These technical capabilities have greatly enhanced the usefulness of cancer registry data for epidemiologic studies of environmental risks. The same technology has been applied with studies of access to care and utilization of cancer screening facilities.[32,33]

Under the National Program of Cancer Registries [NPCR], this is the reason that addresses are linked to census tracts.[34] Assigning case addresses to specific census tracts involves a procedure called address-matching. Cancer incidence data that is geographically referenced may be used to study cancer occurrence in very small areas; and it may be used to

integrate social and demographic characteristics recorded with the decennial census (e.g., years of education, median household income). The capacity to analyze geographic data has become a major component of the cancer epidemiologist's armarium for surveillance studies.

Glossary

Additional information on the vocabulary of epidemiology may be found in the Dictionary of Epidemiology.[33]

- *Classification of subjects:* Study subjects must be able to be distinguished or classified with respect to the study factors (exposure and endpoint) of interest. How the study question is phrased does not matter. That is, you may ask either "Do persons with a certain exposure experience a different pattern of disease than do persons without that exposure?" Or you may ask "Do people with a specific disease have a history of a certain exposure more so than persons without the disease?" The same four groups will always be formed.

- *Comparison groups:* In some disciplines (e.g., biology or chemistry), true "control" groups (those without any exposure other than that of the study) may be possible. People may not be so manipulated; thus a true control group is never actually attained in epidemiology. Rather, persons that represent the general population or background situation are used as a *comparison* to the study group.

- *Confounder:* This term refers to a factor that is known to be associated with the occurrence of a health event. As an example, most health events vary by age, race, sex, etc. If such a known risk factor is not taken into account, the study results may be "confounded" (mixed up), so that an effect due to the study exposure may not be distinguishable from the already known factor (e.g., race, sex). In the study's analysis, the influence of a confounder can be separated from the effects of the study factor; also, two factors can be analyzed together for combined effects.

- *Exposure:* This term may refer to an ambient environmental factor (e.g., air pollution), to a factor in the individual's environment (e.g., smoking and diet), or to personal characteristics (e.g., age, race, and sex). In general, an exposure is considered a precedent factor associated with a likelihood of one experiencing some health event or endpoint.

- *Endpoint:* Usually this term refers to an undesirable health event, as the occurrence of disease or death. Yet it could represent a beneficial event as well (e.g., recovery from an illness or healing of a wound). In general, an endpoint is the health consequence of some exposure. To view the exposure-endpoint relationship as being a cause and effect sequence is unrealistic in epidemiology. Exposure-endpoint associations imply a risk relationship, not certain causation.

- *Epidemiological reasoning:* A three-step sequence is used in epidemiological reasoning: (1) determination of an association between an exposure and an endpoint, and (2) formulation of a biologic inference (i.e., a hypothesis) about that relationship, and then (3) the hypothesis is tested.

- *Matching:* This is a design strategy, used in epidemiology to make the study groups as comparable as possible. For example, if the study groups are made to be comparable with respect to age, any difference between them cannot be due to the influence of age. Matching can be for the whole study group or for individuals. Individual matching may be "1 to 1", or "k to 1," which means that more than one comparison person is selected for each study subject.

- *Nested:* Nesting combines two study designs to get the best of both choices: more data, quicker, and at lower costs.

- *Person-years:* For study designs where subjects are followed through time, each person contributes a *person-year,* for each year of participation. For example, a group of 100 persons, studied from January 1, 1970, to December 31, 1979 (10 years), contribute 1000 person-years to the study.

- *Risk:* This term expresses the relationship between the health experience *observed* for the study group and what would have been *expected* on the basis of the comparison group's health experience. When this value is expressed as a ratio (risk = observed/expected), it is a measure of the strength of association that exists between an exposure and an endpoint. It may be shown as a decimal fraction (e.g., 1.5) or multiplied by 100 to give a percentage (i.e., 150%). Risk may imply either an adverse (>1.0) or a beneficial (<1.0) relationship; no risk is shown by a value of 1.0.

- *Statistical techniques:* The general premise behind statistics is the use of information gained from a *sample* that is a subset of a larger group, in order to make statements about that larger group. This larger audience of persons (whom the sample represents) is the *population* of interest. Statistical methods are important to epidemiology; they are used to help distinguish between a "real" association and one that results from chance. These methods are influenced by the number of subjects used for the calculations.

Appendix I - Sample Data for Statistical and Survival Analyses

Sample data (Contrived: Childhood Leukemia Experience)

Case Number	Age Years	Race	Type of Sex	Date of Leukemia	Date of Diagnosis	Status at Last Contact	Interval Last Contact	Years
1	7	B	M	AML	12/72	4/73	D	0.3
2	5	W	M	AML	8/75	2/76	D	0.6
3	6	B	M	AML	9/77	8/78	D	0.9
4	11	W	M	AML	6/75	5/76	D	0.9
5	7	B	F	ALL	5/77	3/78	D	0.9
6	14	W	M	AML	10/73	2/75	D	1.3
7	9	B	M	AML	4/78	10/79	D	1.5
8	6	W	M	ALL	8/76	5/78	D	1.8
9	5	B	M	ALL	3/72	1/74	L	1.9
10	8	W	F	AML	7/77	10/78	D	2.2
11	3	W	M	ALL	5/74	10/76	D	2.4
12	6	W	M	ALL	4/73	12/75	D	2.7
13	2	B	M	ALL	11/70	9/73	L	2.9
14	10	W	M	AML	6/73	6/76	A	3.0
15	6	B	M	ALL	1/75	1/78	A	3.0
16	4	W	F	ALL	8/73	8/76	A	3.0
17	1	W	M	ALL	9/74	9/77	A	3.0
18	3	B	M	ALL	5/76	5/79	A	3.0
19	5	B	F	ALL	2/76	2/79	A	3.0
20	4	W	M	ALL	8/75	8/78	A	3.0

Abbreviations:

Race:	W = White B = Black
Sex:	F = Female M = Male
Type Leukemia:	AML = Acute Myelocytic Leukemia
	ALL = Acute Lymphocytic Leukemia
Status:	D = Deceased L = Lost to follow-up A = Alive

STUDY QUESTIONS

1. What type of data is stage-at-diagnosis?
   A. Nominal
   B. Ordinal
   C. Interval/ratio
   D. Continuous

2. Which of these estimates of risk is characteristic of the case-control study design?
   A. Chi-square
   B. Relative risk
   C. SMR
   D. Odds Ratio

3. The enormous technological advance in population-based surveillance due to the emergence of GIS represents what sort of implications for cancer registry data reporting.
   A. Studies over time
   B. Mapping of cases to study 'place' effects
   C. Studies of treatment outcomes with gastric studies
   D. International studies of cancer among migrants

4. Registrars may encounter which form of a cohort study in a hospital-based setting.
   A. Screening for breast cancer.
   B. A case-control study for a rare cancer
   C. A historical cohort for occupational exposure
   D. A clinical trial for a new medication

5. Incidence differs from prevalence because it
   A. Includes new and active cases, at a point in time
   B. Includes living and deceased cases of disease at a point in time
   C. Is based on morbidity only, not fatal cases over a period of time
   D. Includes only new cases of disease, over a period of time

6. The epidemiologist's triad of causation is represented by these three components:
   A. Agent, host, environment
   B. Person, place and time
   C. Observe, hypothesize, test
   D. Primary, secondary, tertiary prevention

7. If you are told to produce a frequency polygon showing the decline in annual mortality from cancer over the last ten-years, how will you recognize the correct figure made by your computer program?
   A. It will be a line chart
   B. It will have bars extending from the left axis
   C. It will have bars extending from the abscissa
   D. It will have incidence rates on the x-axis

8. Using tests in parallel to increase the effectiveness of screening for disease means..?
   A. Using one test, then another and a person must fail all of them
   B. Using more than one test and a person must fail the majority
   C. Increasing the prevalence by selecting a high risk population
   D. Using one test, then testing those who are 'positive' with a second test

9. This study design features randomization, and all of the subjects have disease.
   A. Clinical trial
   B. Community Trail
   C. Case-Control Study
   D. Historical Cohort Study

10. Some times the change in the coding scheme for disease (e.g., with death certificates or hospital records) leads to a systematic error in assigning people to disease categories, this is:
    A. A form of misclassification bias.
    B. A form of selection bias.
    C. Differential for exposed versus non-exposed persons.
    D. Damn stupid, and plain, bad luck for the investigator.

11. Presuming that you wish to compare the rate of lung cancer to annual cigarette sales, by county, in your state. Which statistical test would you perform for a simple measure of the agreement between these two values, while also limiting the impact of the extreme values that might be found for rates in some of the smaller population counties?
    A. Pearson's Correlation Coefficient
    B. Spearman's Correlation Coefficient
    C. Linear Regression
    D. Logistic regression

12. *In Situ* fraction of cancer is considered a 'national chronic disease indicator' for progress with cancer control. If you wanted to compare the proportion of breast cancer cases diagnosed at the *in situ* stage for your county to that of the state, to assess the need for [or benefit from] local screening activity, what statistical test would you apply with the observed and expected cases?
    A. The t-test
    B. Wilcoxson sign-rank test
    C. 1.96 standard deviations
    D. Chi-squared test, one degree of freedom

13. In developing a research protocol, which of the following is NOT a critical consideration?
    A. Internal Review Board [IRB] review of the study protocol.
    B. Protection of privacy for case data.
    C. Additional time it will take for completing paperwork for the study.
    D. Description of the consideration for informed consent or its waiver.

14. In testing two survival rates for their difference, it is common to compare median survival e.g., the curves of cumulative survival reach 50%. Which is the appropriate test for assessing the statistical significance of these two values when making such a comparison?
    A. Z - test
    B. t - test
    C. Chi-squared
    D. Correlation coefficient

15. If you were asked to find the 'expected' cancer cases for a particular county, you might call an epidemiologist or statistician for assistance. To request the appropriate calculation, what sort of 'standardization' would you request?
    A. Age-standardization
    B. Directly Standardized rates
    C. Joinpoint analysis
    D. In-direct Standardization

16. Many states present their cancer in percentiles, e.g., quartiles, or quarters of the county-specific rates. National statistics often use deciles [10%] fractions for their county-level mortality maps. For a state with 100 counties, what would a cancer incidence map with shading by quintiles mean?
    A. 10% of the counties would be shown as 'High'
    B. 20% of counties would be shaded as 'Very Low'
    C. Five of the counties would be call 'High'
    D. You cannot tell without the state rate and standard deviation.

17. As cancer mortality rates are dropping in the United States, which is the best explanation of this pattern?
    A. Deaths occurring later in life reduce the age-adjusted rate.
    B. Deaths occurring earlier in life reduce the age-adjusted rates.
    C. More minority populations reduce the cumulative rates.
    D. Incidence rates are rising so there is a greater prevalence of cancer.

18. Assume the national cancer incidence rate for lung cancer is 65.5/100,000 [standard error = 2.34]; the state rate is 97.6/100,000 [standard error = 3.74] and your county rate was 102.4/100,000 [standard error = 5.42]. You want to do a one-tailed test at the $p < 0.05$ level of significance, of the evidence for your county being statistically significantly higher than these other two referent groups. How many standard error units would you use for your comparison?
    A. 1.96   cumulative area remaining under the curve = 0.025
    B. 0.05   cumulative area remaining under the curve = 0.495
    C. 1.282   cumulative area remaining under the curve = 0.10
    D. 1.645   cumulative area remaining under the curve = 0.05

REFERENCES

1. Moore DS. *Statistics: Concepts and Controversies.* New York, NY: W.H. Freeman Company; 1985
2. Duncan RC, Knapp RG, Miller III MC. *Introductory Biostatistics for the Health Sciences.* New York, NY: John Wiley and Sons; 1983.
3. Steel RGD, Torrie JH. *Principles and Procedures of Statistics: A Biometrical Approach,* 2nd ed. New York, NY: McGraw-Hill Book Co; 1980.
4. Dixon WJ, Massey Jr. FJ. *Introduction to Statistical Analysis.* New York, NY: McGraw-Hill Book Co; 1969.
5. Kaplan E, Meier P. Nonparametric estimation from incomplete observations. *Journal of the American Statistical Association.* 1958; 53:457-81.
6. Gordis L. *Epidemiology.* Philadelphia, Penn: WB Saunders Company; 1958; 1996.

7. Kleinbaum DG, Kupper LL, Morgenstern H. *Epidemiologic Research: Principles and Quantitative Methods.* Belmont, Calif: Wadsworth Publishing, 1982.

8. Fleming ST, Scutchfield FD, Tucker Tc. *Managerial Epidemiology.* Chicago, Ill; Health Administration Press; 2000.

9. Hennekens CH, Buring JE. *Epidemiology in Medicine.* Boston, Mass: Little, Brown and Co.; 1987.

10. Calle EE. Criteria for selection of decedent versus living controls in a mortality case-control study. *American Journal of Epidemiology.* 1984; 120:635-42.

11. Pearce N, Checkoway H. Case-control studies using other disease as controls: problem of excluding exposure related diseases. *American Journal of Epidemiology.* 1988; 127: 851-6.

12. Wacholder S, Silverman DT. RE: Case-control studies using other disease as controls: problems of excluding exposure related cases. (Letter). *American Journal of Epidemiology.* 1990;132: 1017-18. [Note also authors reply.]

13. Schlesselman JJ. *Case-Control Studies: Design, Conduct, and Analysis.* New York, NY: Oxford University Press; 1982.

14. Mantel N, Haenszel W. Statistical aspects of the analysis of data from retrospective studies of disease. *Journal of the National Cancer Institute.* 1959; 22: 719-48.

15. Friss RH, Sellars TA. *Epidemiology of Public Health Practice,* 2nd ed. Aspen Press; 1999.

16. Houk VN, Tacker SB. Registries: one way to assess environmental hazards. *Health and Environmental Digest.* 1986; 1(1):5-6.

17. Thacker SB, Berkelman RL. Public health surveillance in the United States. *Epidemiologic Reviews.* 1988;(10):164-90.

18. Schulte PA, Kaye WE. Exposure registries. *Archives of Environmental Health.* 1988;43(2): 155-161.

19. The Centers for Disease Control and Prevention. *Comparison.* Atlanta, Ga: US Department of Health and Human Services, CDC; Veterans Health Study, Sept. 1989.

20. Sackett DL. Bias in analytic research. *Journal of Chronic Disease.* 1979;32:51-63.

21. Jemal A, Thomas A, Murray T, Thun M. Cancer statistics. *CA- A Cancer Journal for Clinicians.* 2002. 52(1):23-45.

22. Doll R, Peto R. *The Causes of Cancer: Quantitative Estimates of Avoidable Risks of Cancer in the United States Today.* New York, NY: Oxford University Press; 1981.

23. Aldrich TE, Leaverton PE. Sentinel event strategies in environmental health. *Annual Reviews of Public Health.* (14):205-17.

24. Centers for Disease Control and Prevention (1995). *A National Program of Cancer Registries: At a Glance, 1994-1995.* Atlanta, Ga: US Department of Health and Human Resources; 1995.

25. Hully SB, Cummings SR, Browner WS, Grady D, Hearst N, Newman TB. *Designing Clinical Research: An Epidemiological Approach.* 2nd ed. New York, NY: Lippincott Williams, and Wilkins; 2001.

26. Thacker SB, Berkelman RL. Public health surveillance in the United States. *Epidemiologic Reviews.* 1988; (10): 164-90.

27. Rutstein DD, Mulan RJ, Frazier TM, Halperin WE, Melius JM, Sesito P. Sentinel Health Events occupational: A basis for physician recognition and public health surveillance. *American Journal of Public Health.* 1984; 39:1054-62.

28. Miller RW. Area wide chemical contamination: lessons from case histories. *Journal of the American Medical Association.* 1981; 245: 1548-51.

29. Rutstein DD, Berenburg W, Chalmers TC, Child CC, Fishman AP, Perrin EB. Measuring the quality of medical care: a clinical approach. *New England Journal of Medicine.* 1976; 294:582-88.

30. Aldrich TE, Sinks T. Cancer Clusters: What to know and what to do. *Cancer Investigation.* 2002; 20:810-16.

31. Hanchette CL, Schwartz GG. Geographic patterns of prostate cancer mortality: evidence for a protective effective of ultraviolet radiation. *Cancer.* 1992; 70:645-53.

32. Howe HL, Lehnerr M, Qualls RY. Using Central Cancer Registry data to monitor progress in early detection of breast and cervical cancer (Illinois, United States). *Cancer Causes and Control.* 1995; 6(2):155-63.

33. Aldrich TE, Andrews KW, Liboff AR. Brain cancer risk and EMF: assessing the geomagnetic component. *Archives of Environmental health.* 2001; 56(4):314-19.

34. Last JM. *A Dictionary of Epidemiology.* Pub. New York, NY: Oxford University Press: 1983.

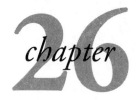

REPORT GENERATION

Karen S. Phillips
BS, CTR

INTRODUCTION

Before discussing the principles of data reporting, it is appropriate to review the fundamental reasons for the existence of registries. Population-based central registries are receiving increased attention because scientists are still searching for the causes of cancer. Hospital-based registries exist for a similar reason: because a cure has not been found. Investigators are continuing to search for effective treatments. In other words, there is still much to be learned from careful analysis and reporting of cancer data.

The purpose of cancer registries is to provide information that would otherwise not be available: cancer incidence, treatment, and outcomes. The demanding and complex process of collecting accurate, complete and timely data often obscures the compelling need to make the data available. A registry that neglects to provide frequent reports, even when they have not been requested, is a registry that is likely to find its resources threatened.

The days are gone when registrars could meet their data usage obligation to generate reports by producing an annual report and two studies of quality and outcomes each year. As early as 1986, Greenwald et al. wrote, "We think that any registry—hospital, local, regional, or national—must devote at least as much time, resources, and talent to its use for research and control purposes as it does to data acquisition, computerization, and publication of annual reports. Otherwise, it is doubtful that the registry investment is being optimally used."[1]

Distribution of meaningful data ultimately provides the only employment security for a registry staff. Medical and administrative hospital staff are often unaware of the breadth and depth of clinical and marketing statistics available from the registry. A registrar's *primary responsibility* is to identify and present interesting or anomalous features of the data for further use and interpretation.

Patient demographics, referral patterns, hospital service area, and allocation of resources can be identified and monitored by using registry data. The purpose of collecting these data is to utilize the information to assist medical and administrative staff to manage patients and deliver needed services more effectively.

Cancer registries have more thorough policies for disease-oriented casefinding than any other disease or product line within the hospital. They are therefore better prepared to assess caseload and resource use than any other service. Since cancer is likely to be the number one product line in most hospitals at the beginning of the new millennium, registrars have an obligation to report their institutions' experience frequently and thoroughly.

What does the future hold for registries? Clearly, the roles of registrars and functions of registries are undergoing rapid change. The dramatic positive effect of computerization in reducing the drudgery of follow-up letter production is already apparent. Similarly, less time will be needed for abstracting as computerized interfaces with other databases permit automatic downloading of more data items. The nationwide move toward standardization of data elements and procedures frees registrars from time-consuming data conversions and problems of data incompatibility.

On the other hand, there will be increased emphasis on quality control and timely (if not concurrent) abstracting and follow-up, and dramatic increases in report requests. There will be no time for collecting and managing data items that are not regularly incorporated into studies.

The Commission on Cancer (CoC) has traditionally required that the Cancer Program Annual Report contain comparisons with available regional, state, or national data. The CoC now requires comparisons between the National Cancer Data Base and hospital-designed studies of quality and outcomes.[2] The Joint Commission on Accreditation of Healthcare Organizations now routinely asks about use of "reference" databases in the healthcare facility and incorporates quality indicators into the accreditation process.

Use of clinical guidelines and outcome measures, and other methods of comparing the outcome of care and resource use, are standard. Subjects that affect higher-quality, more efficient, and cost-effective patient care are popular topics for cancer registry reports. Accurate assessment of the need for new or reduced facilities, staff, and services requires comparisons with other facilities. Frequent market-share studies that address information important to the cancer program's service area and target populations are essential.

OBJECTIVES OF THIS CHAPTER: GETTING THE BIG PICTURE

The overall purpose of this chapter is to challenge the way registrars have traditionally viewed data management; that is, changing from a primary focus on data collection to an emphasis on generating meaningful information for a wide spectrum of audiences. Each data element should be part of a planned analytical report pertinent to administration, medical staff, or a centralized database (usually a state registry). Other chapters in this text address data use, statistical methods, quality control, and other vital topics. This chapter reviews the selection, retrieval, quality analysis and interpretation, presentation, and comparison of cancer data. Suggestions for effective written and verbal communication are included.

DATA SELECTION

The first step in providing useful data is to examine the needs of the intended audience. The recipient of cancer data determines selection of the data items, the type of analysis performed, and the optimal style of presentation. Both inside and outside the healthcare industry, targeting information to the specific audience is critical to communicating the intended message. An overview of report-writing steps is shown in Figure 26-1.

Quality management of patient care by medical professionals requires technical information such as diagnostic evidence, extent of disease, treatment modalities, performance status, co-morbidities, recurrence, and long-term survival. Data are commonly grouped by site, morphology, stage, and treatment combinations. Comparisons with scientific literature and patterns of care studies are preferred. Accuracy and completeness requirements are usually 80 to 90%.

Cancer data managers realize that administrators need hard evidence to justify the expenditure of resources for research, staffing, equipment, and physical facilities. Reports emphasizing profit and loss (margin), market share, and planning for the future encourage administrators to value the registry. Although financial data are not usually collected by cancer registries, the occasional interface with the billing and accounting data can provide excellent marketing opportunities for registrars. Financial and market share analysts need current data that are grouped by referral source, patient demographics, resource use, and treatment outcome. Their interest is in comparisons with other databases, changes over time, and public image. Although the need for data

Figure 26-1

Overview of Report-Writing Steps

1. Identify the audience.
2. Define in detail the questions posed for the study.
3. Clarify how the data are intended to be used. What should happen as a consequence of the study?
4. Determine the period the study is to cover and the time frame allowed for completion.
5. Assign responsibility for completion of each step in the preparation and review of the study.
6. Identify the data items and codes to be collected.
7. Specify the statistical methods and resources required for analysis.
8. Define the cases to be included in the study.
9. Collect the data.
10. Perform quality control checks of the data.
11. Prepare the preliminary report for review.
12. Outline the options for action based on the study results.
13. Publish and distribute the final report.
14. Document resulting actions taken and the outcome of those actions.

accuracy is always important, it is not as rigorous for administrative reports as that required for medical decisions in patient care. Meeting administrative needs for cancer data is the registrar's most reliable form of job security.

The public needs a clear understanding of available services, what to expect from staff, and the impact of treatment on the everyday lives of patients. Patients and their families, as well as potential patients, have little technical background but are intensely curious about medical procedures and their own roles in medical decision-making.

The registry should always retain samples of reports developed for each type of audience. The key to effective reporting is tailoring information to the specific request. A safe rule of thumb is to underestimate the knowledge of cancer in every audience. Complete, concise explanations of all terms are necessary to ensure accurate interpretation by even the most technical audience. Additional suggestions for responding to data requests are listed in Figure 26-2.

Figure 26-2

Suggestions for Responding to Data Requests

- Advertise the services and data available in the cancer registry.
- Be user-friendly. Respond to requests quickly, accurately, and completely.
- Ensure that the question being answered is the one that was asked—use a study request form to set query parameters.
- Always approach the information requested from the user's perspective. Seek a full and complete understanding of how the final report will be used.
- Always verify the data before presenting it to anyone.
- Scrutinize the output carefully and compare the items being analyzed in a variety of ways to ensure that any resulting recommendations being made are based on fact, not artifact.
- Present material with visual impact-charts, graphs, and tables, rather than lists.
- List the registry as the source of the information and include the registry's phone number and email address for those who want further information.

DATA RETRIEVAL

The first step in data retrieval is to clarify the questions posed by the request. Even the most specific requests for information can be ambiguous to registrars who are familiar with the complexities of coding issues. Posing specific questions can identify potential problems; for example, questions that cannot be answered with the registry's existing database and thus require extensive additional data collection effort. There is no substitute for careful scrutiny of the report request by an experienced registrar.

If, for example, a marketing department employee is interested in increasing the number of profitable breast cancer treatments at the facility, she may ask, "How many breast patients did we see last year?" The registrar needs considerable clarification, including:

- Last calendar year, last fiscal year, or last complete year of registry data
- All breast patients, including benign, borderline, in situ, and malignant
- All stages of disease, or only in situ and localized?
- All breast patients this facility diagnosed, treated, or consulted
- Inpatients, outpatients, and patients seen only in staff physician offices
- Whether patient received all of first course of treatment, part of first course, or subsequent treatments there
- Patients under active follow-up. For what period?
- How will the data be used?
- Are simple frequencies adequate, or are other details about the cases needed?

- What additional potential questions will the data be expected to answer? When are the data needed?
- What is the requested format of the data—electronic or paper? Delivered by email, fax, USPS, or other?

Other questions that may arise include the following:

- Will the study involve all cases meeting the study criteria or a random sample?
- Is comparison data needed? From what region or database?
- Are survival statistics required? Observed, adjusted, or relative?

For each report request, it is important to clarify and clearly describe the criteria for selecting cases and the data elements to be displayed or counted. Novice data analysts often confuse the questions of "Who do we want to study?" with "What do we want to know?" These statements represent the difference between selecting the population and identifying the details about each case to be described.

A report request form that poses questions about the criteria for each study is useful. It should list the data items collected by the registry and an explanation of coding policies for each item. Jargon and terms not generally understood outside the registry should be avoided or clearly defined. Examples of frequently misinterpreted definitions include the terms *analytic, definitive treatment, first course, adjuvant, stage,* and *survival.*

A thorough examination of site groupings, morphology groupings, staging schemes, classes of case, and treatment types and combinations is critical. The registrar's knowledge of, and experience with, the complex details involved in data collection over several years cannot be overestimated. These issues are thoroughly addressed later in this chapter.

Having clearly defined the questions and the timeframe for the study, one can estimate resources required for data collection, analysis, review, publication, and distribution.

QUALITY CONTROL

Before further discussion of data analysis, a few words about data quality are in order. Fundamental to making registry reporting useful is ensuring that data quality is as high as possible. No database can tout 100% accuracy, but verifiable levels of quality are imperative. Quality control is a continuous process involving every member of the cancer data team. The Commission on Cancer suggests several procedures, including rigorous documentation and involvement of physicians in the quality assessment process, but the best way to improve data quality is to *use* the data. In other words, the very process of generating reports will enhance data quality.

Every good study generates more questions than it answers. Registrars typically find that the "first run" for a report shows multiple inconsistencies in the data. The raw data always indicate several cases that should be re-examined for accuracy. The registrar should be vigilant about obvious mistakes in the data, but should also watch for what is *missing* in the data. For example, any field with more than 10% of codes specifying "unknown," "not otherwise specified," "other," "none," or blank should be suspect. Can this bias the result? Nothing substitutes for the registrar's knowledge and common sense when watching for implausible results.

The quality of data in cancer registries unarguably improves with their use. Reporting encourages quality; quality encourages reporting.

Chapter 21 in this textbook is devoted entirely to quality control procedures, but a few ideas are so fundamental to report writing that they bear repeating here. Completeness of casefinding, current follow-up, and thorough documentation of registry policies and coding procedures are paramount in quality data collection. Differences in coding practices over the years and among individual registrars should always trigger extra vigilance.

To remain constantly aware of data quality issues, registrars should become familiar with studies of cancer data across the nation. These are published by state or regional central registries, the National Cancer Institute's SEER Program, the CoC's National Cancer Data Base, the American Cancer Society, the North American Association of Central Cancer Registries, and other scientific sources.

DATA ANALYSIS AND INTERPRETATION

This section provides general guidelines and considerations for the analysis of registry data; statistical principles are addressed in other chapters of this text. Although registrars must be cautious in drawing conclusions about the appropriateness of medical care, they are uniquely qualified to assess the data for validity. The registrar should question data reliability and reproducibility. It is the registrar's obligation to recognize not only anomalies in the data but also departures from standard patterns of care and outcomes.

There are special considerations when studies involve examination and comparison of treatment options. For example, whether the patient received chemotherapy may not affect the outcome of care as much as whether the patient received a full course of chemotherapy. Amount, number of cycles, and duration of treatments should be considered when examining radiation therapy patterns as well.

Methods of calculation used for survival data and other statistical methods should be carefully selected. Only statistics calculated by similar methods can be meaningfully compared. Every report should contain an introduction from the registrar describing the type and number of cases studied and the time period covered. Reports should also contain a description of cases that were excluded from the study, such as in situ lesions or unknown primaries. The registrar must ensure that clear explanations of technical terms are included with the results of all studies.

Registry procedures that affect conclusions from the data must be described. For example, reportability policies, casefinding completeness, currency of abstracting and follow-up, and consistency of coding interpretations must be made clear at the time of data analysis. When interpreting results of data covering long time periods, changes in diagnostic, staging, and treatment patterns should be considered. Registrars should also be wary of overinterpretation of data when small sample sizes (generally fewer than 10 to 30 cases) are used.

Registrars should be aware of the possible influences of case mix on data analysis. The population of patients served by a healthcare facility can influence interpretation of the data. For example, in areas where the proportion of elderly patients is greater than in the population at large, more comorbid conditions can be expected, retirees may have more than one residence, and referral patterns may be affected. All of these factors influence data interpretation.

Similarly, race, socioeconomic conditions, occupation, geographic setting, and the effect of recent cancer control efforts such as smoking cessation interventions and screening programs may affect the outcome of studies. Patterns of diagnosis and treatment options, and outcomes of care, may be markedly affected by patient choice, cultural mores, and availability of convenient medical facilities. Interpretation of such factors should accompany the registrar's analysis. In fact, it is generally presumed that differences in outcome between two groups of patients are more likely the result of differences between patient groups than of differences in care.

As noted previously, although initial results of any study should be viewed cautiously, it is to be expected that most studies will generate more questions than answers. However, the additional questions are generally more focused and better defined.

DATA PRESENTATION

The persuasiveness and meaning to the audience of accurate data depend on the use of carefully chosen data presentation methods. Data can be presented as raw data or as measures of central tendency. They can be tabulated, grouped, or represented graphically. Raw data are usually included in reports only when further interpretation by the audience is solicited. Measures of central tendency—mean, median, and mode—are described in Chapter 25, Statistics and Epidemiology. Because tables and graphs add to audience appeal and enhance clarity and promote understanding of the data, they should be used often.

Tables

Tables present and summarize detail that would be cumbersome in narrative form. Exact values and comparisons among several variables are easier to interpret in tables.

Rows and columns in a table should be surrounded by as much white space (unprinted) as possible. Instead of using grid lines to divide cells, consider using white space instead. Shading or textured background can also be used for variety. If words are used in tables, keep them short. Numbers should be aligned on decimal points. Avoid leaving blanks in any cell; instead enter a zero, a dash, or NA (not applicable). Subtotals are often useful to summarize categories of data within tables; subtotals can be shown at the top or bottom of the column. In any case, registrars should strive for an uncluttered look that leads the eye both horizontally and vertically.

Tables take a variety of forms, but all have common requirements. Each must be accurately and completely labeled so that the information depicted in the table can stand on its own, without additional narrative. Labels should explain not only what is depicted, but why it is important. Lettering in labels should be easily readable; avoid stacked lettering or numbering. The source of the data and the number of events or cases being reported (n) should always be clearly evident.

Titles should tell who is represented by the data, what items are being shown, where the data were generated, and what time period the data cover. Subtitles add descriptive information. Footnotes add important detail that may not be obvious in the body, such as the source of the data, explanation of jargon, abbreviations, and references.

The simplest kind of table is a one-way classification showing only one variable, shown in Figure 26-3. Tables can also take the form of two-, three-, or even four-way tables (Figure 26-4) showing multiple variables. For example, a table might depict the distribution of breast cases by cell type, stage, menopausal status, and estrogen receptor status.

Figure 26-3
Example of a One-Way Table

St. Anonymous Hospital
2003 *Breast Cancer Stage at Diagnosis*

Summary Stage	Frequency
Local	157
Regional	122
Distant	56
Unknown	23
Total	358

Figure 26-4

Example of a Four-Way Table

2003 Colon and Rectum Cancers
Treatment by Race, Stage, and Cell Type

RX	Black N = 98					White N = 666				
	None	Surg	RT	Chem	Other	None	Surg	RT	Chem	Other
Stage 1										
Adeno	8	22	—	—	—	10	113	3	—	—
Other	—	2	—	—	—	—	14	—	—	—
Total	8	24	—	—	—	10	127	3	—	—
Stage 2										
Adeno	3	10	9	2	—	3	74	75	41	4
Other	1	—	1	—	—	—	8	16	6	1
Total	4	10	10	2	—	3	82	91	47	5
Stage 3										
Adeno	2	5	5	4	1	1	57	55	29	6
Other	—	2	2	1	—	—	4	5	8	1
Total	2	7	7	5	1	1	61	60	37	7
Stage 4										
Adeno	4	3	4	3	2	8	32	17	41	6
Other	1	—	—	1	—	1	8	4	12	3
Total	5	3	4	4	2	9	40	21	53	9
Total	**19**	**44**	**21**	**11**	**3**	**23**	**310**	**175**	**137**	**21**

Reporting more than four variables usually results in a table that is difficult to interpret. For more detail on tables and other graphic presentation methods, the reader is referred to SEER Book 7.4

Graphics

Although narrative and tables have an important role in the presentation of data, reports also commonly display data in a variety of graphic formats. When a succinct sentence or two describes the outcome of data analysis, graphics are not necessary. A statement that "Forty % of the population in this service area is over the age of 65," requires no additional visual elements. Graphics are, however, a clear way to summarize detail, show relationships, illustrate trends, and make comparisons.

It is no accident that children learn to read by looking at pictures. Visual memory is often our most acute type of memory. Educators have long recognized that we learn about 10% from the words we hear, 40% from the way they are said, and 50% from what we see.

Graphics are neither merely cosmetic nor optional. Numbers are intangible and often boring; graphs allow quick interpretation of the data. The attention-grabbing elements of graphics keep the audience interested in the data. They persuade, add credibility, dramatize important points, and add meaning to the message by condensing detailed information.

With the steady evolution of technology, enhanced sophistication of computerized graphics packages, better photocopying, and breakthroughs in desktop publishing, impressive graphics are simple and inexpensive. Easy-to-use software is available to any registrar who wishes to generate professional-looking graphs.

Graphics are often called charts. Commonly in publications, graphs and charts are consecutively numbered and referred to as Figures (e.g Figure 1, and narrative lists without graphics are referred to as Tables). The kinds of graphs or charts a registrar should choose depend not only on the data but also on the type of audience. Figure 26-5 shows common types of charts. Registrars are encouraged to review the medical literature that their audiences read and note the types of charts that are most often used. Typically, technical audiences prefer graphics and are more sophisticated at interpreting complex charts.

All figures must be labeled with the same attention to *who, what, when,* and *where* that is required in tables. Additional rules of thumb suggest that x-axis (horizontal) labels be placed horizontally and describe categories, often independent variables. Y axis (vertical) labels are also placed horizontally and show amount or frequency often dependent variable. For example, in survival graphs, the independent variable of years survived is normally presented on the x-axis, and the dependent variable, percent surviving, is shown on the y-axis. Legends or keys explain the symbols or colors used.

Line graphs are most effective in showing trends and changes over time. Most line graphs show an increment of time on the x-axis and the amount, frequency, or percentage on the y-axis. When showing more than one line on a single chart, use different symbols with matching lines, or use matching symbols with different lines. Generally, no more than four lines should be depicted on a single chart.

The most common use of line charts in registries is to show survival data. Each line should start at 100% on the y-axis and at time zero on the x-axis. Lines should be stopped (truncated) when fewer than 10 patients begin the interval because, in such a small sample, the death of just one patient produces a dramatic (and misleading) drop in the line.

Bar charts are most effective when comparing size or amount of a variable. Bar charts can show differences in the magnitude of one item at various points in time, such as the number of localized breast cancers diagnosed by year. Bar charts are not as effective as line graphs in showing differences in size over time; in other words, trends. Bars can be filled or shaded with a pattern or color to show differences among categories. The width of the bars should be kept the same within the chart; bars or groups of bars should be separated by spaces. Adjacent columns should contain related or comparable data groups. Three dimensional depictions should generally be avoided because perceptions of the magnitude of y-axis values can be misleading.

Bars can be either vertical or horizontal. Horizontal bar charts, in which the x-axis is vertical and the y-axis is horizontal, are useful when depicting many categories, such as frequency by site. A broken scale on the vertical axis is recommended when the values produce a large blank area in the chart, but the scale should always start at zero.

Special kinds of bar charts include grouped columns (shown in Figure 26-6), stacked columns, 100% columns, component band, and paired. An example of grouped columns might be four groups of bars, with each group representing a year and each bar representing a stage of breast cancer. The number of columns in each group should generally be limited to four.

Stacked columns (Figure 26-7), also called subdivided or component columns, show parts of a whole, where the length of the column is the sum of the totals in the segments. All bars in a 100% bar chart (Figure 26-8) are the same length, and information in each bar is shown as a percentage of a whole. Paired bar charts (Figure 26-9) have two y-axes, with the 0 point in the center of the graph. These are often used to show simultaneous distributions by site in both males and females.

Histograms (Figure 26-10) are used to show frequency distributions in bar form. They look different from bar charts because they have no space between bars, and they are always vertically oriented. Histograms are used for continuous variables, such as age or tumor size, and can show counts or percentages. When added together, the heights of the bars represent the total number, or 100%.

Figure 26-5
Common Types of Charts and Their Uses

Text	concepts and principles
Line	trends over time
Bar	frequency at any given time
Histogram and frequency polygon	frequency of continuous variables
Pie	parts of a whole, percentages
Pictorial	eye-catching effects

Figure 26-6

Example of a Grouped Bar Chart

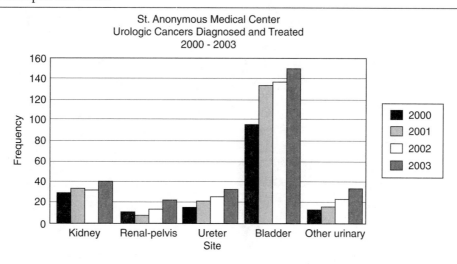

Figure 26-7

Example of a Stacked Bar Chart

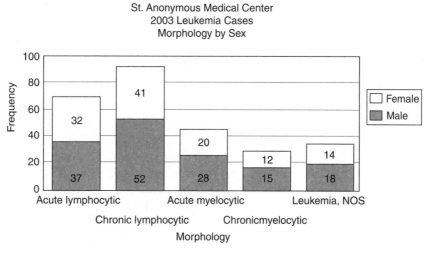

Figure 26-8

Example of a 100% Bar Chart

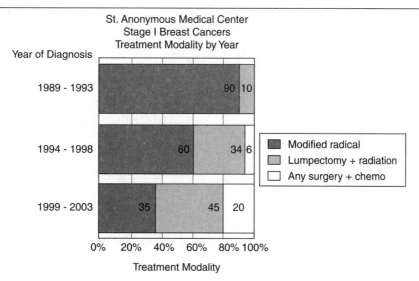

Figure 26-9
Example of a Paired Bar Chart

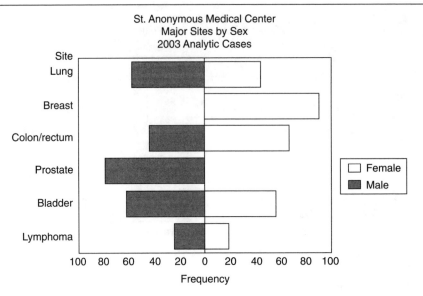

Figure 26-10
Example of a Histogram

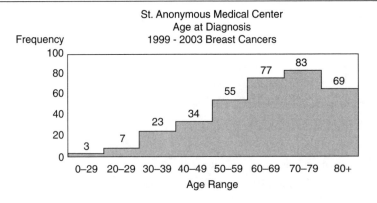

Histograms are useful when it is more important to show the distribution of a variable than absolute numbers. *Frequency polygons* (Figure 26-11) provide a different format for histogram data. A line connects the top midpoint of each bar. If the area beneath the line is shaded, the chart is often called an area chart. Frequency polygons allow data from several histograms to be shown on the same chart.

Pie charts provide a clear method of showing parts of a whole; that is, percentages. Limiting the pie chart to no more than six slices, or wedges, with the smallest wedge comprising no less than 2% of the whole, is a good guideline. Slices can be "exploded," or pulled out, to emphasize one component. Paired pie charts are useful for comparing percentages of the same whole under differing conditions or

during two different time frames. Three-dimensional pie charts are attractive but should be used cautiously, because the relative size of the slices can be easily misread.

Pictorial charts make use of symbols that are, in the viewer's mind, strongly associated with the message of the chart. For example, using symbols of beds of various quantities effectively shows the lengths of stay required by several types of surgery. The profusion of symbols included in graphics, word-processing, and spreadsheet software attests to the popularity of this graphic method. Care should be used to select symbols that are simple and easy to identify, even in small print. Amount or volume is conveyed by the number of symbols, not their size. Although they are eye catching, use of symbols may

Figure 26-11

Example of a Frequency Polygon

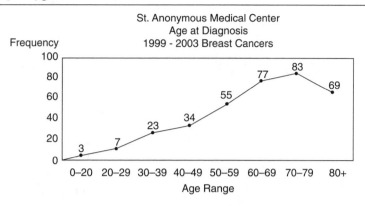

not be considered as "scientific" as traditional line, column, bar, and pie methods. Pictorial charts are also commonly used in registry reports as anatomic drawings and maps.

Anatomic drawings are helpful in identifying segments of organs with different characteristics of malignancy or staging, such as colon, brain, or head and neck sites. Care should be taken to select anatomic drawings that are simple, clear, and directly applicable to the message.

Maps are often used in annual reports to visually represent patient service referral patterns. Dot maps make location of cases or events in a geographic area easy to interpret, but they are often difficult to construct. Shaded maps are easier to create than dot maps and so are used more commonly, with differences in shading indicating varying concentrations of cases or events. The data displayed should usually make use of rates, rather than counts, to show the relationship between occurrences and population density. In either case, maps should be simple and easy to understand. Remember, the purpose of all graphics is to make the message more quickly and more clearly understood.

Using Color in Graphs

The sophistication of graphics software and the falling prices of color printers bring color graphics within the reach of every registry. Color should always be considered whenever the resources are available. Advertising and marketing executives have long recognized that color commands attention. The instant market for color screens on our telephones and global positioning systems is clear evidence of the power of color.

Color increases comprehension, adding an extra dimension to the message. To keep the message clear, however, avoid using both color and pattern in the same graph. No more than six or seven colors should be used in a single graph, and the combination of colors (sometimes called the palette) should be consistent over a series of graphs.

Choose colors conservatively, keeping in mind the meanings often associated with specific colors (see Figure 26-12). For example, use white, blue, or black for the background. Avoid red and green combinations for members of your audience who may be color-blind; avoid red and blue combinations because it is difficult to focus on both colors simultaneously.

Figure 26-12

The Meanings of Colors

- *Red:* danger, stop, risk, heat
- *Dark blue:* conservative, calm
- *Light blue:* cool, youthful
- *Green:* positive, organic, growth, go
- *White:* pure, clean, and wholesome
- *Black:* serious, unyielding
- *Gray:* integrity, neutrality
- *Brown:* rustic, solid, wholesome
- *Yellow:* warm, energetic, cheerful
- *Gold and other metallics:* elegant, enduring
- *Orange:* emotional, energetic
- *Purple:* youthful, contemporary, regal
- *Pink:* youthful, girlish, and delicate
- *Pastels:* soft, childlike

Colors can also vary widely in their luminescence, which is the amount of light a color reflects. Luminescence should be considered when selecting colors. For example, yellow on a bright blue background provides contrast, but is difficult to read because the two have similar luminescence. The goal should be to draw attention to the message, not to the colors or complex graphics.

Following are some general recommendations for effective charts:

- Consider including both percentage and frequency on any chart. Percentages make trends and comparisons easier to identify but can be misleading in studies involving small numbers.
- In black and white graphics, use of reverse type (white letters on a black or gray background) effectively emphasizes important points. Use clear contrasts in shades of gray.
- When rows and columns do not add up to 100%, provide an explanation.
- Use a variety of graphic styles to keep the readers' interest.
- Confine each chart to a single page. Graphics that overlap pages are difficult to interpret and to align.
- Intersperse graphs with text. Keep the text that refers to the graph on the same page or a facing one.
- Make sure that the data agree with the narrative.
- Avoid repeating the same information in two graphs or in the graph and the accompanying narrative.
- Thoroughly define the units used, the total number of cases or events described, the statistical or other methods used, and special terminology or abbreviations.
- Information in a chart, as in narrative text, should flow from left to right and from top to bottom.
- Charts should usually be oriented horizontally (landscape), rather than vertically (portrait).

The message of the graph should be easy to describe in a single simple sentence. No one wants to *study* a graph. Graphs should make data more easily and more quickly understandable. If a graph is difficult to interpret at a glance, it is probably too complicated. The guiding principle in both designing graphics and developing narrative is clarity .

DATA COMPARISON

One of the long-standing requirements for cancer program approval by the CoC is a review of registry data that includes comparison of hospital data with regional, state, or national aggregate data. In today's competitive healthcare industry, the quest for ever more cost-effective delivery of quality care requires comparisons among institutions. The Joint Commission on Accreditation of Hospital Organizations' (JCAHO) emphasis on clinical indicators has further spurred interest in monitoring and comparing specific elements that influence quality of care.

In the registry, comparison of hospital administrative and clinical data with outside databases has never been more important. A report that contains comparison data is a report with added credibility. Possible sources of comparison information include the following:

- State and regional registries periodically publish aggregate data; many will provide special comparative studies at a registrar's request. The usefulness of the data depends on how current and complete the central registry's database is. Central registries vary considerably in their responsiveness to report requests.
- Most major vendors of registry software offer comparative data to their customers. They vary in sample size, frequency of updates, and whether data are immediately available to the registrar.
- *Cancer Facts and Figures* is an annual publication of the American Cancer Society found at www.cancer.org which provides estimates based on National Cancer Institute SEER data. Little data on treatment and stage are included in this publication, however.
- The National Cancer Data Base aggregated by the CoC in conjunction with the American Cancer Society publishes summary statistics on selected cancers that cover over 50% of the cancer cases in the United States. Data cover 1985 to the present. This is not a population-based registry; it is a convenience sample of cases voluntarily submitted by hospital-based registries. It is an excellent source of treatment and stage data. National Cancer Data Base information can be accessed in the Cancer Programs area of the American College of Surgeons' website. www.facs.org/cancer.

- *Manual for Staging of Cancer,* The AJCC Cancer Staging Manual is developed by the American Joint Committee on Cancer and published by Springer. The manual provides survival data by stage on selected sites.
- MEDLINE and other databases are available through the National Library of Medicine at www.nlm.nih.gov. They are a good source of information from clinical trials and studies of survival based on treatment options.
- PDQ, an abbreviation for Physician Data Query, a database available through the National Cancer Institute, is found on the web at www.nci.nih.gov. Updated monthly, PDQ includes extensive information on all major cancer sites and types, treatments, and ongoing clinical trials, as well as directories of physicians and organizations involved in state-of-the-art research and cancer care.
- CancerFax is a free service providing access to current PDQ information summaries through a fax machine. Dial 301-402-5874 on a fax machine's handset and follow the instructions.
- *Cancer Incidence in North America,* abbreviated CiNA+, available at http://www.naaccr.org, is published by the North American Association of Central Cancer Registries. It provides access to incidence data on major and minor cancer sites (including pediatric groups) for North America, the United States, and Canada, with individual state- or province-specific data available. The on-line system is a flexible interactive query system that offers a choice of custom designed tables, charts (multi-line graphs, pie charts, or bar graphs), and maps.
- According to their website at http://seer.cancer.gov, the SEER Program of the National Cancer Institute has information on more than 2.5 million cancer cases in their database. Approximately 160,000 new cases are accessioned each year within the SEER catchment areas. SEER data, tools to analyze the data, publications, and resources are available free of charge" One of the SEER publications titled, *Cancer Statistics Review,* is published annually, providing data on incidence, mortality, and survival and histologic distribution by site, race, and sex. This publication contains population-based data from about 14% of the United States population. The data are three or more years old. Treatment information is not included.

Registrars should become familiar with the sources listed above. These and other pertinent links can be found on the NCRA website at www.ncra-usa.org. Each source contains a thorough description of the source of data, data collection guidelines, and statistical methods employed. Footnotes and aids to interpreting the data enable registrars to group and analyze data in a way that allows valid comparisons. Registrars can then decide whether comparative data are available for the question their study proposes. If not, perhaps the study plan can be modified. Registrars can prevent repeated regrouping of data by deciding at the outset which source of comparative data is most appropriate. It is sometimes useful to employ two, three, or even more comparison databases to underscore a strong message.

Just as there are no perfect databases, no perfect comparative data source exists. Concerns about using comparative data sources can be minimized with the proper precautions. Among the potential pitfalls, consider the following questions:

- Does the comparative database represent a population of patients that is similar to this registry?
- Regional differences among populations (for example, in age, geographic setting, socioeconomic status, or culture) can influence comparisons, especially in treatment and survival. Areas with active screening programs may show higher rates of early cancers. Changing referral patterns can produce wide variations in local data.
- Does the comparative database use population-based data? If not, how are estimates made? Is the sample size of the comparison database large enough to ensure that it accurately represents the population?
- If the database uses population estimates from the United States, individual states, or regions, what are the sources and procedures used to report census data?
- How complete is the casefinding in the comparative database? Casefinding is rarely 100% complete. Are the missing cases random, or are they likely to somehow affect the data? Do the sources of casefinding overlap? What is the coverage of outpatient settings? For some sites, such as prostate and melanoma, a lack of outpatient accessions can seriously affect the data.
- Is there an adequate mechanism in place to identify duplicate cases in the comparative database? Duplicate cases can occur within a single

institution or among institutions that share patients, staff, or data.

- What is the reference date of the comparison database? Are data available from the years addressed by the proposed study? If not, perhaps years can be grouped. For example, if hospital data are available for 1988 through 1990, and comparison data are available only for 1989, valid conclusions can probably be drawn.
- Are the data in the comparison database current enough? Is follow-up and cause-of-death information as current as data in the proposed study?
- Does the comparison database use standard methods of statistical analysis, data collection, and coding? Have these policies changed during the period of the study? For example, how are the 2001 changes from ICD-O-2 to ICD-O-3 and from SEER Summary Staging 1977 to SEER Summary Staging 2000 handled? If AJCC staging is cited, do changes among editions affect the data? Are there other assumptions or estimates made in the description of the comparison data-base that seem unusual or that might affect coding accuracy?
- In the case of survival data, does the reference database report observed, adjusted, or relative survival? Is follow-up information current at 90%? Are calculations done by actuarial, Kaplan-Meier (product moment), or other methods?
- Does the comparison database report imprecise codes—unknown, none, blank, or not otherwise specified? Caution should be exercised if the proportion of imprecise data is greater than 10%.

When the registrar is satisfied that the comparison database is indeed appropriate for the proposed study, other questions arise. Are the two databases that will be compared similar in their policies for grouping data? Consider the following issues:

- Ambiguous terms: do both databases follow the same definitions for including cases identified?
- Benign, uncertain, and borderline tumors: are these excluded?
- Non-melanoma localized basal and squamous skin cancers of nongenital sites: are these excluded?
- Class of case: are standard definitions observed by both databases, especially with respect to cases seen in outpatient settings?

- Rules for defining multiple primaries: SEER rules are not in complete agreement with the rules of the Commission on Cancer and International Association of Cancer Registries (IACR). Do both databases use the same definitions?
- Paired sites: to code laterality, are definitions identical?
- Multiple bladder lesions: most definitions count only one bladder cancer per patient, despite the number and timing of subsequent lesions.
- In situ lesions: there is considerable variation in policies among available databases. For example, SEER excludes all in situ cancers except bladder; CoC includes all but cervix. Are the study's policies compatible with the comparison data?
- Lymphomas: are non-Hodgkin and Hodgkin lymphomas grouped together? Are extranodal lymphomas counted as lymphomas or as primary cancers of the extranodal site?
- Melanomas: are ocular and cutaneous melanomas grouped together or separately? How are other extracutaneous melanomas handled?
- Brain and central nervous system: are these sites grouped together or separately? Are any benign brain tumors included? Do the two databases agree on this issue?
- Pediatric cancers: do the two databases agree on whether pediatric neoplasms are included with adult cancers?
- Hematopoietic groups: how are multiple myelomas and plasma cell dyscrasias such as alpha heavy chain disease grouped?
- Ill-defined sites: is a separate category included for these sites?
- Unknown primaries: are they listed separately, or excluded entirely?
- Head and neck sites: these sites are often grouped together. If this is the case, are the groupings the same? Is larynx included?
- Digestive sites: is the distal third of the esophagus grouped with stomach? Are colon and rectum primaries grouped together? Does this group include anus?
- Lung: are non-small- and small-cell lung primaries grouped together or separately?
- Sex: are male breast cancers included with female breast cancers?
- Intent: do the terms *palliative* and *curative* affect whether treatment is recorded?

- First course: is the definition limited to planned therapy to be included in the first course? For example, is a five-year course of Tamoxifen for breast cancer considered a continuation of first-course hormone therapy?
- Definitive therapy: does this include excisional biopsies? Are granulocyte-colony-stimulating factors included in immunotherapy (biological response modifiers)? Are investigational drugs included in chemotherapy, hormone therapy, and immunotherapy?
- Adjuvant therapy: is the definition inclusive of all combination modalities, or does adjuvant treatment apply only to patients who have no clinical evidence of disease?
- Stage: which staging schemes are used- SEER Summary Stage 1977, SEER Summary Stage 2000, SEER Extent Of Disease, clinical TNM, pathologic TNM, best TNM or collaborative stage?
- Intervals for grouping data: for example, are ages grouped 1-10, 11-20, 21-30, or are they grouped in five-year or other increments?
- Rare cancers: are there sufficient numbers of cases in both databases to permit valid conclusions about procedures, treatment combinations, recurrence, and survival? Can several years be grouped together to yield sufficient numbers?

The preceding list is not meant to be all-inclusive. It simply illustrates the spectrum of important and complex considerations required when comparing data from more than one source.

WRITTEN COMMUNICATION SKILLS

Few skills are more important to success than the ability to clearly express ideas and explain information in writing. Cancer data managers are certainly no exception. Few authors are satisfied that their writing skills are adequate. In fact, improving written communication skills is a life-long endeavor. The key to success is practice. The ultimate goal is clarity.

An excellent opportunity for practice involves generating one-page "fact sheets" for cancer conferences. Although brief, fact sheets offer the opportunity to highlight a single site or topic using several techniques—short descriptions, succinct tabulations, and one or two graphics.

The next step in practicing writing skills might result in two- or three-page reports for cancer com-

mittee or other administrative meetings. *Whether or not these reports are solicited,* they serve to establish the registry as the cancer information center of the facility. Such reports could include the following:

- Number of new cases added during a given time period and total number of cases in the registry
- Number of follow-up letters mailed and received
- Rates of physician staging by site
- Rates of compliance with College of American Pathologists protocols
- Analysis of clinical indicators or clinical guidelines
- Registry goals met and projected for the coming months
- Results of quality control activities, such as number of charts reviewed
- A list of casefinding sources
- Registry participation in other cancer program activities
- A copy of the Request Log or other evidence of data provided to others

Producing an annual report, participating in CoC-designed special studies or conducting an in-depth study of outcomes should be the culmination of a year's practice with smaller, less ambitious writing projects. Registrars should be encouraged to obtain a comprehensive reference book (such as *The New York Public Library Writer's Guide to Style and Usage*) and take classes to improve writing skills.

Essential components of a report typically include an acknowledgments section, introduction, body (often including methods and results), discussion (often including conclusions), summary, glossary, and references. Additional elements for lengthy reports may include a cover, title page, table of contents, list of figures and tables, preface, abstract or summary, and appendices.

With the availability of sophisticated word processing software, formatting attractive reports is no longer a stumbling block. Ample blank space, often called white space, should surround the text to lead the eye and to emphasize important points. Margins should be at least one inch on all sides, with larger margins when bindings, titles, graphics and tables, page numbering, footnotes, or other additions to the text are used. Margins in graphics and text should be consistent throughout the document.

Word processing software packages also provide easy access to spell checking, dictionaries, thesauruses, formatting styles, and printing options. Similarly, spreadsheet software offers flexibility in data manipulation and presentation styles. Registrars should become thoroughly familiar with one or more word processing and spreadsheet and presentation packages and use all the features that ensure professional-looking documents. Consider including links to appropriate websites and collateral databases.

The report-writing process can be summarized in the following steps:

1. Determine the audience's level of prior knowledge and preferred style.
2. Define the purpose and significance of the report.
3. Clarify the desired result of the report in one or two sentences.
4. Develop an outline of content making sure to
   —explain the significance of the report;
   —thoroughly describe methods used to gather and analyze data;
   —summarize findings;
   —recommend a plan of action based on the findings.
5. Write the first draft.
6. Solicit review and comments from others.
7. Revise.
8. Proofread at least three times, checking both data and text.
9. Print the report.
10. Be creative about extent of report distribution.

Ten additional rules of technical writing, effectively summarize guidelines for writing style:

1. Be brief. Avoid repetition. Authors should write as though they are being charged a fee for every word.
2. Use first or second person to keep sentences lively. Leave the reader feeling as though he or she has been personally addressed.
3. Use active verbs. Passive verbs create impersonal, dull, and often overly "wordy" text.
4. Select words carefully. Use precise words with unmistakable meanings. Make frequent use of a dictionary and a thesaurus. Write in the present tense to convey immediate relevance of the message. Vary sentence structure and length to keep the audience's attention.
5. Choose short words over long ones. A clear message requires concise wording.

6. Avoid fad words and slang. Overuse of current "buzzwords" can turn off an audience.
7. Use jargon only when necessary and explain it. Never assume that the audience has the same technical vocabulary as a registrar. What is perfectly clear to one audience may be incomprehensible jargon to another.
8. State the message positively. An upbeat tone enhances the power of communication.
9. Delete meaningless modifiers and phrases. Make relevant points in as few words as possible.
10. Write plainly—readers will appreciate it.

A typical weakness of written material is lack of focus. The guiding principle of report writing can be summarized by what is known as the "KISS" Principle—Keep It Short and Simple. Clarity of message can be easily obscured by verbosity and jargon. Practice is always the key to improvement.

ORAL COMMUNICATION SKILLS

The idea of standing before a group to make a verbal presentation is intimidating to many registrars—and completely paralyzing to some. However, a registrar's role as a member of the cancer committee and as a spokesperson for the cancer program mandates development of effective speaking skills.

Fear of public speaking is perfectly natural. Effective strategies for overcoming this fear involve observation of role models, thorough preparation, and practice. Registrars often combat their fear through participation in other professional activities. State and regional registry associations, the local chapter of the American Cancer Society, and informal committee work within the office setting provide role models and nonthreatening forums for gaining confidence in verbal presentations.

There is no more potent strategy for a good oral presentation than intensive preparation. Registrars by their very nature are thorough and well organized. Therefore, making careful preparation for a verbal presentation is natural for them. Effective oral skills are not dramatically different from writing skills; practice is the key. Everyone gains confidence after making several successful presentations.

A careful assessment of the audience is essential. Can you provide material at the technical level that is directly relevant to their immediate needs?

Physicians and administrators typically appreciate brevity more than any other quality. Concisely presented material with a crystal clear message is essential. Remember that top-level administrative staff may spend as much as 40% of their time in meetings, and physicians always have patients waiting. Neither group is tolerant of verbosity.

What does the audience want? Is the intent of the presentation merely to inform, or is it necessary to persuade or motivate them to action? Precisely what ideas should they take away from the presentation? What do you want the audience to do as a result? State these goals in three or four succinct sentences. Keep material brief and pertinent. The message should be unmistakable.

Make an outline of your presentation that lists no more than five to ten major points. To this outline, then, add relevant details. A complete script can be helpful but should not be used during the presentation. Reading verbatim from a script will bore and annoy the audience. It is one of the most common criticisms of speakers.

The outline can be used to develop effective supporting visuals—slides and handouts. Another common criticism of speakers is that their visuals are unreadable. A slide or overhead should be limited to six lines, with no more than six words per line. More detailed supporting information can be provided in handouts, which should be prepared whenever possible to provide the audience with information for future reference. Participants and their colleagues who may have been unable to attend will appreciate meaningful resource material long after the oral presentation is forgotten.

The introduction to the presentation should clearly state the purpose and major points. The body of the address must be concise and relevant. A summation of the talk should reiterate the main points and desired results. In other words, tell them what you are going to say, say it clearly, and tell them what you just said.

Human beings are wonderfully expressive creatures. We give hundreds of cues as we speak. Choosing the correct words is important, but it is not enough to ensure a successful presentation. Posture, appearance, expression, body language, and tone of voice can all convey warmth and enhance credibility, adding to the message and its effectiveness. An expressive, natural voice and a well-chosen vocabulary are essential. Conservative, unaffected gestures and variety in voice tone and rhythm can help retain audience interest and enhance credibility. Try to convey the impression that you are sharing useful information from first-hand experience, rather than lecturing or delivering a recitation of facts.

A logical progression of information from a relaxed speaker invites audience participation. When members of the audience interrupt the presentation to relate additional information or to ask questions, the value of the information you are presenting is confirmed.

It is important to make frequent eye contact with members of the audience. Watch people for clues that interest may be waning. A change of tone, posture, or expression can make all the difference in recapturing the audience's attention. The speaker who is thoroughly in command of his or her material is a speaker who is free to concentrate on the audience and respond to the slightest cue. This is sufficient reason to refine, polish, and practice a presentation until its delivery is second nature. Registrars who take the time to prepare thoroughly soon find that making presentations can be enjoyable. The sense of accomplishment and the resulting recognition are ample rewards.

SUMMARY

The cancer registry can achieve a reputation as the facility's oncology information center—the first place to call when cancer data or resources are needed. One way to foster this reputation is to assume that at least a bit of summary data should be provided at every opportunity—every public or professional gathering of people interested in oncology. Converting data into useful information and disseminating it through effective written and oral reports is the principal reason for the existence of cancer registries.

STUDY QUESTIONS

1. What is the first step in selecting the data to be included in a report?
2. Name three sources of information about cancer that a registrar should review as examples of report generation.
3. What are four influences of hospital-specific case mix on data analysis?

4. Titles of tables and charts should answer what four questions?
5. Give three features of a comparative database that may affect whether it may be suitable for your benchmarking purposes.
6. What is the most important key to effective technical writing?

REFERENCES

1. Greenwald P, Sondik EJ, Young JL. Emerging roles for cancer registries in cancer control. *Yale Journal of Biology and Medicine.* 1986; S9: 561-66.
2. *Commission on Cancer Cancer Program Standards 2004.* Chicago, Ill: American College of Surgeons; 2003: 25.
3. Fritz A, Roffers S, eds. In: National Cancer Registrars Association *Marketing Cancer Information and Services.* Alexandria, Va: NCRA; 1995.
4. Shambaugh EM, Young J, Zippin C, et al. In: *Self-Instructional Manual for Cancer Registrars,* Book 7. *Statistics and Epidemiology for Cancer Registries.* Bethesda, Md: National Institutes of Health, National Cancer Institute; 1994. NIH Publication No. 943766.
5. Effective Use of Graphics (Speakers Bureau Topic). Chicago, Ill: Commission on Cancer, American College of Surgeons; 1994.
6. Fritz AG. *Writing for Registrars: A Manual of Style for Annual Reports and Other Cancer Registry Technical Writing.* Rockville, Md: ELM Publications; 1987.

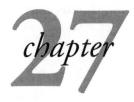

DATA UTILIZATION

Suzanna S. Hoyler
BS, CTR

Karen Malnar
RN, CTR, CCRC

INTRODUCTION

The rapidly changing healthcare environment has increased the need for current, accurate, complete data on which to base decisions. Hospitals are merging, private-practice physicians are joining physician networks, the payor base is moving toward managed care, and more and more oncology treatment is given in ambulatory care settings. As institutions actively evaluate their services, the need for data on which to base decisions is paramount.

The cancer registry contains an extremely valuable commodity-accurate, complete, readily available oncology data. These data can help hospital staff and community leaders make key decisions regarding patient care, institution services, staffing, and community outreach programs. Registry data are useful in planning, monitoring, and evaluating a myriad of programs and services at the institution and in the community at large.

Currently there is no government regulation of the use on cancer registry data. However, institutions with cancer programs approved by the Commission on Cancer of the American College of Surgeons are required to document the usage of registry data and are encouraged to use the data to identify performance improvement projects.[1]

USES OF ONCOLOGY PATIENT DATA

Historically, registry data have been used to review clinical care and outcomes. Increasingly, registry data is used for program planning and evaluation, the marketing of oncology services, financial analysis of treatments, fund-raising, and grant proposals. Data in the cancer registry include patient demographics, diagnosis and stage at initial diagnosis, treatment, and survival. Physician and hospital referral patterns are also available. (Refer to Chapter 13 for information on data sets and data items.)

Administrative Planning and Marketing

The registry's data answer the questions *who, what, when,* and *how many.* Trends (increases or decreases) in oncology patient population, as well as the status of the current oncology population, can be shown. Data that are helpful in preparing a business plan or monitoring existing services include the past and current cancer caseload (both inpatient and outpatient); use of clinical and ancillary services such as the infusion center, radiation oncology, and radiologic tests; distribution of patient insurance plans; patient referral areas; physician usage; patient satisfaction; the most common cancers; and stage at initial diagnosis. These data allow the administrator to quantitatively measure changes in the program.[2,3]

The graph in Figure 27-1 illustrates a hypothetical hospital, "General Hospital," with an increasing cancer caseload. The total number of cancer cases being initially diagnosed or treated at the hospital has increased since 1996. A further review (Figure 27-2) of the same data shows that the number of cases initially diagnosed and treated at the hospital has increased from 490 cases in 1996 to 709 cases in 2001, while the number of cases diagnosed elsewhere and referred to the hospital for either first course of treatment or for recurrences has declined slightly. The number of patients who were initially diagnosed at General Hospital and elected to have their initial treatment elsewhere also declined. Because the implications of these data for the hospital are far-reaching, the changes should be evaluated.

Washington Hospital Center (WHC) in Washington, DC, used data from its registry to help plan its Cancer Institute, an ambulatory outpatient building in which all programs for oncology patients are centralized. WHC continues to use overall registry data to monitor trends in caseload, use of services, and referral patterns and site-specific data and sites of recurrence to evaluate staffing needs.

When data are used for administrative purposes, information may be summarized by the institution's fiscal year instead of the calendar year;[4] this makes for easier comparison with financial data. On the other hand, the calendar year is useful for clinical, marketing, and fund-raising purposes. The timeline for grants can be either the fiscal or calendar year, but numbers of patients should be given instead of percentages.

Oncology data can be used in the oncology product line business plan and the monitoring and evaluation of existing oncology programs and staffing. Data can also be used in marketing, oncology services planning, fund-raising, and grant proposal writing. Table 27-1 outlines which data items are most helpful.

The number of new cancer cases seen at the hospital, the stage at initial diagnosis, patient location, and referral patterns are useful in planning marketing campaigns.

Figure 27-1
General Hospital's Annual Cancer Caseload

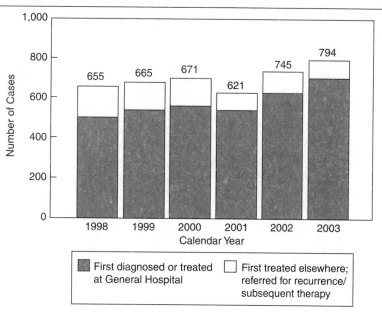

Source: Cancer Registry, 2004

Figure 27-2
General Hospital's Trend in New Cancer Cases

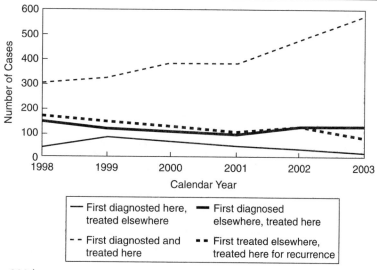

Source: Cancer Registry, 2004

Financial Analysis

Registry data linked with financial data are used to estimate the cost of diagnosing, treating, and following cancer patients. The patient's health record number and the admission or discharge date in the financial and the registry databases can be linked with the diagnosis. Once site-specific cases (for example, stage II breast cancer) are identified, costs can be analyzed by Current Procedural Terminology (CPT4) and Diagnosis Related Grouping (DRG) codes.[5] This capability is useful in developing global pricing agreements for the managed care market.[6]

Table 27-1
Summary of Oncology Data and Uses

Oncology Data	Administrative Planning			Clinical Care	Community Programs	Cancer Control	Cancer Research
	Program Evaluation	Facility Usage	Referral Patterns				
Annual cancer caseload	X	X	X	X	X	X	X
Class of case	X	X	X	X	X	X	X
Patient demographics							
Age, race, sex	X	—	X	X	X	X	X
Current residence (city, state, ZIP code, county)	X	—	X	—	X	X	X
Residence at diagnosis	—	—	X	—	X	—	X
Cancer diagnosis (site and histology)	X	X	X	X	X	X	X
Stage at initial diagnosis (severity of illness)	X	—	—	X	X	X	X
Treatment							
Type of treatment (first or subsequent)	X	X	—	X	X	X	X
Course of therapy (first or subsequent)	—	—	—	X	—	—	X
Consultations (referrals)	X	X	X	X	—	—	—
Where treatment given (location)	X	X	X	X	—	—	X
Physicians involved in case	X	X	X	X	X	X	X
Follow-up							
Recurrences	X	X	X	X	—	X	X
Cancer status	—	—	—	X	—	X	X
Survival	X	—	—	X	X	X	X
Referrals							
Referring hospitals	X	X	X	X	X	X	X
Hospitals referred to	X	X	X	X	—	X	—
Referring physicians	X	—	X	X	X	X	X
Patient satisfaction	X	—	—	X	X	X	X

When global pricing agreements are developed, practice patterns can be reviewed and clarified as the global pricing agreement is defined. This may also indicate areas in which critical pathways and other monitors of quality care should be developed. Critical pathways describe a detailed care plan for patients.[7] Once the critical pathway is implemented, cost and length of stay can be continuously monitored.[8]

In addition, registry data can identify whether patients received all their therapy at the institution or whether some treatment was given at another institution. The financial impact of patients going to other institutions for treatment can be analyzed.

Clinical Care

Clinical care is the realm in which registry data have historically been used the most. Because the cancer diagnosis (site and histology), stage, treatment, and survival are recorded for each case, patient care is easily categorized, as shown in Figures 27-3, 27-4, 27-5, and 27-6. Comparison with national data enables

Figure 27-3

General Hospital's Prostate Cancer Cases—Distribution by AJCC Stage at Initial Diagnosis

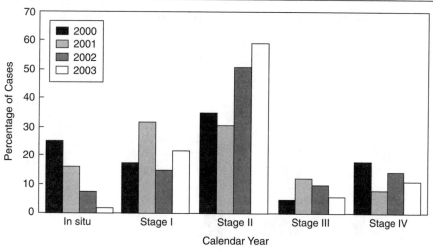

Source: Cancer Registry, 2004

Figure 27-4

General Hospital's Prostate Cancer Cases—First Course of Therapy, 2000 and 2003

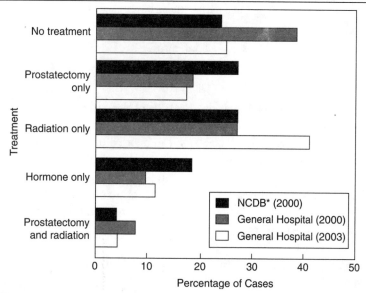

Source: Cancer Registry, 2004
Note: The "no treatment" category includes transurethral resection of the prostate.
National Cancer Data Base Annual Review of Patient Care 2002.

Figure 27-5
General Hospital's Prostate Cancer Cases—Trends in Treatment

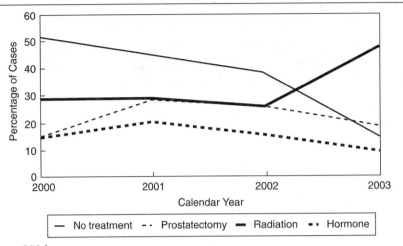

Source: Cancer Registry, 2004

Figure 27-6
General Hospital's Radiation Oncology Referrals for Breast Cancer Cases—2003

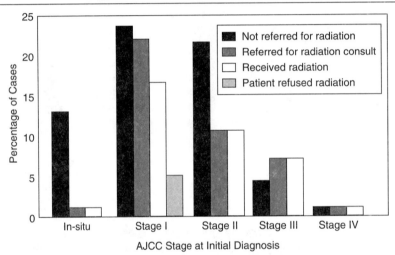

Source: Cancer Registry, 2004
Note: Unstaged cases excluded.

the staff to identify deviations from national or regional standards of care. Both areas of excellence and outliers in patient care can be identified (see Figures 27-4 and 27-5). Site-specific data show the types of oncology cases diagnosed or treated at the institution, the physicians' diagnostic and treatment referral practices, and which treatments the patients elect to receive.[9] These data can lead to the establishment of clinical pathways, which describe acceptable ways to diagnose and manage a disease. Table 27-2 lists a typical site-specific analysis.

The data may be used to evaluate clinical pathways or practice parameters. Cases that meet the cri-

teria of the pathway under development can be identified. As pathways are developed, the registry data can be used to monitor compliance. Table 27-3 illustrates the number of pediatric neuroblastoma cases on protocols at General Hospital. Although 16 of 51 patients are not entered on protocols, only 3 patients actually refused the protocol; 13 patients were ineligible or no study was available.

Cancer Control

As institutions form partnerships with local health departments and other health organizations to

Table 27-2
Typical Site-Specific Analysis

- Distribution by age, race, and sex
- Distribution by subsite
- Distribution by histology
- Distribution by AJCC stage at initial diagnosis and race
- Treatment referral patterns by stage at initial diagnosis
- First course of therapy by stage at initial diagnosis
- Five-year survival by stage

implement cancer control programs, data from the registry can be used to plan and monitor the effect of the programs. Using baseline data—for example, primary site, age at initial diagnosis, race, size of tumor, stage at initial diagnosis (see Figure 27-3), and five-year survival—from the registry, intervention programs can be developed. Analysis of several years of data shows trends in the hospital's population. Caution must be exercised if only the hospital's data are being reviewed. Although this gives a profile of patients seen at the institution, it may not be applicable to the community population at large.

Outcome measures for breast and cervical cancer based on data collected in cancer registries have been identified. For breast cancer, these focus on the stage at initial diagnosis and tumor size; for cervical cancer, stage at initial diagnosis is used. The outcome measures for breast cancer are listed in Table

27-4. Three of the four can be obtained by reviewing registry data. Many of these measures are easy to apply because they are simple proportions and do not require population data.[10]

As data on screening, prevention, and early detection trials become available, stage at initial diagnosis can be monitored to determine the effectiveness of the cancer control programs.

Cancer Research

Cancer registry data play an important role in retrospective studies[12] and case identification for researchers. Detailed information on patient demographics, initial diagnosis, cancer site and histology, extent of disease, treatment, recurrence, and survival provides the baseline for many studies. Using these data, the researcher can collect information not available in the registry database. Most registry software programs can write ASCII (machine readable) files so that the data can be loaded into other database management systems for analysis.

Specific cases to be included in retrospective studies can be identified through the registry's database. If a research grant proposal is to be submitted, data on potential eligible cases can be derived from a historical review of previous years' case loads. In addition, most registries maintain a list of suspense cases. These are cases that need to be reviewed for inclusion in the registry and are usually identified within one to four weeks of diagnosis. The suspense file represents another pool of cases for the researcher to use in prospective studies, in which early case identification is important.

Table 27-3
Pediatric Neuroblastoma Cases on Protocols at General Hospital

International Staging System	On Protocol	Not on Protocol	Total Patients N	%
1	3	2	5	9.8
2	1	3	4	7.8
3	11	2	13	25.5
4	19	3	22	43.1
4S	1	5	6	11.8
Unstageable	0	1	1	2.0
Total = N (%)	35 (69%)	16 (31%)	51	100.0

Reason patients not on Protocol:
No study available 9
Patient not eligible for study 4
Patient refused study 3

Table 27-4
Breast Cancer Control Outcome Measures[9]

- Proportion of all breast cancers of known stage diagnosed at an in situ stage
- Proportion of all invasive breast cancers of known stage diagnosed at a localized stage
- Average annual age-specific and stage-specific breast cancer incidence rates
- Proportion of localized female breast cancer diagnosed with a tumor size less than 2 cm in diameter (of all cases known stage and known tumor size)

If an institution participates in clinical trials, site-specific data on the number of cases, the stage at initial diagnosis, and the type of recurrence should be reviewed. (See Table 27-5.) These data are helpful in determining what trials should be made available to patients or how many patients might be eligible for a trial.

Community Uses

Community groups can only use registry data if institutional policies regarding the release of the data are in place and observed. Whether it is the American Cancer Society's local unit office, the public health department, a church, or the area hospice, data from the registry allow these local community leaders to "zero in" on the cancer occurrence in their area. Examples for General Hospital are shown in Figures 27-7 and 27-8. The number of cases by site by year; the stage at initial diagnosis; geographic location of patients; and age, race, and sex distributions are useful to these social agencies. Community screening events, public education programs, support groups, survivors' day programs, or hospice programs can be planned. For example, the American Cancer Society public education committee and the local health department would be interested in trends in staging or increases or decreases in the numbers of cancer patients diagnosed with a particular cancer at an institution. When combined with other data from area hospitals or freestanding centers, such information may indicate that screening programs or clinic services should be planned or evaluated.

Registry data are extremely useful in targeting populations for specific events, such as living cancer patients for a National Cancer Survivors Day program or a memorial service for the families of expired patients. Because the registry is required to accession any patient diagnosed with or treated for cancer in the institution, a list of oncology patients, their addresses, and their status, living or expired, is readily available. Registry data can only be used in this manner if the follow-up rate is above the target of 90 percent[1] and information on expirations is posted immediately.

Registry databases can also be used to target oncology patient populations for studies. In 1995, the Commission on Cancer's Cancer Liaison Program, the American Cancer Society, and the National Cancer Registrars Association wanted to survey cancer patients and their families on access to, use of, and satisfaction with available support services from community providers. The study was conducted through institution-based cancer committees and the patients' managing physicians. Cancer registrars were asked to identify a sampling of their living patients to whom a health survey could be mailed. Institutions who elected to participate used their registry databases to identify cohorts of patients to participate in the study.

Other uses of registry data include new program planning and evaluation of existing services. For example, site-specific information on the type and number of stage III and stage IV cancers and the patient geographic referral area are useful to a hospice agency or home healthcare agency planning new services or service areas.

Professional Education

Site-specific oncology data can be used to plan continuing medical education activities, as well as topics for presentation at the meetings. Presentation and analysis of data at conferences can serve as a major part of an oncology program's continuous quality improvement program. Recommendations from the conference can be forwarded to the cancer committee and quality assurance department at the institution for action. At one institution, a cancer fact sheet was prepared for each cancer conference. The fact sheet highlighted a single cancer site and included data on the hospital's annual case load, as well as distributions by anatomic site, age group, race and sex, stage, and five-year survival.[11]

Public Education

Public awareness and education are accomplished by using informational brochures, fact sheets, newslet-

Table 27-5
General Hospital's 2003 Cancer Cases

Site	Total N	%	Class of Case Analytic	Nonanalytic	In Situ	I	II	III	IV	Unknown	NA
Head/Neck	39	5.0	37	2	0	10	3	8	11	5	0
Tongue	11	1.4	10	1	0	7	0	1	1	1	0
Larynx	12	1.5	12	0	0	2	1	4	4	1	0
Other head/neck	16	2.0	15	1	0	1	2	3	6	3	0
Digestive organs	143	18.2	108	35	3	12	23	20	38	12	0
Esophagus	11	1.4	11	0	0	3	1	1	3	3	0
Stomach	16	2.0	13	3	0	1	1	4	5	2	0
Colon	79	10.1	55	24	2	4	17	9	18	5	0
Rectum	10	1.3	9	1	1	1	1	4	1	1	0
Pancreas	13	1.7	10	3	0	3	1	1	4	1	0
Other digestive	14	1.8	10	4	0	0	2	1	7	0	0
Lung	92	11.7	86	6	0	18	10	26	27	5	0
Bone	8	1.0	8	0	0	2	3	0	0	3	0
Connective Tissue	18	2.3	15	3	0	3	4	6	1	1	0
Skin, other	16	2.0	15	1	0	4	2	0	0	9	0
Melanoma, all sites	15	1.9	12	3	2	6	2	2	0	0	0
Kaposi's sarcoma	17	2.2	15	2	0	0	0	0	0	0	15
Breast	99	12.6	83	16	10	31	27	13	1	1	0
Genital, female	91	11.6	83	8	27	29	4	10	10	3	0
Cervix uteri	41	5.2	36	5	21	9	2	3	0	1	0
Corpus uteri	28	3.6	28	0	2	18	0	4	2	2	0
Ovary	12	1.5	10	2	0	1	0	3	6	0	0
Other, female	10	1.3	9	1	4	1	2	0	2	0	0
Prostate	119	15.1	103	16	0	23	63	4	12	1	0
Urinary organs	28	3.6	25	3	2	5	13	1	4	0	0
Bladder	14	1.8	13	1	2	5	6	0	0	0	0
Kidney and other urinary	14	1.8	12	2	0	0	7	1	4	0	0
Brain and CNS	12	1.5	0	12	0	0	0	0	0	0	0
Thyroid	10	1.3	8	2	0	3	2	1	2	0	0
Leukemia	8	1.0	8	0	0	0	0	0	0	0	8
Non-Hodgkin lymphoma	27	3.4	24	3	0	13	0	0	9	2	0
Multiple myeloma	14	1.8	10	4	0	0	0	0	0	0	10
Primary unknown	13	1.7	13	0	0	0	0	0	0	0	13
All other	17	2.2	16	1	0	7	3	1	3	2	0
Total	786	100	669	117	44	166	159	92	118	44	46

Figure 27-7

Five Most Common Cancers for Area Residents Seen at General Hospital—2003

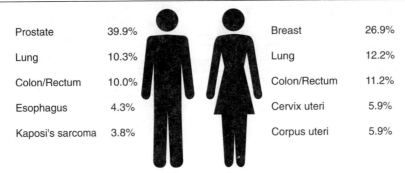

Prostate	39.9%		Breast	26.9%
Lung	10.3%		Lung	12.2%
Colon/Rectum	10.0%		Colon/Rectum	11.2%
Esophagus	4.3%		Cervix uteri	5.9%
Kaposi's sarcoma	3.8%		Corpus uteri	5.9%

Source: Cancer Registry, 2004

Figure 27-8

Profile of Area Residents Seen at General Hospital—2003

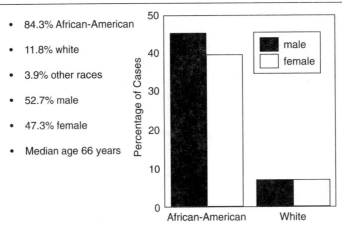

- 84.3% African-American
- 11.8% white
- 3.9% other races
- 52.7% male
- 47.3% female
- Median age 66 years

Source: Cancer Registry, 2004
"Other races" are excluded from graphic.

ters, and exhibits that promote the institution's screening clinics, availability of clinical trials, multidisciplinary programs, support groups, and other activities. When data from the registry are incorporated into the brochures, the public will know what types of patients are seen at the hospital. The brochures serve as a marketing tool for the oncology product line. Data such as age, race and sex distributions, patient referral areas, most common cancer sites, and trends in stage and treatment are valuable. For example, registry data could be displayed in a public fact sheet[3,11] alongside the American Cancer Society recommendations, risk factors, warning signs, and a listing of the institution's support programs.

Through the hospital's speakers bureau and public relations department, the institution's oncol-ogy data can be made available to civic, social, and religious organizations, as well as to the media (television, radio, and print). Use of local cancer statistics makes the stories in health segments on television and radio and in newspapers more relevant to their audience.

OUTCOME MEASURES

As patients move through the healthcare system, measuring the impact of care delivery is paramount. Historically, stage of disease at initial diagnosis and survival time has been the two principal outcome measures. Stage at initial diagnosis is used as an indicator for cancer control programs. Other data that should be used to measure outcome are recurrence rates, disease-free intervals, and therapy referral patterns.

If clinical pathways are in place, registry data can be used to help measure compliance with them. Ongoing monitoring of pathways can help identify issues in resource consumption, length of stay, and quality of care.[8] The National Comprehensive Cancer Network (NCCN) has developed clinical practice guidelines for the major cancers. These guidelines are available on the web.[16]

Other issues regarding outcome can be identified through development of oncology indicators. Indicators can be designed to assess the quality of care in an institution. For example, the indicator "patients undergoing treatment for primary care of the female breast cancer with the stage of tumor designated by a managing physician" focuses on the use of staging, which helps determine treatment.[12] Table 27-3 shows whether General Hospital's pediatric patients were put on protocols. The indicator being measured is "all children with neuroblastoma should be placed on protocol."

When yearly follow-up letters are mailed to patients, patients are asked if they have any comments or concern that they would like to share. Many patients use this as an avenue to praise staff and services or to air complaints.[13] Patient follow-up letters can be redesigned to include targeted patient satisfaction questions. Although the results are not statistically valid, such a survey does provide administrators and clinicians a method of ongoing monitoring.

INTERPRETATION AND EXPLANATION OF ONCOLOGY DATA

Many of the different data items in a registry are used in more than one way. What follows is an explanation of how to use the most common elements and the limitations in using them, if any.

Annual Cancer Caseload

The annual cancer caseload reflects the number of new cancer cases seen in an institution for diagnosis or treatment of primary cancer. It includes cases being initially diagnosed and those with recurrences. This number is usually reported by calendar year and is based on the data item "date first contact." The data can also be calculated by fiscal year by using the

admission or discharge date instead of the accession year.

Monitored over time, the totals show overall gain or loss in new cancer cases. Figure 27-1 shows six years of data for General Hospital. From 1996 through 1998, the number of new cancer cases was constant. In 1999, there was a 7.5 percent decrease in cases, which could be the result of a physician retiring, institutional facilities being closed or renovated, or lack of equipment or staff to treat a certain type of cancer. Data from 2000 and 2001 show increased cases. This increase might be due to new oncology facilities, new equipment in radiation oncology, or a new oncologist on staff. Increases or decreases in numbers should be explained.

The annual cancer caseload total should not be used to indicate or monitor use of services and facilities or the total number of visits by cancer patients. Cases are counted only when they initially present to the institution. For example, a patient diagnosed with breast cancer in April 2001 and who had numerous visits for radiation therapy during May and June 2001 would only be represented once in the total. A patient initially diagnosed in 1998 and who presents with a recurrence for the same primary in 2001 would only be counted in the 1998 annual accession total. The 2001 information would be detailed as a follow-up to the original diagnosis and treatment of the patient's primary.

Class of Case

The data item class of case shows the role that the institution plays in the patient's diagnosis and treatment. Cases are coded as to where the initial diagnosis or treatment occurs. The codes are further categorized as analytic or nonanalytic cases for reporting clinical outcomes. Analytic cases include those cases that were initially diagnosed or treated at the institution. Nonanalytic cases include those referred to the institution for recurrence or subsequent therapy. Nonanalytic cases are usually excluded from any survival analysis. Many institutions do not collect nonanalytic cases since the Commission on Cancer does not require them[17]. Use of data in clinical reporting focuses on analytic cases, because the hospital's staff are deciding or performing the treatment.

For administrative uses, all cancer cases seen at the institution should be reported. This includes both analytic and nonanalytic cases. Trends over time, usually five years, show a unique picture of the oncology product line.[3] The data shown in Figure 27-1 have been further refined in Figure 27-2. The class, or type, of case is shown for six years. Cases initially diagnosed and treated at the institution have continued to increase, and account for 89% of all cancer cases seen in 2001 (709 of 794 cases). Analytic cases represent the patients first diagnosed at the institution and treated elsewhere, first diagnosed and treated at the hospital, and cases initially diagnosed elsewhere that were referred to the hospital for treatment. In 1996, analytic cases accounted for 75% of the cases; in 2001, 89%.

The number of patients being diagnosed at the hospital and electing to be treated elsewhere has declined from 40 patients in 1996 to 15 in 2001. These patients represent lost opportunities. The reasons for patients electing to be treated elsewhere should be monitored over time. The number of cases that have recurred has also decreased over time, while the number of cases diagnosed elsewhere and referred to the institution for therapy has shown a slight decrease. This could indicate that physicians not on staff are not referring to the institution or that a managed care contract requires patients to go elsewhere. A developing cancer program should monitor these figures.

Patient Demographics

Demographic data are important in assessing the institution's patient population. They are used to identify patients for prevention trials, develop support groups, market the oncology product line, plan community outreach programs, write grant proposals, and evaluate patient care. Data collected include current address (street, city, state, ZIP code, county of residence, and telephone number), birth date, age at initial diagnosis, and race. Race and Spanish origin fields must be combined to identify minority patient populations.

Diagnosis—Primary Site and Histology

The primary site, identifying the patient's cancer, is the most often-used data item in the registry. This code allows site-specific data to be easily identified. For cancers such as melanoma, Kaposi's sarcoma, Hodgkin's and non-Hodgkin lymphoma, leukemia, multiple myeloma and other blood disorders, as well as many pediatric cancers, both the site and histologic codes must be reviewed to obtain an accurate count of the number of cases. For example, a lymphoma of the stomach (Cl6) has a different site code than a lymphoma arising in a lymph node (C77).[17] By using the site and histology codes, all lymphomas can be reported together. The site distribution in Table 27-5 has been categorized in this manner.

Monitoring the site distribution is an important element in administrative use of oncology data. The yearly site distribution is used in analyzing the need for new programs, ordering equipment, or changing staffing patterns. The five or ten most common cancers should be monitored.

Stage Distribution

The stage, or extent, of disease at initial diagnosis is a key indicator for the types of staff, equipment, and services that should be available for patients. Institutions that have large numbers of cases diagnosed in advanced stages usually need to have more advanced equipment and more specialists on staff than institutions with a predominance of early stage cases. Staging data are extremely helpful to community outreach departments, hospice, and home healthcare agencies.

Treatment

The patient's initial treatment is recorded for each analytic case, regardless of where it is administered. The treatment is classified by whether the patient received the treatment or refused it. The exact treatment, such as lumpectomy with axillary node dissection and radiation therapy for a stage I breast cancer, is recorded. By combining the treatment data with the diagnosis and stage at initial diagnosis, site-specific treatment patterns are determined in what was recommended versus what patients actually received.

Information on referral patterns can be established by reviewing the various treatment fields (surgery, radiation, chemotherapy, hormonal, endocrine therapy, biological response modifier, and other cancer-directed therapy) and where the treatment was done. Some software packages record the exact location of treatment. This allows the administrator to monitor which treatments are done at the institution and which are referred out, as well as changes over time.

By using data on both first course of therapy and subsequent therapy for a stated time period, the administrator can monitor the types of services being used. Data on subsequent therapy may not be complete.

Follow-Up

Survival data are based on the date of last follow-up. Registries located in institutions with cancer programs approved by the Commission on Cancer of the American College of Surgeons or in states with central registries that collect follow-up data are required to obtain information on patients until they expire. Follow-up is usually done on a yearly basis.[1] From the follow-up data, the patient's status (living or expired) is obtained. The information is then used to calculate survival and disease-free intervals.

Recurrence

The patient's first recurrence, including date and site, is recorded. This information is used to calculate disease-free interval. It is also useful in evaluating the need for physician specialists. However, it may be incomplete and not as accurate as date of last follow-up.

Physician Referrals and Usage

As each case is abstracted, the managing physician and other physicians (such as the surgeon, radiation oncologist, or medical oncologist) who participate in the care of the patient are recorded. These data are then used to determine physician activity (such as cancer distribution, service usage, and types of cases—such as early stage versus late stage at diagnosis).

If the registry software tracks referring physician, it is important to note which staff physicians refer to other staff in addition to which nonstaff physicians refer to the institution.

Hospital Referrals

These data items allow administrators to review which hospitals refer patients to the institution and to which institutions the hospital refers patients. These fields need to be combined with analysis of class of case and the treatment fields to give a clear picture of the referral patterns for a hospital.

Patient Satisfaction

The registry is required to annually assess the status of all analytic cases in the registry. Normally, this is done by reviewing charts to see if the patient has been back to the institution or by writing to the patient's managing physician. If new information is not obtained by these methods, then a letter may be sent directly to the patient. The cancer committee approves policies regarding when and if patients are contacted. Follow-up letters to patients normally ask for comments that can be used to help identify areas of excellence and areas that should be improved.[13]

ISSUES IN DATA USE

Release of Data

Institutional policies determine whether the cancer registry staff, the cancer committee (or its designee), or the institutional review board (IRB) approves requests for information. Requests may range from the numbers of cancers seen during a specific time period to a list of all breast cancer patients treated at the hospital. Although aggregate numbers do not breach the patients' or physicians' confidentiality, a list of patient names and addresses or a list of physicians who treat cancer patients would do so in many institutions. The registry must have written policies that are compliant with healthcare privacy laws. Another chapter in this textbook discusses release of data, including HIPAA. A record of all requests for data should be kept and available for review by the institution's cancer committee or other appropriate hospital staff.

Comparison of Data

A clear definition of the data must accompany any data used in a report. If the institution's data are being compared with other data, several issues such as data definitions, methods used in analysis, and time frames[6] must be addressed. When the comparison is done, the same data definitions and criteria must be used for both sets of data.[14] Everyone knows that apples should not be compared to oranges, and the registrar should keep in mind that Granny Smith apples should not be compared to Winesap apples. (Refer to the Statistics & Epidemiology chapter and Report Requests chapters for more information.)

SUMMARY

Innovative uses of registry data are important to the survival of the registry. The registrar must understand the oncology data and the needs of the audience. Data must be produced routinely and accurately in a timely fashion.[15] The registrar must meet the needs of the targeted audience. Comparison of the institution's data with other available data gives the institution a benchmark against which to measure its own performance.

Every opportunity must be used to distribute reports that feature oncology data. Guidelines must be in place for sharing data with sources outside the institution. Sources within and outside the hospital should look to the registry for their oncology data needs.

A priority must be placed on using registry data. Increasing use of data makes the registry a valuable tool for the institution.

STUDY QUESTIONS

1. What data elements should be used in a report to an administrator who is doing research on the possibility of starting a community mobile mammography unit?
2. What type of report should be given to the medical staff if they are anticipating the recruitment of a pediatric oncologist?
3. What data items are needed to link registry data with the financial department?
4. What data items are needed by an outside researcher who is writing an article on breast cancer in the community?
5. What approvals process is necessary to give the researcher the requested data?

REFERENCES

1. Commission on Cancer. *Cancer Program Standards.* Chicago, Ill: American College of Surgeons; 2003: 25, 47-48.
2. Gilden KM. The challenge of cancer marketing. *Seminars in Oncology Nursing.* 9(1):52.
3. Fritz AG. Administrative and marketing data from your registry. *Oncology Issues.* 9(5): 17-19.
4. Hoyler SS. Increase the Demand and Use of Registry Data. *The Abstract.* 21(1): 6-8.
5. Schau K, Mohnsen ME, Fritz A. Using registry data to assess differences in reimbursement. *The Abstract.* 19(3): 16-19.
6. Wodinsky HB, Didoklar MS, Cohen SP. New technology assessment: cryosurgery as a Case Study. *The Journal of Oncology Management.* 3 (1):3 2-3 7.
7. American Health Information Management Position Statement. "Issue: Clinical Practice Guidelines and Critical Paths-Role of HIM Professional." February 1994.
8. Hawkins J, Goldberg PB. Planning, implementing and evaluating a chemotherapy critical pathway. *The Journal of Oncology Management.* 3(2):24-29.
9. Michels DK. Outcomes assessment—a product of comprehensive follow-up. *The Abstract.* 19(13):7.
10. Roffers SD, Austin DF. Cancer registry data measures for breast and cervical cancer control: definitions, applications, and analyses. *The Abstract.* 19(3):13-15.
11. Coke DE. Making yourself visible by marketing your product line. *The Abstract.* 20(1):4-9.
12. Clive RE, Kearny M, Menck H, Hoyle SS. Using cancer registries to collect oncology clinical indicators-beta test site experience. *Journal of Oncology Administration.* 1993; 2(5): 17-30.
13. Harding J, Snow CS, Patee G. Managed care: using cancer registries in clinical quality improvement. *Journal of Registry Management.* 22(1):5-13.
14. Chen VW. Should we or shouldn't we compare cancer incidence rates among registries? *Cancer Incidence in North America.* 1988-1991; 1995: V-5.
15. Potts M, Hafterson JL. Increasing data usage at central and hospital registries. *The Abstract.* 20(1):15-16.
16. National Comprehensive Cancer Network (NCCN). Practice Guidelines in Oncology, Version 2. 3/15/02. NCCN (website).
17. Commission on Cancer. *Facility Oncology Registry Data Standards.* Chicago, Ill: American College of Surgeons; 2002: 3, 7.

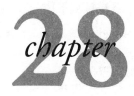

CANCER PROGRAM ANNUAL REPORT

M. Asa Carter
CTR

INTRODUCTION

Whether a cancer program serves a single institution or a central registry, producing an annual report provides the registry an opportunity to highlight the past year's accomplishments with a statistical summary of the cancer program's experience. The annual report serves as a valuable historical document for the cancer program's activities.[1] The report can be a source to present the facility's experience with outcomes, comparison to regional or national data, or a tool to market the cancer program to the community at large, state and local legislators, and healthcare providers.

Previously, Commission on Cancer (CoC)-approved cancer programs were required to meet certain expectations for responsibility, content, timeliness, and distribution of the cancer program annual report.[2] *Cancer Program Standards 2004* eliminated the requirements for content and publication which will afford the cancer committee the flexibility to craft an annual report that is meaningful and useful to the facility.[3] Some cancer programs have other specific requirements directed by their governing bodies. In either case, the authors may choose to include additional elements or distribute the report beyond the minimal requirements.

An annual report can be published simply to meet the governing body's requirements, or it can be used for other purposes. The style, content, and budget for the annual report depend on which of these approaches is chosen.[4,5]

REQUIREMENTS OF THE COMMISSION ON CANCER

Beginning January 1, 2004, CoC-approved cancer programs are no longer required to publish an annual report.[2] The cancer committee may continue the annual reporting process and determine the content and publication time frame.[2] The committee often delegates the preparation of the text to an annual report team or subcommittee. The cancer registry staff and one or more physician members of the committee are often appointed to this team or subcommittee. Other members representing departments or areas providing care to cancer patients as well as a representatives from public relations or marketing may be selected. The cancer committee's involvement in the preparation of the annual report should be documented in cancer committee minutes.

COMPONENTS

In addition to the text of a report, other components can add impact, meaning, and detail to the document. Of the possible components of a hospital cancer program annual report listed in Table 28-1,[4] some are not necessary for certain styles of annual reports. Key components are briefly discussed in this chapter.

Report Cover

The purpose of the annual report can affect the choice of cover style, size, and shape. Regardless of the report's intended use, the cover should be recognizable, attractive, and durable. A printer or the facility's public relations department can offer advice on the most desirable choice. The design of the front cover is important since it provides the first impression of the entire cancer program and its data.[4]

Institutions may wish to use a logo as part of the cover design. There may also be institutional standards or policies for printed materials. The same cover design may be used each year for consistency. If it is, recipients will recognize the report and look forward to reviewing the information. Also, the expense of special artwork can be reduced. On the

Table 28-1

Components of a Cancer Program Annual Report

- Report cover (front and back)
- Title page
- Executive summary or abstract
- Preface or foreword
- Table of contents
- Lists of tables and figures
- Introduction
- Cancer program activity report
- Cancer committee member listing
- Cancer registry activity report
- Cancer registry data presentation
- Primary site table
- In-depth report on major site(s)
- Glossary
- Acknowledgments
- References
- Appendices
- Data for administrators
- Other sections specified by the cancer committee
- Binding

other hand, when using the same cover, recipients may not realize that a new report containing updated information is published each year. This situation could be remedied by varying the color of ink or cover stock each year.

The back cover should be the same color and paper quality as the front cover. The institution name, address, city, state, and telephone number (including the registry extension, if applicable) should be placed on the back cover.

Title

The title of the annual report should reflect its scope. Cancer Program Annual Report or a similar title should reflect the entire program, not just the registry.[4] The title should state both the year of the publication as well as the year for which data are summarized.

Title Page

The title page is the first right-hand page of the report, inside the front cover. In addition to the title, this page should include the names of the authors, the name and address of the facility, and the date of publication. Figure 28-1 is a suggested format for an annual report title page.

Figure 28-1
Sample Title Page

2004 Cancer Care Progress Report

2003 Cancer Registry
Statistical Review
Institution Name
Address
City, State

Published December 2004
by Institution (Name)
Cancer Committee

The title page may be set in larger type than the text. Graphic identifiers (such as hospital logo) should be reserved for the cover of the report. The person or persons who prepared the report should be acknowledged in the text, the acknowledgment section, or inside the back cover.

Executive Summary or Abstract

This section summarizes the report content and highlights important facts or conclusions. It provides essential information for readers who may not read the entire report. The summary should be less than one page long and should describe the intent of the publication, objectives of the report, observations or findings in summary form, conclusions, and any recommendations made as a result of the report. The cancer committee may choose to include the summary in a cover letter rather than in the report itself.

Preface or Foreword

A preface or foreword should be placed before the body of the text begins. These components are usually not necessary for a traditional annual report; if included, however, the preface should describe any special circumstances surrounding the preparation of the report, its intended audience, and the format. Report contributors can be acknowledged in the preface if an acknowledgment section is not included. A foreword is sometimes written by someone other than the authors in order to enhance the report's credibility or to encourage recipients to read it.

Table of Contents

The table of contents should be on a right-hand page and as close to the beginning of the report as possible, after the title page, preface or foreword, and summary or abstract (if included). It should precede the introduction, which is usually considered part of the body of the report.

The table of contents should be as complete as possible, listing the page number and heading for each section in order, exactly as they appear in the text. Only the first page number of each section should be listed.

List of Tables and Figures

A list of table and figures can be included in an annual report. If the report is brief, the tables and figures can be listed in the table of contents with the section headings. If there are numerous figures and tables, a separate page following the table of contents should be prepared.

Report Introduction

An introduction provides readers with information in addition to what is included in the summary or abstract. It can contain a dedication; the history of the program and registry; a statement of goals, purposes, and philosophy; and introductory data on the cancer program.

Cancer Program Activity Report

The cancer program activity report should summarize all the activities of the cancer program for the reporting period, not just those of the cancer registry and cancer committee. The cancer committee may elect to include additional information such as related events occurring after the reporting period (calendar year) or current goals; however, minimal requirements must be met for the actual reporting period.

The activity report should include a statement of goals and achievements met during the past year and goals proposed for the coming year. The accomplishments of all departments, sections, or groups involved in the care of cancer patients should be included. Include facts and figures as part of the narrative. Suggested content for an annual report is listed in Table 28-2, Anatomy of an Annual Report.[4,5]

It requires skill and creativity to present the activities for the year in such a way that the reader's interest is sustained. A midpoint must be found between superficial mention of activities and tedious detail.[4,5] Statistics should be presented using interesting and meaningful methods.[4]

Cancer Committee Member Listing

Including a roster of cancer committee members in the annual report is a good way to recognize the members for their work during the year. The members should be listed by discipline, specialty, or department. Usually, the cancer committee chair's name is placed at the beginning of the list and indicated as the chair. Both physician and nonphysician members should be included in the list.

Cancer Registry Activity Report

A variety of information can be included in the annual report regarding registry activities. Items that can be included in the registry activity summary are shown in Table 28-2.[4,5] The registry telephone number and location should be listed prominently in the report so that additional information can be requested.

Cancer Registry Data Presentation and Primary Site Table

A statistical summary may include a distribution of primary sites, as well as tables or graphs highlighting the most common sites. The inclusion of comparison data using the National Cancer Data Base (NCDB) benchmark reports or other national, state, or regional data enhances the facility information. A brief narrative statement that ties the data to the management of cancer in the institution may be included with the statistical summary.[3] The narrative can include the stage of cancer at diagnosis and treatment for the cancers in the statistical analysis. For example, the stage at diagnosis can be correlated with screening programs, new diagnostic equipment, or expansion of services.[3]

Data Comparison

There are a number of sources available for comparing registry data, including state or central registries and the Surveillance, Epidemiology, and End Results (SEER) program. The American Cancer Society publishes a review of SEER data in their annual publication Cancer Facts and Figures.

The on-line NCDB hospital comparison benchmark reports enable CoC-approved cancer programs to obtain customized data comparison to local, regional, or national data for user-designed data requests. Summary comparison data is also provided to the public through the public version of the NCDB benchmark reports.

When data are compared, any statistical or demographic differences in the databases should be noted. Use caution when comparing institutional data with population-based registry data because of differences in patient referral trends or demographics.[4,6]

The statistical analysis must be interesting, meaningful, and accurate. Graphics charts and illus-

Table 28-2
Anatomy of an Annual Report

Ideas for Content of Annual Report
- Cover design and content
- Characteristics: theme, layout, binding type, print style and graphics
- Acknowledgments or Dedication
- Table of Contents with page numbers include tables and figures
- Introduction/Foreword/Preface/Executive Summary
- Message from the administrator
- Message from the cancer committee chair
- Components of cancer program with phone numbers and location
- Organizational chart
- Departmental reports, diagnostic, therapeutic, support, research

Medical staff	Social services/support groups
Nursing staff	Nutritional services
Treatment modalities available	Rehabilitative services
Cancer registry	Pastoral services
Diagnostic services	Screening programs
Quality assurance activities	Hospice
Research activities	Community involvement
Membership in cooperative groups	Volunteer efforts

- List of cancer committee members by specialty or responsibilities within the committee
- Goals and objectives of the cancer program
- Historical information on program development
- Current year achievements
- Future plans
- Glossary and abbreviations used in the report
- References cited in report or bibliography

Highlights of Cancer Program Activities During this Year
- New equipment and/or facilities
- Use of diagnostic, treatment, and support services
- Honors received by committee members
- Professional education completed by committee members
- New board certifications
- Papers published
- New professional specialties recruited
- New institutional memberships in professional associations
- Special recognition of the program by community and media
- Community education programs
- Screening programs
- Smoking cessation programs
- Cancer Awareness Month activities: April of each year
- Fund-raising activities
- Gifts and services contributed by volunteers

Cancer Conferences
- Sites covered
- Topics of didactic lectures

(continued)

Table 28-2
(continued)

- Number and specialties of participants
- Instructions for scheduling a patient for cancer conference review

Other Administrative Data

- Admissions and discharges by major site groupings
- Percent of total hospital caseload that is cancer-related
- Marketing goals and objectives set and/or met
- Consultations by specialty
- Length of stay
- DRG assignment distribution
- Oncology unit admissions
- Number of readmissions
- Hospitals referred from and hospitals referred to
- Patient and tumor status at discharge
- Follow-up sources
- Outpatient service utilization

Summary of Cancer Registry Activities

- Narrative summary
- Total cases in registry (with trend)
- Increases or decreases in case load
- Goals and objectives for the year
- Changes in staff
- Participation in public and professional education programs
- Descriptions of registry usage
- Special reports and projects
- Patient care evaluations completed
- Follow-up rate report
- Primary sites by stage
- Most common sites
- Distributions by sex and age
- Distribution by class of case

Site Studies

- Comparison with regional, state, or national data
- Narrative by cancer committee
- Distributions (tables or graphs)
  sex and age
  stage
  histology
- Outcomes of diagnostic tests (ERA/PRA, CEA, PSA, etc.)
- Treatment combinations
- Survival rates
- Description of program's referral area
- Maps or graphics by county, zip code
- Size and demographic characteristics of population served
    age and sex

Reprinted with permission by the National Cancer Registrars Association, Marketing Cancer Information and Services. Originally developed by Karen Phillips, CTR.

trations are useful to convey the message quickly and concisely.[4] Each type of graphic format has particular advantages in displaying information, and each has its own set of guidelines.[4] Refer to other chapters in this textbook for specific information regarding data presentation.

In-Depth Report on Major Site

Beginning January 1, 2004, cancer committees in CoC-approved programs are required to analyze patient outcomes and disseminate the results of the analysis. This information can be disseminated through the cancer program annual report by including an in-depth report of at least one major site.(2) The in-depth report must include outcomes data and comparison to the cancer experience reported to the NCDB. Analysis of patient survival is the preferred outcome; however other outcomes may be selected at the discretion of the cancer committee.

Many publications are available that explain survival statistics and presentation. The most recent edition of the Cancer Staging Manual, by the American Joint Committee on Cancer Cancer, provides a useful explanation of survival data.[7] Another practical source for learning about survival statistics is the SEER Program Self-Instructional Manual, Book 7: Statistics and Epidemiology for Cancer Registries.[6]

Cancer programs with less than five years of registry data may omit survival information from the in-depth analysis. However, they can report other outcomes information such as statistics on recurrence rates, the disease-free survival period, or make observations about sites such as lung, pancreas, and adult acute leukemia, where prognosis is poor.[3,4]

A physician member of the cancer committee provides an overall narrative analysis or critique of the major-site data. Descriptive statistics must be presented in appropriate graphic, tabular, or narrative form. If more than one site is presented, various graphics and charts should be used to display the data.[3]

Glossary

A glossary, or list of terms and definitions, is a useful addition to an annual report. It can help readers who are not familiar with the technical jargon of oncology or the registry. The definitions should be brief and clear. The glossary is usually placed toward the back of the report.

Acknowledgments

The acknowledgment section should include the names of individuals who contribute to the preparation of the annual report. The acknowledgments need not be effusive, but should indicate the reason for the individual's participation in the project. The acknowledgment section should be near the end, before appendices or references. A copy of the annual report should be given to each person mentioned.

References and Bibliography

Any data taken from another source must be identified. A reference list makes it easier for the reader to obtain additional information from the source. The bibliography should be consistent in style and content. Citations should be numbered consecutively in the text, and the list of references presented in numeric order in a separate section at the end of the text.

Appendices

Usually an appendix contains supplemental data or reference tables that are large or disrupt the flow of text in the body of the report. As an example, the appendix may reproduce staging forms or criteria for sites discussed within the report. The appendices are placed at the end of the report.

Data for Administrators

Administrators and planners are interested in data that describe the population using hospital services. Core data items of the registry abstract (such as sex, age, and place of residence) may reflect changes in the institution's service, or catchment area.[4] This information can be used to develop marketing strategies for the facility. Items such as the follow-up source can be used to track care after discharge. Insurance payor source and other financial data have become increasingly important to administrators; however, care should be exercised when releasing administrative and financial information to the general public.

Other Sections

The purpose of the report and its target audience (whether it is for physicians, administrators, or the general public) affect the style and content of the report. The report must be written for its primary audience. Information for a secondary audience can be included as long as it does not interfere with the primary message of the report.[4]

Many institutions include pictures of the institution or personnel, maps, descriptions of services, and telephone numbers for departments serving the cancer patient. Some institutions phrase the descriptive section of the report (cancer program activity summary) so that it will remain accurate for several years. This section is printed separately from the report of cancer registry activities and statistical analysis. In this way, a current registry report (noting any changes in the cancer program summary) can be inserted into a pocket at the back of the information packet each year, without the need to reprint the entire piece.[5] A pocket can be included in the front to hold brochures, information (such as specific cancer site or treatment descriptions), or newsletters for physicians or patients. For example, the cancer registry may choose to develop a pamphlet describing the follow-up service with a change-of-address card and include this in the pocket of the report.[4]

Binding

The binding affects the design of the cover, the layout of text, the amount of necessary postage for distribution, and the total cost of the publication. There are many types of binding available in a wide range of prices. The type of binding should be decided early in the report-planning process because it affects other aspects of report production.

TIMELINE

In the past, the CoC required that the annual report be distributed by November 1 of the following year. This deadline no longer applies and the data may be more meaningful if presented earlier. Many cancer programs target June or July as the publication date.

A production timeline should be developed for completing all components and tasks associated with the annual report. Delegation and monitoring completion of assignments is a primary role o the annual report team. If another department such as public relations is involved in the production, efforts and timelines must be coordinated. A checklist can assist with tracking timelines and projects.

Departmental narratives can be delegated to department heads or other individuals. Guidance on format, subject matter, and length of contribution

should be provided. A copy of the previous year's report can be helpful to these individuals. A reasonable amount of time should be given to the contributors for completion of their assignments.

The registry staff should compile the data for the physicians who write the narratives on the registry data and major site(s). The statistical summary should be provided to the physician with an appropriate timeline for completion. It may be wise to meet with the physician(s) to determine the type of information and presentation style desired before preparing the graphics and tables.

BUDGET

A production budget should be prepared and approved for the annual report. The items that appear in Table 28-3 are factors that should be considered when developing an annual report budget.

The CoC does not specify the production requirements for the annual report. Some facilities may choose to have the report professionally printed or typeset by a commercial printer. Other facilities may prefer to print the annual report in-house or post the information on a hospital intranet or Internet website. The most important consideration is that the data be clear, concise, and accurate. Many software programs are available to produce professional-quality reports while substantially reducing expenses.

SUMMARY

Though no longer a Commission on Cancer requirement, most CoC-approved cancer programs publish an annual report. Other governing bodies may have requirements for the annual report. The components

Table 28-3
Factors Affecting an Annual Report Budget

- Number of pages
- Size and quality of paper
- Number of ink colors
- Binding
- Method of production
- Number of copies
- Number of illustrations
- Mailing and distribution costs

and scope of the report can vary, as long as requirements are met. The annual report serves as a valuable historical document for the cancer program's activities.

The purpose of the report and the target audience must be established before production begins, because they affect style, content, timelines, and budgets. Institutions may have policies for published material that should be incorporated into the annual report.

A review of annual reports from other cancer programs may reveal ideas for future annual reports. Annual reports can have the same appearance each year or change periodically. The format and style can change along with the annual report's purpose or the cancer program's scope.

STUDY QUESTIONS

1. Name four factors that can affect the budget of an annual report.
2. In programs approved by the Commission on Cancer, who is responsible for analyzing outcomes that may be included in the annual report?
3. Name two databases that can be used to compare registry data in a cancer program annual report.
4. What department or person is usually appointed as the coordinator of the cancer program annual report?

REFERENCES

1. Creech, CM, Scarlett PB, Watkins SA. *Guidelines for Preparing a Hospital Cancer Program Annual Report,* 2nd ed. The American Cancer Society, California Division, Inc.; 1986.
2. Commission on Cancer. *Cancer Program Standards 2004.* Chicago, Ill: American College of Surgeons; 2003.
3. Commission on Cancer. *Standards of the Commission on Cancer, vol. I: Cancer Program Standards.* Chicago, Ill: American College of Surgeons; 1996.
4. Fritz AG, *Writing for Registrars: A Manual of Style for Annual Reports and Other Cancer Registry Technical Writing.* Rockville, Md: ELM Publications; 1987.
5. Jolitz G, Increasing data usage. In: Fritz A, Roffers S, et al., eds. *Marketing Cancer Information and Services.* Lenexa, Kan: National Cancer Registrars Association; 1995.
6. Shambaugh, EM, Young JL, Zippin C, et al. Statistical inference. In: National Cancer Institute. *Self-Instructional Manual for Cancer Registrars, Book 7: Statistics and Epidemiology for Cancer Registries.* Bethesda, Md: National Institutes of Health, National Cancer Institute; 1994. NIH Publication No. 94-33766.
7. Greene FL, Page DL, Fleming ID, et al., eds. *AJCC Cancer Staging Manual,* 6th ed. American Joint Committee on Cancer. New York, NY: Springer-Verlag; 2002.

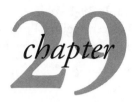

chapter 29

DEPARTMENT OF DEFENSE AND OTHER FEDERAL REGISTRIES

Raye-Anne Dorn
CTR

Betty Nielsen
RHIT, CTR

Judy Tryon
CTR

Patricia Babin
RHIT, CTR

INTRODUCTION

The foundations of medicine may have been laid in Greece around 500 BC, but no actual recording of diseases was published until the late sixteenth and seventeenth centuries.[1] The need for reliable cancer statistics became increasingly apparent during the early twentieth century, when in 1915 Frederick L. Hoffman, a statistician for the Prudential Insurance Company of America, published a compilation of cancer statistics from around the world.[2] Hoffman was instrumental in having the US Census Bureau analyze cancer mortality of the United States for the 1914 data.

Ongoing interest and isolated studies into the disease process eventually led to a declaration of war on cancer by Richard Nixon in 1971. Since then, billions of dollars have been spent on education, treatment, and research. Fundamental to any research was the need to develop databases for long-term acquisition and validation of knowledge about the different disease processes in human patients.[3] The federal government has become the leader in the data collection arena, maintaining registries in all branches of the military establishment, the Department of Veterans Affairs, the National Institutes of Health, and the Indian Health Service.

CANCER REGISTRIES

Cancer registries are by far the most numerous of the databases maintained within the federal system. The Department of Defense administers, through the respective branches of the armed forces, registries for the tracking of cancer incidence at all of its military hospitals. A summary of cancer programs within the federal government is shown in Table 29-1.

Programs at federal institutions are similar in nature to their nongovernmental counterparts. The guidelines established by the Commission on Cancer (CoC) of the American College of Surgeons Approvals Program and the National Cancer Institute's Surveillance, Epidemiology, and End Results (SEER) Program are followed. Approval by the CoC is desirable and encouraged.

Although the data collection methods and the external approval standards are the same as for the private sector, the major difference between federal cancer registries and nongovernment registries is in the way the programs are established. Within the federal environment, programs are established by direc-

Table 29-1

Cancer Registry Programs Administered by the Department of Veterans Affairs

	Total Programs	CoC*-Approved Programs
Veterans Affairs	103	53

Cancer Registry Programs Administered by the Department of Defense

Department	Total Programs	CoC*-Approved Programs
US Army	28	10
US Air Force	41	4
US Navy	23	4

Note: This table only includes the Department of Defense and Department of Veterans Affairs. It does not include Federal entities such as National Institutes of Health and Indian Health Service.

* Commission on Cancer of the American College of Surgeons

tive from a central, national headquarters.[4,5,6] General direction and guidance are provided. The actual implementation and establishment of these directives are left to the institution, thereby enabling them to preserve their autonomy and flexibility.

DEPARTMENT OF DEFENSE CANCER REGISTRIES

Following the National Cancer Act of 1971, the military community joined in the war on cancer, and in 1986 established the Automated Central Tumor Registry (ACTUR), a database which was developed to identify Department of Defense (DoD) patients diagnosed with malignancies. The Air Force, Army, and Navy have all joined to mandate the use of ACTUR by all facilities that diagnose, treat, and/or conduct follow-up of cancer cases.[4,5] In 1989, following design and development of the software, a number of service facilities were designated as ACTUR sites, and cases were entered into the system for tracking. Since its inception, the ACTUR system has undergone multiple upgrades and changes designed to bring the program in line with the American College of Surgeons (ACoS) and North American Association of Central Cancer Registry

(NAACCR) standards. ACTUR gives us total connectivity, allowing us to have read-only access to all patients with a cancer diagnosis within the DoD arena. As of September 30, 2002, there are a total of 258,463 cases in the database. Data is sent from ACTUR to the various state registries to meet federal reporting standards.

The Armed Forces Institute of Pathology (AFIP) administers the ACTUR program for the Department of Defense's three military services (Army, Air Force, and Navy). The ACTUR program is a component of the Defense Eligibility and Enrollment Reporting System (DEERS) program, which is used to establish eligibility for DoD services. This also allows DoD registrars access to patients' addresses (active duty/retired military) as they move around the country, which is extremely helpful in follow-up.

While the DoD cancer programs follow the guidelines of the ACoS CoC and the NCI SEER programs, they differ from those in the private sector in several ways. The Department of Defense requires data sets that are military-specific, such as branch of service, sponsor SSN, active duty status, exposure to Agent Orange, participation in Desert Storm, etc. The database is linked through ACTUR and DEERS.

Most of our DoD Registries fall under a clinical service rather than medical records; thus providing a closer working relationship between physician and tumor registrar. DoD registries may come under the Department of Surgery, Pathology or Oncology. Registrars also keep a convenience file of all patients with their cancer data. This is because inpatient and outpatient files in the military hospitals are generally maintained for two to five years. At that point in time and with no activity, they are sent to St. Louis, the DoD medical record repository. When active duty military patients are transferred to another assignment location, the outpatient records of the active duty patients and their families are transferred to the military medical facility at that location.

Another difference in DoD tumor registries is that our first point of contact for follow-up is the patient because of the constant rotation and transfer to other facilities of our physicians. The patient is informed by letter after initial diagnosis, explaining the tumor registry, and a questionnaire and privacy act statement are enclosed to be signed and returned to the registry. At many facilities, an informational pamphlet which gives a more in-depth description of

a tumor registry, including clinic phone numbers and American Cancer Society groups is also provided to newly diagnosed cancer patients.

Direction on how the DoD cancer program is maintained is provided by the DoD ACTUR Coordination Committee, composed of various military service representatives, DEERS personnel, and civilian service appointed CTR consultants. Committee members provide input based on their service-specific requirements.

Although DoD registries differ from civilian facilities, we are all working toward one common goal—early diagnosis and prevention of cancer through research and compassion toward our cancer patients.

SPECIALTY REGISTRIES

The federal government maintains many other different types of registries whose goal is to collect diverse data sets in compliance with both national law and the public interest. Registries such as the National Cancer Institute's SEER Program have been actively collecting, analyzing, and distributing data since 1973,[7] and some VA facilities have been doing so since the 1950s.

Registries for HIV and AIDS, diabetes, spinal cord injuries, prostheses, pacemakers, Agent Orange exposure, radiation exposure, Persian Gulf Syndrome, bone marrow transplantation, organ donor recipients, mammography, cervical screening, benign colon polyps, burn patients, and laryngectomies are actively maintained. Training in the specialized data collection methods of these programs parallels the training needed for becoming a cancer registrar. Certification from an organization such as the National Cancer Registrars Association (NCRA) is encouraged. The need for specialized databases continues to grow as the federal government increases its interest in providing information for new and ongoing research.

To be at the cutting edge of technology and research is the unifying common goal within the federal registry communities. The various departments of the federal government have research and development offices that are expanding the role of computer applications in medical care. Telemedicine, conferencing, and fully integrated computer systems maintaining electronic health records, complete with images that can be sent from station to station, allow for the sharing of patient information at a speed of millions of bytes of information per second. Information- and technology-sharing agreements between the various departments provide greater flexibility in long-term care and longitudinal studies.

SUMMARY

Albert Gelhorn, in a presentation to the World Health Organization in 1963, said that cancer was no longer the most lethal of chronic diseases but the most chronic of lethal diseases, and that the benefit of successful research was not the prevention of death, but the enrichment of life. In any research field, quality data are paramount. The fundamental basis for this data collection is the registry, and as the major user of this information, the federal government has become the prime developer of cancer and other specialty databases. The Department of Defense has established a tumor registry program and mandated software (ACTUR) to use in cancer reporting to meet federal statutes. The service branches follow certain guidelines and have the authority to develop requirements which are service-specific, i.e., Air Force, Army, and Navy. Becoming a registrar in the federal government offers personal challenges and opportunities plus the advantage of being on the cutting edge of technology.

STUDY QUESTIONS

1. Name three departments of the federal government that have registries.
2. Name the three military service branches.
3. Name a military-specific data set.
4. Name five different types of registries.
5. What is the acronym for the military tumor registry software program?
6. What is the main difference between federal registries and their private counterparts?

REFERENCES

1. Shimkin MB. Contrary to nature. *National Institutes of Health (NIH) Report 76-720.* Washington, DC: US Government Printing Office; 1977.
2. Hoffman FL. *The Mortality from Cancer throughout the World.* Newark, NJ: Prudential Press; 1915.
3. DeVita VT, et al. *Cancer Principles and Practice of Oncology,* vol. 1, 2nd ed. Philadelphia, Penn: J. B. Lippincott; 1985: 153.
4. MEDCOM Reg (Medical Command Regulation) 40-1, Ft. Sam Houston, San Antonio, TX: US Army; 1996.
5. Air Force Instruction 44-110. Washington, DC: US Air Force; 1996.
6. *Criteria and Standards for VA Oncology Programs.* VA Reg M9, Chapter 9, Appendix 9D, Change 12. Washington, DC: Department of Veterans Affairs; 1992.
7. Shambaugh EM, ed. *SEER Self-Instructional Manual for Tumor Registrars, book 1,* 2nd ed. Bethesda, Md: National Cancer Institute; 1994.

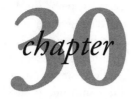

PEDIATRIC CANCERS

Frederick B. Ruymann
MD

Marla K. Moloney
MD

Lisa J. Wise
CTR

INTRODUCTION

The early diagnosis of malignancy in children and adolescents requires a knowledge of presenting signs and symptoms and perseverance by the physician responsible for primary care. As in the medical diagnosis of adults, there is no substitute for a thorough history and physical examination. Perhaps the best explanation for a physician overlooking the correct diagnosis has been given by Dr. Lewis Barness, in his textbook *Handbook of Pediatric Physical Diagnosis,* in which he states,

"More is missed by not looking than by not knowing. Few doctors miss diagnoses because of ignorance; errors are caused by careless omission of simple procedures."[1]

Pediatric or childhood cancers refer to those occurring in patients 0 to 14 years, sometimes including those who are 15 years old. For descriptive purposes these childhood malignancies are sometimes further subgrouped into ages 0 to 4, 5 to 9 or 10 to 14. Incidence, treatment, response, and survival are sometimes constructively categorized by age subgroup.

The twelve most common complaints associated with 85 percent of childhood malignancies have been summarized by Dr. Mark Nesbit and are found in Table 30-1.[2] It is interesting to note how commonplace these complaints are among otherwise healthy children. Perhaps the most subtle presentation is that of acute leukemia, which may include

fever, leg pain, limp, and nonspecific symptoms of not feeling well, known as malaise.[3] These symptoms frequently mimic those seen with the flu and are often dismissed. A brain tumor can also have an insidious presentation with symptoms of headache and vomiting, typically worse in the morning. A complete work-up for a brain tumor—after one or two episodes of headache and increasing vomiting, however—would not be appropriate. Rather, it is the persistence of symptoms that should prompt the primary care physician to refer the patient for further studies or consultation.

Hodgkin lymphoma may appear as a swollen lymph node that does not resolve with antibiotics. The only sign of an abdominal mass such as Wilms tumor of the kidney, neuroblastoma in an adrenal gland, or a retroperitoneal rhabdomyosarcoma may be a protuberant abdomen, which may occur as a normal finding in a growing child. Retinoblastoma, a malignant tumor of the retina, is the most common familial tumor of childhood and often presents as a white spot or white reflex in the eye (leukocoria) of a child seen on a flash photograph (Figure 30-1).

EPIDEMIOLOGY

Genetic and Environmental Factors

Cancer kills more children than any other disease: more than asthma, diabetes mellitus, cystic fibrosis, congenital anomalies, and AIDS combined. The

Table 30-1
Common Chief Complaints Given by Parents that Suggest a Pediatric Cancer

Chief Complaints	Suggested Cancer
Chronic drainage from ear	Rhabdomyosarcoma, Langerhans cell histiocytosis
Recurrent fever with bone pain	Ewing sarcoma, leukemia
Morning headache with vomiting	Brain tumor
Lump in neck that does not respond to antibiotics	Hodgkin disease or non-Hodgkin lymphoma
White dot in eye	Retinoblastoma
Swollen face and neck	Non-Hodgkin lymphoma, leukemia
Mass in abdomen	Wilms tumor, neuroblastoma, hepatoma
Paleness and fatigue	Leukemia, lymphoma
Limping	Osteosarcoma, other bone tumors
Bone pain	Leukemia, Ewing sarcoma, neuroblastoma
Bleeding from vagina	Yolk sac tumor, rhabdomyosarcoma
Weight loss	Hodgkin lymphoma

Reprinted with permission from P. A. Pizzo and D. G. Poplack (eds.), *Principles and Practices of Pediatric Oncology,* 2nd ed., 1993, p. 106.

Figure 30-1
Leukocoria in a Five-Month-Old with Bilateral Retinoblastoma

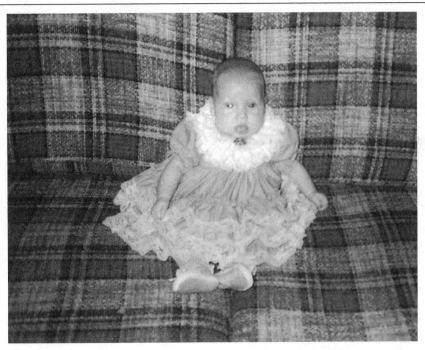

incidence of malignancy in children from age 0 to 14 is 14.5 per 100,000, relatively low compared with the 549.6 and 416.1 incidences in adult male and female populations, respectively.[4] In general, genetic and familial factors are believed to have a greater influence on the occurrence of malignancies in children than environmental factors. As more is learned about the inheritance and molecular biology of familial cancer syndromes, we may find that genetic factors are more important than presently thought in adult cancers.

For example, it has been hypothesized that an early presentation of rhabdomyosarcoma, a common soft tissue malignancy of muscle origin, in a child is more likely to occur in a family with a genetic predisposition to the breast sarcoma syndrome Li-Fraumeni Syndrome.[5,6,7] The interaction of genetic and environmental factors may also explain the reason for one adult developing lung cancer after 15 years of smoking and another having no problems after 40 years of smoking. The inconsistent findings for cigarette smoking as a breast cancer risk factor may also be an example of individuals having similar environmental exposures but different genetic susceptibilities.[8]

One of the most common gene changes in human tumors is alteration of the p53 tumor sup-pressor gene.[9] The normal p53 gene stops cell proliferation and permits cells with DNA damage to undergo repair. When both copies (alleles) are inactive due to deletion or mutation, the normal restraint on proliferation by a tumor suppressor gene is lost.

In children, malignancies of endothelial and epithelial surfaces, such as adenocarcinomas and squamous cell carcinomas, are relatively rare. Children more commonly have tumors of mesenchymal, neural, and germ cell origin, such as sarcomas, leukemias, and teratomas, respectively.[10] Sarcomas have the capacity for early hematogenous spread (metastasis) and local lymph node extension. The highly malignant small cell lung carcinoma in adults behaves much like a child with an unfavorable alveolar rhabdomyosarcoma,[11,12,13,14] with early extension through the bloodstream to distant metastatic sites.

Congenital anomalies have a high association with many childhood tumors. This has been shown in leukemias, Wilms tumor,[15] rhabdomyosarcoma,[16] and Ewing sarcoma of bone.[17] Marina, Bowman, Pui, and Crist have published an excellent summary of existing conditions and associated tumors, as shown in Table 30-2.[18] For example, neurofibromatosis is an autosomal dominant

Table 30-2
Conditions Associated with Increased Risk of Childhood Cancer

Conditions and Primary Sites Associated Tumors

Conditions:	Primary Sites Associated Tumors:
Cutaneous syndromes	
Nevoid basal cell carcinoma syndrome	Basal cell carcinoma
Familial trichoepithelioma syndrome	Esophageal squamous cell carcinoma
Tylosis (palmar-plantar keratosis)	Basal and squamous cell carcinoma, melanoma
Xeroderma pigmentosum	Squamous cell carcinoma
Albinism	Soft tissue sarcomas, carcinoma
Werner syndrome (adult progeria)	Basal and squamous cell carcinoma
Epidermodysplasia verruciformis	Squamous cell carcinoma
Polydysplastic epidermolysis bullosa	Squamous cell carcinoma, mucous membrane carcinomas
Dyskeratosis congenita	
Familial atypical mole, malignant melanoma syndrome	Melanoma, breast cancer, colon cancer, leukemia, lymphoma, sarcoma
Neurocutaneous syndromes	
Neurofibromatosis	Brain, pheochromocytoma, neuroblastoma, medullary thyroid carcinoma, Wilms tumor, leukemia, rhabdomyosarcoma, neurosarcoma
Tuberous sclerosis	
von Hippel-Lindau disease	Brain, pheochromocytoma, hypernephroma
Chromosomal syndromes	
Down syndrome (trisomy 21) Klinefelter's syndrome (47 XXY) Female XY mosaicism (47 XO/46 XY) 13q-syndrome llp-, aniridia-Wilms tumor syndrome t(3,8)	Leukemia
	Breast cancer, leukemia, lymphoma, teratoma
	Gonadoblastoma
	Retinoblastoma
Bloom syndrome	Wilms tumor
Fanconi's anemia	Renal cell carcinoma
Ataxia-telangiectasia	Leukemia, lymphoma, colon cancer, squamous cell carcinoma
	Leukemia, hepatoma, squamous cell carcinoma
	Leukemia, lymphoma; Hodgkin disease; brain, gastric, ovarian cancers
Primary immunodeficiency syndromes	
X-linked agammaglobulinemia (Bruton)	Lymphoma, leukemia, brain
X-linked lymphoproliferative disease (Duncan)	Lymphoma
Severe combined immunodeficiency	Lymphoma, leukemia
Wiskott-Aldrich syndrome	Lymphoma, leukemia, brain
IgA deficiency	Lymphoma, leukemia, brain, gastrointestinal
DiGeorge syndrome	Brain, oral squamous cell carcinoma
IgM deficiency	Lymphoma
Basal cell carcinoma, medulloblastoma, Rhabdomyosarcoma	

(continued)

Table 30-2 *(continued)*
Conditions Associated with Increased Risk of Childhood Cancer

Conditions:	Primary Sites Associated Tumors:
Gastrointestinal syndromes	
Polyposis coli	Colon cancer
Gardner's syndrome	Colon, soft tissue, bone, thyroid, adrenal cancers
Turcot syndrome	Colon cancer, brain
Peutz-Jeghers syndrome	Gastrointestinal, ovarian, breast cancers
Inflammatory bowel disease	Colorectal cancer
Miscellaneous	
Hemihypertrophy	Wilms tumor, hepatoma, adrenocortical carcinoma
Renal dysplasia	Wilms tumor
Sporadic aniridia	Wilms tumor
Beckwith-Wiedemann syndrome	Gonadoblastoma
Gonadal dysgenesis	Testicular cancer
Cryptorchidism	Testicular cancer
Multiple endocrine adenomatosis type I (Wermer's syndrome)	Schwannoma
	Thyroid carcinoma, pheochromocytoma
Multiple endocrine adenomatosis type 11 (Sipple's syndrome)	Chondrosarcoma
	Lymphoma
Enchondromatosis	Leukemia
Chediak-Higashi syndrome	Adrenocortical, testicular, mesodermal, neurogenic cancers
Shwachman syndrome	
21-hydroxylase deficiency, congenital adrenal hyperplasia	Liver cancer
	Liver cancer
Galactosemia	Liver cancer
Hereditary tyrosinemia	Liver cancer
Type I glycogen storage	Liver cancer
Hypermethioninemia	Liver cancer
Alpha-1-antitrypsin deficiency	
Familial cholestatic cirrhosis of childhood	

Reprinted with permission from G. P. Murphy, W. Lawrence, and R. E. Lenhard, (eds.), American Cancer Society *Textbook of Clinical Oncology,* 2nd ed., 1995, pp. 525-26.[36]

congenital syndrome of hyper- and hypo-pigmentation occurring in one in 3,000 persons with cafe-au-lait spots and multiple neurofibromata.[19] These individuals have an increased risk for malignant schwannomas, rhabdomyosarcoma, leukemia, and brain tumors in childhood, as well as a spectrum of malignancies in their adult years.[20,21] It has been estimated that 25% of individuals with neurofibromatosis will develop cancer in their lifetime.[20]

Two major explanations have been proposed for these observations. One is that the congenital anomaly observed with the malignancy is influenced by a common molecular event. The example of sporadic aniridia in association with Wilms tumor

(known as Miller's Syndrome) is probably consistent with a common molecular event. The second hypothesis is that an environmental factor such as a teratogenic agent may also be carcinogenic. Maternal ingestion of the hormone diethylstilbestrol (DES) in early pregnancy has been associated with a rare vaginal adenocarcinoma in female offspring.[22,23] Curiously, an increase in malignancy has not been reported in the male offspring of mothers taking DES during pregnancy.[24]

Central nervous system tumors have been described in children of parents who have had work-related exposures to carcinogens.[25,26] Radiation, a major carcinogen and teratogen, has been associated with an increased incidence of leukemia in survivors of the atomic bomb,[27,28,29] as well as a spectrum of congenital anomalies. This increased risk for leukemia also extends to in utero fetuses whose mothers are exposed to radiation. Amazingly, however, the risk has not been shown to be transmissible to a second generation of children conceived after the radiation exposure. These observations suggest a remarkable and poor understanding of recovery from, and protective mechanisms against, potential germ cell mutations.[30,31]

Second Malignant Neoplasms

An increased incidence of second malignant neoplasms (SMN) was reported by Mosijcsuk and Ruymann in survivors of childhood leukemia.[32] A later study by Neglia and coworkers in the Children's Cancer Group (CCG) showed that survivors of childhood leukemia who had received cranial radiation had an increased incidence of central nervous system tumors.[33] These tumors were usually high-grade gliomas. A paper from the Late Effects Study Group showed that the most common SMN developing in previously irradiated sites is a bone sarcoma whereas the most common SMN unassociated with radiation is leukemia.[34] Osteogenic sarcoma has been shown to follow radiation therapy for retinoblastoma or soft tissue sarcoma. Females diagnosed with Hodgkin disease and treated with radiotherapy are reported to have a risk of breast cancer 75 times higher than the general population.[35]

Due to the increased incidence of SMNs, therapeutic programs are being modified. One of the major efforts of the refinement in treatment of childhood lymphocytic leukemia has been to eliminate the need for cranial radiation prophylaxis in low-[36] and intermediate-risk[37,38] patients. Strategies for eliminating cranial radiation in children with high-risk ALL have included the increased use of intrathecal and intravenous chemotherapy. Current therapy for Hodgkin disease has also evolved to include regimens that seek to limit alkylating agents and decrease radiotherapy exposure.[39]

Long-Term Effects

Improvements in survival for individuals diagnosed with pediatric malignancies have coincided with an upsurge of interest in the area of long-term effects. With so many children surviving their primary malignancy, the effects of treatment received on quality of life becomes clinically important. One study utilizing neuropsychological testing demonstrated that from 40% to 100% of long-term survivors of childhood brain tumors had some form of cognitive deficit. These deficits not only encompass intelligence quotient, but also areas of visual/perceptual, learning abilities, and adaptive behaviors.[40]

Another prospective study looked at the treatment factors affecting cognitive outcome. The child's age, mainly as it related to radiotherapy, affected outcome. The use of whole brain radiotherapy also affected outcome, especially in children less than seven years of age. The extensiveness of tumor resection and chemotherapy had no bearing on intellectual outcome.[41] Patients under two years of age treated with surgery and chemotherapy fared better intellectually than patients treated with surgery and radiation.[42]

Kaleita reviewed studies of the Children Cancer Group from 1972 to the present to ascertain major developments with CNS-directed therapy and its effect on neurobehavioral outcomes. His research showed that if cranial radiotherapy is excluded, modern ALL treatment is not associated with major cognitive impairment. The trend, however, in ALL therapy to include more potent oral steroids and direct CNS administration of neurotoxic agents necessitates further neurobehavioral research in this area.[43]

The Childhood Cancer Survivor Study (CCSS) is a recent retrospective study with over 18,000 participants nationwide designed to ascertain the effects of a cancer diagnosis. The cohort consists of patients diagnosed with a malignancy between 1971 and 1986. A multitude of areas of interest are being studied; these areas range from effects on intellectual function to marital relationships to health insurability. The results of these studies will soon be released.

Chemotherapy

Chemotherapy itself has been shown to be a carcinogen, which has led to the expression, "A drug that cures cancer may also cause a cancer." Alkylating agents, in particular, have been implicated in promoting SMNs in patients cured of their initial cancer. Alkylating agents cause injury to deoxyribonucleic acid (DNA), similar to that caused by radiation therapy. Young patients with Hodgkin disease who received an alkylating agent in their treatment program have been reported to have a significantly increased risk of developing an SMN.[44] Alkylating agents may increase the risk of leukemia by fourteen-fold in survivors of childhood cancer.[45] Interestingly, Cyclophosphamide, a drug that is activated by the liver to a nitrogen mustard-like product, has not conclusively been associated with an increased risk for SMNs in survivors of ALL.[33]

Another class of cancer chemotherapy agents associated with secondary malignant neoplasms is that of the topoisomerase inhibitors.[46] Topoisomerases are DNA repair enzymes. The podophyllotoxin VP-16 is a topoisomerase II inhibitor, and high cumulative doses have been associated with the development of acute myelocytic leukemia (AML) and myelodysplastic syndrome (MDS). The cumulative rate of treatment related AML/MDS is 3.2% at 6 years in patients who have received epipodophyllotoxins,[47] which is similar to the 4% risk for leukemia at 10 years in survivors of pediatric Hodgkin disease.[44] The delay-time latency for VP-16 associated SMNs is relatively short, averaging 33 months, when compared with the more extended risk for SMNs in survivors of Hodgkin lymphoma.[46]

The National Cancer Institute (NCI) is conducting an extensive epidemiologic investigation of podophyllotoxin associated SMNs, which will utilize molecular biology techniques to analyze chromosomal defects, particularly of 11q23.[47] Preliminary studies from the Intergroup Rhabdomyosarcoma Study Group (IRSG) suggest that the risk for AML and MDS in patients receiving VP-16 and alkylating agents on the IRSG-III study is about 1% and somewhat lower than other reports.[48]

The prolonged daily use of oral methotrexate, an anti-folic acid agent, has been associated with hepatic fibrosis and the development of hepatocarcinomas.[49] Intermittent oral Methotrexate, however, commonly used in the maintenance phase of therapy for ALL, seems less prone to cause hepatic fibrosis.

Viral Agents

Several viruses have been implicated in childhood cancers. Hepatitis B has been associated with the development of hepatocarcinomas in older children and adolescents.[50,51,52,53] The Epstein-Barr virus (EBV), which causes mononucleosis, has been implicated in lymphoepitheliomas and lymphomas. It seems that some sort of unique susceptibility, timing, or associated genetic vulnerability would be required in these cases, since EBV infections are so ubiquitous. Children and adolescents who survive the infectious complications of HIV have been found, like their adult counterparts, to have an increased risk for lymphoproliferative malignancies.[54,55] Very recent epidemiologic studies suggest that the influx of people into a previously isolated community increased the risk for new cases of acute lymphocytic leukemia in children and non-Hodgkin lymphoma (NHL) in adults.[56,57] These observations strongly suggest a viral trigger for both ALL and NHL that should be studied further.

Ethnic Factors

Ethnic variability in the incidence of childhood cancers has been well described. The most striking example is seen in the lower incidence of ALL in blacks compared with whites.[58] The incidence of non-rhabdomyosarcoma has been found to be lower in both blacks and Chinese.[59,60,61,62] In contrast, nasopharyngeal carcinomas are disproportionately more common in individuals from South China and Northern Africa.[63,64] Survival rates are also reported to be significantly different among children of different ethnicities. Theories for these disparities include socioeconomic status, access to medical treatment, compliance, and genetic differences.[65]

Gender

A male predominance has been observed in many malignancies including acute leukemia, rhabdomyosarcoma, non-Hodgkin lymphoma, neuroblastoma, osteosarcoma, and hepatic malignancies.[58,59,66,67,68,69] Although Hodgkin lymphoma is more common in males under 10 years of age, the incidence in teenagers and young adults is equal in both sexes.[70] Both thyroid cancers and non-gonadal germ cell tumors, however, are more common in girls than in boys.[71,72]

Age

Childhood cancers have a tendency to cluster in certain age groups.[73] This is illustrated in Table 30-3, which shows the incidence of childhood cancer by age groups in 4756 cases from the Columbus, Ohio, Children's Hospital Cancer Registry (CCHCR) from 1945 through 2000. These data are consistent with published series and support the following observations: acute lymphocytic leukemia (ALL) incidence peaks at 3 to 4 years of age; only 9% of non-Hodgkin lymphoma (NHL) occurs in children under 2 years of age; non-RMS sarcoma is relatively uncommon in children between 5 and 10 years of age; only 8% of osteosarcomas occur in children under 7 years of age; and thyroid malignancies are extremely rare in children under 5 years of age. The median age at diagnosis in hepatoblastomas and hepatocellular carcinoma is less than 1 year and 9 years, respectively. As can be seen in Table 30-3, the incidence of childhood cancer is lowest in children 9 to 10 years of age.

SPECIFIC MALIGNANCIES

The Columbus, Ohio, Children's Hospital Cancer Registry (CCHCR) database reflects published national and international statistics and is alluded to throughout this chapter. The CCHCR database spans a 55 year reporting period. The major specific malignancies in the CCHCR series are shown in Figure 30-2. The most common childhood malignancies are discussed in the following section.

Leukemias

Acute leukemias comprise 33% of the CCHCR series and are the most common malignancy. Leukemias can be most easily categorized into acute lymphocytic leukemia (ALL), acute myelocytic leukemia (AML), and other varieties including myelodysplastic syndrome (MDS). MDS represents a unique preleukemic state in which the bone marrow shows progressive deterioration in red cell production, platelet formation, and white cell

Table 30-3
Incidence of Childhood Cancer by Age Group, Children's Hospital, Columbus, Ohio, 1945-2000

Type	< 1	1-2	3-4	5-6	7-8	9-10	11-12	>13	Total	Percent
Osteosarcoma/Bone	0	0	1	9	9	11	18	71	119	2.5
Ewing/Bone	0	1	2	4	10	8	11	36	72	1.5
Bone/Other	1	0	0	1	2	4	1	9	18	0.4
CNS/Supratentorial	24	51	50	28	30	32	44	68	327	6.9
CNS/Infratentorial	21	81	83	102	89	57	45	65	543	11.4
CNS/Spinal cord	2	8	3	8	2	8	4	9	44	.9
Gonadal/Ovary	0	2	0	0	1	8	5	8	24	.5
Gonadal/Testis	2	12	1	0	0	1	0	7	23	.5
Germ-cell/Nongonadal	19	10	3	0	4	8	5	9	58	1.2
Malignant histiocytosis	21	10	3	0	2	0	0	3	39	.8
Wilms tumor	39	73	61	31	18	3	3	4	232	4.9
Kidney/Other	0	0	1	1	1	1	3	4	11	.2
Leukemia/ALL	31	240	298	166	106	66	54	116	1077	22.7
Leukemia/AML	29	43	32	25	13	15	16	58	231	4.9
Leukemia/Other	10	16	13	2	4	4	8	15	72	1.5
Liver	17	19	5	4	3	2	1	9	60	1.3
Lymphoma/Hodgkin	0	2	8	12	12	12	30	95	171	3.6
Lymphoma/NHL	1	19	30	32	30	26	27	62	227	4.8
Neuroblastoma	109	112	54	25	7	4	3	7	321	6.8
Retinoblastoma	44	44	12	2	1	0	0	0	103	2.2
Rhabdomyosarcoma	23	28	24	17	22	11	17	35	177	3.7
Soft-tissue/Other	17	15	13	4	5	8	14	70	146	3.1
Skin	2	2	1	1	3	1	3	7	20	.4
Thyroid	0	0	0	4	7	7	7	10	35	.7
Other malignant tumors	3	6	3	2	1	3	11	32	61	1.3
Benign/Borderline tumors	81	84	56	49	59	44	64	108	545	11.5
Totals	496	878	757	529	441	344	394	917	4756	

Figure 30-2
Summary of 3,967 Cases by Type, CCHCR, 1945–1994

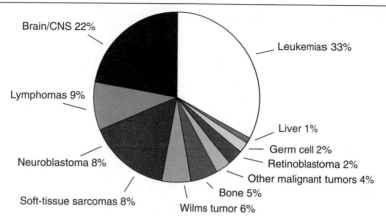

maturation. In time, MDS may progress to AML. Seventy-eight percent of the patients in this series had ALL and 17% had AML. This ratio of 4:1 is the exact opposite of the types of acute leukemia seen in adults.[74] The third most frequent leukemia in children is chronic myelocytic leukemia (CML), which accounts for 5% of the CCHCR patients. Acute leukemias are the predominant leukemia in children and by convention are defined as having over 25% malignant blasts in the bone marrow.[75,76]

Many children with acute lymphocytic leukemia (ALL) lack peripheral blood findings. In 14% of the cases, the hemoglobin (red cells) may be normal; in 29%, the platelet count may be normal; and in 34%, the white count may not be elevated.[77] Despite the relatively high number of patients with a nearly normal complete blood count, the majority (57 percent) of children presenting with ALL will have 85 percent or more of their normal bone marrow replaced with leukemia cells.[77]

The French-American-British (FAB) morphological classification of acute leukemia is the standard.[76] In this classification, leukemias are named according to their predominant malignant cell. In the FAB classification, which is summarized in Table 30-4, acute lymphocytic leukemia is divided into three categories based on the Wright stain characteristics of the predominant lymphoblast. The FAB classification is useful in diagnosis, treatment, data analysis, and presentation. It can also help with the determination of prognosis.

In the FAB classifications, there are eight categories of AML. A battery of surface markers supplement the Wright stain and cytochemical stains in classifying acute leukemias. The surface markers are most efficiently quantified using cell sorter (flow cytometry) technology to analyze a large population of bone marrow cells in a very short time. These supplemental techniques have made investigators aware of hybrid leukemias that have markers from two or more cell lines.[78] Hybrid leukemias are emerging as a major diagnostic challenge and cause of treatment failure.[36,78] Two cytogenetic abnormalities have been associated with an unfavorable diagnosis in ALL: Philadelphia chromosome (t[9;22] [q34;q11]); t(4;11) (q2l;q23) and hypodiploid (forty-four or fewer chromosomes at diagnosis). With the average cure rate surpassing 80% in childhood ALL, detection and development of specialized treatment of lymphocytic leukemias with subsets of myeloid leukemia markers will become even more critical to further improving the rate of cure in ALL.

Prognostic factors and the risk of relapse are considered when establishing a therapy plan for leukemias. For ALL, these include the white blood cell count at diagnosis (with a higher count predictive of a poorer outcome), age at diagnosis, sex, organomegaly (hepatomegaly or splenomegaly), and chromosome abnormalities in the leukemic blasts. Patients older than 12 months and younger than 10 years of age have a better outcome. Girls have a better prognosis because boys can have testicular relapse and a higher frequency of T-cell ALL. Certain cytogenetic abnormalities are associated with poor prognosis, including t(4;11) and a positive Philadelphia chromosome. Certain genetic aberrations may be associated with favorable prognostic features such as chromosome 12p aberrations.[79] The prognostic

Table 30-4

Classification of Childhood Leukemias by French-American-British (FAB) Criteria

FAB Designation	Percent of Total	Prominent Features
ALL		
L_1	84	Small blasts with scanty cytoplasm, homogeneous nuclear chromatin, regular nuclear shape, and inconspicuous nucleoli
L_2	15	Large blasts with increased cytoplasm, irregular nuclear shape, and prominent nucleoli
L_3	1	Large blasts with finely stippled and homogeneous nuclear chromatin, regular nuclear shape, prominent nucleoli, and very deep basophilia of cytoplasm with vacuolation
AML		
M_0	2	Minimal myeloid differentiation
M_1	18	Poorly differentiated myeloblasts with occasional Auer rods
M_2	29	Myeloblastic with differentiation and more prominent Auer rods
M_3	8	Promyelocytic with heavy granulation and bundles of Auer rods
M_4	16	Myeloblastic and monoblastic differentiation in various proportions
M_5	17	Monoblastic
M_6	2	Erythroleukemic with bizarre dyserythropoiesis and megaloblastic features
M_7	8	Megakaryoblastic with bone marrow fibrosis

Reprinted with permission from the *American Cancer Society Textbook of Clinical Oncology,* 2nd ed., G. P. Murphy, W. Lawrence, and R. E. Lenhard (eds.), 1995, p. 502.

factors for AML have been less clearly defined, but M3 (promyelocytic) and M2 (well-differentiated AML) have more favorable prognoses.[80]

Chemotherapy is the standard treatment for acute leukemias. Treatment regimens are generally classified into induction, consolidation, delayed intensification and maintenance phases. Induction therapy is administered to induce or achieve remission or reduction in bone marrow blasts to less than 5 percent. Then a more intensified treatment, consolidation therapy, is administered. Prophylactic therapy of the central nervous system (CNS) is also given to all patients with ALL who have a high risk of CNS relapse. Prophylactic therapy consists of intrathecal chemotherapy with or without cranial irradiation to prevent CNS leukemia. After one or two courses of delayed intensification, maintenance therapy, or continuation treatment is given to all patients for two to three years. During the treatment period and upon conclusion of therapy, bone marrow and cerebrospinal fluid examinations can be performed to assess the status of medullary or extramedullary disease.

Complications of bleeding and infection are more common in children with AML because the platelet and granulocyte precursors are directly affected by leukemias of the myeloid cell lines of the marrow.[81] AML has been shown to follow a different cell kinetic pattern than ALL.[82,83] Once this was learned, doctors changed both the timing and intensity of chemotherapy to attack the AML blasts, thereby reducing the need for maintenance chemotherapy in AML without compromising cure.[83]

A relapse or return of leukemia can occur anywhere in the body. The most common sites of relapse are the bone marrow, CNS, and testes. Relapses usually occur during treatment or within 2 years after completion of therapy but have been reported up to 10 years later. Treatments for relapses will usually include combinations of chemotherapy, radiotherapy, and bone marrow transplantation.

Brain Tumors

Tumors of the central nervous system (CNS) make up 22% of the CCHCR series. These tumors represent a diverse group of diseases requiring different treatment approaches for better survivals. Children with brain tumors are usually operated on by pediatric neurosurgeons. With better diagnostic equipment and surgical technology, tumors are removed more completely, resulting in lower morbidity and mortality rates.

Tumors below the tentorium, which separates the posterior fossa from the cerebral hemispheres, account for 60% of the brain tumors in the series, which is exactly the opposite of the distribution of brain tumors in adults. Two-thirds of infratentorial tumors in children and adolescents are evenly divided between astrocytoma and medulloblastoma, followed by ependymoma (9%), malignant neoplasms not otherwise specified (21%), and miscellaneous tumor types (2%). Malignant neoplasms in the brain stem are often not biopsied due to location and technical difficulties. Forty percent of CNS tumors are either supratentorial (35%) or in the spinal cord (5%). Brain tumors located above the tentorium in the CCHCR series include astrocytoma (60%), malignant neoplasms not otherwise specified (12%), miscellaneous (11%), primitive neuroectodermal tumor (PNET) (9%), and ependymoma (8%).

Tumors of the brain arising from the supporting, or glial, cells are known as gliomas. The term *astrocytoma* has also been given to these tumors to describe their star-like extensions into the surrounding tissue. Astrocytomas, or gliomas, make up the largest group of brain tumors in children.[84,85] Gliomas can be graded from 1 to 4 in the Daumas-Duport et al classification with excellent reproducibility.[86] Grade 4 is the most malignant glioma, which is also known as glioblastoma multiforme,

and contains areas of necrosis with marked nuclear atypicality and anaplasia. The World Health Organization (WHO) system classifies glioblastoma multiforme in a separate category.[87] The higher the grade of a glioma, the poorer the survival rate. An association between age and mutation frequency in malignant glioma has been reported. Children greater than 3 years of age at diagnosis have a higher frequency of P53 mutations, indicating the possible existence of at least two pathways for the molecular origin of gliomas.[88]

Medulloblastomas are tumors of neural crest origin and are one of the several malignancies of childhood described in Table 30-5 as blue cell tumors. Medulloblastomas have the ability to spread throughout the subarachnoid space, causing "drop" metastasis to the spinal cord and cauda equina. An additional and unique characteristic of medulloblastomas is the ability to escape from the central nervous system and metastasize to bone or bone marrow. The expanded designation of PNET in recent years has shifted more brain tumors into this category.[89] Medulloblastomas occurring above the tentorium are usually designated as PNETs. In general, there is better survival with infratentorial medulloblastomas than with supratentorial PNETs.

Ependymomas originate in or near the ependymal cells that line the ventricular system, central spinal canal, and filum terminale. Most ependymomas are intracranial and are found in the posterior fossa. Spinal cord ependymomas are rare. Ependymomas range from well differentiated to anaplastic and usually spread contiguously into adjacent tissue. Systemic metastasis occurs but is rare.

The Chang staging classification is designed for medulloblastomas.[90,91] This classification evaluates the extent of the tumor and metastatic disease. In general, there is no other widely accepted staging

Table 30-5
Common Blue Cell Tumors of Childhood

Common Sites	Unique Sites
Neuroblastoma*	Wilms tumor
Ewing sarcoma/PNET of soft tissue and bone*	Medulloblastoma/PNET*
Rhabdomyosarcoma	Retinoblastoma*
Non-Hodgkin lymphoma	
Acute lymphoblastic leukemia	

*Neural markers

system for brain tumors. Detection of tumor cells in the cerebrospinal fluid by cytospin technology was first used in acute leukemia and has proved of great importance in staging brain tumors in children and adolescents. It allows the extent of disease to be summarized as either local or distant.

Therapy and its duration for brain tumors depends on type of tumor, its differentiation and location, staging, and other prognostic factors. Molecular and cytogenetic characteristics are supplementing the histologic characteristics in determining prognosis. Complete resection of the tumor is almost always attempted, if possible, and is followed by radiation, chemotherapy, or a combination of the two. Survival of patients with brain tumors is higher in children and adolescents than adults.

Lymphomas

Lymphomas are malignancies of lymphoid tissue and are most easily divided into two major categories: Hodgkin lymphoma and non-Hodgkin lymphoma.

Hodgkin disease is generally an indolent, slowly progressing malignancy characterized by the presence of a unique, multi-nucleated malignant cell known as the Reed-Sternberg cell.[92,93,94] Hodgkin disease is subclassified into four histological subtypes based on the presence of fibrosis and the prevalence of lymphocytes. Decreased lymphocytic infiltration is associated with advanced disease and a poorer prognosis. Hodgkin disease can originate in any lymphoid tissue including the spleen, liver, lung, bone marrow, and other extranodal sites, as well as lymph node groups above and below the diaphragm.

The non-Hodgkin lymphomas (NHL) have many histological subclassifications. Because the nomenclature has been revised, cases of NHL accessioned into registries prior to 1990 may require an updated pathology review. Perhaps the two most helpful subclassifications of NHL are lymphoblastic and nonlymphoblastic NHL. The overlap between lymphoblastic NHL and ALL of childhood was designated as lymphoma-leukemia by the (CCG) in the 1980s and 90s. In a series of patients with more than 25% lymphoblasts in the bone marrow and other criteria of lymphoma-leukemia, more intensive therapy has resulted in improved survival.[95] NHL in children with fewer than 25% blasts in the bone marrow is usually treated as a lymphoma, with generally excellent results.[96]

The nonlymphoblastic NHL subset contains several groups of higher-risk lymphomas, such as Ki-1+, large cell anaplastic lymphoma.[97] In a CCG study assessing the treatment of disseminated non-lymphoblastic NHL, the addition of daunomycin to standard COMP (cyclophosphamide, vincristine, methotrexate, and prednisone) therapy did not improve prognosis. Current studies are utilizing short duration intensive chemotherapy.[98] Results of a study published on Ki-1 anaplastic large-cell lymphoma demonstrated effective treatment with short-pulse chemotherapy.[99] NHL often undergoes leukemic transformation. About 15% of recurrent NHL presents as ALL.

Burkitt lymphoma, first described by Dr. Dennis Burkitt in Kenya, Africa, is the major subclassification of nonlymphoblastic NHL in children. Burkitt lymphomas may have cell kinetics similar to AML and respond best to intensive, "blitzkrieg" chemotherapy that takes advantage of the tumor cells' vulnerability during DNA synthesis, the S phase of cell cycle.[100] Burkitt lymphoma cells can divide every 36 to 48 hours, resulting in a fulminant illness with an enormous tumor-cell burden. The two presentations of Burkitt lymphomas have been informally named after the geographic areas where these descriptions were first made. Massive cervical node and jaw involvement has been termed African Burkitt, and the more disseminated presentation with an abdominal mass and malignant peritoneal and pleural effusions has been termed American Burkitt. Titers for Epstein-Barr virus can be positive in either clinical presentation, but are more likely to be elevated in the African variety. These observations have suggested a different epidemiologic mechanism in the two presentations.[101,102]

A third and increasingly common presentation in Burkitt lymphoma has been as an acute abdomen.*[103] Burkitt lymphoma in the small or large bowel can mimic acute appendicitis. It can also present with iron deficiency due to chronic gastrointestinal blood loss. An intra-bowel wall tumor mass may cause the telescoping of the large or small intestine on itself, which is known as an intussusception. This complication is associated with cramping abdominal pain and blood loss. In the CCHCR series, Burkitt lymphoma accounted for 65% of malignancies in the small or large intestine (see Table 30-6). In marked contrast with adults, only 7% of pediatric intestinal malignancies are adenocarcino-

Table 30-6

Malignancies of the Small and Large Intestine in Children

Histology	Number	Percent	Mean Age in Years	Age Range
Burkitt lymphoma	38	65	8	2-16
Other malignant lymphoma	5	9	10	3-16
Carcinoid	11	19	12	1-17
Adenocarcinoma	4	7	13	11-16
TOTAL	58	100		

mas. A recent review of Burkitt Lymphoma over fifty years suggests that the incidence of this form of NHL is increasing.[104]

The present staging system used for Hodgkin disease is commonly known as the Ann Arbor staging classification.[94,105] Beyond the dichotomy of localized and disseminated, there is presently no universally accepted staging system for non-Hodgkin lymphomas. Dr. Sharon Murphy recommended a four-stage system that expanded on the localized and disseminated theme for NHL while at St. Jude Children's Research Hospital in Memphis, Tennessee.[106]

Treatments vary for lymphomas (Hodgkin and non-Hodgkin) and depend on histologic type. A biopsy should be done to confirm the diagnosis. Surgery may often accomplish a complete resection in intestinal NHL. Systemic chemotherapy is effective in improving survival for NHL,[107,108,109] and should be administered in all patients regardless of stage or histologic diagnosis. The duration of chemotherapy for NHL has progressively decreased due to the findings of group clinical trials.[110,111,112] Radiotherapy, chemotherapy, or a combination of the two are effective in the treatment of Hodgkin disease. Treatment for Hodgkin disease is usually determined by extent of disease rather than histologic subtype. Imaging may be substituted for a staging laparotomy in Hodgkin disease.

In a current therapeutic Hodgkin Lymphoms (HL) study, females are being treated differently due to their lower risk of gonadal dysfunction and to offset their increased risk of developing a second malignancy. Because females are almost twice as likely to develop a SMN following HL treatment, chemotherapy is being substituted for radiotherapy in rapid responders.[113] Most chemotherapy regimens for children and adolescents with HL have eliminated nitrogen mustard, which has also been associated with an increased risk of SMN.

Neuroblastoma

Neuroblastoma occurred in 8% of the CCHCR series (Table 30-3) and is tied with soft tissue sarcomas as the fourth most common childhood malignancy. Like medulloblastomas, neuroblastomas are small blue cell tumors arising from neural crest ectoderm. The usual site distribution of neuroblastomas is the adrenal glands and the region of the sympathetic ganglion chains, which run in two parallel posterior lines on either side of the midline. A "dumbbell" tumor may arise in the retroperitoneum or posterior mediastinum and extend through the intervertebral foramen and either up or down the spinal canal. The CCHCR had 321 cases of neuroblastoma, of which 65% were adrenal or abdominal, 22% thoracic, and 3% head and neck. An additional 6% occurred in the pelvis in sites near the organ of Zuckerkandl at the aortic bifurcation. In 4%, the primary site could not be determined.

Using conventional histology in combination with molecular-biological techniques, it has been possible to identify favorable and unfavorable features of neuroblastoma based on histology, patient age,[114,115] N-myc amplification,[116,117] cellular DNA content,[118] and neuropeptide receptors.[119] Neuropeptides are chains of protein building blocks that act on nerve cells. Functional neuropeptide receptors are increased in neuroblastomas with a favorable prognosis. The upgrading of this expression by gene therapy has been suggested by O'Dorisio and coworkers at the Columbus, Ohio, Children's Hospital as a means of improving survival in poor-prognosis tumors.[119] Hyperploidy of cells compared to diploidy has been associated with a better response to chemotherapy.[118,120] Neuroblastomas with

N-myc amplification behave aggressively and have a higher likelihood of early treatment failure.[120]

Neuroblastomas usually produce epinephrine and norepinephrine, which increase the urinary excretion of catecholamines such as vanillylmandelic acid (VMA) and homovanillic acid (HVA). These compounds can be detected in the urine by high-pressure liquid chromatography.[121,122] Recently, mass urine screening of very young children in Japan and Canada almost doubled the number of patients diagnosed with neuroblastoma in those countries.[123,124]

It remains to be seen whether patients diagnosed with advanced stage disease or a poorer prognosis at an earlier stage will experience an improved survival as a result of mass screening.[123,124] Apparently, many of the neuroblastomas detected by urine screening would have matured asymptomatically to a mixed ganglioneuroblastoma and eventually to a completely benign ganglioneuroma. Traditionally, most neuroblastomas with amplified N-myc oncogene and low expression of neuropeptide receptors have had a mortality rate exceeding 90% regardless of *age*. In a 45 year review of the CCHCR experience, Rauck (Termuhlen) and colleagues found statistically no improvement in the survival of patients with advanced-stage neuroblastoma from 1972 to the present.[125]

The (CCG) and the Pediatric Oncology Group (POG) had different staging systems for neuroblastoma; Dr. Audrey Evans of the Children's Hospital of Philadelphia developed the Evans Staging System for Neuroblastoma, which was adopted by CCG for staging.[126] Dr. Ann Hayes of St. Jude Children's Research Hospital in Memphis, Tennessee, was primarily responsible for the classification system adopted by POG.[127] The Children's Oncology Group, has recently chosen to utilize a common international staging system.[128]

The treatment modalities used in the management of neuroblastoma are surgery, chemotherapy, and radiotherapy. Treatment regimens depend upon extent of disease and other prognostic factors. Extent of surgery appears to be a significant predictor of patient outcome.[129] Radiotherapy is beneficial to patients with lymph node involvement. A recently conducted, multi-institutional study in CCG revealed that autologous bone marrow transplant in combination with chemotherapy and retinoic acid improved event-free survival among children with high risk neuroblastoma versus chemotherapy alone.[130]

Soft Tissue Sarcomas

Soft tissue sarcomas are tumors of mesenchymal origin arising in virtually any site or organ. These tumors are separated into two main groups: rhabdomyosarcomas (RMS) and non-rhabdomyosarcoma (non-RMS). RMS is the most common childhood soft tissue sarcoma, followed by undifferentiated soft tissue sarcoma (UND-STS).[131,132,133] The four classical forms of childhood RMS are embryonal, botryoid, alveolar, and pleomorphic. The pleomorphic type of RMS has recently been shown to be an anaplastic variant of embryonal RMS.[134,135] Soft tissue sarcomas have a better outcome in children between the ages of one and ten than in infants, adolescents, and young adults.

Rhabdomyosarcoma and Undifferentiated Sarcomas

The RMS and UND-STS are best treated according to protocols developed by the Intergroup Rhabdomyosarcoma Study Group (IRSG). The Soft Tissue Sarcoma Committee of the Children's Oncology Group (COG) is currently completing the fifth generation study (IRSG-V). RMS have skeletal muscle origin and constitute 55% of soft tissue sarcomas in children and adolescents.[12,136] The UND-STS have no characteristic immunohistochemical staining or molecular markers. Alveolar RMS and UND-STS constitute, respectively, 20% and 7% of patients on IRSG-I, -II, and -III studies. Both alveolar RMS and UND-STS histology have unfavorable prognoses.[137,138] Alveolar RMS is associated with a translocation of chromosomes 2 and 13.[139] A subset of alveolar RMS have a translocation between chromosome 1 and 13. The primary tumor site, histologic classification, and stage are key prognostic factors in RMS. Tumors arising in the orbit and genitourinary regions, excluding the bladder and prostate, have better outcomes whereas primary sites in the intrathoracic and retroperitoneal areas have poorer prognoses.

Assessment of the extent of disease for these tumors is important for prognosis and treatment. The IRSG has also developed a clinical grouping and TNM staging system. Extensive studies are required at diagnosis in all soft tissue sarcomas to identify the extent of disease, so that accurate staging can be determined. A pretreatment TNM staging system is being used to plan therapy. Site, tumor size, nodal involvement, and presence of metastases are assessed. The postsurgical clinical grouping developed by the IRSG has proven extremely effective in identifying low, intermediate, and high-risk patients. This clinical grouping is based on the extent of resection in addition to the presence or absence of metastatic disease and is used to plan radiotherapy.[140] Immunologic and molecular studies are also being conducted as part of IRSG-V with primary objectives being to aid in the diagnosis and provide additional prognostic information.[141]

Function-preserving surgery is recommended for patients with rhabdomyosarcoma. Radiotherapy is presently recommended for all sites with microscopic residual disease and for completely resected tumors over 5 centimeters in size in unfavorable sites. Ruymann and Grovas have recently reviewed the treatment of soft tissue sarcomas.[142]

Ewing Sarcoma Group of Tumors

Ewing sarcoma was originally described in bone. These tumors, however, can also arise in soft tissue. Whether in bone or soft tissue these tumors, which have a common translocation, are now known as the Ewing sarcoma group of tumors and share a common translocation t(11;22). Immunohistochemical stains show these tumors to be primitive neural ectodermal tumors or PNETs. It is sometimes difficult for clinicians to determine whether the primary site of Ewing sarcoma is bone or soft tissue. Magnetic resonance imaging can be very helpful in determining the site of origin. PNETs also occur in the central nervous system; PNETs originating in the CNS should not be analyzed with PNETs of bone and soft tissue.

PNETs of soft tissue, also known as extraosseous Ewing sarcomas, have shown a treatment response comparable to embryonal RMS using surgery, chemotherapy, and radiotherapy in IRSG-I, -II, and -III.[140,143,144] As of 1995, these soft tissue sarcomas are being treated with multiagent chemotherapy under the direction of the Ewing committee of the COG.

Other Soft Tissue Sarcomas

Except for EOEs, PNETS, and UND-STS, most non-RMS have not been well studied in a cooperative group setting. Non-RMS soft tissue sarcomas are not common; some of these sarcomas, such as malignant fibrous histiocytomas have been associated with prior irradiation for a previous primary tumor.[145] Non-RMS soft tissue tumor types, other than the ones previously described, also include fibrosarcomas, neurofibrosarcomas, malignant fibrous histiocytomas, synovial sarcomas, hemangiopericytomas, alveolar soft part sarcomas, leiomyosarcomas, and liposarcomas. Other soft tissue sarcoma types are even more rare than the ones listed.

There is no widely accepted staging classification to assess the extent of disease for non-RMS soft tissue sarcomas. Some clinicians and institutions use the pretreatment (TNM) staging and clinical grouping classifications developed by the IRSG. Attempts at complete surgical resection of a primary RMS will usually improve the prognosis.[146,147,148,149,150] The roles of multiagent chemotherapy and radiotherapy in non-RMS are being studied by the COG.

Wilms Tumor and Other Kidney Tumors

Wilms tumor, or nephroblastoma, is the most common malignant tumor of the kidney in children. It is an embryonal malignancy that almost always arises in the kidney, although extrarenal Wilms tumors can very rarely occur in the retroperitoneum, pelvis, or inguinal canal. Some researchers have proposed that extrarenal Wilms tumors arise from extrarenal displacement of metanephric or mesonephric remnants.[151] Wilms tumor can be classified into favorable and several unfavorable histological variants. Unfavorable histology is demonstrated by the presence of anaplastic tumor cells and is associated with a high rate of relapse and death.[152] Multidisciplinary therapies developed by the National Wilms Tumor Study Group (NWTSG) over the past twenty-five years have been highly successful in converting a 20 to 25% survival in 1959[153] to 90% survival in 1989.[154]

Wilms tumor behaves much like a sarcoma. In its more immature forms, it is a typical small blue cell tumor. Tumor cell identification has not usually been a diagnostic problem in the kidney. Clear cell sarcomas and rhabdoid tumors of the kidney can usually be identified by their unique histology.[155,156] These two tumor types are now being treated with more intense sarcoma-like therapy lasting 24 weeks on the NWTSG-5 study. Congenital mesoblastic nephroma occurs in very young children. It is a low-grade malignant tumor of the kidney that is also known as

Bolande's tumor.[157] It is usually treated by simple nephrectomy.

About 5 to 10% of Wilms tumors are bilateral. For this reason, preoperative imaging of both kidneys must be performed. At surgery, the opposite kidney is palpated, examined, and sometimes biopsied. Beckwith has described a unique histological pattern that suggests a potential bilateral tumor.[158] Even if a second tumor is not present at the time of initial diagnosis, it will usually occur within two years of the initial tumor.[159,160] Patients with Wilms tumor have an increased incidence of renal anomalies including horseshoe kidney, in which both kidneys are united at their lower poles.[161]

A refined version of the NWTSG staging system is used for Wilms tumor and is based on clinical imaging and surgical resection. Bilateral Wilms tumors are designated as Stage V. Treatment for Wilms tumor is based on the extent of disease and tumor histology (favorable or unfavorable).

Wilms tumor was the first malignant solid tumor in children to be treated with chemotherapy.[162] The survival rate has risen from 20% to 90% two years after diagnosis.[163] This is due to the therapeutic approach modified over the course of three decades based on the results of four NTWGS studies. This therapeutic approach includes prompt surgical resection, followed by chemotherapy or radiotherapy, depending on the stage and histology. The primary strategy in approaching a patient with a bilateral Wilms tumor is to utilize multiagent chemotherapy, limited surgery, and minimal radiotherapy to conserve renal function. A major objective of the NWTSG has been to develop treatment regimens that cause less acute and long-term morbidity.[164]

A torrent of molecular-biological studies was unleashed by the observation that homologous deletions on 11p were common to three embryonal tumors of childhood: Wilms tumor, embryonal rhabdomyosarcoma, and hepatoblastoma.[165] These findings seem related to observations in Beckwith-Wiedemann Syndrome (BWS) that show an increased risk for a variety of malignancies including bilateral Wilms tumor, hepatoblastoma, and adrenal cell carcinomas.[166,167] Neuroblastoma has also been associated with BWS.[168] This genetic disorder is associated with a homologous deletion on the short arm of chromosome 11 more precisely, at 11p13. Ongoing molecular biological investigations using tumor and constitutional DNA are in progress.[169] In the near future, routine molecular studies should be available to complement the pathological diagnosis of existing or potential bilateral Wilms tumor and assist in detecting patients with atypical, mild BWS.[170,171,172] The consequences for children of patients with bilateral Wilms tumor and BWS are presently unknown.

In a pilot study, Grundy and colleagues, using pathologic material from NWTSG-3 and -4, have shown an unfavorable prognosis for loss of heterozygosity of 16q and 1p markers.[173] In contrast, loss of heterozygosity for 11p markers and duplication of 1q were not associated with an unfavorable outcome. These molecular differences, in addition to the prognostic importance of tumor cell DNA content, are under prospective evaluation in NWTSG-5 and may provide a basis for stratified therapy in the future.

Bone Sarcomas

Sarcomas of the bone can be classified into three major categories: osteosarcomas, Ewing sarcoma, and other. The CCHCR series had 57%, 34%, and 9% of these three types of sarcoma, respectively. The median age for osteosarcoma is 14 years and 12 years for Ewing sarcoma of bone. About 40% of patients with osteosarcoma have tumors in the proximity of the knee, compared with 27% in Ewing sarcoma of bone.[174,175] Ewing sarcoma of bone tends to appear in a greater variety of sites than osteosarcoma. For both osteosarcoma and Ewing sarcoma, the average prognosis for a distal tumor is better than for a proximal, more central tumor. Primary Ewing sarcomas occurred in flat bone in the CCHCR series three times as often as did osteosarcomas. Delay in the correct diagnosis of more than three months results in a poorer prognosis for survival.[176] Traumatic injuries and concern about osteomyelitis are two of the more common reasons for delay in diagnosis.

Both Ewing sarcoma and osteosarcoma have major risks for microscopic pulmonary metastases, which are probably present at diagnosis in over 80 percent of the cases. Hematogenous metastases to other bones may also occur at diagnosis but are more common in recurrent disease. Bone marrow metastases are very rare in osteosarcoma but relatively common in Ewing sarcoma of bone.

There is no uniform staging classification for bone tumors. The extent of disease for these tumors can be evaluated by tumor site, confinement within the cortex, and whether metastatic disease is present.

Osteosarcomas are not particularly radiosensitive, which leaves the modalities of surgery and multiagent chemotherapy as the primary treatments. In Ewing sarcoma of bone, all three modalities are effective. The dose intensity of doxorubicin has been shown to be an important determinant of favorable outcome for both osteosarcoma and Ewing sarcoma.[177] Limb salvage surgery in osteosarcoma has been used over the past twenty years to maintain a functional extremity.[178,179,180,181,182] More recently, this technique is also being applied to Ewing sarcoma of bone.[183] A child with an immature skeleton poses several challenges in limb-salvage surgery that may be solved with techniques of rotation plasty and expandable endoprostheses.[184]

Liver Tumors

The two most common primary malignancies of the liver in the CCHCR series were hepatoblastoma (57%) and hepatocarcinoma (32%). The former

occurred at a median age of less than 1 year in the CCHCR series; hepatocarcinoma had a median age of 9 years. Alphafetoprotein (AFP) is a protein made by fetal hepatocytes that serves as a biological marker for hepatoblastoma. AFP is an excellent guide to the presence of active disease. The rate of response to chemotherapy and surgery can be assessed by a decline in the level of AFP.[185] A syndrome of hemihypertrophy and virilization has been reported in about 3 percent of patients with hepatoblastoma, who secrete increased amounts of human chorionic gonadotropin (B-HCG).[186,187] Gonadotropins can cause precocious virilization in males and breast development in females (Figure 30-3).

Alphafetoprotein is a useful tumor marker in both hepatocellular carcinomas and hepatoblastoma.[188,189,190] Hepatocellular carcinomas are associated with a variety of environmental agents including hepatitis B,[51] treatment with androgens,[191] aflatoxins,[191,192] and hepatotoxic drugs such as methotrexate.[49] The incidence of hepatocarcinoma should decrease with the widespread use of

Figure 30-3
Precocious Virilization in a Male Infant

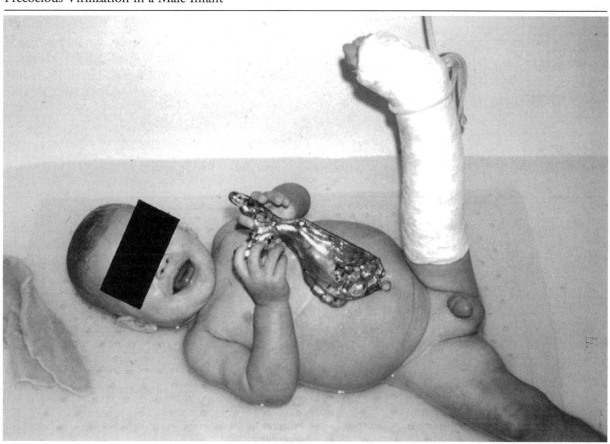

hepatitis B vaccine and avoidance of provocative exposures.

In the CCHCR series, both hepatoblastoma and hepatocarcinoma had metastatic disease at diagnosis in a quarter of the cases. Ninety percent of the metastases were pulmonary. Appropriate studies should include a bone scan with CT scan of the chest and abdomen to evaluate resectability.

There is no universally accepted staging system for liver tumors. The most often used staging of liver tumors is based on extent of tumor resection.[193]

Surgical resection of malignant hepatic tumors in children and adolescents is the primary determinant of long-term survival.[194,195] If surgical resection is not possible and the tumor is confined to the liver, the patient should be evaluated for a liver transplant.[196] Embryonal sarcomas of the liver are not presently eligible for the IRSG-IV study. These tumors are very rare, amounting to only six cases in the CCHCR series. Surgery and sarcoma-like chemotherapy are recommended treatments. Surgical resectability of the malignancy is the primary objective. Multiagent chemotherapy may facilitate delayed resection in liver tumors and improve the survival of patients found initially to be unresectable.[197,198,199]

Germ Cell Tumors

Germ cell tumors may be either gonadal (45%) or extragonadal (55%) in children, as experienced in the CCHCR study. The most common sites of extragonadal germ cell tumors in the CCHCR series are the pelvis and brain. The distribution of extragonadal germ cell tumors in children and adolescents is shown in Figure 30-4, with a female/male ratio of 1.7:1. The gonadal germ cell tumors, in contrast, have a female/male ratio of 1:1. An elevated alpha-fetoprotein (AFP) is usually present in germ cell tumors and is a valuable index of tumor response and continued remission. However, some of the malignant non yolk sac components of complex germ cell tumors do not produce AFP.

A major epidemiologic association in germ cell tumors has been abnormalities in the X-chromosome.[200] Both males and females with X-chromosome defects are thought to be at a significantly increased risk for a germ cell malignancy.[200]

The most widely accepted staging system for germ cell tumors is the one used by COG. There are separate systems for nongonadal tumors, ovary tumors, and testis tumors. The extent of disease is the best prognostic factor for these tumors.

Members of COG are collaborating in an Intergroup Germ Cell Study. The major chemotherapy treatment programs being used are derivatives of the Einhorn regimen and utilize Cisplatinum, VP-16, and Bleomycin.[201] The replacement of Vinblastine, another common agent traditionally employed, with VP-16 has led to diminished neuromuscular toxicity and better efficacy.[202] Metastatic germ cell tumors in children had a relatively high five-year survival rate of 47% in the CCHCR series.

Figure 30-4
Distribution by Type of Nongonadal Germ Cell Tumors, Columbus, Ohio, Children's Hospital Cancer Registry, 1945–1994

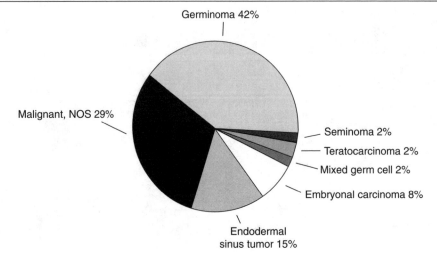

Although seminomas primarily originate from the testes, in our series 2% of nongonadal germ cell tumors were seminomas but were found in the retroperitoneum.

Retinoblastoma

Retinoblastoma, a primitive neuroectodermal tumor, is the most common primary ocular malignancy in children and arises in retinal cells. As seen in Table 30-3, it is primarily diagnosed in children under 3 years of age. The most common sign presenting is leukocoria, a white spot on the eye, which prompts parents to take the child to the physician. Leukocoria, illustrated in Figure 30-1, has been termed "cat's eye reflex." In 20-30% of newly diagnosed cases, retinoblastoma presents with bilateral disease. Trilateral disease can occur when the pineal gland of the brain is involved along with bilateral retinal disease.[203]

Retinoblastoma can be either hereditary (40%) or nonhereditary (60%).[204] If there is familial history, retinoblastoma is usually diagnosed earlier, the risk for bilateral disease and other malignancies is higher, and the chromosomal abnormality is probably a germinal mutation. The sporadic, nonhereditary type arises when two somatic mutations are present in the retinal cell. If family history is positive, genetic counseling should be recommended to the family. The major risk for second malignant neoplasm (SMN) may be related to genetic factors rather than to radiation per se. The most common SMN for retinoblastoma patients with the hereditary type is osteosarcoma, which can occur outside the field of radiation.[205] Second malignant neoplasms found within the radiation field are usually sarcomatous. Also, the prognosis depends on tumor size, location, and stage of disease. A clinical staging classification by Reese Ellsworth,[206] based on extent of intraocular disease, is widely accepted. This classification evaluates the potential for ocular preservation, rather than survival, and does not classify metastatic disease.

In addition to seeing an ophthalmologist, retinoblastoma patients should be referred to a radiation oncologist and medical oncologist for consultation. Treatment considerations should include the unilaterality or bilaterality of disease, level of visual acuity, and extent of intraocular and extraocular disease. Eyes with extensive retinal destruction or neurovascular glaucoma are enucleated, with an attempt to resect as much of the optic nerve as possible. Treatment modalities include irradiation, photocoagulation, and cryotherapy, in order to preserve sight. In the past, chemotherapy has been used only in advanced disease; however, clinical trials are in progress to evaluate its efficacy for early stage disease. Extreme care is taken by radiotherapists to minimize injury to less severely affected or normal eyes.

Langerhans Cell Histiocytosis

Langerhans cell histiocytosis (LCH), a borderline malignancy,[207] has been monitored by the CCHCR for the past fifty years.*[208] This tumor constitutes a proliferation of histiocytes, eosinophils, and lymphocytes. The histiocytes have been identified as being of the Langerhans cell type with Birbeck granules. Eosinophilic granuloma, Hand-Schuller-Christian syndrome, and Letterer-Siwe Syndrome are clinical variations of LCH. LCH is the preferred designation over the older terminology of histiocytosis X. The letter "X" was used to designate the so-called X-bodies occurring in the Birbeck granules on electron microscopy. The site of origin is the reticuloendothelial system, but solitary or multiple lesions occur in bone, skin, soft tissue, lymph nodes, spleen, liver, and bone marrow.

A borderline behavior classification has been given to Langerhans cell histiocytosis by the World Health Organization.[209] LCH has been designated Class I by the LCH International Society Classification.[207] The classification system relates this disease to the normal histocytic cell subsets. Recent studies suggest that LCH is a clonal neoplastic disorder with highly variable biologic behavior.[210] Fatality occurred in 6 percent of CCHCR cases; a majority of the fatalities were in children under 2 years of age with bone marrow involvement who would be classified as having Letterer-Siwe syndrome. Right heart failure as a consequence of pulmonary fibrosis and hypoxemia is usually progressive and fatal in a small number of patients. Patients with only bone involvement have negligible mortality. Morbidity, however, is quite common and includes scoliosis with vertebral body involvement, growth hormone deficiency following hypothalamic or anterior pituitary extension, and diabetes insipidus with posterior pituitary disease.

Liver involvement is common in systemic LCH of the Letterer-Siwe type. Hepatomegaly may not be noted on physical examination. Treatment consists mainly of surgery, low-dose radiotherapy, and chemotherapy. Corticosteroids, vinblastine, methotrexate, VP-16, and cyclophosphamide have been associated with improving disease. Modest success with bone marrow transplants has been reported. The spontaneous regression of this tumor without any therapy makes interpretation of any treatment difficult unless a control group is used.

PEDIATRIC CLINICAL TRIAL GROUPS

Cooperative, interinstitutional, antileukemic programs began in 1955 when two national groups were formed. Acute Leukemia Group A dealt exclusively with children; Acute Leukemia Group B treated patients in all age groups. Through their cooperative investigations, chemotherapy was found to be effective in treating leukemia in children. Similar multiagent treatment regimens were developed for adults with leukemia. During the 1960s, chemotherapy was extended to the common solid tumors of children. Treatment was initially given to children whose cancers had recurred or progressed following surgery and radiation therapy. Some pediatric malignancies responded to the chemotherapy, so clinical studies were initiated using chemotherapy in conjunction with surgery and radiation in multidisciplinary trials.[211]

Acute Leukemia Group A changed its name to the Children's Cancer Study Group and later became known as the Children's Cancer Group (CCG). Acute Leukemia Group B became the Cancer and Leukemia Group B (CALGB). Another group, the Southwest Cancer Study Group, began in 1956 and created pediatric and adult divisions in 1971. In 1973, this group changed its name to the Southwest Oncology Group (SWOG) to reflect the multidisciplinary activities of the group. In 1980, the pediatric division of SWOG elected to separate and combine with the former pediatric section of CALGB to establish the Pediatric Oncology Group (POG).[212] The National Wilms Tumor Study Group was established in 1970 as the first intergroup study for a specific malignancy. In 1972, CCG and the two pediatric divisions of SWOG and CALGB combined their efforts in studying rhabdomyosarcomas and formed the Intergroup Rhabdomyosarcoma Study Group.

In 2001, the major North American pediatric clinical trials groups, including the Children's Cancer Group (CCG), the Pediatric Oncology Group (POG), the National Wilms Tumor Study Group (NWTSG), and the Intergroup Rhabdomyosarcoma Study Group (IRSG) joined forces to focus their unified efforts in seeking a cure for cancer. The cooperative group—Children's Oncology Group (COG)—was formed. COG includes over 250 institutions in the United States, Canada, Australia, and New Zealand.

Clinical Oncology Trials

The development of multidisciplinary treatment programs in pediatric cancers involves careful quantification of toxicity, response, and disease status. If a tumor is to be measured at specific intervals, the method of measurement must be prescribed beforehand in a written protocol. Similarly, the successive development of a single agent in a Phase I trial and its later inclusion in a multiagent, randomized Phase III trial requires great care and carefully written documentation (see Table 30-7). These issues and many others such as quality of life and long-term follow-up are reviewed by Drs. Brigid Leventhal and Robert Wittes in their excellent monograph, *Research Methods in Clinical Oncology.*[213]

The importance of sound statistical support in making decisions on toxicity and efficacy requires

Table 30-7
Phases of Development of a New Treatment

- Phase I Agents selected for evaluation on the basis of broad activity in preclinical screens are tested on humans so that the toxicity and the maximum tolerated dose in humans can be established.

- Phase II Drugs are tested in the appropriate number of patients with measurable disease and with specific diagnoses to determine whether or not a drug has effect against a particular tumor type. Generally, the tests are performed at doses that are about 80% of the maximum tolerated dose.

- Phase III The therapy is tested in a way that provides a quantitative estimate of the contribution it might make to the treatment of a particular disease.

Modified from Leventhal and Wittes, *Research Methods in Clinical Oncology,* p. 2.[213]

that the cooperative group statisticians be involved during the initial planning of any study. This ensures selection of the appropriate design and analysis with which to answer the study questions. Constructive criticism from all members of the multidisciplinary team is essential. An assessment of feasibility is based on the type of analysis being performed and represents the basic foundation of any clinical trial.

The 250 institutions that make up the Children's Oncology Group require registration of all children and adolescents with malignancy, regardless of whether the patients were officially on a group-sponsored study. Because the group treats greater than 90% of children and adolescents with malignancy in the United States and Canada, this database serves as an excellent source for planning new studies and developing hypotheses for epidemiologic investigations. Required registration increased the collaboration of cooperative group clinical research associates with pediatric cancer registrars locally and at the national level. This collaboration is helpful in case-finding, staging, treatment, and follow-up.

In cooperation with the National Cancer Institute, the pediatric study groups were pioneers in the era of multidisciplinary team management and clinical investigation of multimodal therapies. The successful treatment of cancer in children is a product of over 45 years of clinical trials by the cooperative groups.

STAGING OF PEDIATRIC CANCERS

Pediatric cancers are best staged according to the national clinical trial groups with which individual institutions participate.[214,215] Most pediatric hospitals treating large numbers of children with malignancies are members or affiliates of the Children's Oncology Group. Pediatric cancers are exempt from the staging requirement set by the Commission on Cancer (CoC) of the American College of Surgeons, which says that cancers must be staged using the current edition of the American Joint Committee on Cancer (AJCC) *Manual for Staging of Cancer* in approved cancer programs.

The latest edition of AJCC *Manual for Staging* is appropriate to use for certain childhood cancers.[216] These include non-Hodgkin lymphoma, nasopharyngeal carcinomas, skin cancers, and thyroid cancers.

The Children's Oncology Group and its antecedent cooperative groups have developed inter-

nationally accepted staging classifications for rhabdomyosarcomas, bone tumors, germ cell tumors, hepatoblastoma, and Wilms tumor. The FAB classification is commonly used for the acute lymphoblastic and myelocytic leukemias. Refer to the specific malignancies discussed in this chapter for tumor specific staging.

ANALYSIS OF CHILDHOOD CANCERS

Adult cancers are analyzed by site, which is appropriate because they are often of epithelial cell origin. In contrast, pediatric cancers are usually nonepithelial in origin and vary considerably in histologic type at any given site.[217] If pediatric cancers were analyzed by site, as are adult cancers, many types of malignancies would be lumped together for statistical analysis. This would be misleading because most types of pediatric malignancies have multiple sites and different tumors at the same site with variable prognoses.

Neuroblastomas, for example, originate in the adrenal glands in the retroperitoneum, sympathetic ganglia in the posterior mediastinum, the aortic body in the neck, and other paraganglia such as the organ of Zuckerkandl located in the retroperitoneal space at the bifurcation of the aorta. The incidence of neuroblastoma should be reported as one tumor type, regardless of site; however, investigators must be able to analyze neuroblastoma by both site and histology. This example also applies to other pediatric tumors.

Traditionally, pediatric malignancies have been primarily analyzed by type rather than site. Grouping the relatively small number of pediatric cases by diagnosis facilitates analysis. Subset analyses using unique histological subgroups and age subgroup have also proved especially useful in Wilms tumor, rhabdomyosarcoma, neuroblastoma, and virtually all solid tumors. When the molecular-biological signature of a particular subset becomes characterized, more or less intensive treatment can be tailored to a relatively small number of cases.

To meet data standards set by the Commission on Cancer of the American College of Surgeons, hospital cancer registries must use the latest edition of the *International Classification of Diseases for Oncology (ICD-O)* for coding the topography and morphology of each registered tumor.[209,218] Occasionally, an investigator will request a report by a particular site or even a histological subtype. Most reports and comparisons of data in the Surveillance, Epidemiology and End Results (SEER) Program database and other interinstitutional studies are based on traditional pediatric histological subgroups.

Many central registries and international publications use the Manchester (UK) Children's Tumour Registry classification scheme for classification of cancer in children.[219] This classification system is divided into twelve main diagnostic groups containing several subclassifications. Each diagnostic group contains a list of the ICD-O morphology codes that should be included for reporting purposes. The Manchester classification scheme is workable for central, state, and national registries that employ computer programmers. It is not, however, especially practical or functional for the average hospital cancer registrar with no background in computer programming.

Problems can arise for hospital cancer registrars in analyzing childhood cancers because traditional pediatric groupings have a great variety of morphologies that fit into different ICD-O classifications. The Columbus, Ohio, Children's Hospital (CCH) has developed a pediatric tumor-grouping system for hospital registrars that can be used in addition to the ICD-O topography and morphology at the time of abstracting.[220,221] With the CCH Pediatric Grouping System, the hospital registrar can easily, without programming, produce a variety of reports by selecting a pediatric grouping. Investigators can then compare data with greater flexibility, identify groups of particular interest more precisely, and still maintain the ability to distinguish certain rare conditions. Table 30-3 shows the CCH Pediatric Grouping System using the CCHCR data by age groups. The CCH Pediatric Grouping System has been shared with other institutions and is currently in use at several large pediatric hospitals and has been incorporated into certain **cancer registry software programs.**

The hospital tumor registrar must have the capability of producing reports in various age groups that differ from those used by adult hospital cancer registries. An important factor for pediatric investigators in using their hospital cancer registry data is to determine the age groups of the study. This facilitates comparisons with central, state, national, or international databases. Many large pediatric databases, such as SEER, include only cases from 0 through 14 years of age. Most Children's Oncology Group treatment programs cover the pediatric-

young adult group from 0 to 21 years of age. The current Ewing studies study includes individuals up to 30 years of age.

When designing the data set for a hospital pediatric cancer registry, the cancer committee must consider including data items such as cytogenetics, prognostic classifications, FAB classification, associated congenital anomalies, molecular analyses, and other areas of special interest. Investigators are increasingly using molecular and cytogenetic endpoints in defining risk group. Pediatric hospital cancer registries need software systems that can easily add supplemental data constructs without excessive manipulations.

MOLECULAR ANALYSIS AND FUTURE TREATMENT STRATEGIES

Molecular analysis is a promising area of research that may guide the therapeutic management of pediatric tumors. Brain tumors have conventionally been stratified utilizing histologic and clinical factors. However, with the advent of molecular analysis, distinct subgroups of brain tumors with very different prognoses have been identified among histologically comparable lesions.[222] In NHL, tumor stage and tumor burden have traditionally been used as prognostic factors to select the length and intensity of treatment. The presence or absence of adhesion molecules or aberrant proteins, such as soluble CD30 and anaplastic lymphoma kinase are being studied as potential prognostic factors.

Current research is attempting to measure initial response to therapy utilizing flow cytometry, positron emission tomography, and molecular studies.[223] Soft tissue sarcomas are classified by histologic appearance and chromosomal abnormalities, many sarcomas exhibit chromosomal translocations that create fusion genes. These identifiable fusion genes are a promising resource which may aid in diagnosis, prognosis, and treatment.[224] In ALL, the TEL/AML1 fusion gene is the most common chromosomal abnormality and is associated with a good prognosis.[225] Ongoing and future clinical cooperative trials will explore this expanding area of research and attempt to determine the role of molecular analysis on risk assignment and therapeutic management. It is hoped that these molecular fingerprints will provide targeted therapies which will exploit areas of molecular vulnerability and prove less toxic than present treatments.

CONCLUSION

The survival of children and adolescents with cancer has been dramatically improved by the pediatric cooperative group clinical trials in cooperation with the National Cancer Institute using multiagent chemotherapy and multidisciplinary care. The average survival for all malignancies in children and adolescents ranges from about 50% in AML to over 90% in Wilms tumor (see Table 30-8). Accurate assessment of tumor histology has been at the heart

Table 30-8
Trends in Survival for Children under Age 15 Comparing Surveillance, Epidemiology, and End Results Program (SEER) of the National Cancer Institute and Columbus, Ohio, Children's Hospital Cancer Registry Data, 1960–1990.

	Five Year Relative Survival Rates (Percent)					
	Year of Diagnosis					
Type	1960–1963[†]	1970–1973[†]	1974–1976	1977–1979	1980–1982	1983–1990
All types*						
SEER[1]	28	45	55	61	65	68
CCH	26	48	51	63	63	74
Acute lymphocytic leukemia						
SEER[1]	4	34	52	67	70	73
CCH	1	40	59	75	73	93
Acute myeloid leukemia						
SEER[1]	3	5	14	26	22	28
CCH	0	0	12	10	36	47
Wilms' tumor						
SEER[1]	33	70	74	77	86	88
CCH	50	81	82	85	100	90
Brain and other nervous system						
SEER[1]	35	45	54	56	55	60
CCH	49	58	43	49	56	65
Neuroblastoma						
SEER[1]	25	40	52	53	52	57
CCH	33	54	42	50	45	59
Bone and joint						
SEER[1]	20	30	54	52	55	59
CCH	67	23	57	33	36	55
Hodgkin's disease						
SEER[1]	52	90	79	83	91	90
CCH	67	57	89	100	100	92
Non-Hodgkin lymphomas						
SEER[1]	18	26	45	50	62	70
CCH	42	17	56	42	75	73

[1]Source: Wingo PA, Tong T; Bolden S., Cancer Statistics 1995. CA-A Cancer Journal For Clinicians: Volume 45(1), January/February, 1995.

*Excludes basal and squamous cell skin cancer and in situ carcinomas except bladder.

[†]Rates are for whites only.

of this progress. With evolving technology, pathological assessment has progressed from the interpretation of histological patterns with conventional stains to immunohistochemical staining and advanced molecular techniques. The molecular biological signature of a solid or circulating tumor will be increasingly critical in defining prognosis and treatment, as well as providing targets for translational strategies.

Cancer registrars should have simple (but expandable) tumor classification systems that permit multivariant analyses using age, sex, site, and ethnicity, in addition to histology. Prognostic factors will also be increasingly based on chromosomal, ploidy, and molecular biological studies. The register must have the capability of incorporating these variables, in addition to those for family history of malignancy, associated congenital anomalies, familial syndromes (for example, neurofibromatosis), and pertinent follow-up events to further enhance the available data on survivors of childhood cancer. Retrospective analyses of these variables will be increasingly important in evaluating treatments that minimize risk and maximize the rate of cure for children and adolescents with cancer.

STUDY QUESTIONS

1. Identify and describe two factors thought to cause childhood cancers.
2. Adult cancers are mainly of endothelial and epithelial surfaces, adenocarcinoma, and squamous cell carcinoma. What are the common types of childhood cancer?
3. Name the national clinical trial group presently studying childhood cancers in the United States and Canada.
4. When analyzing childhood cancers, what is the major difference between adult and childhood cancers?
5. Identify and describe one factor associated with second malignant neoplasms in survivors of childhood cancers.

REFERENCES

1. Barness LA. *Handbook of Pediatric Physical Diagnosis*. Philadelphia, Pa: Lippincott-Raven Publishers; 1998: 1, 3.
2. Nesbit ME Jr. Clinical assessment and differential diagnosis of the child with suspected cancer. In Pizzo PA, Poplack DG, eds. *Principles and Practice of Pediatric Oncology*, 2nd ed. Philadelphia, Pa: J. B. Lippincott Company; 1993: 106.
3. Miller DR. Hematologic malignancies: leukemia and lymphoma. In Miller DR, Baehne RL eds. *Blood Diseases of Infancy and Childhood*, 6th ed. St. Louis, Mo: C.V. Mosby; 1990: 604-721.
4. Ries LAG, Eisner MP, Kosary CL, et al, eds. *SEER Cancer Statistics Review. 1973-1999*. Bethesda, Md: National Cancer Institute. 2002; *http://seer.cancer.gov/csr/1973_1999*.
5. Li FP, Fraumen JR Jr., Mulvihill JJ, et al. A cancer family syndrome in 24 *kindred Cancer Research*. 1988: 48; 5358.
6. Strong LC, Stine M, Norsted TL. Cancer survivors of childhood soft-tissue sarcoma and their relatives. *Journal of the National Cancer Institute*. 1987; 79: 1213.
7. Malkin D, Li FP, Strong LC, et al. Germ-line p53 mutations in a familial syndrome of breast cancer, sarcomas, and other neoplasms. *Science*. 1990; 250: 1233-38.
8. Ambrosone CB, Freudenheim JL, et al. Cigarette smoking, N-Acetyletransferase 2 genetic polymorphisms, and breast cancer risk. *JAMA*. 1996; 276 (18): 1494-1501.
9. Harris CC. p53: at the crossroads of molecular carcinogenesis and risk assessment. *Science*. 1993; 60: 477-511.
10. Sutow WW. General aspects of childhood cancer. In Sutow WW, Fernbach DJ, Viett TJ, eds. *Clinical Pediatric Oncology*, 3rd ed. St. Louis, Mo: C.V. Mosby; 1984.
11. Enterline HT, Horr RC. Alveolar rhabdomyosarcoma: a distinctive tumor type. *American Journal of Clinical Pathology*. 1958; 29: 356.
12. Raney RB, Hays DM, Tefft M, Triche TJ. Rhabdomyosarcoma and the undifferentiated sarcomas. In Pizzo PE, Poplack DG, eds. *Principles and Practices of Pediatric Oncology*, 2nd ed. Philadelphia, Pa: J. B. Lippincott; 1993: 769-94.
13. Enzinger FM, Shirak M. Alveolar rhabdomyosarcoma: an analysis of 110 cases. *Cancer*. 1969; 24: 18-31.
14. Seidal T, Mark J, Hagman B, and Angervall L. Alveolar rhabdomyosarcoma: a cytogenetic and correlated cytological and histological study. *Acta Pathologica, Microbiologica et Immunologica Scandinavia*. 1982; [A] 90: 345-54.
15. Breslow NE, Beckwith JB. Epidemiological features of Wilms tumor: results of the National Wilms Tumor Study. *Journal of the National Cancer Institute*. 1982: 68(3); 429-36.
16. Ruymann FB, Maddux HR, Ragab A, et al. Congenital anomalies associated with rhabdomyo-

sarcoma: an autopsy study of 115 cases. A report from the Intergroup Rhabdomyosarcoma Study Committee. *Medical and Pediatric Oncology.* 1988: 16; 33-39.

17. McKeen EA, Hanson MR, Mulvihill JJ, Glaubidger DI. Birth defects with Ewing sarcoma. *New England Journal of Medicine.* 1983; 309: 1522.

18. Marina NM, Bowman LC, Pul CH, Crist WM. Pediatric solid tumors. In Holleb AI, Fink DJ, Murphy GP, eds. *American Cancer Society Textbook of Clinical Oncology,* 2nd ed. Atlanta, Ga: American Cancer Society; 1995: 525-51.

19. Smith DW. Neurofibromatosis syndrome. In Smith DW, Jones KL. *Recognizable Patterns of Human Malformation-Genetic, Embryologic and Clinical Aspects,* 3rd ed. Philadelphia, Pa: W B Saunders Company; 1982: 377-79.

20. Hope DG, Mulvihill JJ. Malignancy in neurofibromatosis. In Riccardi VM, Mulvihill JJ, eds. *Advances in Neurology,* Vol. 29: *Neurofibromatosis (Von Recklinghausen's Disease).* New York, NY: Raven Press; 1981.

21. Yang P, Grufferman S, Khoury MJ et al. Association of childhood rhabdomyosarcoma with neurofibromatosis type I and birth defects. *Genetic Epidemiology.* 1995: 12(5); 467-74.

22. Herbst AL, Scully RE. Adenocarcinoma of the vagina in adolescence: a report of 7 cases including 6 clear-cell carcinomas (so-called mesonephromas). *Cancer.* 1970; 25: 745-57.

23. Melnick S, Cole P, Anderson D, Herbst A. Rates and risks of diethlystibestrol-related clear-cell adenocarcinoma of the vagina and cervix: an update. *New England Journal of Medicine.* 1987; 316: 514-16.

24. Cosgrove MD, Benton B, Henderson BE. Male genitourinary abnormalities and maternal diethylstilbestrol. *Journal of Urology.* 1977; 117(2): 220-22.

25. Kwa S, Fine L. The association between parental occupation and childhood malignancy. *Journal of Occupational Medicine.* 1980; 22: 792-94.

26. Peters J, Preston-Martin S, Yu M. Brain tumors in children and occupational exposure of parents. *Science.* 1981; 213: 235-37.

27. Bizzozzero OJ Jr., Johnson KG, Ciocco A. Radiation-related leukemia in Hiroshima and Nagasaki, 1946-64, 1: distribution, incidence and appearance in time. *New England Journal of Medicine.* 1966; 274: 1095-1101.

28. Folley JH, Borges W, Yamawak T. Incidence of leukemia in survivors of the atomic bomb in Hiroshima and Nagasaki, Japan. *American Journal of Medicine.* 1952; 13: 311-21.

29. Moloney WD. Leukemia in survivors of atomic bombing. *New England Journal of Medicine.* 1966; 253: 88-90.

30. Jablon S, Kato H. Childhood cancer in relation to prenatal exposure to atomic-bomb radiation. *Lancet 2.* 1970: 1000-1003.

31. Kato HW, Schull WJ, Neel JV. A cohort-type study of survival in the children of parents exposed to the atomic bombings. *American Journal of Human Genetics.* 1966; 18: 339-73.

32. Mosijczuk AD, Ruymann FB. Second malignancy in acute lymphocytic leukemia: a review of 33 cases. *American Journal of Diseases of Children.* 1981; 135: 313-16.

33. Neglia JP, Meadows AT, Robison LL, et al. Second neoplasms after acute lymphobiastic leukemia in childhood. *New England Journal of Medicine.* 1991; 325: 1330-36.

34. Meadows AT, Baum E, Fossati-Bellani F, et al. Second malignant neoplasms in children: an update from the Late Effects Study Group. *J Clin Oncol 3.* 1985: 532-538.

35. Bhatia S, Robison L, Oberlin O, et al. Breast cancer and other second neoplasms after childhood Hodgkin disease. *The New England Journal of Medicine.* 1996; 334: 745-51.

36. Pui CH. Childhood leukemias. In Murphy GP, Lawrence W, Lenhard RE. eds. *American Cancer Society Textbook of Clinical Oncology,* 2nd ed. Atlanta, Ga: American Cancer Society; 1995: 501-23.

37. Turbergen DG, Gilchrist GS, O'Brien RT, et al. Prevention of CNS disease in intermediate-risk acute lymphoblastic leukemia: comparison of cranial radiation and intrathecal Methotrexate and the importance of systemic therapy: a Children's Cancer Group report. *Journal of Clinical Oncology.* 1993; 11(3): 520-26.

38. Tubergen DG, Gilchrist GS, O'Brien RT, et al. Improved outcome with delayed intensification for children with acute lymphoblastic leukemia and intermediate presenting features: a Children's Cancer Group phase III trial. *Journal of Clinical Oncology.* 1993; 11(3): 527-37.

39. Wolden S, Lamborn K, Cleary S, et al. Second cancers following pediatric Hodgkin disease. *J Clin Oncol.* 1998; 16: 536-544.

40. Glauser TA, Packer RJ, et al. Cognitive deficits in long-term survivors of childhood brain tumors. *Child's Nerv Sys.* 1992; 7:2-12.

41. Ellenberg L, McComb J, et al. Factors affecting intellectual outcome in pediatric brain tumor patients. *Neurosurgery.* 1987; 21(5): 638-644.

42. Chen BH, Packer JR, et al. Brain tumors in children under 2 years: treatment, survival and long-term prognosis. *Pediatr Neurosurg.* 93; 19: 171-179.

43. Kaleita T. Central nervous system-directed therapy in the treatment of childhood acute lymphoblastic leukemia and studies of neurobehavioral outcome:

Children's Cancer Group Trials. *Current Oncology Reports.* 2202; 4: 131-141.

44. Meadows AT, Obringer AC, Marrero O et al. Second malignant neoplasms following childhood Hodgkin Disease: treatment and splenectomy as risk factors. *Medical and Pediatric Oncology.* 1989; 17: 477-84.

45. Tucker MA, Meadows AT, Boice JD Jr., et al. Leukemia after therapy with alkylating agents for childhood cancer. *Journal of the National Cancer Institute.* 1987; 78: 459-64.

46. Whitlock JA, Greer JR, Lukens JN, Epipodophyllotoxin-related leukemia: identification of a new subset of secondary leukemia. *Cancer 68.* 1991: 600-604.

47. Smith MA, Rubenstein L, Cazenave L, et al. Report of the cancer therapy evaluation program monitoring plan for secondary acute myeloid leukemia following treatment with Epipodophyllotoxins. *Journal of the National Cancer Institute.* 1993; 85(7): 554-58.

48. Heyn R, Khan F, Ensign LG, et al. Acute myeloid leukemia in patients treated for rhabdomyosarcoma with Cyclophosphamide and low-dose Etoposide on Intergroup Phabdomyosarcoma Study III: an interim report. *Medical and Pediatric Oncology.* 1994; 23: 99-106.

49. Ruymann FB, Mosijczuk AD, Sayers RJ. Hepatoma in a child with Methotrexate-induced hepatic fibrosis. *JAMA.* 1977; 238: 2631-33.

50. Gasser RW, Judamier G, Nedden DZ, et al. Primary hepatocellular carcinoma with hepatitis B virus infection in a 16-year-old noncirrhotic patient. *American Journal of Gastroenterology.* 1983; 78: 305-308.

51. Shafritz DA, Shouval D, Sherman HI, et al. Integration of hepatitis B Virus DNA into the genome of liver cells in chronic liver disease and hepatocellular carcinoma. *Studies in percutaneous liver biopsies and post-mortem tissue specimens. New England Journal of Medicine.* 1981; 305: 1067-83.

52. Brechot C, Pourcel C, Louise A, et al. Presence of integrated hepatitis virus DNA sequences in cellular DNA of human hepatocellular carcinoma. *Cancer.* 1984; 54: 1360-63.

53. Shimoda T, Uchida I, Miyata H, et al. A 6-year-old boy having hepatocellular carcinoma associated with hepatitis B surface antigenemia. *American Journal of Clinical Pathology.* 1980; 74: 827-31

54. Shad A, Bhatia K, Hamdy N, et al. Pediatric HIV associated non-Hodgkin lymphomas. *Proceedings of the Annual Meeting of The American Association of Cancer Researchers.* 1994; 35: A1140.

55. Levine AM, Shibata D, Sullivan-Halley J, et al. Epidemiological and biological study of acquired immunodeficiency syndrome-related lymphoma in the county of Los Angeles: preliminary results. *Cancer Research.* 1992; 52(19): 5482s-84s.

56. Reynolds T. Is childhood leukemia the price of modernity? Editorial Journal of the *National Cancer Institute.* 1995; 87(8): 560-63.

57. Kinlen LJ, Dickson M, Stiller CA. Childhood leukemia and non-Hodgkin lymphoma near large rural construction sites, with a comparison with Sellafield nuclear site. *British Medical Journal.* 1995; 310: 763-68.

58. Fraumeni JR, Wagoner JK. Changing sex differentials in leukemia. *Seminars in Oncology.* 1985; 12(2):80-91.

59. Young JL Jr, Miller RW. Incidence of malignant tumors in US children. *Journal of Pediatrics.* 1975; 86: 245-58.

60. Fraumeni, JF, Glass AG. Rarity of Ewing sarcoma among US negro children. *Lancet 1.* 1970: 366-67.

61. Lindin G, Dunn JE. *Ewing sarcoma in negroes.* Lancet. 1970; 1: 1171.

62. Li FP, Tu JP, Liu FS, et al. Rarity of Ewing sarcoma in China. *Lancet.* 1980; 1: 1255.

63. Cammoun M, Horener GV, Mourali N. Tumors of the nasopharynx in Tunisia. An anatomic and clinical study of 143 cases. *Cancer.* 1974; 33: 184-92.

64. Ho HC. Nasopharyngeal carcinoma in Hong Kong. In Muir CS, Shamugaratnan K, eds. *Cancer of the Naso-Pharynx: A Symposium Organized by the International Union Against Cancer,* monograph series, Vol. 1. Copenhagen, Denmark: Munksgaard; 1967: 58-63.

65. Bhatia S, Sather H, et al. Ethnicity and survival following childhood Acute Lymmphoblastic Leukemia (ALL). Proceeding of ASCO 1999, 18: 568a (#2190).

66. West R. Childhood cancer mortality: international comparisons 1955-1974. World *Health Statistics.* 1984; 37: 98.

67. Kinnier-Wilson LM, Draper GJ. Neurobastoma its natural history and prognosis: a study of 487 cases. *British Medical Journal.* 1974; 3: 301-307.

68. Mann RB, Jaffe ES, Braylan RC, et al. Non-endemic Burkitt lymphoma. *New England Journal of Medicine.* 1976; 295; 685-91.

69. Dahlin D, Coventry M. Osteogenic sarcoma: A study of six hundred cases. *Journal of Bone and Joint Surgery, American Volume.* 1967; 49: 101-10.

70. Leventhal GB, Donaldson SS. Hodgkin Disease. In Pizzo PA, Poplack DG eds. *Principles and Practice of Pediatric Oncology,* 2nd ed. Philadelphia, Pa: J. B. Lippincott; 1993: 577-94.

71. Altman PR, Randolph JC, Lilly JR. American Academy of Pediatrics surgical section survey-1973. *Journal of Pediatric Surgery.* 1974; 9: 389-98.

72. Chrousos GP. Endocrine tumors. In Pizzo PA, Poplack DG, eds. *Principles and Practice of Pediatric Oncology*, 2nd ed. Philadelphia, Pa: J. B. Lippincott; 1993: 889-912.

73. Robison L. General principles of the epidemiology of childhood cancer. In Pizzo PA, Poplack DG, eds. *Principles and Practice of Pediatric Oncology*, 2nd ed. Philadelphia, Pa: J. B. Lippincott; 1993; 3-10.

74. Pui CH. Childhood leukemias. In Murphy GP, Lawrence W, Lenhard RE, eds. *Textbook of Clinical Oncology*, 2nd ed. Atlanta, Ga: American Cancer Society; 1995: 501-23.

75. Bennett JM, Catovsky D, Daniel MT, et al. French-American British (FAB) Cooperative Group: The morphological classification of acute leukemias-concordance among observers and clinical correlation. *British Journal of Haematology*. 1981; 47: 553-61.

76. Bennett JM, Catovsky D, Daniel MT, et al. French-American-British (FAB) Cooperative Group proposals for the classification of acute leukemias. *British Journal of Haematology*. 1976; 33: 451-58.

77. George SL, Fernbach DJ, Vietti TJ, et al. Factors influencing survival in pediatric acute leukemia: the SWCCSG experience 1958-1970. *Cancer*. 1973; 32: 1542-53.

78. Wiersma SR, Ortega J, Sobel E, et al. Clinical importance of myeloid-antigen expression in Acute Lymphoblastic Leukemia of childhood. *New England Journal of Medicine*. 1991: 324(12); 800-808.

79. Kanerva J, Niini T. Loss at 12p detected by comparative genomic hybridizatiooo (CGH): association with TEL-AML1 fusion and favorable prognostic features in childhood Acute Lymphoblastic Leukemia (ALL). *Med Pediatr Oncol*. 2001; 37: 419-425.

80. Woods WG, Ruymann F, Lampkin BC, et al. Aggressive intensification treatment may abrogate the need for maintenance therapy in children with acute nonlymphocytic leukemia (ANLL). Blood. 1987; 70(5): 241a.

81. Pizzo PA. Infectious complications in the child with cancer, I. Pathophysiology, II. Management, III. Prevention. *Pediatrics*. 1981; 98: 341, 513, 534.

82. Wells JR, Woods WG, Buckley JD, et al. Treatment of newly diagnosed children and adolescents with acute myeloid leukemia: a Children's Cancer Group study. *Journal of Clinical Oncology*. 1994; 12(11): 2367-77.

83. Lampkin BC. Cell kinetics as related to treatment of patients with acute nonlymphoid leukemia. *American Journal of Pediatric Hematology/Oncology*. 1985; 74(4): 358-72.

84. Duffner RI, Cohen ME, Myers MH, Heise HW. Survival of children with brain tumors. SEER Program, 1973-1980. *Neurology*. 1986; 36: 597-601.

85. Farwell JR, Dohrmann GJ, Flannery JT. Central nervous system tumors in children. *Cancer 40* (1977): 313-32.

86. Daumas-Duport C, Scheithauer B, O'Fallon J, et al. Grading of astrocytomas: a simple and reproducible method. *Cancer*. 1988; 62: 2152-65.

87. Zulch KJ. Histologic typing of tumours of the central nervous system. *International Histological Classification of Tumours*, no 21. Geneva, Switzerland: World Health Organization; 1979: 17-57.

88. Pollack IF, Finkelstein SD, et al. Age and TP533 mutation frequency in childhood malignant gliomas: results in a multi-institutional cohort. *Cancer Research*. 2001; 61: 7404-7407.

89. Burger RC, Scheithauer BW. Tumors of the central nervous system. *Atlas of Tumor Pathology*, 3rd series, fascimle 10. Washington, DC: AFIP; 1993: 193-221.

90. Harisiadis L, Chang CH. Medulloblastoma in children: a correlation between staging and results of treatment. *International Journal of Radiation Oncology, Biology, Physics*. 1977; 2: 833.

91. Laurent JP, Chang CH, Cohen ME. A classification system for primitive neuro-ectodermal tumors (medullobastoma) of the posterior fossa. *Cancer*. 1985; 56 (7 Suppl): 1807-1809.

92. Sternberg C. Uber eine Elgenartige unter dem Bilde der Pseudoleukamie Verlaufende Tuberculose des Lymphatischen Apparates. *Zeitschrift fur Heilkunde*. 1898; 19: 21-90.

93. Reed DM. On the pathological changes in Hodgkin Disease, with especial reference to its relation to tuberculosis. *Johns Hopkins Hospital Reports*. 1902; 10: 133-96.

94. Kaplan HS. *Hodgkin Disease*, 2nd ed. Cambridge, MA: Harvard University Press, 1980.

95. Gaynon P, Steinherz P, Bleyer WA, et al. Superiority of intensive therapy for children with acute lymphoblastic leukemia (ALL) and unfavorable presenting features. *Lancet*. 1988; 2(8617): 921-24.

96. Wollner N, Burchenal JH, Exelby P, et al. Non-Hodgkin lymphoma in children: a review of 104 cases. In Sinks LF, Godden JO, eds. *Conflicts in Childhood Cancer. An Evaluation of Current Management*. New York, NY: Liss; 1975: 179-223.

97. Ribeiro RC, Pui CH, Murphy SB, et al. Childhood malignant non-Hodgkin lymphomas of uncommon Histology. *Leukemia*. 1992; 6(8): 761-65.

98. Sposto R, Meadows A, et al. Comparison of long-term outcome of children and adolescents with disseminated non-lymphoblastic non-Hodgkin lymphoma treated with COMP or Daunomycin-COMP. *Med Pediatr Oncol*. 2001; 37: 432-441.

99. Reiter A, Schrappe M, et al. Successful treatment strategy for Ki-1 anaplastic large-cell lymphoma of childhood: a prospective analysis of 52 patients enrolled in three consecutive Berlin-Frankfurt-Munster Group studies. *J Clin Oncol.* 1998; 12: 899-908.

100. Magrath I, Janus C, Edwards B, et al. An effective therapy for both undifferentiated (including Burkitt) lymphomas and lymphoblastic lymphomas in children and young adults. *Blood.* 1984; 63: 1102-11.

101. Epstein MA, Achong BG, Barr YM. Virus particles in cultured lymphoblasts from Burkitt lymphoma. *Lancet 1.* 1964: 702-703.

102. Lenoir G, Philip T, Sohier R. Burkitt-type lymphoma: EBV association and cytogenetic markers in cases from various geographical locations. In Magrath IT, O'Conor G, Ramot B. eds. *Pathogenesis of Leukemias and Lymphomas: Environmental Influences.* New York, NY: Raven Press; 1984: 283-95.

103. Bethel C, Bhattacharyya N, Hutchison C, Ruymann F, et al. Alimentary tract malignancies in children. *Journal of Pediatric Surgery.* 1997; 32(7): 1004-3.

104. Tang JY, Kahwash S, Hutchison C, Rauck AM, Ruymann FB, Newton WA. Burkitt lymphoma in children: a 50-year experience at a single mid-Ohio, USA institution. *International Journal of Pediatric Hematology/Oncology.* 1999; 6(3): 199-207.

105. Carbone PP, Kaplan HS, Husshoff K, et al. Report of the committee on Hodgkin disease staging classification. *Cancer Research.* 1971; 31: 1860-61.

106. Murphy SB. Classification, staging and end results of treatment of childhood non-Hodgkin lymphomas: dissimilarities from lymphoma in adults. *Seminars in Oncology.* 1980; 7: 322-39.

107. Murphy SB, Fairclough DI, Hutchinson RE, Berard CW. Non-Hodgkin lymphoma of childhood: an analysis of the histology, staging, and response to treatment of 338 cases at a single institution. *Journal of Clinical Oncology.* 1989; 7: 186-93.

108. Link MR, Donaldson SS, Berard CW et al. Results of treatment of childhood localized non-Hodgkin lymphoma with combination chemotherapy with or without radiotherapy. *New England Journal of Medicine.* 1990; 322: 1169-74.

109. Brecher M, Murphy SB, Bowman P, et al. Results of Pediatric Oncology Group (POG) 8616: a randomized trial of two forms of therapy for stage III Diffuse, small noncleaved cell lymphoma in children. *Proceedings of the Annual Meeting of the American Society of Clinical Oncologists.* 1992; 11: A1167.

110. Meadows AT, Sposto R, Jenkin RDT, et al. Similar efficacy of 6 and 18 months of therapy with four drugs (COMP) for localized non-Hodgkin lymphoma of children: a report from the Children's Cancer Study Group. *Journal of Clinical Oncology.* 1989; 7: 92-99.

111. Sullivan MP, Brecher M, Ramirez I, et al. High-dose Cyclophosphamide-highdose Methotrexate with coordinated intrathecal therapy for advanced non-lymphoblastic lymphoma of childhood: results of a Pediatric Oncology Group Study. *American Journal of Pediatric Hematology/Oncology.* 1991; 13(3): 288-95.

112. Cairo MS, Krailo M, Hutchinson R, et al. Results of a phase II trial of "French" (F) (LMB-86) or "Orange" (O) (CCG-Hybrid) in children with advanced nonlymphobastic non-Hodgkin lymphoma: an Improvement in survival. *Proceedings of the Annual Meeting of the American Society of Clinical Oncology.* 1994; 13: A1336.

113. CCG 59704—Pilot Study for the Treatment of Children with Newly Diagnosed Advanced Stage Hodgkin Disease: Upfront Dose Intensive Chemotherapy. Background Section. Study Chairperson: Kelly, Kara; 1999.

114. Shimada H, Chatten J, Newton W, et al. Histopathologic prognstic factors in neuroblastic tumors: definition of subtypes of ganglioneuroblastoma and an age-linked classification of neuroblastomas. *Journal of the National Cancer Institute.* 1984; 73: 405-16.

115. Joshi V, Cantor A, Altshuler G, et al. Age-linked prognostic categorization based on a new histologic grading system of neuroblastomas. A clinicopathologic study of 211 cases from the Pediatric Oncology Group. *Cancer.* 1992; 69: 2197-2211.

116. Brodeur GM, Seeger RC, Schwab M, et al. Amplification of N-myc in untreated human neurobastomas correlates with advanced disease stage. *Science.* 1984; 224: 1121-24.

117. Brodeur G, Seege R. Gene amplification in human neurobastomas: basic mechanisms and clinical implications. *Cancer Genetics and Cytogenetics.* 1986; 19: 101-11.

118. Look AT, Hayes FA. Cellular DNA content as a predictor of response to chemotherapy in infants with unresectable neurobastoma. *N Engl J Med.* 1984; 311: 231-5.

119. Qualman SJ, O'Dorisio MS, Fleshman D, et al. Neuroblsatoma: correlation of neuropeptide expression in tumor tissue with other prognostic factors. *Cancer.* 1992; 70(7): 2005-12.

120. Look AT, Hayes FA. Clinical relevance of tumor cell ploidy and N-myc gene amplification in childhood neurobastoma. *J Clin Oncol.* 1991; 9:581-591.

121. Gitlow SE, Bertani LM, Rausen A, et al. Diagnosis of neuroblastoma by qualitative and quantitative

determination of catecholamine metabolites in urine. *Cancer.* 1970; 25: 1377-83.

122. Laug W, Siegel S, Shaw K, et al. Initial urinary catecholamine metabolite concentrations and prognosis in neurobastoma. *Pediatrics.* 1978; 62: 77-83.

123. Woods WG, Lemieux B, Leclerc JM, et al. Screening for neuroblastoma (NB) in North America: The Quebec Project. *Progress in Clinical and Biological Research.* 1994; 38S: 377-82.

124. Tsuchida Y, Kaneko M, Takeda T, et al. Therapy and prognosis of neuroblastoma: the Japanese experience. In Sawada T, Matsumura T, Kizaki Z, eds. *Proceedings of the 3rd International Symposium on Neurobastoma Screening.* 1993; 193-98.

125. Rauck AM, Newton WA, O'Dorisio MS, et al. Neuroblastoma (NB), a tumor modified by therapy (analysis of clinical pathologic data from 291 patients treated from 1945-1992). In Sawada T, Matsumura T, Kizaki Z, eds. *Proceedings of the 3rd International Symposium on Neuroblastoma Screening.* 1993; 189-92.

126. Evans AE, D'Anglo GH, Randolph J. A proposed staging for children with neurobastoma. *Cancer.* 1971; 27: 374-78.

127. Hayes FA, Green A, Husfu HO, et al. Surgicopathologic staging of neuroblastoma: prognostic significance of regional lymph node metastases. *Journal of Pediatrics.* 1983; 102: 59-62.

128. Brodeur GM, Seeger RC, Barrett A, et al. International criteria for diagnosis, staging and response to treatment in patients with neurobastoma. *Journal of Clinical Oncology.* 1988; 6: 1874.

129. Haase GM, O'Leary MC. Aggressive surgery combined with intensive chemotherapy improves survival in poor-risk neuroblastoma. *Journal of Pediatric Surgery.* 1991; 26(9): 1119-1124.

130. Matthay KK, Villablanca JG, et al. Treatment of high-risk neurobastoma with intensive chemotherapy, radiotherapy, autologous bone marrow transplantation, and 13-Cis-Retinoic Acid. *N Eng J Med.* 1999; 341: 165-173.

131. Young JL Jr., Miller RW. Incidence of malignant tumors in US children. *Journal of Pediatrics.* 1975; 86: 254-58.

132. Raney B Jr. Soft-tissue sarcoma in adolescents. In Tebb CK. *Adolescent Oncology.* Mt. Kisco, NY: Futura Publishing; 1987: 221-40.

133. Young JL Jr., Ries LG, Silverberg E, et al. Cancer incidence, survival and mortality for children younger than 15 years. *Cancer.* 1986; 58: 598-603.

134. Ruymann F, Kodet R, Newton W, et al. Decreased survival in children with anaplastic embryonal rhabdomyosarcoma. A report of the Intergroup Rhabdomyosarcoma Study Committee of CCG &

POG. *Proceedings of the Annual Meeting of the American Society of Clinical Oncology.* 1993; 12: A1441.

135. Kodet R, Newton WA, Hamoudi A, et al. Childhood rhabdomyosarcoma with pleomorphic-anaplastic features: a report of the Intergroup Rhabomyosarcoma Study. *American Journal of Surgical Pathology.* 1993; 17(5): 443-53.

136. Ruymann F, Newton W, Hutchison C, et al. Non-rhabdomyosarcomatous soft-Tissue tumors of children and adolescents: types, stage, and survival seen over a 45-year period. *Official Program and Scientific Proceedings of The American Society of Pediatric Hematology/Oncology Seventh Annual Meeting.* Chicago, Ill. 1994; 3: 24.

137. Shimada H, Newton WA, Soule EH, et al. Pathology of fatal rhabdomyosarcoma, report from Intergroup Rhabdomyosarcoma Study (IRS-I and IRS-II). *Cancer.* 1987; 59: 459.

138. Ruymann FB, Asmar L, Ramu N, et al. Undifferentiated soft-tissue sarcomas and alveolar rhabdomyosarcoma: major unfavorable histologies with improved survival in a review of Intergroup Rhabdomyosarcoma Studies 1, 11, and III. Manuscript in preparation.

139. Douglass EC, Valentine M, Etcubanas E, et al. A specific chromosomal abnormality in rhabdomyosarcoma. *Cytogenetics and Cell Genetics.* 1987; 45(3-4): 148-55.

140. Maurer HM, Beltangady M, Gehan EA, et al. The Intergroup Rhabdomyosarcoma Study-I; a final report. *Cancer.* 1988; 61: 209.

141. Qualman SJ, Coffin CM, et al. Intergroup rhabdomyosarcoma study: update for pathologists. *Pediatric and Developmental Pathology.* 1998; 1: 550-561.

142. Ruymann FB, Grovas A. Progress in the diagnosis and treatment of rhabdomyosarcoma and related soft tissue sarcomas. *Cancer Investigation.* 2000; 18(3): 223-241.

143. Crist W, Gehan EA, Ragab AH, et al. The third Intergroup Rhabdomyosarcoma Study. *Journal of Clinical Oncology.* 1995; 13(3): 610-630.

144. Maurer HM, Gehan EA, Beltangady M, et al. The Intergroup Rhabdomyosarcoma Study-II. *Cancer.* 1993; 71(5): 1904-22.

145. Laskin WB, Silverman TA, Enzinger FA. Post-radiation soft-tissue sarcomas. An analysis of 53 cases. *Cancer.* 1988; 62: 2330-40.

146. Rao BN, Etcubanas EE, Horowitz M, et al. The results of conservative management of extremity soft-tissue sarcomas in children. *Proceedings of the Annual Meeting of the American Society of Clinical Oncologists.* 1986; 5: 266.

147. Brizel DM, Weinstein H, Hunt M, et al. Failure pattern and survival in childhood soft-tissue sarcomas. *Proceedings of the American Society of Therapeutic Radiation Oncology.* 1988; 29: 183.

148. Carli M, Perilongo GI, Paolucci E, et al. Role of primary chemotherapy in childhood malignant mesenchymal tumors other than rhabdomyosarcoma. Preliminary results. *Proceedings of the Annual Meeting of the American Society of Clinical Oncology.* 1986; 5: 208.

149. Olive D, Flamant F, Rodary C, et al. Responsiveness of non-rhabdomyosarcoma malignant mesenchymal tumors (NRMMT) to primary chemotherapy (CT). *Proceedings of the 20th Meeting of SIOP.* Trodheim, Norway. 1988: 118.

150. Pratt CB. Clinical manifestations and treatment of soft-tissue sarcomas other than rhabdomyosarcoma. In Maurer HM, Ruymann FB, and Pochedly C, eds. *Rhabdomyosarcoma and Related Tumors in Children and Adolescents.* Boca Raton, Fl: CRC Press; 1991: 426.

151. Coppes MJ, Wilson ECG, Weitzmann S. Extrarenal Wilms tumor staging, treatment, and prognosis. *Journal of Clinical Oncology,* 1991; 9: 167-174.

152. Beckwith JB, Falmer NF. Histopathology and prognosis of Wilms tumor. Results from the National Wilms Tumor Study. *Cancer.* 1978; 41: 1937-48.

153. Klapproth HJ. Wilms tumor: a report of 45 cases and analysis of 1,351 cases reported in the world literature from 1940 to 1958. *Journal of Urology.* 1959; 81: 633-47.

154. D'Angio GJ, Breslow N, Beckwith JB, et al. Treatment of Wilms tumor. Results of the third National Wilms Tumor Study. *Cancer.* 1989; 64(2): 349-60.

155. Haas JE, Palmer NF, Weinberg AG, et al. Ultrastructure of malignant rhabdoid tumor of the kidney-a distinctive renal tumor of children. *Human Pathology.* 1981; 12: 646-57.

156. Beckwith JB, Norkook P, Breslow N, et al. Clinical observations in children with clear cell sarcoma (CCS) of the kidney. Abstract. *Proceedings of the American Association of Cancer Researchers.* 1986; 27: 200.

157. Bolande RP, Brough AJ, Izan RJ. Congenital mesoblastic nephroma of Infancy. *Pediatrics.* 1967; 40: 272-78.

158. Beckwith JB, Weeks DA. Congenital mesoblastic nephroma. When should we worry? *Archives of Pathology and Laboratory Medicine.* 1986; 110: 98-99.

159. Beckwith JB, Palmer NF. Histopathology and prognosis of Wilms tumor. Results from the National Wilms Tumor Study. *Cancer.* 1978; 41: 1937-48.

160. Beckwith JB. Wilms tumor and other renal tumors of childhood: a selective review from the National Wilms Tumor Study Pathology Center. *Human Pathology.* 1983; 14: 481-92.

161. Miller RW, Fraumeni JF, Manning MD. Association of Wilms tumor with aniridia, hemihypertrophy and other congenital malformations. *New England Journal of Medicine.* 1964; 270(18): 922-28.

162. Farber S. Chemotherapy in the treatment of leukemia and Wilms tumor. *JAMA.* 1966; 198: 826-36.

163. NWTS-5: Treatment of Relapsed Patients. A National Wilms Tumor Study Group Phase II Study. Background Section, Study Chairperson: Green, Daniel; 1995.

164. Evans AE, Norkook P, Evans A, et al. Late effects of treatment for Wilms tumor. *Cancer.* 1991; 67: 331-36.

165. Koufos A, Hansen MF, Lampkin BC, et al. Loss of alleles at loci on human chromosome 11 during genesis of Wilms tumor. *Nature.* 1984; (10)309: 170-72.

166. Beckwith JB. Macroglossia, omphalocele, adrenal cytomegaly, gigantism and hyperplastic visceromegaly. *Birth Defects: Original Article Series.* 1969; 5: 188-96.

167. Cavenee WK. The Beckwith-Wiedemann Syndrome: lessons for developmental oncology. Review. *Serono Symposia Publications from Raven Press.* 1991; 83: 11-23.

168. Sirinelli D, Silberman B, Baudon JJ, et al. Beckwith-Wiedemann Syndrome and neural crest tumors. A report of two cases. *Pediatric Radiology.* 1989; 19(4): 242-45.

169. Rainier S, Dobry CJ, Feinberg AP. Loss of imprinting in hepatoblastoma. *Cancer Research.* 1995; 55(9): 1836-38.

170. Elliot M, Bayly R, Cole T, et al. Clinical features and natural history of Beckwith-Wiedemann Syndrome: presentation of new cases. *Clinical Genetics.* 1994; 46(2): 168-74.

171. Matsumoto T, Kinoshita E, Maeda H, et al. Molecular analysis of a patient with Beckwith-Wiedemann Syndrome, rhabdomyosarcoma and renal cell carcinoma. *Japanese Journal of Human Genetics.* 1994; 39(2): 225-34.

172. Henry I, Puech A, Austruy E, et al. Towards the gene(s) for Beckwith-Wiedemann Syndrome and associated tumors in 11p15. *Proceedings of the Annual Meeting of the American Society of Clinical Oncology.* 1992; 11: A226.

173. Grundy PE, Telzerow PE, Breslow N, et al. Loss of heterozygosity for chromosomes 16q and 1 p in

Wilms tumors predicts an adverse outcome. *Cancer Research*. 1994; 54: 2331-33.

174. Meyers PA. Malignant bone tumors in children: Osteosarcoma. *Hematology/Oncology Clinics of North America*. 1987; 1(4): 655-65.

175. Meyers PA. Malignant bone tumors in children: Osteosarcoma. *Hematology/Oncology Clinics of North America*. 1987; 1(4): 667-73.

176. Evans RG, Nesbit ME, Gehan EA, et al. Multimodal therapy for the management of localized Ewing Sarcoma of pelvic and sacral bones: a report from the second Intergroup Study. *Journal of Clinical Oncology*. 1991; 9(7): 1173-80.

177. Smith MA, Ungerleider RS, Horowitz ME, et al. Influence of Doxorubicin dose intensity on response and outcome for patients with osteogenic sarcoma and Ewing sarcoma. *JNCI*. 1991; 83: 1460-1470.

178. Carter SR, Grimer RJ, Sneath RS. A review of 13 years experience of osteosarcoma. *Clinical Orthopaedics & Related Research*. 1991; 270: 45-51.

179. Ogihara Y, Sudo A, Fujinami S, et al. Current management, local management, and survival statistics of high-grade osteosarcoma. Experience in Japan. Review. *Clinical Orthopaedics & Related Research*. 1991; 270: 72-78.

180. Tsuchiya H, Tomita K. Prognosis of osteosarcoma treated by limb-salvage surgery: the Ten-Year Intergroup Study in Japan. *Japanese Journal of Clinical Oncology*. 1992; 22(5): 347-53.

181. Ma ZT, Li HG. Limb-salvage surgery for osteosarcoma. *Chinese Medical Journal*. 1994; 107(11): 854-57.

182. Cara JA, Canadell J. Limb salvage for malignant bone tumors in young children. *Journal of Pediatric Orthopedics*. 1994; 14(1): 112-18.

183. Jurgens H, Exner U, Gadner H, et al. Multidisciplinary treatment of Ewing sarcoma of bone: a 6-year experience of a European cooperative trial. *Cancer*. 1988; 61: 23-32.

184. Finn HA, Simon MA. Limb-salvage surgery in the treatment of osteosarcoma in skeletally immature individuals. Review. *Clinical Orthopaedics & Related Research*. 1991; 262: 108-18.

185. Pritchard J, da Cunha A, Cornbleet NA, et al. AlphaFetoprotein (AFP) monitoring of response to Adriamycin in hepatobla toma. *Journal of Pediatric Surgery*. 1982; 17: 429.

186. Murphy ASK, Vawter GF, Lee ABH, et al. Hormonal bioassay of conadotropin-producing hepatoblastoma. *Archives of Pathology and Laboratory medicine*. 1980; 104: S13-17.

187. McArthur JW, Toll GD, Russfield AB, et al. Sexual precocity attributable to ectopic gonadotropin secretion by hepatoblastoma. *American Journal of Medicine*. 1973; 54: 390-403.

188. Nomura F, Ohnishi K, Tanabe Y. Clinical features and prognosis of hepatocellular carcinoma with reference to serum alpha petroprotein levels. *Cancer*. 1989; 15:64(8): 1700-1707.

189. Melia WM, Bullock S, Johnson PJ, et al. Serum ferritin in hepatocellular carcinoma-a comparison with AlphaFetoprotein. *Cancer*. 1983; 51: 2122-25.

190. Matsumato Y. Response of AlphaFetoprotein to chemotherapy in patients with hepatoma. *Cancer*. 1974; 34: 1602-1606.

191. Johnson FL, Feagler JR, Lerner KG, et al. Association of androgenic-anabolic steroid therapy with development of hepatocellular carcinoma. *Lancet*. 1972; 2: 1273-76.

192. Wogan GN. Diet and nutrition as risk factors for cancer. *International Symposium of the Princess Takamatsu Cancer Research Fund*. 1985; 16(3): 10.

193. Evans AE, Land VJ, Newton WA, et al. Combination chemotherapy in the treatment of children with malignant hepatoma. *Cancer*. 1982; 50: 821-26.

194. Exelby P, Filler RM, Grosfeld JL. Liver tumors in children in the particular reference to hepatoblastoma and hepatocellular carcinoma: American Academy of Pediatrics Surgical Section Surgery-1974. *Journal of Pediatric Surgery*. 1975; 10(3): 329-37.

195. Randolph JG, Altman RP, Arensman RM, et al. Liver resection in children with hepatic neoplasms. *Annals of Surgery*. 1978; 187(6): 599-605.

196. Koneru B, Flye MW, Busittil RW, et al. Liver transplant for hepatoblastoma. *Annals of Surgery*. 1991; 213(2): 118-121.

197. Munro FD, Simpson E, Azmy AF. Resectability of advanced liver tumours in children after combination chemotherapy. *Annals of the Royal College of Surgeons of England*. 1994; 76(4): 253-56.

198. Ortega JA, Krailo MD, Jaas JE, et al. Effective treatment of unresectable or metastatic hepatoblastoma with Cisplatin and continuous influsion Doxorubicin chemotherapy: a report from the Children's Cancer Study Group. *Journal of Clinical Oncology*. 1991; 9(12): 2167-76.

199. King DR, Ortega J, Campbell J, et al. The surgical management of children with incompletely resected hepatic cancer is facilitated by intensive chemotherapy. *Journal of Pediatric Surgery*. 1991; 26(9): 1074-81.

200. Shu XO, Nesbit ME, Buckley JD, et al. An exploratory analysis of risk factors for childhood malignant germ-cell tumors: report from Children's Cancer Group (Canada, United States). *Cancer Causes and Control*. 1995; 6: 187-98.

201. Einhorn LH, Donohue JP. CisDiamminedichloroplatinum, Vinblastine and Bleomycin: combination

chemotherapy in disseminated testicular cancer. *Annals of Internal Medicine.* 1977; 87: 293.

202. Williams S, Birch R, Einhorn L, et al. Treatment of disseminated germ-cell tumors with Cispaltin, Bleomycin, and either Vinblastine or Etoposide. *NEJM.* 1987; 316: 1435-40.

203. Holladay DA, Holladay A, Montebello JF, et al. Clinical presentation, treatment, and outcome of trilateral retinoblastoma. *Cancer.* 1991; 67: 710-15.

204. Knudson AG. Mutation and cancer: statistical study of retinoblastoma. *Proceedings of the National Academy of Sciences of the United States of America.* 1971; 68: 620-23.

205. Draper GJ, Saunders, DM, Kingston JE. Second primary neoplasms in patients with retinoblastoma. *British Journal of Cancer.* 1986; 53: 661-71.

206. Ellsworth RM. The practical management of retinoblastoma. *Transactions of the American Ophthalmological Society.* 1969; 67: 562-32.

207. Ladisch S, Jaffe ES. The histiocytoses. In Pizzo PA, Poplack DG, eds. *Principles and Practice of Pediatric Oncology,* 2nd ed. Philadelphia, Pa: J. B. Lippincott; 1993: 617-31.

208. Grovas A, Grossman N, Hamoudi A, et al. A Fifty Year Experience with Langerhans Cell Histiocytosis in a Single Hospital. Abstract accepted for presentation at the Eleventh Annual Meeting, The Histiocyte Society, September 30-October 3, 1995, Alexandria, Virginia.

209. Percy A, Van Holten V, Muir C. *International Classification of Diseases for Oncology,* 2nd ed. Geneva: Switzerland; World Health Organization, 1990.

210. Willman CL, Busque L, Griffith BB, et al. Langerhans cell histiocytosis (histiocytosis X)-a clonal proliferative disease. *New England Journal of Medicine.* 1994: 331(3): 154-60.

211. Hammond D. Management of childhood cancer. Guest editorial. *CA-A Cancer Journal for Clinicians.* 1990; 40(6) : 325-26.

212. Personal Communication with Pediatric Oncology Group (POG) Operations Office.

213. Leventhal BG, Wittes RE. *Research Methods in Clinical Oncology.* New York, NY: Raven Press; 1988.

214. American College of Surgeons Commission on Cancer. *Standards of the Commission on Cancer, Vol.*

1, *Cancer Program Standards.* Chicago, Ill: The Commission; 1996: 58.

215. Clive RE. Cancer department news. *American College of Surgeons Commission on Cancer Newsletter.* 1994; 5(3): 3-5.

216. Beahrs OH, Henson DE, Hutter RVP, Kennedy BJ, eds. American Joint Committee on Cancer, *Manual for Staging of Cancer,* 4th ed. Philadelphia, Pa: J. B. Lippincott; 1992.

217. Birch JM, Marsden HB. A classification scheme for childhood cancer. *International Journal of Cancer.* 1987; 40: 620-24.

218. American College of Surgeons Commission on Cancer. *Cancer Program Manual.* Chicago, Ill: The Commission; 1991: 8.

219. Marsden HB. The classification of childhood tumours. In Parkins DM, Stiller CA, Draper GJ, et al, eds. *International Incidence of Childhood Cancer.* New York, NY: Oxford University Press; 1988: 9-16.

220 Puymann FB, Hutchison CL, Newton WA, Disbro AE. The need for development of a common system to analyze childhood cancers. The Abstract, *Journal of the National Cancer Registrars Association.* 1994; 21(1): 26-27.

221. Ruymann FB, Hutchison CL, Newton WA. The Need for the Development of a Common Grouping System to Analyze Childhood Cancers. Official program and Scientific Proceedings of The American Society of Pediatric Hematology/Oncology Seventh Annual Meeting, Chicago, Ill, 1994; Vol. 3: 24.

222. Pollack I, Biegel J, Yates A, et al. Risk assignment in childhood brain tumors: the emerging role of molecular and biologic classification. *Current Oncology Reports.* 2002; 4: 114-122.

223. Weitzman S, Suryanarayan K, Weinstein H. Pediatric Non-Hodgkin Lymphoma: Clinical and Biologic Prognostic Factors and Risk Allocation. *Current Oncology Reports.* 2002; 4: 107-113.

224. Qualman S, Morotti R. Risk assignment in pediatric soft-tissue sarcomas: an evolving molecular classification. *Current Oncology Reports.* 2002; 4: 132-130.

225. Jamil A, Theil K, Kahwash S, Ruymann F, et al. TEL/AML-1 fusion gene: its frequency and prognostic significance in childhood acute lymphoblastic leukemia. *Cancer Genetics and Cytogeneticas.* 2000; 122(2): 72-8.

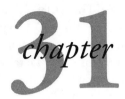

chapter 31

THE NATIONAL CANCER DATA BASE

Andrew K. Stewart
MA

PURPOSE

The National Cancer Data Base (NCDB) was established to serve as a comprehensive clinical surveillance resource about cancer care in the United States. The NCDB was the first national database used to track and compare the treatment of most types of cancers. Working in conjunction with other activities of the Commission on Cancer (CoC), the purpose of the NCDB is to improve the quality of cancer care by providing physicians, cancer registrars, and others with the means to compare their management of cancer patients with the way in which similar patients are managed in other cancer care centers around the country. The NCDB resides in and is operated by the CoC of the American College of Surgeons (ACoS).

OVERVIEW

The forerunner to the CoC, the Cancer Campaign Committee, was founded in 1913 and was charged with "conducting a study of the efficacy of surgery and radiation therapy in the management of gynecologic cancers." By 1922, the CoC was formally established. Currently the CoC is a group of multidisciplinary professionals dedicated to the mission of reducing cancer morbidity and mortality through education, standard-setting and monitoring the quality of cancer care. The National Cancer Data Base is a means toward the active monitoring of cancer care in the United States.

The American Cancer Society (ACS) and the CoC of the ACoS have maintained a long-standing partnership in the fight against cancer. The ACS and the ACoS jointly fund the activities of the NCDB. The NCDB was established in 1989 by these two organizations to provide important information to individuals and institutions interested in the care of cancer patients. The NCDB is a nationwide, institutionally-based, oncology data set that currently captures 75% of all newly diagnosed cancer cases in the United States annually holds information on almost 15 million cases of reported cancer diagnoses for the period 1985 through 2001, and continues to grow. Data on all types of cancer are tracked and analyzed. Data collected include patient characteristics, tumor staging and histology characteristics, type of first course treatment administered, and disease recurrence and survival informa-

tion. These data elements are submitted to the NCDB from CoC-approved cancer program registries using nationally standardized data transmission formats. Data confidentiality is of prime importance and the NCDB has proactively worked to continually ensure and maintain compliance with the Health Insurance Portability and Accountability Act (HIPAA) of 1996 privacy regulations established by the Federal Government in 2003. Data residing in the NCDB can be linked to other reference data sources, such as US census files to provide aggregate estimates of various socio-economic variables such as family income and educational achievement, or American Hospital Association (AHA) files to obtain specific hospital characteristics. Data in the NCDB can be analyzed and reported in a variety of ways. Most importantly for comparative analyses. For example, to examine patterns of care to evaluate if and how treatment patterns vary regionally or over time.

ORGANIZATION

The CoC of the ACoS operates under the guidance of three standing committees: the Committee on Approvals, the Committee on Cancer Liaison (Physicians), and the Quality Integration Committee. The Quality Integration Committee (QIC) is the central advisory panel that guides and assists in the prioritization of the work conducted by the National Cancer Data Base staff. The Committee is concerned with, and represents the CoC in matters addressing the progress and direction of research and continuing education as it pertains to improving the care of cancer patients. The Committee directs and oversees the activities of the Disease Site Teams that include conducting research using NCDB resources, developing focused studies and educational interventions, and evaluating quality of cancer registry data. The committee members are selected from the CoC membership. Surgical specialties should be representative of the College Fellowship. Multidisciplinary balance, programmatic goals, potential member interests, and geography are considerations. Preferably, members are actively involved in cancer-related activities through clinical practice, approved cancer programs, research activities, or by association with professional groups supporting cancer programs. Members of the QIC are responsible for: 1) identification, recommendation, and approval of the membership composition of the CoC's DSTs; 2) the review and prioritization of the proposals put forth by the DSTs based on merit; 3) setting goals and priorities of the research programs of the CoC ; and 4) overseeing the activities of the DSTs.

The CoC has formulated 13 DSTs to meet the national demand for ongoing assessment of the quality of cancer care. Team members may be selected from the CoC membership and member organizations. Surgical specialties are representative of the College Fellowship. Multidisciplinary balance, programmatic goals, potential member interests, and geography are considerations. Preferably, members are actively involved in cancer-related activities through clinical practice, approved cancer programs, research activities, or by association with professional groups supporting cancer programs. The purpose of the DSTs is to: 1) conduct research using NCDB resources; 2) develop focused studies; 3) develop educational interventions including program content and recommending speakers; 4) evaluate quality of cancer registry data; and 5) collaborate with other national leaders and agencies in cancer care. The DSTs include colorectal, head and neck, liver, pancreas, thoracic oncology, upper GI, colorectal, sarcoma, melanoma, breast, gynecologic oncology, thyroid and parathyroid, urology, and brain/CNS. Several member organizations of the CoC, including the American Society for Clinical Oncology, the Society for Surgical Oncology, the American Society for Therapeutic Radiology and Oncology, the American College of Radiology, the College of American Pathologists, and the Central Brain Tumor Registry of the United States have been instrumental in nominating national experts to these teams. Each DST is provided administrative and analytic support by NCDB staff.

DATA CYCLE

The NCDBs data cycle consists of three parts: 1) an Annual Call for Data, 2) data processing which includes edit checks and writing case records to the CoC's data warehouse, and 3) data analysis and evaluation. All documentation described below is maintained for the current and most recent Calls on the NCDB page of the ACoS website: www.facs.org.

Call for Data

The annual Call for Data is sent electronically to all CoC-approved cancer programs. These cancer programs diagnose and/or treat approximately 75-80% of all cancer patients in the United States. The call for data is issued in the autumn of each year. Specific instructions are provided outlining case submission transmission file specifications and data format requirements. These guidelines are consistent with the North American Association of Central Cancer Registries (NAACCR) data transmission specifications established for the most current data year requested in the Call for Data. In addition, instructions are provided describing how registries can prepare, validate, and complete their data submission.

Data are requested for four years at the time of each Call for Data, in order to facilitate obtaining the most recent data available as well as follow-up recurrence and survival data for previously reported patients. For example, in the fall of 2003, the Call for Data requested that cases for the years 2002, 1997, 1992, and 1987 be submitted to the NCDB. The 2002 cases were the most recently abstracted and completed case records available that hospital registries could provide at that time. Case records from 1997 were used to update those previously reported and included 5-year follow-up information, cases from 1992 were used to update previously reported records and included 10-year follow-up information, and the 1987 cases provided 15-year follow-up data.

Data are received from CoC-approved cancer program registries via the secured CoC Datalinks web application. Upon receipt of a data file the corresponding registry is notified via e-mail confirming receipt of the transmission. As data files pass through the sequence of data edit reviews and case writing to the CoC's data warehouse additional email notifications are generated informing each respective registry of the status of their data submission. The NCDB monitors the participation of hospitals, tracking the accuracy and frequency with which data submissions are made, as well as checking for unexpected fluctuations in site-specific caseloads.

Data submission to the NCDB is a requirement of the CoC approvals program. Standard 3.6 of the CoC *Cancer Programs Standards 2004* specifies that a complete data for all analytic cases are submitted to the National Cancer Data Base (NCDB) in accordance with the annual Call for Data. Although this requirement has been in place since 1996 it was infrequently monitored. Starting with cases reported for 2002 cancer program participation in the Call for Data and compliance with Standard 3.6 will be automatically included in the facility's Survey Application Record (SAR) for review and use at the time of the program's next scheduled survey. The web-based reporting application employed by the NCDB simultaneously updates the SAR as data files are received, edited, and written to CoC's databases.

Data Edits

In advance of transmitting data files to the NCDB, CoC-approved cancer program registries are advised to use the most current NCDB EDITS metafile to pre-edit their data transmission file to ensure that submitted records are of the highest possible quality. The NCDB EDITS metafile for each Call for Data is made available on the NCDB web page three to four months in advance of the deadline for data submission. The NCDB EDITS metafile utilizes standardized and nationally accepted data edits and can be used using GenEdits, free software available from the Centers for Disease Control. Instructions for using the NCDB metafiles and EDITS software are available on the NCDB web page.

Once data files are received, each case submitted undergoes three parallel editing processes. Each of these steps employs the same NCDB metafile made available to registries to pre-edit their data transmission file.

The first editing process evaluates the quality of the data reported for each case. With each Call for Data specified edits, both single items and inter-item combinations, are checked for validity. Cases that fail certain specified single and inter-item "rejection edits" will be automatically excluded from further processing and will not be written to the CoC's data warehouse. At minimum these "rejection edits" include edit failures associated with the codes reported in the data items: Accession Number; Postal Code at Diagnosis; Birth Date; Date of 1st Contact; Date of Diagnosis; Tumor Morphology; Primary Site; Sequence Number; Sex; and Sex/Primary Site. Other additional "rejection edits" may also be included.

The second editing process is applied to all cases that did not fail any of the previously mentioned "rejection edits." Records are evaluated and scored

depending on which and how many of the specified single and inter-item edits a case fails. Cases that accumulate a data quality score equal to or greater than 200 points are subsequently rejected and are not written to the CoC's data warehouse. Cases with a data quality score of 0 are considered problem-free, while those with a score between 1 and 199 should be reviewed, corrected, and resubmitted in accordance with Standard 3.7 of the CoC *Cancer Program Standards 2004*. The data quality score assigned to each case is recorded as part of the case record in the CoC data warehouse. Documentation providing specific information describing edit names and the data quality score associated with each edit is posted on the NCDB web page and is made available when the NCDB metafile is released.

Standard 3.7 of the CoC *Cancer Programs Standards 2004* specifies that "cases submitted to the NCDB for the most recent accession year requested meet the established quality criteria included in the annual Call for Data." This standard requires CoC-approved cancer program registries to resolve errors which result in rejected records and to correct any other errors leading to the assignment of a data quality score of greater than one for all case records submitted for the most recent accession year. For example, in the Call for Data requesting cases for the years 2002, 1997, 1992, and 1987, Standard 3.7 applies to cases for the year 2002. Resolution of edit errors and data quality problems for cases from the remaining three years, though advised and strongly encouraged, is not required.

The third editing process includes the production of an edit report for each of the years included in every data transmission made by a CoC-approved cancer program registry. These reports specify the exact nature of any identified edit errors or warnings and should be used by registries to review particular elements of its registry database, thus providing both the cancer program and the CoC with better quality data. The hospital data edit reports are posted electronically and are made available to each respective facility registry using the secured CoC Datalinks Web application. The electronic posting of each edit report is accompanied by information specifying the receipt date of the submission, the total number of records received in the submission file, the number of records rejected and the number of records identified as having quality problems. In addition, a summary site/stage table showing the distribution of all quality accepted records by ICD-O topography code and AJCC Stage Group is generated to serve as a mechanism by which registries can confirm and validate the type and number of cases received and processed as part of their data submission. Registries are notified via email upon completion of the editing process, summary information describing the status of the edits review of their data submission is provided in the notification.

Writing Cases to the CoC Data Warehouse

The CoC data warehouse is maintained on a dedicated Oracle server. Individually edited and data quality scored records are written to the CoC data warehouse as soon as the editing process is complete. Each case is assigned a contextual code that is used in the duplicate case-elimination process. Cases are written to the CoC data warehouse after a primary key search is performed. This key is based on the specific code values made up of the CoC Facility Identification Number (FIN) of the submitting registry, the accession and sequence number of the case, and the year portion of the data item "Date of 1st Contact." One of two types of merges is applied at this stage. If a match is found, depending upon the data quality score of the two cases, a case update is performed. If no match is found, the case is added to the database as a new case. Once a record is written to the database a second key search is performed to identify clinical duplicates, instances in which the same patient is reported by more than one registry. When clinical duplicate cases are identified the contextual code assigned to each case is used to flag one of the two, or more, cases for use in aggregate analysis. The remaining cases are preserved for use in generating registry specific reports.

Data Analysis and Evaluation

Case records reported to the NCDB are maintained in the CoC data warehouse in such a way as to maximize the analytic utility of the data, whether this be for aggregate analytic purposes or for generating hospital based benchmark reports. All the data collected by the NCDB is frequently utilized in the analytic work and report generation conducted by the NCDB, however much of the basic framework for this work is informed by the following set of co-variates.

Over 15 years of data are maintained by the NCDB. This longitudinal depth allows for the systematic evaluation of changing patterns of diagnosis and disease presentation and first course therapy by diagnosis year.

The NCDB bases much of its analysis and reporting by disease site. There are 61 NCDB analytic disease sites and every case reported to the NCDB is assigned to one of these categories. All cases reported with ICD-O morphology codes 9590–9948 are assigned to the appropriate hemic or lymphatic site. The remaining cases are assigned to the appropriate site group depending upon the specified combinations of topography and morphology codes (Table 31-1). Tumor morphology, including tumor histology, behavior and grade, are coded for each case reported to the NCDB. Codes describing tumor histology are reported to the NCDB using either the International Classification of Diseases for Oncology, 2nd edition, 1990 (ICD-O-2), if diagnosed prior to 2001, or the 3rd edition, 2000 (ICD-O-3), if diagnosed 2001 or later. Cases diagnosed prior to 2001 that have not been converted forward to ICD-O-3 standards are converted as part of the process of writing cases to the CoC data warehouse, the reported ICD-O-2 morphology codes are retained.

Analyses utilizing patient characteristics typically involve consideration of age, gender, and race. Patient age is typically categorized into 5- or 10-year age ranges, depending upon the analytic task. Adult cases are defined as those aged 16 or higher at the time of diagnosis. Cases reported as men or women are retained for most analytic work, cases reported as hermaphrodites or transsexuals are infrequently encountered. Patient race/ethnicity is computed using a combination of the race codes and reported information describing Spanish/Hispanic heritage and is frequently reported as White, African American, Hispanic, Native American, Asian/Pacific Islander (API), and Other/Unknown. Additional racial/ethnic information can be imputed using a combination of coded race and place of birth information depending upon the analytic task. Additionally, certain socio-economic measures can be employed such as insurance status, and aggregate measures of family income and educational status. The latter two measures are derived from published United States census data and matched to NCDB case records based on the reported zip code of residence at the time of diagnosis for each case.

Table 31-1
NCDB Analytic Site Groups

Anatomic System	Anatomic Site	ICD-O-2/3 Topography Code	ICD-O-2/3 Histology Code
Head and Neck	Lip	CD00.0-C00.9	8000-9582
	Tongue	C01.9-C02.9	8000-9582
	Salivary Glands	C07.9-C08.9	8000-9582
	Floor of Mouth	C04.0-C04.9	
	Gum and Other Mouth	C03.0-C03.9, C05.0-C05.9, C06.0-C06.9	8000-9582
	Nasopharynx	C11.0-C11.9	8000-9582
	Tonsil	C09.0-C09.9	8000-9582
	Oropharynx	C10.0-C10.9	8000-9582
	Hypopharynx	C12.9, C13.0-C13.9	8000-9582
	Other Oral Cavity and Pharynx	C14.0, C14.2-C14.8	8000-9582
Digestive System	Esophagus	C15.0-C15.9	8000-9582
	Stomach	C16.0-C16.9	8000-9582
	Small intestine	C17.0-C17.9	8000-9582
	Colon	C18.0-C18.9, C26.0	8000-9582
	Rectosigmoid Junction	C19.9	8000-9582
	Rectum	C20.9	8000-9582
	Anus	C21.0-C21.8	8000-9582
	Liver	C22.0	8000-9582
	Intrahepatic Bile Duct	C22.1	8000-9582
	Gallbladder	C23.9	8000-9582
	Other Biliary	C24.0-C24.9	8000-9582
	Pancreas	C25.0-C25.9	8000-9582
	Retroperitoneum	C48.0	8000-9582
	Peritoneum, Omentum, Mesentary	C48.1-C48.2	8000-9582
	Other Digestive	C26.8-C26.9, C48.8	8000-9582
Respiratory System	Nose, Nasal Cavity, Middle Ear	C30.0-C31.9	8000-9582
	Larynx	C32.0-C32.9	8000-9582
	Lung, Bronchus - Small Cell Carcinoma	C34.0-C34.9	8040-8045
	Lung, Bronchus - Non-Small Cell Carcinoma	C34.0-C34.9	8012-8035, 8046-8576
	Lung, Bronchus - Other Types	C34.0-C34.9	8000-8011, 8580-9582
	Pleura	C38.4	8000-9582
	Trachea, Mediastinum, Other Respiratory	C33.9, C38.1-C38.3, C38.8, C39.0-C39.9	8000-9582
Bones and Joints	Bones and Joints	C40.0-C41.9	8000-9582

Table 31-1
(continued)

Anatomic System	Anatomic Site	ICD-O-2/3 Topography Code	ICD-O-2/3 Histology Code
Soft Tissue and Heart	Soft Tissue and Heart	C38.0, C47.0-C47.9, C49.0-C49.9	8000-9582
Skin (non-epithelial)	Melanoma - Skin	C44.0-C44.9	8720-8790
	Other Non-Epithelial Skin	C44.0-C44.9	8120-8713, 8800-9582
Breast	Breast	C50.0-C50.9	8000-9582
Female Genital System	Cervix	C53.0-C53.9	8000-9582
	Uterus	C54.0-C54.9, C55.9	8000-9582
	Ovary	C56.9	8000-9582
	Vagina	C52.9	8000-9582
	Vulva	C51.0-C51.9	8000-9582
	Other Female Genital	C57.0-58.9	8000-9582
Male Genital System	Prostate	C61.9	8000-9582
	Testis	C62.0-C62.9	8000-9582
	Penis	C60.0-C60.9	8000-9582
	Other Male Genital	C63.0-C63.9	8000-9582
Urinary System	Bladder	C67.0-C67.9	8000-9582
	Kidney and Renal Pelvis	C64.9, C65.9	8000-9582
	Ureter	C66.9	8000-9582
	Other Urinary	C68.0-C68.9	8000-9582
Eye and Orbit	Eye and Orbit	C69.0-C69.9	8000-9582
Brain, Nervous System	Brain	C71.0-C71.9	8000-9523, 9540-9582
	Other CNS	C71.0-C71.9	9530-9539
		C70.0-C70.9, C72.0-C72.9	8000-9582
Thyroid/Endocrine	Thyroid	C73.9	8000-9582
	Endocrine	C37.9, C74.0-C74.9, C75.0-C75.9	8000-9582
Hemic and Lymphatic	Hodgkins Lymphoma	Any	9560-9667
	Non-Hodgkins Lymphoma	Any	9590-9569, 9670-9719
	Plasma Cell Tumors	Any	9731-9734
	Leukemia	Any	9800-9948
Other and Unspecified	Other and Unspecified	All other cases not otherwise specified above	

Cases reported to the NCDB are staged using the AJCC staging system. In many analyses pathologic stage group information is used whenever possible, supplemented by clinical stage group information when pathologic is unknown. This method is used to minimize the number of cases under analysis without an AJCC stage designation. The stage grouping utilized in analysis are sensitive to the disease site under review and the AJCC Cancer Staging Manual in use at the time the case was diagnosed. The introduction of the Collaborative Staging System, starting with cases diagnosed in 2004, presents new opportunities to analytically evaluate and describe the extent of disease reported at the time of diagnosis and will complement the NCDB past reliance on physician based staging information.

The NCDB is particularly interested in treatment patterns. The first course of treatment represents the combination of treatment modalities used in the management of the disease. Surgery is among the principal recognized treatment modalities for cancer and includes the local excision or resection of the primary tumor. The type and description of surgical procedures are specific to the reported ICD-O primary site of disease, and have been clearly defined and described in CoC coding manuals, including the DAM, ROADS, and FORDS. Radiation, which includes beam radiation, brachytherapy, or radioisotopes, and systemic therapy, separately reported as chemotherapy, hormone therapy, or immunotherapy (biological response modifiers) are also reported to the NCDB and included in the analysis of treatment patterns. In some instances no treatment is provided to certain cases. For many analyses cases are categorized using one or a number of the following specified descriptions of first course treatment: surgery alone; radiation alone; chemotherapy alone; hormone alone; surgery plus radiation; surgery plus chemotherapy; surgery plus hormone therapy; surgery plus BRM (immunotherapy); surgery, radiation plus chemotherapy; surgery, radiation plus hormone therapy; surgery, radiation, chemotherapy plus hormone therapy; radiation plus chemotherapy; radiation plus hormone therapy; other specified treatment modalities (which may include surgery, radiation, chemotherapy, hormone therapy, and/or immunotherapy); and no treatment. Treatment modalities are reported depending upon the disease site and stage of disease under review, some treatment management strategies are used in the treatment of one type of disease but not of another. Similarly, management of disease may depend upon its stage of presentation, thus excluding certain treatment modalities from analytic review.

Data can be analyzed geographically. Typically this is performed using the state or the seventeen ACS divisions in which the reporting hospital is located. Alternatively, United States census regions (Northeast, Atlantic, Southeast, Greatlakes, South, Midwest, West, Mountain, and Pacific) can be used to provide a broader set of regional areas for analysis. Furthermore, facility characteristics, based on one or a combination of the scope of resources and services available and case volume can be used to review patterns of diagnosis, patient care and outcomes.

Outcomes, or survival analysis, are performed by computing observed or relative survival rates, depending upon the focus of the analytic task. Observed survival rates are computed using the actuarial method, compounding survival in one-month intervals from the date of diagnosis, with death from any cause as the recognized endpoint. Relative survival rates are the ratio of the observed survival rate to the expected survival rate of persons of the same sex, age, and racial or ethnic background. Expected survival rates are computed in single-year increments using the most recent life-expectancy tables published by the National Center for Health Statistics. Using this methodology, the relative survival rates become risk-adjusted for the demographic variability in patient populations, and can be calculated in the absence of specific and reliable cause of death information for each patient. Outcomes analyses also include the application of multivariate survival techniques, particularly the use of Cox regression techniques which model the relative risk of patient survivorship based on one or more co-variates.

DATA CONFIDENTIALITY

The NCDB is committed to ensuring the strictest adherence to the CoC's policies on data confidentiality and has implemented all the appropriate policies, procedures, and information systems to comply with the rules and regulations concerning privacy of patient data under the HIPAA and is in compliance with the final regulations released in August 2002. The CoC has entered into a "business associate" (BA) agreement with each approved cancer program and as such functions as an organization that performs activities such as quality assurance and improvement or accreditation functions for a covered entity ('160.103). In this function, the NCDB collects a limited data set from CoC-approved cancer program registries. A limited data set is defined as one which <u>does not include any</u> of the 14 following data elements: name; street address; phone/fax numbers; email addresses; social security number; certificate or license numbers; vehicle identification numbers; URLs or IP addresses; full face photographs; medical record numbers; health beneficiary numbers; other account numbers; devise identifiers or serial numbers; and biometric identifiers.

Under these guidelines, the NCDB assures: 1) all covered entities that any and all data that may lead to the identity of the any patient, research subject, physician, other person is strictly privileged and confidential; 2) no patient, physician, or facility will be identified in published results; 3) data will be received, stored, analyzed, and reported in accordance with the confidentiality requirements as set down by HIPAA; and 4) secure data repositories will be used at all times.

DATA QUALITY

Data are reported to the NCDB from a variety of facilities—from very large academic/research institutions to medium and small sized community facilities. A great number of people trained in a variety of ways and coming to registry abstracting, coding and information systems work from a wide array of backgrounds are participating, directly or otherwise, in the submission of data to the NCDB. Because of the importance of these data, both for local review and use of the data and for broader aggregated cancer research, to promote the improvement of the quality of cancer care, data quality is essential. All reports, publication, and information disseminated using data entered into the NCDB are affected by their quality. Therefore, it is mandatory that the data be assessed on a regular basis to ensure their reliability. The primary method employed by the NCDB for doing this is the establishment and regular monitoring of the data quality scores and edit errors generated as part of the data submission process.

In addition to data edit reports, further studies must be performed to assess the impact of available data quality evaluation and monitoring tools that are currently applied to data reported to the NCDB. Various types of re-abstracting studies have been done to satisfy this need. However, additional statis-

tical approaches are being developed to monitor various parameters on an ongoing basis.

The data reporting and quality requirements set fourth in the CoC *Cancer Program Standards 2004* represent an ongoing commitment by the CoC to maintain quality assurance efforts by the NCDB. In addition, the introduction of a programmatic standard that case abstracting be performed or supervised by a CTR (Standard 3.1) is further demonstration of the CoC's recognition of the qualitative contribution certified cancer registry professionals bring to the task of accurate and consistent case abstracting and coding. Finally, the ongoing requirement that CoC-approved cancer programs conduct studies evaluating quality and outcomes (Standard 8.1) provide opportunities for cancer programs to document carefully designed and thoroughly executed internal reviews of the quality of registry data.

REPORTS AND PUBLICATIONS

Benchmark Reports

A set of Web-based Benchmarking applications have been developed to promote access to NCDB data by the general public, researchers, and clinicians. The benchmark reports have been released in two formats. One release is explicitly designed to facilitate public use. The other targeted for use by CoC-approved cancer programs as a tool by which to evaluate and compare the cancer care delivered to patients diagnosed and/or treated at their facility, these reports are provided as a direct benefit of their CoC approvals status.

The public benchmark reports are limited in scope to the eleven most commonly diagnosed and treated solid tumors in the United States. Users are provided access to data for six diagnosis years and can design queries using data from any one or a combination of three types of hospitals (small community, comprehensive community, and academic/teaching facilities), and specify a geographic region or state to narrow the scope of their analysis. As many as three co-variates (including patient age, ethnicity and sex; tumor histology and stage; first course therapy and type of surgical resection) are available for users to define the type of information they wish to review. No facility identifiers are included as part of this application, and queries which return aggregated data from fewer than 6 facilities are suppressed to ensure facility confidentiality. Since its release in mid-March of 2002, the public benchmark reports have been well received, on average, 80 queries per weekday are received. Breast cancer, followed by non-small cell lung cancer, colon, and prostate cancers are the most frequently reviewed disease sites and account for approximately two-thirds of all queries. These reports are updated annually as subsequent NCDB Call for Data cycles are completed.

Also available for public use is a companion survival reporting tool. This application provides site-specific AJCC stage stratified observed survival rates for the same 11 disease sites. Similar to the reports describing patient characteristics, tumor characteristics, and first course therapy the application allows users to specify the hospital type and geographic region of interest. Data from the two most recent diagnosis years (with available five-year follow-up data) are used to calculate the rates available in this application. This application attracts, on average, 40 queries per weekday. Breast cancer and non-small cell lung cancers are the most frequently queried disease sites.

The Hospital Comparison Benchmark Reports are similar in design to those reports available to the public, but provide authorized users with more options and control over the generation of desired reports. Access to these reports is limited to authorized persons affiliated with CoC-approved cancer programs. These reports contain data starting with the diagnosis year 2000 and have expanded as subsequent NCDB Call for Data cycles are completed. In contrast to the public benchmark reports described above, these reports include data on each of the NCDB analytic disease sites, with the exception of cancers of other and unspecified sites which are not included. Users are allowed greater control over the type of cases selected and have a longer list of co-variates from which to select. These include patient insurance status, an aggregate measure of median family income, tumor behavior, and more detailed information on the type of radiation and/or systemic therapy administered as part of the first course of therapy. While the public benchmark application only allow users to generate aggregate reports the Hospital Comparison reports provide users with three options: 1) show data reported to the NCDB from their own cancer registry; 2) show aggregated data; 3) display a comparative report that contains data reported from the users—hospital registry along side with aggregated data. Aggregated data can be provided based on the users selection of hospital characteristics. In addition, facilities which are part of cooperative or corporate systems, such as Veterans Administration hospitals, hospitals that are members of the Children's Oncology Group (COG), or a for-profit system of hospitals can compare their performance with that of other facilities in the same system. Specific geographical regions, either states or American Cancer Society Divisions, can also be used to further refine queries submitted to this application. Similar to the benchmark reports available to the public, breast, non-small cell lung, colon, and prostate are the most frequently queried cancers.

In addition, site-specific AJCC stage stratified observed survival rates for all disease sites are also available to authorized persons affiliated with CoC-approved cancer programs. Due to methodological restraints hospital specific survival rates are not provided as part of this application. In many instances the number of cases reported from any one hospital may be quite small, limiting the generalizability of the computed rates for many types of cancer. Work is ongoing to develop meaningful and useful hospital specific outcomes reports.

These "point and click" applications allow data to be displayed as tables, bar graphs, or pie charts. Hospitals can view their own data, and then compare their patient mix, treatment patterns, and outcomes to peer groups (facilities similar to their own) or to different types of facilities. They can also review state, region, or national norms for treatment patterns and outcomes. These reports should enable physicians and registrars at cancer treatment facilities to identify patterns of care in their own institution that differ significantly from patterns in similar institutions or differ from state, regional or national norms. Such information can be useful for identifying issues for quality improvement studies, a requirement of the *CoC Cancer Program Standards 2004* (Standard 8.1). The information may also be useful for planning and marketing purposes.

Publications

Over 250 peer-reviewed journal articles have been published using data submitted to the NCDB. Articles have broadly been focused on the clinical surveillance of patterns of care and outcomes for almost all disease sites. The CoC's Disease Site Teams are charged with the development and execution of focused surveillance and review projects. The analysis stemming from these projects will result in the publication of additional peer reviewed articles. The dissemination of information maintained by the NCDB is limited only by the number of reporting tools, analyses and publications that can be produced.

INTERACTIONS WITH OTHER NATIONAL ORGANIZATIONS

Due to its function as a database of reported cancer diagnoses, the NCDB interacts with a number of other groups and organizations. Integral to many of the functions performed by the NCDB is the wide array of relationships maintained with other organizations interested in the surveillance and epidemiology of cancer and cancer care in the United States. These interactions include NCDB and CoC staff participation in coordinated activities involving the American Joint Committee on Cancer (AJCC), ACS, the Canadian Association of Provincial Cancer Registries (CAPCR), the North American Association of Central Cancer Registries (NAACR), the National Cancer Registrars Association (NCRA), the National Program of Cancer Registries (NPCR) of the Centers for Disease Control, and the Surveillance, Epidemiology, and End Results (SEER) Program of the National Cancer Institute. Much, though by no means all, of the cancer surveillance inter-agency activity revolves around the setting of standards for data abstracting and recording and optimal cancer registry management practices.

In addition, membership in the CoC includes 37 national professional organizations. Exhibits have been prepared for display at various medical conventions in order to help promote the profile and work of the NCDB. NCDB staff serve as contact persons for a number of these organizations and are available at conventions to distribute NCDB materials and to answer questions from researchers and other potential users of the database. Among these national professional organizations are: American Society of Clinical Oncology (ASCO); American College of American Pathologists (CAP), Society of Surgical Oncology (SSO); The American College of Radiology (ACR); the American Society for Therapeutic Radiation and Oncology (ASTRO); as well as a number of surgical specialty societies.

One of the missions of the NCDB is to help educate groups and individuals concerned with the development and maintenance of better cancer registry data, and the use and impact of that data.

NCDB staff regularly schedule presentations to various organizations, including cancer registry data managers and other medical and oncology groups. These groups have the potential to use the information recorded in registry databases to manage and direct cancer care in facilities and cancer care centers.

SUMMARY

Since its inception in 1989, the NCDB has collected diagnostic, staging, treatment, and outcomes information on almost 15 million cancer diagnoses. These data have been published and reported on in several formats and have been used by clinicians and hospitals throughout the United States. The uses of the data are many and include significant advances in the utilization of the database as a clinical and facility benchmarking tool. As the database continues to grow and become more widely recognized, it will be used to an even greater extent. Its potential is abundant. With millions of case records at its disposal, the NCDB is enormous and provides a valuable resource for patterns of care information upon which quality improvement can be leveraged at the point of delivery of cancer care in the United States.

Further information is available through the NCDB webpage of the ACoS website at www.facs.org.

STUDY QUESTIONS

1. Name the two groups or bodies that provide the advisory structure for the NCDB and list their respective charges.
2. What tools does the NCDB employ to evaluate data quality in submitted records?
3. What is the formal mechanism instituted between the cancer programs and the ACoS to assure compliance with the privacy regulations?
4. Describe a "limited data set."
5. The NCDB annual Call for Data requests multiple years of data, describe what kind of data is represented in data submitted from "older" years.
6. Name two different methods of survival analysis.
7. Describe two features of the NCDB Hospital Comparison Reports.
8. For what purposes can a cancer program use benchmarking applications?

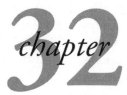

chapter 32

NORTH AMERICAN ASSOCIATION OF CENTRAL CANCER REGISTRIES, INC.

Holly L. Howe
PhD
Executive Director

HISTORY OF NAACCR

In the 1980s, a number of states passed legislation establishing population-based cancer registries. State programs were eager to follow guidelines and procedures of the Surveillance, Epidemiology, and End Results (SEER) Program of the National Cancer Institute (NCI) as this program was world-renowned for excellence in cancer registration. Many states implemented systems that, at a minimum, were able to produce basic surveillance statistics on newly diagnosed cancer patients for the state as a whole, and often for regions within the state (e.g., counties).

In response to the growing number of state registries, the National Cancer Institute (NCI) explored ways to support the new registries and to maximize the usefulness of the data collected across all jurisdictions. In 1987, Drs. Charles Smart and Edward Sondik of NCI convened a meeting with representatives from the American College of Surgeons (ACoS), the American Cancer Society (ACS), and the American Association of Cancer Institutes (AACI).[1] The purpose was to discuss how these organizations could benefit from and assist in the collection of population-based registry data. From that meeting, the American Association of Central Cancer Registries (AACCR) was born.

The first organizational meeting was hosted by ACoS in March 1988, to which representatives from all existing central registries in the United States were invited.[1] AACCR was envisioned as an organization in the U.S. modeled after the International Association of Cancer Registries, with a secretariat and support services provided by NCI. The assembled group endorsed the concept. State registries saw value and opportunity in sharing methods, procedures, and resource materials, and ultimately in improving the information derived from cancer incidence data throughout the United States. A president and five at-large representatives were elected to serve one year to establish bylaws and standing rules for the association. The National Tumor Registrars Association (now the National Cancer Registrars Association (NCRA) and the Association of Community Cancer Centers (ACCC)) joined the four original organizations (ACS, ACoS, AACI, and NCI) as the founding and sponsoring members of AACCR. The bylaws and standing rules were formally adopted in April 1989 at the second meeting of AACCR held in Chicago.

In 1992, AACCR became incorporated in the state of California as AACCR, Inc., a non-profit organization with 501c(3) status. In 1994, the association officially changed its name to the North American Association of Central Cancer Registries, Inc. (NAACCR) to better reflect its broadening membership among the provincial and territorial registries in Canada. Additional national organizations joined as sponsoring members: the American Joint Committee on Cancer (AJCC), the Centers for Disease Control and Prevention (CDC), Statistics Canada, Health Canada, and in 2002, the Canadian Association of Provincial Cancer Agencies (CAPCA). In the late 1990s, ACCC and AACI dropped their membership.

In 1991, NAACCR and CDC began a cooperative agreement to explore the quality and utility of cancer registry data for cancer control initiatives. Through this project, NAACCR partnered with the California Public Health Foundation for fiscal, administrative, and personnel services. The CDC support also enabled support for several other NAACCR activities: the development of uniform cancer registration standards for data collection and of guidelines for registry operations and the printing and distribution of an annual statistical monograph developed by NAACCR volunteers. The statistical publication launched NAACCR into assessment of data quality and implementation of standard approaches in compiling incidence statistics. In 1995, in support of the CDC's National Program of Cancer Registries (NPCR), NAACCR competed for continuing support as a contract for training and quality assurance activities. Through these resources, NAACCR was able to assist both the new NPCR program at CDC and US population-based registries that were not in the SEER program. In the same year, a contract was also awarded to NAACCR by NCI to provide training and quality assurance activities to registries in the SEER program. Both contracts were awarded to the California Public Health Foundation on behalf of NAACCR.

By 1998, NAACCR had matured sufficiently as an organization to act as its own financial agent. The relationship with the California Public Health Foundation was severed and NAACCR competed independently for a CDC cooperative agreement to provide infrastructure support for the organization. In May 1999, an executive director was hired and an executive office was opened in Springfield, Illinois.

By 2002, NAACCR had nine staff and agreements with private consultants for an additional 1.5 full-time equivalents. With this infrastructure, the Secretariat role, provided by NCI, was changed and the Executive Director became an *ex officio* member of the Board and the Executive Office assumed many of the duties of the Secretariat. The bylaws restated the purpose of the organization in 2002 to more accurately embrace its mission: a professional group to develop and promote uniform data standards for cancer registration; provide education and training; certify population-based registries; aggregate and publish data from central cancer registries; and promote the use of cancer surveillance data and systems for cancer control and epidemiologic research, public health programs, and patient care to reduce the burden of cancer in North America.

MEMBERSHIP

All population-based central cancer registries in the United States and Canada are NAACCR members. Membership consists primarily of population-based cancer registries, although four membership categories are available: full, sponsor, sustaining, and individual. Full member organizations are central registries which are population-based registries. Sponsoring members are national organizations involved in cancer control prevention or research. Sustaining members are organizations interested in promoting the purposes of the Association. Individual members are persons who are not currently working in a member organization, but who have demonstrated career and professional commitments and interests that are consistent with or complementary to NAACCR.

NAACCR STRUCTURE

The bylaws and standing rules define NAACCR structure. Although the composition has changed over the years, an elected Board of Directors governs NAACCR. The Board includes the President, President-elect [or Past-president], Treasurer, six Representatives-at-Large, one Sponsoring Member Organization representative, and the Executive Director, as an *ex officio* member. All board members serve a two-year term, except the President-elect and the Past-president, who each serve for one year.

The work of the organization is conducted primarily through an extensive committee structure including 13 standing committees, various sub-committees, *ad hoc* committees, work groups, special task forces, and research groups. Figure 32-1 summarizes the organizational relationship of the Board of Directors, sponsoring members, standing committees, and the executive office. The activities of each standing committee are defined by the standing rules and are:

- *Bylaws:* receives and reviews all proposed amendments to the Bylaws.
- *Data Evaluation and Publication:* gathers data from member organizations, reviews the data, and prepares a publication of cancer incidence and mortality data for North America.
- *Data Use and Confidentiality:* addresses issues related to confidentiality, data use, and privacy legislation.
- *Education:* determines the educational needs of the Association and proposes methods to meet the needs.
- *Information and Technology:* develops the format for exchange of data among members and for the standards to ensure the security and accuracy of transmitted data.
- *Membership:* reviews and approves applications for membership
- *Nominating:* secures candidates for the office of President-Elect, Treasurer, and Representatives-at-Large.
- *Program:* plans the technical program for the Annual Conference.
- *Public Relations and Communications:* compiles and releases the NAACCR newsletter.
- *Registry Certification:* establishes objective certification standards; implements and oversees an annual process to evaluate data collected by central cancer registries; and conducts an annual recognition of those registries meeting certification standards.
- *Registry Operations:* discusses methodological issues relevant to policies, procedures, and operational methods of a central cancer registry and provides models and guidelines for their implementation.
- *Uniform Data Standards:* provides a formal mechanism for reviewing and recommending consensus on proposed changes in data codes or

Figure 32-1
North American Association of Central Cancer Registries (NAACCR) Organization Relationship 2003-2004

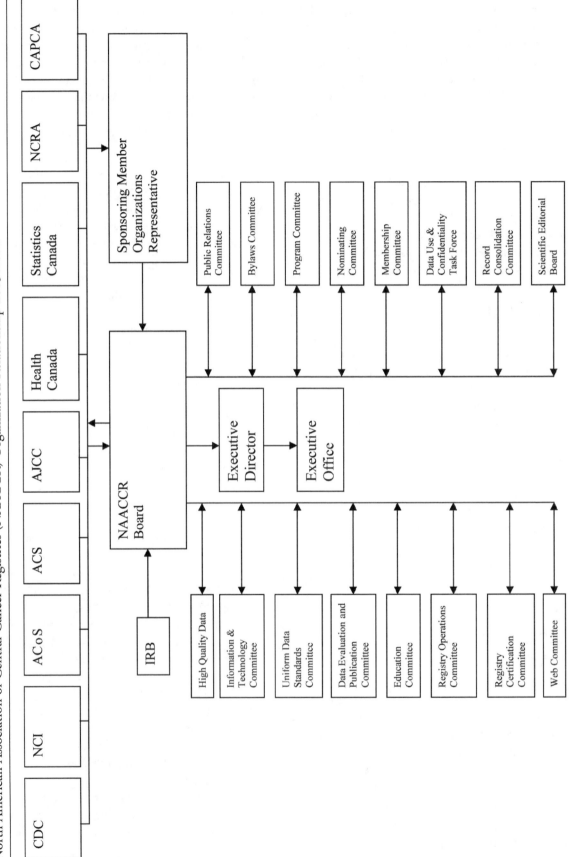

the addition of new items and data edits submitted by NAACCR members to ensure that data remain comparable among all cancer registries, both population- and hospital-based.

- *Web:* oversees and directs the content, format, and functionality of the NAACCR website.

NAACCR GOALS AND OBJECTIVES

In the mid 1990s, NAACCR instituted a management-by-objectives approach to running the organization. The Board of Directors define the major goals of the organization and standing committees develop, and ultimately execute, specific objectives. The goals and objectives have a five-year time frame; they are monitored; and progress and accomplishments are noted annually at the NAACCR business meeting. A current list of goals, objectives, and accomplishments since 1999 are posted on the NAACCR website (www.naaccr.org).

In addition to the five-year goals, short-term, two-year overarching issues are routinely identified by the NAACCR Board and standing committee chairs. Resolution of these overarching needs often requires special task forces involving representatives from all types of NAACCR members and multiple NAACCR committees. During the first two-year cycle, 2001-2002, six priorities were identified and resolution of all six was achieved. The six priorities for the next two-year cycle beginning 2003 are:

1) The need to move toward electronic, real time case reporting from all reporting sources that includes demographic information, disease codes, and pathology results. (Highest Priority)
2) The need to develop guidelines for designating, organizing, and managing the task forces addressing implementation of new or revised standards. (Highest Priority)
3) The insufficient numbers of qualified staff for employment in cancer registries, including both a pool of qualified CTRs and low recruitment into the cancer information management field, and the increasing complexity of the work that has raised the job requirements to a level higher than current job titles, pay scales, and the pool of potential job candidates (even those with a CTR). (Higher Priority)

4) The need to improve interagency collaboration. (Higher Priority)
5) The identification of a method to improve timely implementation of standards revisions and recommendations for best practices registry operations. (High Priority)
6) The value of minimum cancer incidence data set for public health surveillance and if valuable, the variables that should be included. (High Priority)

MAJOR NAACCR ACTIVITIES

The activities of the organization are tied to its goals, objectives, and ultimately its mission statement. The five major groups of activities are:

1. Establish and maintain a consensus of standards for data definitions, variable codes, data exchange formats, measures to assess data quality, and data presentation. The initial thrust of NAACCR was to standardize data definitions, variables, codes, and exchange formats to provide all registries with guidelines and tools to enable collaboration and information exchange and to maximize data comparability. Now, all US cancer registries use standardized record layouts, data definitions, and codes. Standardization activities in the early 1990s expanded to include by 2000 standards for data aggregation, data presentation, and definition of high-quality registry data outcomes.

By the late 1990s, the need for registry operational guidelines was recognized. NAACCR supports the concept that there can be more than one approach to operate a quality registry program; however, it also recognizes that some processes are better and more efficient than others. The guidelines needed to balance a single best practice approach with an awareness of the variety of organizations, structures, laws, and administrative codes that contribute to each registry's uniqueness. The Procedure Guidelines for Registry Operations embraces both concepts. The guidelines are a compendium of procedures for specific registry operations written by work groups of volunteers. About two guidelines are completed each year. To date, these have included, among others, interstate data exchange, case ascertainment, a geographic information system (GIS) Handbook, and death certificate clearance operations.

2. Train and educate registry staff. A variety of education and training opportunities are offered each year. Traditional workshops include regional programs on the fundamentals of central cancer registry operations; an annual program on data processing and electronic data management tools; and programs offered in conjunction with the annual NAACCR meeting, SEER*Stat and SEER*Prep training, an advanced course that addresses topical issues, and a central cancer registries course focusing on design, management and use. Depending on the host and location of the annual meeting, other training opportunities have been offered on topics of interest, e.g., record linkage, medical informatics, or GIS and geocoding, to name themes of recent seminars.

In 2001, NAACCR members developed a four-day course on cancer surveillance, the Cancer Surveillance Institute (CSI). Graduate programs in epidemiology have not to date included curricula on surveillance approaches and methods. Registries report that on-the-job training has been the sole approach to prepare staff to use cancer registry data in routine surveillance activities. The CSI has already expanded into two week-long courses: CSI I will be devoted to Principles and Public Health Applications and CSI II, to Methods and Statistical Approaches. The first CSI II was offered in the spring of 2004.

The NAACCR Education committee has recently focused on training approaches with wider accessibility by not requiring time away from the registry or a travel budget to obtain continuing education. NAACCR has implemented a Mentor Fellowship Program for one-on-one training opportunities to support travel costs for a mentor or a trainee to obtain individualized training on specific registry operation issues. To enhance on-site training opportunities, NAACCR is developing a series of CD-ROMs on central cancer registry operations. All CDs will be widely distributed to central cancer registries for use in local and staff training programs.

3. Certify registries that meet national data quality standards for producing accurate cancer statistics. In 1997, NAACCR instituted a review of member registries for their ability to produce complete, accurate, and timely cancer incidence information. NAACCR registry certification began as an internal process, replacing subjective registry assessments with objective metrics of data quality and completeness. Certificates are awarded to registries that meet the Gold or Silver standards for the data year under evaluation. Specific certification criteria are described in detail on the NAACCR website (www.naaccr.org/filesystem/pdf/finalcriteriaforRegistryCertificationPage.pdf, last accessed November 19, 2003).

From 1997 through 2003, certified registries increased from 23 to 54 throughout the United States and Canada, as shown in Figure 32-2. As part of the annual program, registries are provided individualized feedback on their data submissions and provided detailed output on all certification criteria. It has been a very successful program, recognized internationally and by many entities, including the US Congress, that NAACCR certification is a benchmark of a quality cancer registry program.

4. Evaluate and publish data from member registries. In 2003, NAACCR is working on its 14th annual release of the statistical monograph, *Cancer in North America.* The monograph includes both incidence and mortality statistics for each member registry, as well as combined statistics for the United States, Canada, and North America from registries that meet NAACCR standards of high quality. Data files are submitted voluntarily and evaluated for completeness and quality using standard methods and metrics. Individualized feedback is provided to all registries on common data quality issues, in addition to those that are unique to a registry. When requested, NAACCR staff will work with registries to explain results and to identify operations or methods that could enhance their data in future years.

5. Promote the use of registry data. Data quality, including validity, reliability, and completeness, has improved dramatically since 1987 through the efforts of NAACCR, federal programs in the United States and Canada. These efforts have included extensive training of cancer registrars and allied workers in cancer registries both in reporting facilities and population-based centers. In 1995, Dr. Calum Muir remarked, at the NAACCR annual meeting in San Francisco, that he would prefer "islands of excellence rather than a sea of mediocrity." The maps in Figure 32-2 clearly show that North America is achieving, perhaps what was unthinkable in earlier years, but by 2003 what is feasible, and that is, a sea of excellence. With this achievement comes a responsibility to increase and enhance the uses of cancer registry data. NAACCR produces annually several products from the data submitted, evaluated, and aggregated by the Data and Evaluation Publication Committee. In addition to *Cancer Incidence in North America (CINA),*

Figure 32-2
NAACR Certification for 1995 and 2000

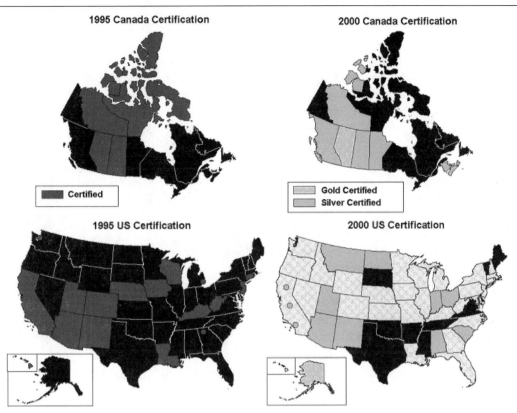

NAACCR also produces *CINA+ Online,* an interactive, flexible, query system on the NAACCR website. This online data resource can be accessed by the public for specific cancer information by year, geography, sex, race, cancer type, age, and by any combination of these variables. Registries are included at their choice and when they meet NAACCR high quality data standards. Data are updated annually with the most recent five-year interval (e.g., 1997-2001 in 2004).

An analytic data file, known as *CINA Deluxe,* may be requested by NAACCR individual researchers or by NAACCR committees engaged in multi-registry research or surveillance projects. NAACCR has developed a detailed set of protocols for users to access the data file, that provide assurances of data security and data confidentiality. Patients' right to privacy is always balanced with the valuable information contained in the file that can be very useful to a growing number of qualified researchers interested in this analytic resource.

NAACCR also organizes special research groups, inviting interested persons to collaborate in producing a set of research and surveillance papers on a particular topic. In the last two years, a monograph on descriptive epidemiology of ovarian cancer has been produced as has a set of manuscripts on breast cancer topics. In addition, a NAACCR research group released a statistical monograph in 2003 on cancer incidence among US Hispanics/Latinos, with information that covers more than 86% of this large and rapidly growing population. The CINA data set enabled ovarian cancer studies that were based on the largest data set of ovarian cancer cases ever assembled, featuring analyses of some rare aspects of this disease such as pediatric ovarian tumors, multiple primaries involving the ovary, and ovarian tumors of borderline (low) malignant potential.

RESOURCES AND SUPPORT FOR ACTIVITIES

Since 1987, NAACCR has provided valuable services and resources to central cancer registries and the entire cancer surveillance community. Because of this, in addition to the outstanding leadership that the organization has been fortunate to attract to elected positions and the breadth of volunteers that commit their time and energy to the activities of the organization, NAACCR has grown and has been successful. Further, cancer registry staff (the people most knowledgeable about the issues) participate in all NAACCR activities: standards development; training; and data aggregation, evaluation, and publication. This participation has had a significant impact on the success of the organization. In 2002, 70 members (of 141 member organizations) had 214 different representatives participating on NAACCR committees, work groups, and task forces, and these numbers grow every year

While NAACCR depends and thrives on its active member participation, it has also been successful in obtaining grants, contracts, and other awards that have enabled many of NAACCR's current activities. Member dues represents a very small proportion of the resources available for NAACCR activities. Sponsoring member organizations not only support the organization through their higher

dues structure, but also through their in-kind contributions to support specific activities. NCI and CDC provide substantial financial support to developing and maintaining the infrastructure, services, and resources that NAACCR provides to the cancer registration community.

STUDY QUESTIONS

1. What four membership categories are available for NAACCR?
2. Name the members of the Board of Directors that governs NAACCR.
3. Name two major groups of activities of NAACCR.

REFERENCES

1. Seiffert J, Young JL. The North American Association of Central Cancer Registries. In Hutchison CL, Roffers SD, Fritz AG, eds. *Cancer Registry Management Principles & Practice.* Dubuque, Iowa: Kendall/Hunt Publishing Company; 1997.

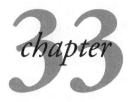

chapter 33

THE SURVEILLANCE, EPIDEMIOLOGY, AND END RESULTS PROGRAM

Carol Hahn Johnson
BS, CTR

PURPOSE

The Surveillance, Epidemiology, and End Results (SEER) Program of the National Cancer Institute (NCI) is an authoritative source of information on cancer incidence and survival in the United States. Prior to 2001, SEER collected and published cancer incidence and survival data from 11 population-based cancer registries and three supplemental registries covering 14% of the United States population. In 2001, four expansion registries were added to the SEER coverage area increasing the coverage to approximately 26%. Because quality control has been an integral part of the SEER program since its inception, the SEER program is considered to be the standard for quality among cancer registries around the world. SEER statistics are frequently quoted in the media and in scientific journals because the SEER database is recognized as the most authoritative source of cancer statistics in the United States.

This national program provides a vital, dynamic measurement of progress in cancer prevention and control. It provides guidance for an array of research, prevention, diagnosis, treatment, and planning efforts. The SEER Program staff act as liaisons and coordinate activities with a number of other organizations involved in cancer surveillance and related disciplines. Activities include setting standards for data collection by cancer registries, providing for the interchange of ideas and tools for cancer surveillance, training and providing educational materials for the credentialing of cancer registrars, leading workshops to provide advanced training in data collection and coding, collaborating in the analysis and reporting of cancer rates, and supporting efforts to expand existing cancer surveillance and to establish new cancer reporting systems.

HISTORY

The National Cancer Institute (NCI) allocated 10% of its initial funding for cancer surveillance in 1937. That funding was used for the "Ten Cities Study" that measured the impact of the national cancer problem using data obtained in 10-selected United States cities. This study later became known as the First National Cancer Survey. The Ten Cities Study was repeated in 1947 (Second National Cancer Survey), and the Third National Cancer Survey (TNCS) was done from 1969 to1971.

The NCI sponsored the End Results Group from 1956 through 1972. The End Results Group was a set of medical school affiliated hospitals throughout the United States. Those hospitals collected survival data on cancer patients diagnosed or treated at their facility.

The National Cancer Act of 1971 launched the nation's "War on Cancer." The act directed the NCI to collect, analyze, and disseminate all data useful in the prevention, diagnosis, and treatment of cancer and report those findings to congress. In an effort to accelerate, enhance, and focus the national cancer effort, a committee of experts recommended collecting both population-based cancer incidence and survival data for the same set of patients on a continuous basis. The SEER Program was established based on that recommendation. SEER was organized from the two earlier NCI programs: the Third National Cancer Survey and the End Results Group.

REPORTING AREAS

SEER Case ascertainment began on January 1, 1973 in the states of Connecticut, Iowa, New Mexico, Utah, and Hawaii and the metropolitan areas of Detroit and San Francisco-Oakland. The metropolitan area of Atlanta and the black rural counties in Georgia were added in 1974-1975, followed in 1980 by the American Indians residing in Arizona. Three additional geographic areas participated in the SEER program prior to 1990: New Orleans, Louisiana (1974-1997; rejoined 2001); New Jersey (1979-1989, rejoined 2001); and Puerto Rico (1973-1989). The NCI also began funding a cancer registry that, with technical assistance from SEER, collects information on cancer cases among Alaska Native populations residing in Alaska. In 1992, SEER added Los Angeles County and four counties in the San Jose-Monterey area south of San Francisco. That expansion increased the coverage of minority populations, especially Hispanics. In 2001, the SEER Program underwent their largest expansion to date. The expansion registries are: The states of Kentucky, Louisiana and New Jersey and Greater California (the regions that did not have an existing SEER contract).

The SEER registry programs are shown on the United States map in Figure 33-1.

Figure 33-1
Cancer Registration in the U.S.—2000

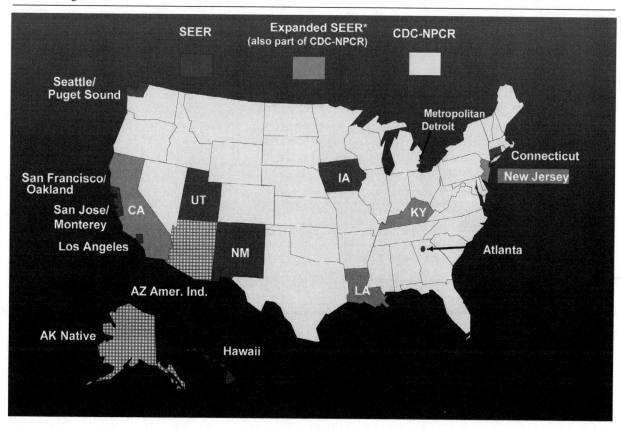

The SEER Program areas were selected for their coverage of populations for which limited data existed, and data quality that meets SEER standards and reporting requirements. For demographic and epidemiologic purposes, the SEER registries are reasonably representative subsets of the United States population. In 2001, they represent about 26% of the United States population, over 65 million people. The SEER areas represent an over-sampling of most minority groups in the United States as shown in Figure 33-2.

By the end of 1999, the national SEER database contained information on over three million cases diagnosed since 1973. Approximately 171,430 new cases are accessioned annually.

GOALS

The SEER Program goals reflect the many aspects and efforts used to measure progress against the cancer burden in the United States.[1] The scope and capabilities of the program are far-reaching. The goals are listed in Table 33-1.

DATA COLLECTION

The SEER Program registry contracts are with nonprofit, medically oriented organizations. The responsibilities of those organizations include casefinding and other duties as shown in Table 33-2.

The registry members collect data on initially diagnosed and treated in situ and malignant neoplasms within their geographic area. Data on newly diagnosed cases include patient demographics, primary site, morphology, diagnostic confirmation, extent of disease, the first course of cancer directed therapy, and death certificate-coded underlying cause of death. Patients are followed on an annual basis from diagnosis to death.

The data set sent to the NCI SEER Program from the registry has no patient identifiers. Once the SEER program receives data, incidence data are

Figure 33-2
SEER Coverage Before/After Expansion

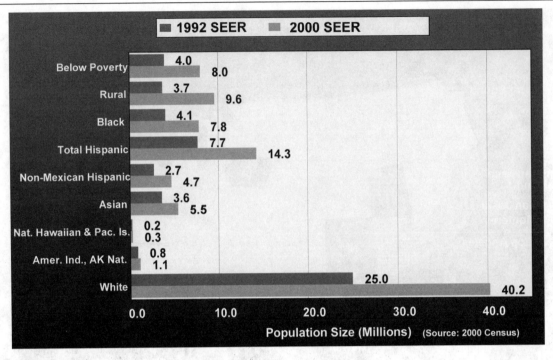

Source: 2000 Census

Table 33-1
Goals of the Surveillance, Epidemiology, and End Results (SEER) Program

- Assemble estimates of cancer incidence, survival, and mortality in the United States, which will be published in the "Report to The Nation."
- Monitor annual cancer incidence trends to identify patterns of cancer occurring in population subgroups defined by geographic and demographic characteristics.
- Provide continuing information on changes over time in the extent of disease at diagnosis, trends in therapy, and associated changes in patient survival.
- Promote studies to identify factors that can be studied and applied to achieve cancer prevention and control such as environmental, occupational, socioeconomic, dietary, and other exposures; screening practices, early detection, and treatment; and determinants of the length and quality of patient survival.
- Promote specialty training in epidemiology, biostatistics, and cancer registry methodology, operations and management.
- Promote research studies measuring progress in cancer control that link information from the biomedical and social sciences.

analyzed along with data on cancer-related deaths from the National Center for Health Statistics. SEER uses this information to determine representative national cancer incidence, mortality, and survival rates by using the data items: primary site, race, sex, age at diagnosis, extent of disease at diagnosis (stage), and other variables. An updated report on cancer trends is prepared and distributed annually in

NCI's *SEER Cancer Statistics Review,* SEER's most visible and frequently consulted publication.[2]

Quality Improvement

SEER's commitment to the quality of its database, field operations, and central management was established in the earliest days of the program.[3] Field

Table 33-2

Responsibilities of Contractors for the Surveillance, Epidemiology, and End Results (SEER) Program

- Maintain a cancer reporting system and abstracted information for resident cancer patients seeking healthcare in facilities in and outside the coverage area.
- Review all death certificates on which cancer is listed as a cause of death for residents dying inside and outside the coverage area.
- Search records of private pathology laboratories, cancer treatment centers, radiation therapy units, nursing homes, health services units that provide diagnostic services, physician providers, and organizations that render extended care and hospice services to ensure complete ascertainment of cancer cases.

monitoring, quality assurance audits, workshops, and liaisons with other government agencies and professional organizations all contribute to the quality of the SEER program. SEER conducts three types of audits: casefinding, reabstraction of data, and reliability studies. The casefinding audits measure the registry compliance with the SEER goal of 95% case ascertainment. Auditors review case finding sources at the hospitals in the region and compare those findings with the regional registry's database. SEER does a random selection of cases for the reabstracting audits. The results of the audits are compared to SEER goals for accuracy on a data item basis. The reabstracting audits measure the quality of the data in the SEER database. All of the abstractors and coders in each registry complete ten abstracts based on the same medical records.

The results of the abstraction and reconciliation measure compliance and comprehension of SEER rules and codes. The results of all of these studies are used to improve the SEER coding manuals, write coding guidelines, and plan educational workshops throughout the following year. The registries are audited one year; the following year is dedicated to quality improvement, identifying any areas that need clarification or revision and producing products to achieve quality improvement. Detailed reports of field studies provide guidance to each member registry including measures of data quality useful in local program management. Each member registry program is responsible for maintaining the integrity and quality of the data. This includes visual and computer edits, periodic casefinding audits to assess completeness of reporting, and reabstracting or recoding audits to assess overall data reliability.

SEER Data Standards

Over the many years of the SEER Program, data standards have been established and the importance

of achieving and maintaining the standards has been impressed upon the registries. SEER standards for various components of a registry's operation are shown in Table 33-3.

Follow-up percentage rates are calculated for all malignant and in situ cases, excluding in situ cervical cancer cases, using all available methods to attain an overall successful followup rate of at least 95%. The standard for those younger than 65 is 85%. Meeting the standard for the group of patients who were less than 20 years of age at diagnosis has proven to be difficult as this is a more mobile group.

An important aspect of completeness is assessing the quality of case ascertainment in hospitals, which have been the primary source of case identification for many years. The registries have state or region specific standards for casefinding in non-hospital settings such as private pathology laboratories, physician's offices and facilities providing same-day health care services both inside and outside the coverage area. Death Certificate Only (DCO) rates are calculated

Table 33-3

Surveillance, Epidemiology, and End Results Program Standards for Various Components of a Registry's Operation

Components	Standard (%)
Follow-up rate:	
All ages	95
20-64 years old	85
<20 years old	85
Case ascertainment rate (hospital)	98
Death certificate only rate (after followback)	1.5

after follow-back attempts have been exhausted. The DCO standard of 1.5% is based on historical efforts (for nearly twenty years) of diligently tracking the cancer information found on the death certificates for cases not previously registered.

Timely reporting is extremely important. One measure of timeliness is to calculate the percentage increase in the number of cases reported for a given calendar year in successive data submissions. The percentage increase or decrease by primary site, along with screening and early detection trends, can help explain changes in cancer incidence. Incidence rate increases for breast and prostate cancer over the past few years have been directly linked to early detection techniques including mammography screening and testing for prostate-specific antigen (PSA).

Data Utilization

SEER data are accessed directly and indirectly by thousands of people each year in printed and computer formats.[4] Incidence, mortality, and survival data are available using various electronic media, including data tapes, diskettes, CD-ROMs, and the Internet. In addition, member registry programs respond to requests for data in printed or computer form and will provide either published or unpublished data representing local aspects of their SEER data. Researchers and health professionals have uti-

lized SEER data for a variety of projects as listed in Table 33-4.

Medical and public health researchers have used SEER data to identify risk groups for research and public health intervention programs. These efforts are shown in Table 33-5.

Many voluntary and advocacy organizations use SEER data to establish program priorities, plan legislative and policy campaigns, and assist in the production of their own cancer statistics. The American Cancer Society uses SEER data to create its statistical reports, including annual state-by-state incidence projections.

The media frequently consult SEER data for background information. SEER findings are newsworthy, and reporters and editors use SEER data to verify cancer incidence and survival statistics and to decide whether to report local cancer trends.

The lay public, including patients, often request information. The callers to NCI's Cancer Information Service (1-800-4-CANCER) receive incidence, treatment, and survival information provided by the SEER Program. The information is also available though NCI's electronic mail (CancerNet) or by facsimile (CancerFax).

International public health organizations use SEER data in their efforts to respond to changing cancer incidence patterns worldwide. Every five

Table 33-4
Variety of Projects Using Surveillance, Epidemiology, and End Results (SEER) Data

- Data have been used as the foundation for studies of changing cancer incidence in immigrant populations and to identify patient variations in cancer risk and survival that are associated with racial, socioeconomic, and urban-rural differences.
- Data have been reviewed when investigating potential links between cancer incidence and a variety of occupational, environmental, and lifestyle-related exposures. Examples are the continuation of cigarette smoking and exposure to chemical dyes that have been implicated as risks for bladder cancer. Among women, the relationships of oral contraceptives, estrogen replacement therapy, and childbearing behaviors to breast cancer have been the subjects of extensive investigation.
- Researchers have also used SEER data to study patterns and outcomes of cancer patient care and to determine the extent to which the general medical community has adopted state-of-the-art cancer treatments.
- Physicians and cancer registrars in hospitals across the country have used SEER data and information in patient management conferences and other groups. Oncologists and other healthcare providers treating cancer patients and cancer survivors often consult SEER data in their daily practice. Medical, public health, and nursing students have been instructed on cancer incidence and survival by SEER sources.
- Researchers and analysts at pharmaceutical and biotechnology firms have used SEER data to guide decisions on cancer-related programs.

Table 33-5

Uses of Surveillance, Epidemiology, and End Results (SEER) Program Data to Identify Risk Groups for Research and Public Health Intervention Programs

- A series of studies suggesting a possible link between cancer and agricultural exposures to pesticides and other agents, culminating in a large-scale investigation of health status, including cancers among farmers
- A national public awareness campaign to combat smokeless tobacco use among adolescents, aimed at educating the public about tobacco-related cancers of the oral cavity and pharynx
- An investigation of illness-related behavior and coexisting disease in older patients with breast, ovarian, cervical, colon, stomach, bladder, and prostate cancers, exploring how chronic diseases such as diabetes, hypertension, and heart disease influence cancer treatment and demonstrating that cancer is frequently treated less aggressively in older patients
- A project that uses SEER data with AIDS case information to describe patterns of cancer incidence, survival, treatment, and other factors among AIDS patients and HIV-infected individuals

---

years, the International Agency for Research on Cancer publishes *Cancer Incidence in Five Continents* and the SEER Program contributes their member programs' data.

SEER PUBLICATIONS

The numerous SEER publications provide valuable resources for the cancer registrar. They can be used for making data comparisons such as age-specific rates and survival statistics. SEER publications are available for use as educational and training materials, morphologic and extent of disease (stage) references, and for registry management including operational data standards. Publications and SEER data are available in a variety of electronic media formats including data tapes, diskettes, CDROMs, and the Internet.[5] Registrars can order available publications on the website.

SEER Stat

The SEER STATCD is available on the website. It contains the public use data file and programs to select data sets and compute survival rates.

SUMMARY

Since 1973, the Surveillance, Epidemiology, and End Results Program has evolved into a national resource and treasure that is used by many people in the United States and throughout the world. Public-use data are available through various electronic media at no cost to those who request the information. Because of the SEER Program, scientists, the

media, the public, and healthcare providers concerned about cancer can measure and report progress, and plan, and target areas for study and intervention. SEER provides an important component in solving the mysteries surrounding cancer and assists in conquering the disease.

Publications are available from SEER by writing to the SEER Program. NCI/DCPC/CCRP/CSB, EPN 343J, 6130 Executive Boulevard, MSC 7352 Bethesda, Maryland 20892-7352. Facsimile: 301-496-9949.

STUDY QUESTIONS

1. What does the acronym SEER stand for?
2. On what date did the SEER Program begin case ascertainment?
3. What is the SEER follow-up rate for cases in which the patient was less than 20 years of age at the time of diagnosis?
4. Which SEER publications would serve as useful resources for cancer registrars?
5. What is the death certificate only (DCO) rate, after followback, allowable for SEER registries?

REFERENCES

1. National Cancer Institute. *Measuring Progress Against Cancer, 20th Anniversary Publication.* Bethesda, Md: The Institute; 1993.
2. Ries LAG, Miller BA, Hankey BF, Kosary CL, Harras A, Edward BK, eds. *Annual Cancer Statistics Review 1973-1992.* Bethesda, Md: National Cancer Institute; 1995.

3. Menck HR, Smart CR, eds. *Central Cancer Registries: Design, Management, and Use.* Langhorn, Penn: Harwood Academic Publishers; 1994.

4. Harras A. Tapping the SEER database. *Cancer Practice.* 1995; 3(3).

5. Shambaugh EM, ed. *SEER Self-Instructional Manuals for Tumor Registrars,* books 1-8. Bethesda, Md: National Cancer Institute; 1977-1999.

6. Percy C, ed. Histology of cancer incidence and prognosis: SEER population-based data, 1973-1987. *CANCER Supplement.* 1995; 75(1).

chapter 34 | CENTRAL CANCER REGISTRIES

Herman R. Menck
MBA, CDP

Jerri Linn Phillips
MA, CTR

INTRODUCTION

Central cancer registries have much in common with hospital registries. This chapter addresses unique aspects of central registries, including types and administration, data set planning, data collection, computerization, quality management, follow-up, incidence and survival rates, other uses, and history of central registries.[1-4] Central registries are, by definition multi-hospital and either population-based[5-7] or hospital (not population-based).[8-12] Numerous non-US population-based registries are also in operation.[13-16]

TYPES OF CENTRAL REGISTRIES

Central registries are definitively described by a combination of primary characteristics including goals and objectives, population coverage, data set used, data recipient, organizational setting, and source of funding.[17-20]

Goals and Objectives:

The goals and objectives of registries include various components:

1) incidence surveillance, such as monitoring incidence rates and trends by age, sex, and race/ethnic group;

2) survival surveillance, such as contributing to the annual SEER survival statistics;[21-23]

3) analytic research, such as contributing cases to be interviewed for etiologic case-control studies;[24]

4) clinical research, such as contributing cases to clinical trials;

5) patient care surveillance, such as contributing case information to national studies of patterns of care;[25-26]

6) professional education for clinicians and others;[27]

7) enumeration of caseload statistics (for administrative and planning purposes) such as Cancer Facts and Figures.[28]

These goals can be focused at the local (state) level, and/or the national level through data submittal to a national data collector such as SEER.[5]

Population Coverage:

Most central registries are population-based and are regional, state, multistate, or national. Ambiguity exists in the use of the term *central,* with some users meaning population-based only when they say central, and others including non-population-based central registries within the term central registry. The geographic area from which the population source of the central registry is drawn is sometimes referred to as its catchment area.

Population-based registries include all cancer cases in a defined geographic area (for example, the state of Illinois) allowing the calculation of incidence and mortality rates. These rates include all cases which are diagnosed in the population at risk. The population from which the cases are derived must be explicitly determined from census or related data. It also means that a case reported from multiple hospitals must be consolidated into one record and only counted once.

Some population-based registries operate at the incidence only level, others are more multipurpose. Incidence-only registries have as their primary goal determination of cancer rates in different groups of people living in their defined geographic area. Various surveillance activities are enabled including the tracking of cancer trends in the population. Necessary requirements include an accurate and complete case count; reasonable timeliness, ranging from nine to twenty-four months after the close of the calendar year; quality control of casefinding and abstracting; and data necessary to categorize patients and tumors into groups for which rates are computed. For these registries, there are generally no treatment data or outcome data. The incidence-only registry provides incidence and trend data for a specific geographic area in order to assess the burden of cancer in that specific geographic area. For example, it has become common for government health agencies to evaluate cancer clusters and suspected cancer problems related to possible environmental contamination using such registry data.

Some population-based registries serve multiple purposes such as combining incidence reporting with survival results, patient care, and various other research and cancer-control activities.[29]

Often the primary objective of a registry supporting epidemiologic research is to get the notification of eligible study subjects to the study manager for survey or questionnaire as quickly as possible.[30] Therefore, the case ascertainment must be ascertained rapidly. Sometimes this necessitates the utilization of a pathology report preceding the slower, traditional medical record-based process. This is often referred to as rapid case ascertainment. An advantage of research derived from population-based patient rosters is the reduction or avoidance of selection bias in casefinding for both demographic and tumor classification purposes. Incomplete casefinding is undesirable because it compromises the generalization of results.

Some central registries are not population-based, but are multihospital registries. Examples of these would be all hospitals using a particular software package or related professional services. Several suppliers of data systems and services pool the data of their client institutions into a single file that can be used for comparative purposes.[8-9] These databases are characterized by the geographic dispersion of their particular clients, but are not representative of all patients in the geographic area.

Another example of a non-population-based central registry is formed by all hospitals which choose to participate in the National Cancer Data Base of the Commission on Cancer.[10] Its data for 1992 included a convenience sample of approximately 53% of US incident (newly diagnosed) cancer cases. Its total case file includes over 3,000,000 cases accessioned from 1985 through 1992.

Some registries operate as central repositories for hospitals from one or more of the military services or the Veterans Administration. An example of one of these military central registries is the Department of Defense, which uses ACTUR[12] as its cancer-reporting software.

Data Sets:

Data set definitions are discussed in greater detail in another chapter of this textbook. Data sets are predominantly influenced by what data are necessary to meet the goals and objectives of the registry, and what available data set standards may prevail.

Data Submittal:

Central registries generally submit their data to some national collection of data. These national data collections are generally maintained by a primary funding source or sponsoring organization. The SEER program's collection of population-based data, and the National Cancer Data Base's[10] collection of hospital data are by far the largest and most well established data bases that have multi-regional, or national coverage. The National Program of Cancer Registries (NPCR) is establishing multi-regional

data collection, and will be a rich national source of information in the future.[6] Thus, a central population-based registry might be a SEER registry, and/or an NPCR registry.

Organization Setting/Funding Source:

A legislative mandate often empowers a central registry to establish and maintain their mechanism for cancer data collection and related surveillance activities, and provides some or all of the necessary funding. The Department of Health within the state or federal government often sponsors central registries. Sometimes they are hosted by a university, a medical or hospital association, or a prominent hospital or medical center.

ADMINISTRATION OF CENTRAL REGISTRIES

The administration of a central registry is a complex matter involving organizational concerns and interrelationships with various outside groups.[30,31]

Legislation, Affiliation, and Governance

Early central registries, which were often based on voluntary participation, were usually started by a core organization, which formed alliances with other interested parties, or a consortium of cancer treatment facilities (e. g., Connecticut, Utah, Los Angeles County). Nowadays, a central registry is usually enabled by a state legislative mandate, whether it started voluntarily or not.[32,33] Both voluntary and legislatively mandated registries take time to be implemented. Many of the initial tasks are easier to accomplish with a legislative mandate. The legislative mandate often specifies operational requirements, provides a process for determining compliance, and establishes funding.[31]

Although some registries were started earlier, the pace of registry-enabling legislation increased greatly during the 1990s. The Surveillance, Epidemiology, and End Results (SEER) Program of the National Cancer Institute (NCI), and the National Program of Cancer Registries (NPCR) of the Centers for Disease Control and Prevention (CDC) are the major funding sources for US central cancer registries. Most states now have statewide, population-based (central) registries as a result of NPCR or SEER funding.[34,36]

In addition to enabling legislation, central registries need the advice and support of a variety of stakeholders, including clinicians from major medical facilities, public health and government officials, epidemiologists, biostatisticians, university and other researchers, local cancer registrar organizations, the Commission on Cancer, the American Cancer Society, and community special interest groups.[37-39] In many respects, a population-based registry is both a monopoly and a public trust and should encourage and enjoy wide participation.

Most central registries have an advisory committee, an executive committee, or a governing board. The functions and responsibilities of these committees vary from giving advice to setting policies. The members of the advisory committee are usually representatives of the various community and state organizations that have alliances with the central registry.

Participation by clinicians from the local major medical facilities fosters cooperation. Public health officials welcome the central registry as an aid in investigating cancer clusters and in performing other surveillance activities. Central cancer registries serve as a valuable source of useful statistical data for epidemiologists and other health researchers. Participation by a key hospital registrar whose facility reports to the central registry can keep the governing committee informed of data collection problems encountered at the hospital level. The organization chart of a central registry often reflects two governance groups at the top—both an advisory committee and the hosting organization's line of authority, such as an official from the state health department.

Staffing

Operation of a central cancer registry is labor intensive. Composition and number of staff depend to a large extent on the goals of the registry, the size (number of cases accessioned), and the nature of the data collection process.[40-45] The goals of the registry determine which data items are collected, the rapidity of data collection, whether follow-up is conducted, and the uses to which the data are put, all of which influence staffing. The geographic area and population covered also affects the cost and method of data collection.

The scientific or medical director often has budgetary responsibility for the central registry and may serve part- or full-time, depending on the size of the registry and the responsibilities entailed. Almost every central registry has a full-time administrative manager or director who is responsible for its day-to-day operation. Most administrative managers have direct casefinding, abstracting, and quality control experience and are well connected with local related professional organizations.

How the processes of quality control, data processing, and statistical analysis are accomplished often depends on the size of a central registry.

Large central registries usually have one or more full-time staff for both quality control and data processing. Due to its specialized nature, the statistical analyses may be done by experts who are members of another department or organizational entity. Registries with smaller budgets may use part-time personnel for these functions.

The number of staff needed for quality control depends on the nature of the data collection, the scope of the data set, and the quality control measures used (such as edits, reabstracting, and casefinding). If the data include treatment and stage, more expertise and time are needed to collect and check them. The requirement that data collection staff be certified by the National Cancer Registrars Association helps to ensure an acceptable level of quality.

A registry's data processing requirements are determined by the type of computer system used to collect, store, and process the data. Computerized systems require software development, maintenance, and support. Development of customized software is time consuming and expensive. Additional functions such as Geographic Information System (GIS), death clearance, report generation, and statistical analyses further define the data processing requirements.

Public relations activities vary from registry to registry. The ability to work with legislators, the medical community, and community interest groups is an important responsibility that should not be overlooked. While some registries have a spokesperson specifically designated for this role, these responsibilities often fall to the medical administrative director.

A 1989 survey of 31 population-based registries included data on the number of full-time equivalent (FTE) employees who were funded and the number of incident cases ascertained annually.[40] Size of caseload for these central registries varied from 1,200 to 83,000 incident cases per year. For these 31 central registries combined, there was a reported average staff ratio of 0.8 FTE per 1,000 incident cases. Reflecting different registry goals and methodologies, there was a wide range of staffing ratios, from a low of 2.5 FTE's for a registry accessioning 20,000 incident cases (0.1 FTE per 1,000 cases) to a high of 42.5 FTE's for 14,000 cases (3.0 FTE'S per 1,000 cases).

Much of the staffing variation relates to the data collection, coding, and processing methodologies employed. Registries collecting data that were already coded and computerized reported lower staff needs for these processes. A 1985 international report on population-based registries also found wide diversity among registration techniques and staffing patterns.[46] For the 61 registries included, there was an average of 1.0 FTE per 1,000 incident cases. Minimal as well as multipurpose central registries were grouped together in this international survey, following a wide range of data collection, coding, and processing methodologies.

In the US survey, several typical central registry job titles were listed, including Medical or Scientific Director/Epidemiologist, Registry/Project Manager, Office/Accounts Manager, Abstractors, quality control, data processing, statistician, coding/processing, research analyst, data entry, and secretarial/clerical. The types and average number of full-time equivalent employees (FTE's) reported are summarized in Table 34-1.

Fifty % of the reported staff were either abstractors or coders/processors. The breadth of necessary staffing

Table 34-1

Full Time Equivalent (FTE) Staffing for Central Registries[40]

	FTE'S	Percent
Director	0.6	4
Registry Manager	0.7	5
Office/Accounts Manager	0.4	3
Abstractor	3.7	27
Quality Control	1.2	9
Data Processing	1.1	8
Statistician	0.5	4
Coding/Processing	3.2	23
Research Analyst	0.3	2
Secretarial	1.1	8
Data Entry	0.9	7
Total	13.7	100

for a central registry is well suggested by the survey. Caution should be exercised in interpreting these past surveys of earlier central registration characteristics.

Budget

Similar to staffing, the most important factors influencing central registry budgets are the number of cases being collected, the amount of data collected per case, and the data collection methods.[40-47] A large state that collects only basic incidence data can probably operate with the same funding as a smaller state that collects a more extensive data set and follows multipurpose processes.

The legislative mandate itself or the administrative policies that govern the mandate with regard to who must report and how they must report also affects the funding necessary for the registry. For instance, the staffing and salary needs of a registry in a state in which institutions are required to submit data to the central registry are quite different from those of a registry in which the registry's staff are required to obtain the data from the institutions.

Even with the most careful planning, adequate funding for the registry can be difficult to obtain. As with many projects, the budgetary allocation can determine the scope of work rather than the other way around. Ideally, it is wise to develop the registry budget for a three or five year period. A central registry's budget is not static, nor is the number of cases; both usually increase over time. If annual increases are not built into the appropriation, the registry may have to absorb the costs of inflation, and the additional workload that occurs with an increase in the number of cases.

The major categories of a central registry's budget include personnel, travel, and data processing costs. There must be an adequate number of well-trained personnel in the registry, and the salaries must be competitive. There must be adequate money for travel within the state or region for professional meetings. On-site training and quality control visits are very important and must be conducted regularly. And finally, the data processing budget must be sufficient to achieve the registry's goals. Whether the data processing functions are performed in-house or are contracted out, data must be entered, edited, aggregated, and reported in some form.

The relationship between incident caseload, FTE Staffing, and dollar cost as reported by central registries is summarized in Table 34-2.

Table 34-2
Incident Caseload, FTE Staffing and Dollar Cost Reported by Several Central Registries

	Incident Cases	FTE Staffing	Cases/FTE	Budget	$/case
1.	15,300	30	510	1,347,367	88
2.	52,000	21.3	2,441	631,650	12
3.	3,900	11.7	333	457,000	117
4.	3,608	3.7	975	102,222	28
5.	13,983	42.5	329	1,139,741	82
6.	28,000	15.0	1,866	620,000	22
7.	16,500	14.9	1,107	660,000	40
8.	15,300	2.5	6,120	122,800	8
9.	3,900	3.2	1,219	105,000	27
10.	37,000	44.2	837	N/A	N/A
11.	83,000	24.7	3,360	721,337	9
12.	57,000	16.5	3,455	650,000	11
13.	7,000	38.4	192	585,449	84
14.	5,000	5.0	1,000	155,000	31
Average	24,392	19.5	1,251	561,351	23

There was an average staff budget of 1251 cases per FTE, and corresponding cost of $23 per incident case in the dollars reported in 1989. It can be seen that there is a wide range from a low of 192 cases per FTE to 6,120 cases per FTE, and the cost ranges from a low of $8 per case to $117 per case. These wide ranges may reflect differences in productivity and cost-effectiveness, but probably more clearly reflect differences in registry goals and objectives.

Security/Confidentiality

Central cancer registries are sizeable databases that store important confidential information about large numbers of patients with cancer.[48-51] To resolve duplicate case reporting, it is essential that specific and precise identifying information be present in the patient record. The storage of this confidential information is justified by the breadth and utility of medical research, patient care surveillance, patient follow-up, and other uses made of the data, but a strong imperative regarding patient confidentiality is created.

Complicating the need for confidentiality is the fact that central cancer registries inherently collect information from a number of different physical locations and transports that data to a central location where it is stored. Hospital data is taken outside the walls of the hospital itself. Traditionally, such abstracted information was often carried manually in automobiles and other transport. Security involved physical protection of the collected data from the hospital to the central registry. In the central registry, physical access to paper records and computer data files were controlled, and password-type access was maintained. The central registry employees sign a security precaution statement when they are employed at the central registry, and those security statements are reviewed annually. Back-up files were stored in locked cabinets.

Until the Internet age, security concerns for central registries focused on controlling physical access to the medical information, either in paper form, or computer files. Security concerns for central cancer registries are changing swiftly as interpretations of the impact of HIPAA (which will be implemented in several phases) are rolled out. Because of the complex nature of HIPAA, interpretations of its requirements are still being proposed and studied.

In a 2001 letter, NAACCR has summarized advice for central registries regarding HIPAA.[52,53]

"To summarize, HIPAA has very little impact on cancer reporting to central cancer registries. Specifically, HIPAA provides for the continuation of reporting identifiable data for reportable diseases to public health entities for the purpose of public health surveillance. Additionally, HIPAA does not obstruct any state law that supports or mandates the reporting of disease or injury for public health purposes. Written informed consent from each cancer patient reported to public health entities is not required under HIPAA; rather hospitals must document that reporting has occurred. This can be done simply for all cancer cases since reporting is mandatory for all cases."

As planning for the more complete compliance with HIPAA proceeds, it is likely that interpretation and implementation at medical centers, central registries, and other related organizations will change. Current insights into HIPAA compliance should be gleaned from cancer registry websites such as NAACCR, and websites specializing in HIPAA itself.

Clearly confidentiality must be a concern to the central cancer registrar.[54]

Ethics

Useful descriptions of ethical concerns for cancer registrars including ethical codes specifically for cancer registrars,[55-58] and those for public health concerns in general[59] have been previously described.

Central registries are generally run under review of the Institutional Review Board (IRB) of the hosting organization.[60] If no IRB is maintained by the hosting organization, an IRB of a likely related organization can sometimes be found. IRB review is concerned with many matters, but ethical concerns garner special attention. The IRB is of fundamental importance in the registry's effort to maintain public trust.

It is prudent for the central registry to have written policies that are IRB approved concerning all possible matters of potential public interest, or ethical concern, and that continuing periodic reviews be scheduled. Many registries include IRB review as a part of the funding solicitation process.

Concerns of the IRB typically include privacy and security of the data, as summarized in Table 34-3.

DATA SET PLANNING STANDARDS

The principles of data set planning have been previously described for the USA,[60-62] and elsewhere;[63] and are covered in more detail in another chapter of this textbook. By consensus of the cancer registration professional community, the Uniform Data Standards (UDS) Committee of NAACCR main-

Table 34-3

Institutional Review Boards (IRB) Concerns Regarding Central Cancer Registries

General
1. Upholding confidentiality and privacy of the data
2. Preservation and securing registry records
3. Disclosure of data only to proper authorities

Minimizing potential risks/harms to the patient
4. Conditions of initial contact with patients
5. Nature of written patient consent for interview, and/or specimen
6. Response to subpoena of registry records

Other ethical concerns
7. Maximizing societal benefits (utility) of registration
8. Maintaining public use samples[59]
9. Ensuring equitable distribution of registry benefits
10. Preserving confidential nature of committees
11. Cooperating with other professions and health service entities
12. Increasing profession's body of knowledge
13. Participating in recruitment, and setting of a good example
14. Planning appropriate levels of quality management
15. Avoiding conflicts of interest
16. Acting in a professional matter

tains responsibility for data set standardization of central cancer registries in the US. Membership of the UDS committee includes representatives of those organizations which have traditionally have been stakeholders in such data set planning, so that everyone's voice is heard. This standardization is documented in a NAACCR *Data Standards and Data Dictionary*,[64] which includes specifications of data items, codes, and storage format.

History of Data Sets

In the early years of central cancer registration, states often developed their data collection rules, definitions, and response sets without detailed regard to what each other—or hospitals—were collecting. The result was multiple definitions and coding rules for concepts as central to cancer registration as primary site and date of diagnosis. There was also a lack of uniformity in the coding of items that have generally shared definitions. For example, the major categories of sex might be represented by M and F, 1 and 2, or 2 and 1 depending on the state. When the codes used to collect items like state or county differed, it was often quite difficult to recognize that a given code supplied by one central registry did not necessarily represent the entity presumed by another. The standardization of data codes developed as central registries were able to share reports for out-of-state patients with the patients' home states, and as software providers confronted the increasingly complex demands from states to provide them with consistent data for hospitals within a given state.

Several organizations have been historically instrumental in developing the *de facto* standard for central cancer registry data item specification in the United States. The Commission on Cancer (CoC) of the American College of Surgeons first added the cancer registry as an approval requirement for hospital cancer programs in 1956 and published its recommended data set in the same year.[65] The 10 Cities Survey, followed by the Third National Cancer Survey (now known as the SEER Program) developed its data set over several decades.[66] Most central cancer registry data originate in the hospital, so SEER's policies influenced hospital and central registry data sets. In the 1970s, concern arose over standardization of hospital data sets. In 1979, at a workshop sponsored by the American College of Surgeons, a comparison of CoC's, SEER's and the Comprehensive Cancer Center Patient Data System's data sets was presented, which provided the impetus for the UDS.[67]

A joint committee of the CoC and SEER was formed in 1983. The California Tumor Registry initially convened it. It was broadened and formalized in 1988 as the Uniform Data Standards Committee of NAACCR. Its work led to increased standardization between the two programs. Although each program had data items unique to itself, a significant number of the data items were the same. For these common data items, a single, standard coding schema was agreed upon and is still maintained.

Each program has continued its own documentation of what is increasingly becoming a mutually agreeable data set. The CoC current data set definition is given in the Facility Oncology Registry Data Standards (FORDS).[68] The most recent version of SEER's coding manual was published in 1998[69] and all revisions can be viewed at the SEER website (www.SEER.cancer.gov). Another standard is for data transfer between states, and similar transfers.[70]

Standard Setters for Central Registries

Standard setters for central registries include a wide range of organizations, notably including the CoC, the American Joint Committee on Cancer (AJCC), SEER, the National Cancer Registrar's Association (NCRA), NPCR, NAACCR, the National Coordinating Council for Cancer Surveillance (NCCCS), and the World Health Organization (WHO).[71]

In addition to these primary standard setters, each of these organizations have liaisons or links to other interested organizations, notably including the College of American Pathologists and the American Cancer Society which has given them an indirect influence on cancer registration standards.

The Commission on Cancer:

The initiation of standards for cancer registration can be traced to 1921 when Ernest Codman, MD, FACS, established the first cancer registry. This bone sarcoma registry and its inherent data set introduced the role of cancer registry data standards for medical care in hospitals and among clinicians.[72]

Building on that beginning, the CoC's activities have included the basic approvals program of US hospitals,[73-76] various education programs, the Cancer Liaison physician network,[77-79] and the National Cancer Data Base (NCDB).[10,80-81]

A hospital cancer registry is a requirement of a Commission-approved cancer program. Compliance with standards for the organization, function, and data elements, including quality assurance, are mandated. This is the primary building block and financial underpinning of data collection for cancer registration in the US.

The Cancer Liaison Physicians form a cancer control/communication network of approximately 2200 surgeons and physicians who are each linked to individual hospitals, and provide oversight for various programs of the hospital cancer program, notably including the cancer registry as well as the use and quality of the data.

The NCDB, a joint project of the CoC and the American Cancer Society, is a resource for benchmarking patterns of cancer management and outcomes based on data available from hospital cancer registries. The data is not population-based. The benchmarks assist hospitals in assessing their services, programs, and performance as compared to established guidelines,

AJCC:

The objectives of the AJCC include the development and publication of schemas or standards to classify cancers, including anatomic staging, multiple prognostic factors, and end results reporting. These coding schemas are designed for use by clinicians for the purpose of treatment selection, estimation of prognosis, and ongoing assessment of cancer control interventions.[82]

In addition, there is a long-established collaboration between the AJCC and the International Union Against Cancer (UICC) T(tumor),N (node), M(metastasis) Staging Committee to ensure that all refinements to the staging schema are consistent and introduced simultaneously to the medical and data management communities.

SEER:

The Surveillance, Epidemiology, and End Results (SEER) Program of the National Cancer Institute (NCI) of the National Institutes of Health (NIH) was established as a population-based registry in accordance with the National Cancer Act of 1971.[5] The program is further described in another chapter of this textbook. There are 10 SEER registries and 4 expansion registries that cover 16 geographic areas. The SEER registries are the source of incidence and mortality rates, survival rates, prevalence estimates, and quality indicators for the covered population. The SEER Program has played a significant role in formalizing cancer registration systems, coding and definition of data items, abstracting rules, and training. Most central and hospital registries can trace some portion of their development, procedural, and reference documentation to the SEER Program. Collaboration between the CoC and the SEER program has continued to refine and realign registration techniques and requirements to reduce the number and significance of data set variations.

NCRA:

The National Cancer Registrars Association was chartered in 1974 "to promote research and education in Cancer Registry administration and prac-

tice."[83] The Association establishes education standards, develops courses of study for registry professionals, disseminates information, and is involved in programs and activities to improve and standardize cancer registration. In 1983, the NCRA initiated a cancer registrar certification program. The credentialing of registry professionals has raised the standards of performance and quality of cancer data management. Today there are more than 3800 Certified Tumor Registrars (CTRs).

NAACCR:

The North American Association of Central Cancer Registries (NAACCR) is the professional organization representing central registries.[84] The organization has played an important role in organizing the standards of the major standard setting groups into a common framework and documenting them. All the major standard setters are represented on NAACCR committees that are charged with the development and maintenance of specific areas of standardization. These include: Data Evaluation and Publications, Data Use and Confidentiality, Education, Information and Technology, Record Consolidation, Registry Certification, Registry Operations, and the Uniform Data Standards Committees.

NPCR:

As cancer registration and the role of the registry professional have evolved, the opportunities to expand the network of registries have expanded rapidly. With the passage of the Cancer Registry Act in 1992, the National Program of Cancer Registries was implemented by the Centers for Disease Control and Prevention (CDC).[6] Through this program, the CDC has developed model legislation and regulations that make cancer reportable and thereby ensure access to the required patient information by qualified registry personnel. The CDC has been the linchpin for the development or expansion of central registries in states not covered by the SEER program. State registries use their data for planning and resource allocation, determination of the efficacy and need for cancer control initiatives, and for the identification of high-risk populations. They also provide incidence and mortality rates as well as prevalence data. Through the CDC and the NPCR standards for completeness, timeliness and quality of data have been developed for state registries.

NCCCS:

The National Coordinating Council for Cancer Surveillance (NCCCS) was formed in 1993 in an effort to define the roles of the major organizations involved in cancer data base management.[85] The council membership includes representatives of the American Cancer Society, American College of Surgeons, American Joint Committee on Cancer, Commission on Cancer (NCDB), Centers for Disease Control and Prevention (NPCR), National Cancer Institute (SEER), National Cancer Registrars Association, National Center for Health Statistics, and the North American Association of Central Cancer Registries. The NCCCS provides oversight of issues in cancer surveillance, including resolution of data set, staging or reporting inconsistencies, identification of new data fields/classifications, development of cancer surveillance processes, and reduction of duplication among the various databases. This forum for dialogue and intervention has further enhanced the uniformity of data standards and reduced the competing demands made on cancer registrars.

WHO:

The standardization of cancer registration for disease classification has been defined by the World Health Organization (WHO). Their publication, *International Classifications of Diseases for Oncology (ICD-O)*[86] was widely accepted as the standard reference for coding topography and morphology. The second edition of the ICD-O[87] was introduced as the standard used by all US cancer registries beginning with malignancies diagnosed on or after January 1, 1992. The third edition was used after January 1, 2001.[88]

Currently the AJCC, CoC, NPCR, and the SEER program are working on a collaborative staging algorithm that will make possible cross translation among the TNM Stage groupings of the AJCC, the Extent of Disease (EOD) system of the SEER Program, and the Summary Stage System.[89] It is hoped that this will eliminate one last area of significant variation in data management standards between different types and networks of cancer registries.

Data Set Content

Central cancer registry data sets are a reflection of the type of registry, its sources of information, its funders and supporters, specific needs of the population served, and the intended use of registry data.[61,62,64,90-92] That is why state central registries may require hospitals to provide information that is not required for COC-approved programs, SEER or NPCR, and not published in FORDS.[90]

Generally, the types of data collected and maintained by central registries are similar to the types collected by hospitals: patient identification, cancer identification, treatment information, follow-up information, and information that describe the nature of the data.

Central registries consolidate information from many sources, including multiple hospitals, physicians' offices and free-standing clinics, pathology and radiology laboratories, nursing homes and rehabilitation centers, coroners' offices and death certificates. To link all of this information correctly requires high quality patient identification detail and the ability to distinguish among slightly disparate descriptions of what may be one or more independent primary cancer. Consequently, central registries collect this information from every facility that is required to report the case. The descriptive demographic and cancer information is also necessary for nearly every use of central registry data. Individual central registries may require additional information specific to their own circumstances. For example, some states collect tribal membership for Native Americans or generation of immigration in addition to race and place of birth. Other registries may collect information regarding patient exposure to potentially cancer-causing natural or accidental events.

A central registry whose sole purpose is to provide rapid identification of changes in cancer incidence that might require intervention does not need any treatment information. However, in reality most registries serve multiple functions and some treatment information is collected. Because nearly every state central registry receives some funding from one of two federal programs, SEER and NPCR, the minimal requirements for collection of treatment information are defined by those standard-setting organizations. Central registries whose data are used for some types of investigative research collect far more extensive treatment information for certain types of cases.

Follow-up activities vary considerably among central registries. Some routinely track recurrence and subsequent treatment; others do not. Some provide feedback about readmission elsewhere to the hospital responsible for following the analytic case, but many cannot due to state confidentiality restrictions. Most central registries perform death clearance to identify patients in the data base who have died, to gather additional information such as cause of death or place of birth if it was not already recorded, and to identify cancer deaths that may not have been reported by any other source. Some states use additional sources of information to determine whether patients otherwise lost to follow-up may still be alive, such as matches to drivers' licenses or Medicare rolls.

Because central registries collect coded information from such a wide variety of sources, and because much of the data used depends on many years of data collection, central registries have a particular need for the kinds of data items that describe the nature of the data. For example, they need to know the type of facility that originated the report, its identity, when the report was submitted, and the coding system version in use for the various items collected (including the primary site, morphology, staging, treatment, cause of death, Census tract, occupation, and history codes). They may also document items that represent data processing steps (which may include the date the report was received, date the edited report was entered into the full database, edit information, or research projects involving the case).

The coding system versions bear special mention because they necessarily are provided by the facilities that report data to the central registry. A "current coding system" version data item describes the form in which the central registry receives the code in a report. It is necessary to interpret the meaning of the code itself. The "original coding system" version item describes the response categories available to the coder when the data item was abstracted and coded. It is used principally in data analysis and is, therefore, fundamental to the operations of central registries. In facility registries, these items can be handled largely behind the scenes by the software, but the registrar may need to enter version information when it changes.

Today, one of the principal requirements in selecting a data set is standardization of the definitions, coding rules, and response sets used. The rule of thumb is if the registry intends to measure something that other registries are using, it should be done the same way. Then, data from multiple central registries can be compared with the knowledge that they mean the same thing. Investigators know the meaning of terms used in published reports will be the same, no matter what registry collected the data. And data from central registries can be combined, as SEER or NPCR combine data from multiple states.

The major standard-setting organizations have been described earlier in this publication. They are called "standard setters" in large part because they are the sources for the codes adopted as shared standards by both central and facility registries. These groups coordinate, principally under the auspices of NAACCR's UDS, to maintain a dictionary of items that provide both contemporary medical relevance and continuity with former codes and definitions from which all types of registries draw items for their respective data sets.

The standard documented by NAACCR includes recommended content for each of six types of registry data sets including:

1. Minimum required for data interchange
2. Incidence data
3. Incidence data plus treatment, detailed staging, and follow-up
4. National Program of Cancer Registries (NPCR) requirements/recommendations
5. Commission on Cancer (American College of Surgeons) requirement/recommendations
6. SEER requirements[64]

These NAACCR recommended contents have been developed to carefully balance the needs and necessary data collection of the hospital registry with those of the central registry. Data set collection is one of several ways in which hospital registries and central registries are closely interdependent. The basic data items needed by central cancer registries are similar but not identical to those of hospital registries, and include those listed in Table 34-4.

In addition to Volume II,[64] NAACCR has also developed a standard to assist in the interstate transfer of data between registries,[76] E-path Reporting,[91] completeness and quality,[92] and recommendations to assist in the use of HL7.[93-95]

Table 34-4
Basic Data Items for Central Cancer Registries

- Patient identification
- Cancer identification
- Hospital-specific (admission dates, class, and analytic status) data
- Stage and prognostic factors
- Treatment: first course and subsequent
- Follow-up and recurrence
- Death
- Specific codes for overriding data edits
- System administration (case completed, changed)
- Special study use
- Patient, hospital, and physician confidential
- Narrative text

Table 34-5
Non-Reportable Cases for the Surveillance, Epidemiology, and End Results Program of the National Cancer Institute

- Malignant neoplasms, NOS (morphology codes 8000-8004) of the skin (C44._)
- Epithelial carcinomas (8010-8045) of the skin (C44._)
- Papillary and squamous cell carcinomas (8050-8082) of the skin (C44._)
- Basal cell carcinomas (8090-8110) of any site except the genital sites-vagina (C52.9), labium majus (C51.0), labium minus (C51.1), clitoris (C51.2), vulva (C51.8-C51.9), prepuce (C60.0), penis (C60.9), and scrotum (C63.2)

CASE ASCERTAINMENT

Reportable List

A central registry's rules for reportability usually include a reportable list, reference date, and rules for residency, multiple primaries, analytic cases, ambiguous terms, and diagnostic confirmation.[96-99]

The reportable list should include all diagnoses that are to be reported and specify which diagnoses are not reportable. The reportable lists for central registries are of course closely interrelated with the reportable lists of hospitals in their reporting area.

Reportable cases for central registries usually include all diseases with a behavior code of 2 (in situ) or 3 (invasive) as identified in the current edition of the *International Classification of Diseases for Oncology (ICD-O-3)*. The SEER Program's reportable list includes all such cases except for the cases listed in Table 34-5. A federal law has been recently passed requiring the reportability of CNS (brain) cancers.[97]

These standards are specified in the NAACCR standards document.[64] Refer to Chapter 6 for a discussion of considerations in developing the reportable list for hospital registries.

Ambiguous Terminology:

A patient has cancer when a recognized medical practitioner states that the patient does. However, there may be times when the diagnosis is vague or inconclusive, such as "probable carcinoma of the lung." Rules have been defined to indicate whether terms

should be considered diagnostic of cancer for the registry's purposes. As stated in the SEER manual[68] the terms that are considered diagnostic of cancer are "apparent(ly)," "appears to," "comparable with," "compatible with," "consistent with," "favor(s)," "malignant appearing," "most likely," "presumed," "probable," "suspect(ed)," "suspicious (for)," "typical of." The terms that are not to be interpreted as diagnostic of cancer (without additional information) are "cannot be ruled out," "equivocal," "possible," "potentially malignant," "questionable," "rule out," "suggests," and "worrisome."

Reference Date:

Central registries adopt and publish their reference (starting) date from which their coverage begins, usually January 1 of a year. All cases diagnosed among area residents on or after the reference date must be included. For population-based central registries, it is required that all cases of cancer occurring in the population residing in the reporting area be entered into the registry, regardless of the place of diagnosis or treatment. Procedures must be in place to achieve the most complete coverage possible within the limits of the resources available.

Residency:

Usually all cancers diagnosed in persons who are residents of the population-based reporting area at the time of diagnoses are reportable. Some central registries may elect to register non-residents to facilitate sharing of data with registries in neighboring areas, to simplify death clearance, and to allow preparation of individual hospital reports that include all of the hospital's cases. Rules should also be in place for handling part-year residents (such as retiree "snow birds"), military personnel, college students, undocumented aliens, or any other group whose residency status might be ambiguous. Whenever possible, rules for determining residency should be comparable to rules used by the Bureau of the Census in determining place of residence, so that numerator definitions will be the same as the definitions for the population at risk when incidence rates are calculated.

Multiple Primaries:

Rules for dealing with multiple primary cancers in the same patient differ somewhat internationally, notably including rules from SEER,[69] IARC,[63] COC[92] and the Canadian CCCR. In the United States most central registries follow the definitions developed by the SEER program and published in The SEER Program Code Manual.[69] These definitions include rules for determining primary site and multiple and subsequent primaries.

Analytic Cases (Class of Case):

Class of case is a data item and concept used by hospital registries to denote whether the case was diagnosed and/or treated at the reference hospital, or has received treatment previously elsewhere. The concept of "analytic" refers to whether the case belongs in a particular analysis cohort or not. Generally central registries are interested in all cases first diagnosed within their residency definition, no matter at which hospital or other facility they were first treated.

Diagnostic Confirmation:

In the past, some central registries elected to register only pathologically confirmed cases. Central registries generally adopt explicit rules for hospitals that report to them to deal with special circumstances, such as whether a hospital should report cancers in patients who are diagnosed in the emergency room only, dead on arrival at the hospital, seen for consultation only, evaluated for cancer but who have no active disease at the time of admission, or seen for treatment but who are transient in the area and only referred for care while passing through or visiting. A list of nonreportable cases is often specified by central registries.

Casefinding (Source of Cases)

The principal source of most cases for a central registry is the hospital, but non-hospital sources are becoming increasingly important. The most common sources are listed in Table 34-6.[98-101] The registry can identify potential sources of cases by contacting the state government agencies that license health care facilities and practitioners, by contacting professional societies and trade associations, and by referring to

Table 34-6
Common Casefinding Sources

- Hospital Sources
    Pathology reports: histology, pathology, autopsy, cytology, and hematology reports
    Health records reports: disease index and daily discharges
    Radiation therapy reports: radiation therapy log and treatment summaries
    Diagnostic radiology reports: nuclear medicine logs and reports
    Outpatient records
    Surgery reports
- Non-hospital Sources
    Outpatient centers
    Independent pathology laboratories
    Radiation and surgery centers
    Physicians' offices, such as oncologists' and dermatologists' offices
    Hospices, nursing homes, Bureau's of Vital Statistics, and coroners' offices for death records
    Out-of-state facilities

---

telephone directories. The intended use of the data should determine when cases must be reported.

Hospital-Registry Sources:

Hospital registries have not always emphasized certain data items that are crucial to a central registry, such as determination of the patient's residency at the time of diagnosis, and hospitals may not be abstracting all cases of interest to the central registry-for example, consultations-only, pathology-only, nonanalytic cases, or carcinoma in situ of the cervix—so requirements must be carefully spelled out.

Because the criteria for which cases should be abstracted may differ between the central registry and reporting hospitals, it is important that the central registry's abstracting requirements be clearly defined. For example, as mentioned above the CoC does not require that hospitals abstract so-called nonanalytic cases, that is, those that were diagnosed and received their entire first course of treatment prior to admission to the reporting hospital. Central registries, however, often require abstracts on nonanalytic cases that are incidence cases for the registry's coverage area.

Sometimes hospital registries abstract cases that are not required to be abstracted by a central registry because the CoC or local cancer committee wants the case to be reportable due to local interest. The central registry must decide whether or not to accept these abstracts if they are submitted by hospitals.

Regular monitoring of completeness of casefinding and abstracting is an essential component of a central registry's quality control plan. Monthly monitoring enables the registry to quickly identify problems and have sufficient lead-time to take corrective action.

Data transmission to the central registry can be via diskette or modem. NAACCR has adopted a standardized format for data exchange, intended as a "second language" that many systems use to share data with each other.[70] Sometimes, a mail-in reporting option is developed for use by small rural hospitals, but confidentiality concerns can limit mail reporting.

Non-Hospital Registry Sources:

For hospitals without cancer registries as well as for nonhospital sources such as clinics, offices of physicians, pathology laboratories, nursing homes, and any other potential sources of cases, the central registry cannot rely on abstracts prepared by a hospital cancer registrar. A successful practice uses "circuit riders," or abstractors who are employed by the central registry, to visit reporting facilities and perform casefinding and abstracting of data in the field.

To the extent that hospitals do not automatically ascertain all cases the central registry requires, the central registry must perform extra casefinding.

Out of Region Cases:

Registries have used various methods to obtain reports on their resident cases that have been diagnosed or treated outside the catchment area. First, referral patterns must be determined. When central registries exist in neighboring areas, formal agreements for exchange of data can be implemented.

SEER central registries are required to provide complete counts of new cases for a calendar year within 20 months of the end of that calendar year. CDC's goal in its National Program of Cancer Registries is that 95% of expected cases be included within six months of the close of the diagnosis year.

Rapid reporting is a consideration when cases are needed for epidemiological protocols, research, or tumor board presentations at hospitals. Using this method, cases are usually identified within 15 to 30 days after diagnosis or hospital admission. For example, the New Hampshire State Cancer Registry requires baseline data on patient, diagnostic, and other information to be reported within 15 days. Other state registries ask hospital registrars to submit electronic pathology abstracts with demographic information, within 15-30 days from the date on the pathology report. The complete information on the patient must be reported within 180 days. This allows cases to be identified rapidly at the Central Registry for inclusion in research studies, but allows more time for the hospital registrars to complete abstracts.

The disadvantages of this method include provision of incomplete information to the central registry, requiring the hospital staff to pull the medical record more than once, and possible duplication in case reporting.

If time is a less important criterion, cases may be reported within three to six months from admission to the hospital. For hospitals participating in the approvals program of the Commission on Cancer, the maximum recommended delay in abstracting is six months calculated from the date of initial diagnosis to the time that the data are available for analysis.

E-path Reporting:

Cancer registration is characterized by pathologic confirmation of diagnoses, thus pathology departments serve as a funnel for the great majority of cancer case ascertainment. Increasingly, high volume pathology laboratories, both independent and hospital, manage their specimen flow, reporting and billing in electronic form.[102]

The need for Rapid Case Ascertainment and a desire for easier, more complete reporting from path labs independent from hospitals, have contributed to the emerging interest in E-path reporting;

The term E-path reporting was first used to connote the concept of automation of cancer casefinding from independent pathology laboratories.[91] Since that time, the major components of E-path reporting, 1) casefinding and 2) electronic transmission to a central registry, have become more broadly described, and some efforts at E-path reporting from hospital pathology labs have been implemented, as well as independent path labs.[30,103,104] Thus, electronic casefinding (with or without external transmission) has emerged as another name for E-path Reporting. E-path Reporting and electronic casefinding are used here synonymously.

In some central registries, circuit riders and/or hospital registrars manually screen all available pathology reports for mention of cancer. This process requires substantial costs in labor and training to be performed well; when done poorly, incomplete and unreliable cancer data may result. In recent years, several factors have increased the desirability of automating this task.

The majority of pathology reports at most pathology laboratories are not cancer-related. The emerging importance of the Health Insurance Portability and Accountability Act (HIPAA) and other security concerns may favor automated review of pathology reports within a secure environment. Avoidance of manual review of these non-cancer cases may be viewed as enhancing protection of confidentiality and therefore patient satisfaction. Also, automated pathologic casefinding offers cost-savings over manual methods, thereby freeing cancer registrars for other key registry functions.

The benefits of E-path reporting can include automated, complete and rapid case-finding, transmission and central registry storage requiring little human intervention, receipt of the complete pathology report in digitized form, with HL7 or other data transmission standards compatibility, improved HIPAA compliance (including encryption, authentication, identification, and complete audit trails for all transactions), lessening of human visual review of non-cancer pathology reports, and decreased pathology hard copy ground transfer.

The automatic nature of this casefinding may potentially obviate the need for routine manual pathology review by central or hospital registry staff. Labor savings of approximately 0.2 FTE for every 1000 incident cases have been estimated.[30,43]

Electronic casefinding without transmission generally includes several discrete steps: 1) extraction of the path report from a Laboratory Information System (LIS), 2) opening of a casefinding dictionary, 3) encoding the various sections of the pathology report into numeric codes, 4) applying specified case selection criteria, 5) parsing of the selected path reports to HL-7 if desired, and 6) writing of the selected pathology reports to a CD-ROM, or other electronic media.

The casefinding dictionary typically includes a list of search terms that appear on reportable cancer pathology reports (e.g. invasive carcinoma, lymphoma). A list of such terms endorsed by NAACCR and is maintained on the NAACCR website. The term *list procedure* is programmed to perform like a human screener. The text of the entire pathology report is scanned for these terms that are indicative of a reportable cancer. The presence of any one of these terms in the pathology report qualifies the report as potentially reportable. Pathology reports that contain none of these words are considered negative for cancer. Screening sensitivities of near 100% with specificity of 75% have been reported.[30]

In addition to electronic casefinding, external electronic transmission typically includes 1) queuing messages to send, 2) establishing an IP Circuit:, 3) exchanging of encryption keys between computers over the Internet, 4) encrypting the path report message, 5) sending the encrypted message over the Internet (the sending computer and receiving computer are typically separated from the Internet by firewalls, which physically separate the computers from the Internet), 6) receiving the message, 7) decrypting the message, 8) electronic storage of the path report in central registry files, and 9) quality control at the electronic casefinding and transmission process.

The design of a particular casefinding process and the enabling software depends on whether electronic transmission is needed, and whether it will occur before casefinding or after. Casefinding systems without external transmission are considerably easier to implement, but are not as automatic.

The total pre-planning effort for E-path implementation, which is in essence an automation task, takes time. Important stakeholders, including information technology, IRB, and pathology laboratory personnel, must be identified and involved.

This preplanning includes various site assessment and preparation tasks, including Laboratory Information System (LIS) file formatting and interface, hardware assessment, and firewall and security protocol planning.

E-path software is typically installed in a PC or server on location at the laboratories. The installation process can be straightforward. The software can possibly share the resources of a single PC or server.

Like other evolutionary steps in cancer registration automation and computerization, the progress of E-path reporting may depend on the availability of cost-effective and transportable E-path software systems. Cooperation of the reporting organization is essential for a successful E-path installation. For registries desiring rapid case ascertainment as well as the other benefits of E-path reporting the investment in development, time and money may be worthwhile.

A major wave of cancer registry automation took place during the late 1980's and 1990's with the emergence of commercially available and central registry supplied, user friendly, PC-based, data management and analysis systems for hospital cancer registries.[105,106] A competitive market has emerged. Perhaps electronic casefinding will turn out to be an extension or continuation of that previous automation evolution.

Death Clearance

Death clearance in a population-based cancer registry includes two processes.[106-110] The first process is to link death records from the state's vital statistics office to registry records in order to obtain death data for previously registered cancer cases. This linkage produces three outcomes: positive matches, possible matches, and nonmatches. The possible matches are manually reviewed to determine whether they are indeed matches. Unmatched death certificates necessitate further evaluation (commonly referred to as "follow-back") to determine whether they meet reportability requirements.

Death clearance requires that the registry work closely with its state's vital statistics office. Routine linkage of death records updates the vital status of the matched cases already in the database. In population-based registries that conduct active patient follow-up, frequent death-record linkage prevents the generation of unnecessary follow-up inquiries.

Vital status and related follow-up information are added to the database for those cases that are absolute matches and those determined by review to be matches. The death-record information is compared with the registry files and consolidated or updated when possible (for example, patient name, including maiden name, social security number or national identification number, race, Hispanic surname or ethnicity, birth date, birthplace). For matched deaths with cancer as a cause of death, it is also important to identify discrepancies between the cancer cause-of-death codes and the diagnosis codes in the registry database.

The second process of death clearance in a population-based cancer registry is the identification of death records that mention cancer as one of the causes of death but do not link with previously registered cases. These cases require follow-back to determine their reportability. For an unmatched cancer death that occurs in a facility that reports to the registry, the presumption is that the case was missed in routine reporting, and a request is made for an abstract to be completed. For cancer deaths that did not occur in reporting hospitals, follow-back must be made to the certifying physician, nursing care facility, or coroner, requesting an abstract or at least minimal history information.

After all follow-back sources have been exhausted and no other information on the case is available, the case is entered or retained on the registry's database as a death certificate only (DCO) case.[108,109]

ABSTRACTING

The abstracting process for central registries is similar to that done by hospital registries. Another chapter in this textbook discusses information on abstracting cases for the hospital registry. Some differences pertain.[99,110-113]

Hospitals with Cancer Registries:

An important underlying central registry decision is whether or not to utilize abstracts prepared by hospital registries in the central registry. There are multiple advantages to doing so. Most obviously, it avoids duplicate work required to abstract the case twice, which can result in a cost saving to the central registry. It makes use of the trained staff working in hospital registries, and reduces the central registry's competition with hospitals for the same limited number of trained registrars.

This method works best when the central registry can standardize the dataset and format that the hospitals are using. The central registry should avoid receiving abstracts in a variety of formats or with varying data sets whenever possible, since a great deal of time will be spent converting and interpreting nonstandard entries.

A comparison of the differences in data set items required by the Commission on Cancer, SEER, and the NPCR has been previously described.[67]

Providing standardized data definitions, abstracting and coding instructions, abstract forms, and even registry software can be one of the most important things a central registry does to achieve complete and accurate data collection. These will all constitute a good foundation for any program of quality control.

When hospital abstracts are utilized, the central registry must plan for a system of quality control. Resources that would otherwise go into case abstraction can be used for abstract review, audits, and training of hospital personnel.

Hospital cancer registries do benefit from having their data incorporated into a central registry. They have the potential of receiving compatible relevant comparison data. The quality of their data will improve through the quality control and training activities of the central registry.

One disadvantage of the use of hospital abstracts is that the central registry has less direct control over the quality and timeliness of the data than they would have if they collected it directly themselves requiring central registry quality review. Any potential problems should be addressed in the registry's planning stages, in any mandatory reporting legislation, and in the budgeting process, with the importance of standardization and a quality control component being recognized from the beginning. For example, standards for timeliness of reporting can be written into mandatory reporting legislation, and even a requirement that hospitals use Certified Tumor Registrars (CTR) can be made.

Hospitals without Cancer Registries:

For hospitals without cancer registries, as well as for non-hospital sources such as clinics, offices of physicians, pathology laboratories, nursing homes, and any other potential sources of cases, the central registry cannot rely on abstracts prepared by a hospital cancer registrar. While it is possible to require abstracting and reporting by other personnel in these sources, it is unlikely that the person doing the registry work will receive adequate training and attention, since these staff, unlike cancer registrars, will have no vested interest in the completeness or accuracy of the data.

The use of "circuit riders" has been mentioned above. While this method can be costly, the central registry can more easily control qualifications, training, and continuity of staff, with increased control over data quality. The central registry can minimize costs by utilizing electronic reporting of casefinding source documents, particularly pathology reports and disease indices, for these facilities. This enables the central registry to perform casefinding procedures centrally for a large geographic region.

Physician Reporting:

Requirements for physician reporting vary by state. Some central registries have active physician reporting because their state law mandates reporting by physicians. Other central registries have developed physician query systems to query physicians on cases identified via pathology reports that are not subsequently reported by a hospital (with or without a cancer registry).

Format of Reporting:

The advantages of permitting or even requiring standardized machine-readable reporting from hospital or non-hospital sources are overwhelming from the central registry's point of view. They are summarized in Table 34-7.

Data transmission to the central registry can be via diskette, modem transmission, or over the Internet. The central registry may choose to establish an electronic reporting standard, which all hospitals must meet, or they may choose to accept the data in a variety of hospitals' and software providers' formats

Table 34-7
The Advantages of Computer-Readable Abstracts

1. Higher quality data available sooner
2. Elimination of separate key entry of cases
3. Possibility of performing extensive data editing via computer at the time the case is being abstracted and the medical record is at hand for making corrections
4. Ease of uploading to the registry's main computer file without the need for extensive conversions or pre-editing, allowing for speedy linkage and retrieval of reported records
5. Decreased time spent in visual editing or quality control, since data items can be presented in identical order, are always legible, can be decoded into English, and checks for validity of codes and consistency among items can be performed via computer before visual editing is begun.
6. Easier to consolidate cases

and perform their own conversions and pre-edits. The former approach is more convenient and less costly for the central registry, while the latter is more convenient for hospitals, which may have adopted a variety of software systems with different data sets and output formats.

If a standard format is chosen, it is recommended that the central registry perform acceptance testing of each system's ability to generate data in the required format and meeting appropriate quality standards.

Registries need to be aware of the manner in which hospital registry software vendors handle changes to coding schemes. For example, some vendors convert data for previous diagnosis years to the coding schemes instituted for the current diagnosis year.

Circuit riding abstractors can be provided with portable computers and standardized software for casefinding and abstracting in the field.

In California, a "mail in" reporting option was developed for use by small rural hospitals. Hospitals with 50 or fewer beds, without registries, located in isolated areas at least one hour's travel from another hospital, were offered the option of having their own staff perform casefinding and then photocopying pertinent parts of the medical record and sending them into the central registry where they are abstracted by registry employees. The central registry audits the hospital's casefinding to ensure that all cases are being submitted. The photocopied records are retained for a short time to allow for quality control and then destroyed.

Reports from Outside the Area:

Registries have used various methods to obtain reports on their resident cases that have been diagnosed or treated outside the catchment area. First, referral patterns must be determined so that the registry can identify areas or facilities where significant numbers of their residents are seen. When central registries exist in neighboring areas, formal agreements can be implemented to allow sharing of resident case reports to benefit both areas. When no central registry exists, or no case-sharing agreement is in place, sometimes agreements can be reached with individual facilities to provide cases. In some instances, a central registry can even send its own staff into facilities outside its area to abstract cases of its residents.

Since datasets and definitions differ among registries, it is important to be aware of idiosyncrasies that can be introduced into the data when including reports from another registry. For example, if Registry A collects Summary Stage and Registry B does not, when Registry B provides cases reports to Registry A on A's residents, Registry A may have a higher-than-expected proportion of cases with stage unknown.

Abstracting Requirements:

Another issue to consider is whether there should be a reduced abstract or data set required by non-hospital reporting sources, such as free-standing cancer centers. A "treatment only" abstract can be more efficient for the reporting facility, while any proliferation of standards will increase the complexity of the central registry's system.

Federal facilities in the central registry's area of coverage may be unwilling or unable to meet any mandatory reporting standards, although they will probably be willing to provide cases in their own format if they already have registries, or to provide the central registry access to records for the central registry's circuit riders to abstract at the central registry's expense. For military facilities, the registry should explore obtaining machine-readable records from the DEERSACTUR system.[12]

Monitoring of Status of Facilities and Completeness of Reporting:

Regular monitoring of completeness of casefinding and abstracting is an essential component of a central registry's quality control. The North American Association of Central Cancer Registries has published a training module on management reports for central cancer registries.[114]

Frequent monitoring, at least monthly, enables the registry to quickly identify problems and have sufficient lead-time to take corrective action. Management reports can be built into the registry's computer system so that reports are automatically generated. The registry will want to monitor progress of all of the activities it is performing itself as well as progress of data collection being performed by reporting sources such as hospital registries. The central registry should expect to process one-twelfth of its annual caseload each month. Types of reports that can prove useful for monitoring are summarized in Table 34-8.

COMPUTERIZATION

Like staffing, planning for computerization is centrally important to the overall functioning of the registry. It affects almost every aspect of registry operation, and almost always involves high tech characteristics requiring specialized expertise. Those responsible for computerization of central registries face a series of decisions or concerns.[46,116,117]

The computer system and its components are generally chosen closely based on the goals and objectives of the registry. For example: will on-line data entry and retrieval be required? Will the registry be a data user itself, or prepare files for use by external biostatisticians, epidemiologists, or others? Is the central registry information system also to subsume the goals of the hospital cancer programs? What hardware, operating system, and software is most compatible with meeting the registry's goals?

Computer System Planning

In the United States it has become increasingly common for central registries to receive computer-readable input from contributing hospitals. Thus the central registry computer system can and probably should be conceived of as an integrated central and hospital registry information system.[105] Each hospital's computer should be capable of operating on its own to meet its hospital registry demands, and of transferring or transmitting its data to the central registry. Hospital computers may communicate with the central registry by teleprocessing or mail.

Table 34-8
Suggested Reports for Monitoring Casefinding, Abstracting, and Processing Status

1. Status reports of review of each casefinding source within a facility.
2. Status reports of progress in screening each type of pathology report within a facility, showing dates, and report numbers screened.
3. Progress reports on follow-back to physicians' offices of cases identified in pathology laboratories. This can be reviewed by primary site and diagnosis year.
4. Reports comparing counts of cases by facility by diagnosis month for the current year against a base year. These reports can also be prepared for selected sites of cancer, especially those that are likely to be diagnosed in outpatient settings.
5. Percent histologically confirmed by facility and for the registry as a whole, by month or year. This may identify facilities or time periods where some casefinding sources have not been reviewed.
6. Distribution by diagnosis year and month of cases submitted during a given month. A high number of incidence cases abstracted in the current month for a previous year may indicate a deficiency in an area of casefinding. The deficiency can indicate either under-reporting or over-reporting for that previous year.

In some states, hospitals report to regional registries that in turn report to the state and national registry, giving rise to four levels of integration. Thus there can be hospital registry systems, networks of hospitals reporting to a central registry, and networks of central registries reporting to a state or national registry. In the case of some larger hospital programs and in multi-hospital registries, several microcomputers are sometimes needed, forming a network within the hospital setting.

Make-or-Buy Decision

Few pre-designed systems with or without a high level of field support are available to a central registry seeking to automate.[117-121] The central registry must therefore weigh advantages and disadvantages of designing, converting or buying a system.

Three major constraints faced when designing a new system are its potential cost, development schedule, and design risk. For these reasons and others, importing or converting a pre-designed system is often seriously considered. The most effective way to look into acquiring a registry information system would be by observing them in operation in functioning registries.

Several circumstances limit transportability of central registry systems. Predefined hardware restraints, data requirements, governance relationships, and the telecommunications mode upon which a given system is based may not be amenable to the needs of a new central registry. Few systems are designed with transportability and universality in mind. More frequently, they are customized for each new user. Some central registry systems have been successfully transported from one central registry to another, with varying degrees of redesign performed by the new registry user.

Conversely, to a large extent, the computer needs of a hospital registry are often largely met by a vendor or a related central registry with an off-the-shelf system.[117,122-126]

Data Editing

Most central registries perform both manual and computerized data editing. Computerized edits typically check for completion of all required fields, allowable range, allowable values, and interfield consistency (such as primary site consistent with gender).[105,127] They can test for invalid entries such as

an unusual site-histology combination, or flag unusual entries for review. It is often desirable or necessary for the central registry computer system to be able to override an edit flag. This increases the complexity of the data system and its usage. Central registry usage may include interrecord editing, or cross-check, of reports about a patient reported from more than one facility. This also adds to the complexity of use of the system. It is in the central registry's interest that comprehensive data-editing routines are built in up-front into the software of those hospitals that contribute data.

NAACCR for central registries, and the Commission on Cancer for hospital registries have standardized data editing.[128,129] NAACCR has also issued instructions,[130,131] downloadable metafiles,[132,133] and narrative descriptions.[134] SEER has also published on the subject of data edits.[135]

Computerized data edits are not in themselves a panacea, but should be used in combination with other quality control techniques that check a number of important factors including completeness of case coverage, overuse of "unknown" codes, and timeliness.

Data Conversion

Because data sets change, at least slightly, over time, conversion of past records to current standards is necessary. Every effort is made to minimize changes as much as possible. Nonetheless important standards such as ICD-O and the AJCC Staging Guides do change as medicine advances and other changes occur.

For data analysis purposes, it is very desirable that all of the years of data in the registry's analytic file be maintained in uniform coding. It is sometimes easier to collect and computerize new cases, an immense task in itself, than it is to handle conversion of past files to current standards. This can be error-prone, and time intensive. Frequently, the most senior registry staff is assigned to this task. SEER has published certain conversion protocols in the form of computer programs and text documents.[136]

Electronic Data Interchange/Data Communications

Electronic Data Interchange (EDI) refers to the linking of computers via telephone lines, or other communication methods. EDI is also sometimes referred to as teleprocessing, data communications, and electric commerce. More recently "e" is added to a wide range of functions to denote electronic Internet methods (e.g., e-commerce). The registry world has been transformed by the Internet, including email, search engines, and many other facilities.[137,138]

EDI may include a simple transfer of data from one computer to another or may involve two-way exchange of data or interactive use of one computer and its files by a second, remote computer.

For those information systems that include and link the central registry and participating hospital registries, EDI with encryption is frequently a necessary requirement. The establishment of a link between a hospital computer and the central registry system is not necessarily a simple or automatic procedure and sometimes entails consultation between IT personnel at the hospital and IT personnel at the central registry. Once effective telecommunication has been established, it often works quite reliably. Such telecommunications require that the central registry either maintain a 7-day, 24-hour capability to handle several linkages at once, or that some process for scheduling of calls be instituted.

EDI can be both the means by which the hospital reports their data and the means by which the central registry provides follow-up information to hospitals. At its best, EDI can save critical time spent on routine registry functions.

Geocoding

For the study of cancer clusters or for other surveillance purposes, it is often desirable to determine the small geographic area, such as the census tract, where the patient resides. In this case, the user codes the census tract of residence. When the patient's address and/or related information is used to infer a geographic location, this geocoding can be an important epidemiologic tool.[139] When geocoding, it is necessary for the user to state the patient's address very explicitly and algorithmically in terms of zip code, street name, street title (Drive, Street, Blvd., and so on), and street direction. Geocoding programs require a large reference file of street names and related information for the specific geographic area concerned, and are therefore quite specialized and complex. In general, when geocoding is performed on a real set of addresses only 70 or 80% are geocod-

able at the census tract level. The remaining 20 to 30% are resolved manually by registry personnel.

In the United States geocoding programs, and their related address files, are usually developed by governmental census efforts.

Record Linkage

An important function of central registries is the ability to combine information from several sources on the same patient; referred to as record linkage.[140] Most central registries have computerized methods for record linkage. Geocoding can be thought of as a specific form of record linkage.

In addition to geocoding, common types of record linkage that a central registry may need to perform include:

- Linking duplicate reports about the same patient in a list of case reports
- Linking of the registry's cases with out-of-state reports
- Linking cancer registry cases to reports of death in death certificate files
- Linking cancer registry cases to cohort lists from special studies[141,142]

Some registries use record linkage for a broad set of other reasons, including linking their cancer patient file with groups of environmentally exposed workers or linking them to Department of Motor Vehicle records to determine whether the patient is still driving, and therefore alive.

It is not unusual for central registries to receive duplicate reports on 20% or more of their cases. Therefore, resolution of the possible duplicates becomes one of crucial importance to incidence-rate calculation. Any central registry in the United States that is not detecting numerous duplicate reports most likely has a troublesome quality control problem. Some linking programs are on-line and interactive, with provision for indicating which computer-selected matches are correct or incorrect as matching proceeds. Others use batch linkages.

Computerized Death Clearance

Central registries use death certificates both as casefinding sources and as sources for date and cause of death for cases already on record.

Customized Output Programs

A primary purpose of central registries is to actively use the data obtained for epidemiologic and other purposes. A wide range of computer output programs are needed for this. Each use of a central registry's data may entail one or more types of output program.

The most basic type of output preparation is some form of patient record selection (list or subfile generation). For many needs, a list of the identified patients is the required output; for example, a list of patients due for follow-up. Patient record selection capabilities are typically built into commercial database systems, but registries that have designed their own file management system must program their own patient record selection and/or subfile extraction.

These lists may be produced in hard copy, or in the form of a subfile. Lists are used for editing, record linkage, and many other purposes. A sort capability is often built into list generating programs.

The next level of output for central registries is based on counts of cases meeting specific criteria in the form of frequency distributions and cross tabulations. A generalized program of counting and cross classifying (for example, comparing age with primary site) is commonly needed. These counting and cross-classifying programs often must also be able to group the individual data values into categories (such as from single years of age into five-year age groups).

Many registries have customized programs for generating follow-up letters. Typically, these programs act on a selected subfile of patient names produced by the list or subfile generator.

Other necessary programs include those for incidence, mortality, and survival rate calculation. Calculation of age-specific and age-adjusted incidence and mortality require population-at-risk data for the geographic area and subpopulations being covered. Notable among these are SEER Stat and SEER Prep for use on SEER and related databases.[143-145]

Survival analysis programs, which use actuarial (life-table) methodology and may provide an age-adjustment (relative), are among the more complicated output programs that are used by central registries. The quality of survival analysis is dependent on good follow-up information. Other special purpose analysis program are available.

QUALITY CONTROL MANAGEMENT OF CENTRAL REGISTRIES

A major requirement for central registries is to maintain a level of quality that supports the uses the registry plans to make of its data.[146-154] The primary quality control concerns of central registries involve two straightforward questions: (1) how complete is case ascertainment, and (2) how complete and accurate are the data that are collected? Data collection, however, is not the only registry activity in need of monitoring. Every aspect of the registry should be considered. Data processing and computer program development can be important contributors to quality. Additional quality concerns should also include timeliness and accuracy of coding and analysis. Several topics in quality control for central registries that have been previously discussed include data editing and detection of unwanted duplicate case reports.

Feedback, communication, and training are also necessary features of a comprehensive quality control program. The results of quality control activities should be communicated effectively to data producers, registry managers, and end users. Front-line abstractors should be aware of the results of their efforts and may be in a favored position to identify the causes of special variations or problems.

The design of an appropriate quality control program must be based on a balance of costs and anticipated benefits. The objectives of a particular registry may influence to some extent the specifics of a central registry's approach to quality control.

The quality challenge registries face, and the potential sources of error, has been previously described, including case-finding (missing cases), abstracting error, coding error, address uncertainties, undetected duplicates, and population-at-risk uncertainties.[155-157]

Quality Control Methods

Various facets of quality review are performed by central registries including:

1. Visual review
2. Case completeness (reabstracting) studies
3. Computerized edit checks
4. Process monitoring
5. Death certificate follow-back
6. Measurement of accuracy
7. Designed experiments

8. Education and training
9. Directly measuring quality

Many registries, using several of these quality activities, seek to achieve registry certification.

Visual Review:

This is the form of quality control most visible to hospital registrars. It involves record-by-record evaluation by visual review. In visual review an inspector examines a sample of abstracts (sometimes all abstracts) for errors. Discrepancies are identified and corrected. Acceptable abstracts are passed along for further processing. Visual review is time-intensive. Problems discovered in visual review are generally resolved before the case can be added to the central registry data base.

Sometimes all abstracts in a batch must be resolved before any records in the batch can be accepted. That procedure is used to guard against systematic problems, some of which may not be detected by the review procedure if the procedure checks only certain records or only certain instances of inconsistencies.

Because acceptance-sampling procedures for visual review evaluate the individual report record, and often result in the need to query the registrar who originally recorded the information, it is most efficient to conduct the review as close to the time the data are entered into the original database as possible.

Re-abstracting Studies:

A somewhat more rigorous quality control process than visual review is the independent reabstracting of the case, and comparison of the reabstracting results to those of the original abstract.[158] Sometimes reabstracting is performed on a randomly selected sample of the cases, and is performed by a second abstractor who is blinded to the original abstract results.

Recoding and reabstracting studies are most often used to assess reproducibility (agreement among data collectors) and validity (agreement with source documents). The objective of a typical reabstracting study is to characterize the degree of agreement between data already in the registry and data reabstracted from source records by a different expert registrar. For each reabstracted case, the codes for each data item either match perfectly or they don't. Mismatches may be further divided into major and minor categories.

Case Ascertainment Audits:

Various sources of cases for a sample period of time are audited to assess comprehensive ascertainment of all reportable cases. NAACCR itself has sponsored such audits. In general all potential sources for the time period must be visited, and this effort is time-intensive, and requires pre-planning.[158]

Computerized Edit Checks:

Automated edit checks that are designed by central registries and incorporated into the facility registry software are especially well suited to that goal.[127-134] The adoption by central registries of standard data items and coding rules has facilitated development of standard edits maintained by NAACCR with input from the standard-setting organizations (editing references). Central registries can use the CDC-designed EDITS software to tailor selection of those edits to fit their data sets, and can add edits for items unique to their own uses. They can be used for all records for a selected period of time or on a sample to establish that the new staff member or procedure being reviewed is functioning as expected.

Data edits are used to eliminate gross inconsistencies but cannot guarantee correctness. Edit checking typically includes checking for allowable codes, range checks, interterm checks, inter-record checks, and sometimes inter-database checks. Edit checks are very cost effective and therefore should be applied to 100% of cases.

Process Monitoring:

Process monitoring involves the tracking of statistical indicators over time to detect changes indicative of a need for intervention.[147] The indicators themselves can be familiar measures: percent of records with edit errors, time lag between hospital admission and submission of the record to the central registry, number of cases submitted every month, percent of unknowns for specific items, and so on. They also can be measures specific to the operations of the central registry: percent of records processed that linked to records already in the data set, time between receipt of the report and its availability to users in the central registry data base. The important point is that process monitoring requires statistical evaluation to determine when the natural variability of these measures moves significantly outside its normal range of variation. When that happens, the central registry will apply its own procedures to identify the probable cause of the change and determine whether or what kind of response is called for. The response may be anything from training, to clarification of a coding rule, to ascertaining that a facility changed its services resulting in a change in the number of types of cases submitted.

The comparison baseline for process monitoring is often set based on historical data. This historic data method compares the number of cases expected (based on previous years or on standard incidence rates) to those observed.

Death Certificate Followback:

The surest method of check on potential missing cases is to manually review all death certificates for the reporting period, and thereafter searching for mention of cancer that may not have previously reported.[108,159] The absence of many new cases found first at death certification is the most rigorous and independent indicator that cancer diagnoses are not being missed in the catchment area.

The death-certificate method uses the percentage of cases reported by death certificate only (DCO) as a measure of incompleteness. Also, the ratio of cancer deaths in a period to incident cancer cases in the same period is compared to ratios from other population-based registries. A central registry can determine any pattern of missing cases by following back the death certificate to determine where the cancer diagnosis was made, and why it was missed.

Automated edit checks have the additional advantage of being fast and inexpensive to apply to all records. Visual review, re-abstracting and re-coding are expensive and time-consuming and are most productive when used under targeted circumstances. For example, they can be used to identify problems faced by new personnel, or raised by new or modified data items or coding procedures, new software or expansion of collection to types of cases formerly not collected.

Designed (Special) Experiments:

Designed experiments are most expensive and time-consuming to central registries and may not have the same direct effect on current data quality obtained from acceptance sampling or process monitoring.[147] However, they are often the most effective method of evaluating the effects of current processes or directing possible changes in procedures. For example, a central registry might use a designed experi-

ment to evaluate the effects of adding a new report source—say physicians who review patient slides in-office instead of sending them to a pathology lab—in terms of case coverage and costs.

Identification of duplicate reports is important to quality and can be challenging in highly mobile populations or in databases where case identifiers are based on self reported information such as name and birth date. Record linkage may be further hindered by legal restrictions related to confidentiality.

In order to be useful and reliable, periodic publication of a central registry's data should follow a consistent format and use accepted statistical procedures. Standardization of methodology can assist in that effort. It is obvious from this discussion that these quality control tools develop "data on data quality," an essential component of a comprehensive quality control program.

Measuring Quality/Certification:

Another method of quality management, which overlaps with some of those mentioned is the direct measurement of the accuracy and completeness of the registry's data. These can then be used as criteria in the certification of registries.[160,161] Several methods have been used to assess completeness of registration including reabstracting, and sample casefinding studies (audits).

NAACCR provides two levels of certification ("gold" and "silver") based on characteristics of the cancer registry data.[162-166] The indicators and the levels required for certification are shown in Table 34-9.

Using the Data:

Epidemiologists, and other analysts often find that using the data, thinking seriously about the findings and their implications lead to useful insights into possible shortcomings of the data, especially where the data's robustness may be questionable. For example, new data edits can be suggested by use of the data, which provides unexpected results.

Population-based rates include not only inaccuracies in the cancer data collected, but uncertainties regarding the populations-at-risk used in calculations. Census enumerations are estimates subject to survey error. These errors can become significant when stratifying the data by age, sex, and race/ethnic group. For example, undercount estimates exceeding 10% have been reported for black males in the 20 to 29 year age groups.

Education/Training:

Several textbooks for central registries have been published[1,2,179] as well as a series of self-instructional manuals.[167] SEER provides training for central registry personnel for the registries they fund.[168-170] The NAACCR education program includes training in introductory and advanced topics in association with its annual conference.[171] In addition, central registries recruit experienced cancer registrars and encourage their staff to obtain certification as cancer registrars.

Central registries often provide regional training for hospital registrars and other interested parties in their region.[172] In addition, other educational opportunities are available for central registry staff.[173-179]

FOLLOW-UP METHODS AND EVALUATION

Purpose of Follow-Up:

The primary purpose of patient follow-up for the central cancer registry is to evaluate the survival of groups of patients according to various parameters such as demographic characteristics, primary site, stage of disease, and first course of therapy.[180]

The central registry and the hospital registry can help each other with follow-up activities. The hospital registrar helps the central registry by sending follow-up information. The central cancer registry may facilitate hospital follow-up by providing information and services; for example, sending follow-up lists to hospitals and physicians, sharing follow-up information, contacting patients, and utilizing follow-up methods that may not be available to hospitals or physicians.

In addition, because the central registry has population-based composite data from all sources, it can calculate population-based survival statistics. These statistics can be used as a reference with which hospitals can compare their data. Finally, the central registry may validate diagnoses or changes in diagnoses that may not have been reported to the hospital.[181]

Active versus Passive Follow-Up:

The central cancer registry may use active or passive follow-up methods. Active follow-up refers to someone, usually a physician or cancer registrar, initiating direct contact with patients to encourage them to see their physician. From a central registry perspective, active follow-up may also include contacts made by hospital registrars with physician's offices.

There are primarily four active follow-up methods used by central registries. First, a list of patients due for follow-up can be sent directly to the physician responsible for patient care. Second, a list of patients due for follow-up may be sent to the hospital that reported the patient. Third, patients due for follow-up may be directly contacted by central registry staff, but any such contacts should be made with the full knowledge of the hospital. Finally, central registries may conduct research programs, and results of patient contacts that ascertain survival can be reported to the central registry.

Passive follow-up refers to methods that do not require registry contact with hospitals, physicians, or patients. Passive methods are used primarily to determine the patient's vital status and current date

Table 34-9
Levels of Certification for Central Cancer Registries

Criterion	Level of Central Registry Certification	
	Silver	Gold
Completeness	>=90%	>=95%
Passing EDITS	>= 97%	>=100%
Death Certificate Only	<=5%	<=3%
Timeliness	within 23 months	within 23 months
Duplicate Reports in Data	<=2/1,000	<=1/1,000
Missing, unknown		
Sex, Age, County	<=3%	<=2%
Race	<=5%	<=3%

last seen alive or date of death. See Table 34-10. These methods usually involve computerized searches or manual review of existing files that may contain the cancer patient's name and the follow-up information. Passive methods are often most easily done by the central registry because they most likely have the appropriate computer capacity and linkage software. There are many possible passive follow-up methods, some of which are listed in Table 34-9.

Passive methods are relatively inexpensive to use and are often time-efficient, but they have limitations. Methods vary in efficiency and cost-effectiveness depending upon the amount and accuracy of the identifying information. Most methods require complex computer programs. Confidentiality may be a problem because computer tapes with names of cancer patients are often provided to the agency with the data to do the linkage. Some methods (such as checking death certificate and DMV records) may not have as high a yield in areas that have high in-and-out migration. Finally, if information is needed about the status of living patients, or if quality-of-life data are needed, passive methods are not usually effective.

Generally, a successful follow-up program in a central registry uses both active and passive follow-up methods. It is not clear what bias exists if only one or a limited number of methods is used. Regardless of methods used, successful registries aim for a low lost-to-follow-up percentage. In reality, there will be losses, so the question is how much loss can be tolerated. In calculating survival statistics, there are no guidelines regarding the percentage that can be lost before the assumptions are violated regarding life-table and other methodologies. Probably the most important assumption is that those lost to follow-up are not different from the rest of the cases being followed.[182] Unfortunately, those that are lost to follow-up may be different. They may have different ages, social class, and health patterns than those who are successfully followed. The kinds of cases lost to follow-up may also be biased with regard to the follow-up methods used.

Patient follow-up can be complex and costly,[183] so hospital and central registries should work together. Cooperation leads to efficiency, accuracy, and high follow-up rates, thus improving patient care and also the accuracy of survival statistics.

SERVICES PROVIDED TO HOSPITAL REGISTRIES BY CENTRAL REGISTRIES

A central registry obtains most of its information from hospitals, and in spite of laws requiring reporting, the central registry's continuing existence is often importantly dependent upon the goodwill and cooperation of hospitals. There are many useful services that a central registry can provide to hospitals in order to encourage their cooperation, including those listed in Table 34-11.

Table 34-10
Passive Follow-up Methods Used by Central Registries

- Linkage with state death certificate files
- Linkage with state motor vehicles records
- Linkage to National Death Index
- Linkage to state health files such as Medicare
- Linkage to national health records such as the Center for Medicare and Medicaid Services
- Review of records of local election boards
- Linkage with hospital discharge summaries
- Review of resident lists in geographic areas
- Linkage to rosters of health plans (HMO's)

Table 34-11
Services Provided to Hospitals by Central Registries

- Feedback on death certificates
- Backup of computerized data (in the event of individual computer or system crashes)
- Edits and quality checks of data
- Assistance in computerizing the hospital registry (providing a backlog of the cases already stored in the central registry and providing workshops and other training)
- Providing participating hospitals with the latest information on all of their patients who have been admitted to other hospitals to determine the total treatment received from all sources
- Ensuring that only one follow-up letter is generated no matter where the patient was accessioned

CALCULATION AND ASSESSMENT OF INCIDENCE RATES

Definition:

One of the primary and unique functions of a population-based registry is to measure the amount or rate of disease in a known geographic area or population. The most commonly used measure of cancer in a population is the incidence rate (IR), defined as the measurement of disease frequency over a specified period of time.[1,184,185] Researchers also use it to determine how the risk of disease varies in different subgroups of the population. The definition of an incidence rate is shown in Figure 34-1.

The numerator includes only newly diagnosed cases during a given time period. The denominator includes only individuals in the same population who are "at risk" for the disease during the same time period. For instance, the incidence rate of prostate cancer in Iowa would only include men in the numerator and denominator. The populations used in incidence rates are generally multiplied by a factor such as 100,000, to create rates expressed in whole numbers, which are easier to use than decimal numbers.

An annual incidence rate is an incidence rate calculated for a one-year period. If the incidence information is combined for several years, an average annual incidence rate can be calculated by dividing the sum of the numerators by the sum of the denominators. This is frequently done to increase the stability offered in several years of data compared to a single year.

Incidence rates are commonly calculated as crude rates, age-specific rates, and age-adjusted rates. Rates that are calculated for a total population (e.g. all ages combined) are called crude rates.

Another measure of disease is prevalence, which includes the total number of cases with a disease at a particular point in time. Unlike prevalence, incidence is not influenced by differences in the survival of cases. Prevalence is a useful measurement, however, for health care planning purposes.

Age-Specific Incidence Rates (ASIR):

Rates that are calculated for subgroups of the population, such as age-group) are called specific rates. Rates for specific age groups are referred to as age-specific rates, and rates for a given cancer site are termed site-specific rates. Rates are further generally calculated separately for men and women (sex-specific) because combining genders hides information.

Age-Adjusted Incidence Rates (AAIR):

A method used to facilitate rate comparison in populations that have different age distributions is to calculate an overall rate and adjust it for age. These rates are known as age-adjusted incidence rates (AAIR's), or sometimes as standardized rates. Three methods are commonly used to age-adjust rates: cumulative incidence, direct standardization, and indirect standardization. Only direct standardization is discussed here.

With direct standardization, we answer the question "What are the rates in a standard population if the age-specific rates in population A and population B were both to occur in the standard population?" In this way, AAIR's can be calculated that are directly comparable because they are derived using the same standard population reference.

Table 34-12 presents an example of the calculation of age-adjusted incidence rates for Asian/Other and Hispanic women in California by the direct method using the 1970 US population as the standard or reference population. The 1970 US standard population, which totals 1,000,000, is shown in column 1. The age-specific incidence rates for breast

Figure 34-1

Definition of a Crude Incidence Rate (IR).

$$IR = \frac{N}{P} = \frac{\text{Number of new cases of disease during a specified time period}}{\text{Number of people at risk in the population during the same time period}}$$

Table 34-12

Example of Calculation of an Annual Age-Specific Incidence Rates (ASIR) and Age-Adjusted Incidence (AAIRíS) Rates for Asian/Other and Hispanic Women in California by The Direct Method Using the 1970 US Standard Population. Female Breast Cancer, Asian/Other and Hispanics Age-Specific Incidence

Age Group	1970 U.S. Standard Population (1)	Asian/Others Average Annual ASIR per 100,000 (2)	Age-Specific Product (3)=(1) x (2)/1,000,000	Hispanics Average Annual ASIR per 100,000 (4)	Age-Specific Product (5)=(1) x (4)/1,000,000
0-4	84,416	0.0	0.00	0.0	0.00
5-9	98,204	0.0	0.00	0.0	0.00
10-14	102,304	0.0	0.00	0.0	0.00
15-19	93,845	0.2	0.02	0.0	0.00
20-24	80,561	2.2	0.18	1.0	0.08
25-29	66,320	5.9	0.39	5.7	0.38
30-34	56,249	20.6	1.16	1.5	1.77
35-39	54,656	50.4	2.75	47.6	2.60
40-44	58,958	91.6	5.40	81.4	4.80
45-49	59,622	149.4	8.91	129.8	7.74
50-54	54,643	155.0	8.47	150.7	8.23
55-59	49,077	157.5	7.73	186.5	9.15
60-64	42,403	154.1	6.53	196.6	8.34
65-69	34,406	196.4	6.76	*255.5*	8.79
70-74	26,789	188.1	5.04	281.1	7.53
75-79	18,871	220.2	4.16	271.5	5.12
80-84	11,241	163.9	1.84	300.3	3.38
85+	7,435	191.7	1.43	247.8.	1.84
	1,000,000		60.77		69.75

Rates, California 1988-1992. Source: California Cancer Registry, Cancer Incidence and Mortality in California by Detailed Race/Ethnicity, 1988-1992. April 1995.27[186]

cancer in Asian/Other women, as calculated in Table 34-6, are listed in column 2. These rates are then multiplied and then divided by 1,000,000, giving a product, shown in column 3. The sum of these products across all age groups is 60.77, the age-adjusted incidence rate for breast cancer in Asian/Other women for 1988-1992, using the 1970 US standard population. Similar calculations are given for Hispanic women in columns 4 and 5 with an age-adjusted rate of 69.75.

The rate for breast cancer, age-adjusted to the 1970 US standard population, is 60.77 per 100,000 per year for Asian/Other women and 69.75 per 100,000 per year for Hispanic women. This implies that, if the 1970 US population had the same age-specific rates as Asian/Other women and as Hispanic

women, there would be an average of 61 cases among Asian/Other women and 70 cases among Hispanic women per 100,000 women in the United States for each year from 1988 to 1992.

Note that the age-adjusted rate for Hispanic women is higher than that for Asian/Other women. Comparison of the crude rates would have shown the opposite conclusion: an incidence of 56 per 100,000 for Asian/Other women compared with 43 per 100,000 for Hispanic women. Comparing crude rates leads to an erroneous conclusion as a result of the age difference of the two populations (the average age of Hispanic women is much lower than that of Asian/Other women).

Choosing a standard population is a matter of judgment. A standard commonly used internationally-ly is the world population. Until recently, the 1970 US population, and populations of the country, state, or other geographic location being studied were frequently used. More recently the 2000 US population has been adopted.[187] It is generally preferable for the age distribution of the standard population to be similar to the age distributions of the study populations. A comparison of the 1970 and 200 standards are given in Table. The 2000 standard population reflects the aging of the US population. Since cancer is age-progressive, this increased weighting of the older age-specific cancer rates will increase age-standardized rates.

Other risk measures are used in population-based epidemiology, including proportional methodologies.[188] Proportional methodologies are useful where populations-at-risk are not available for the subgroups of interest. An example would be the proportional incidence rate (PIR) of lung cancer among spray painters. The PIR would be the proportion of spray painters with lung cancer (cases/all spray painters) divided by the proportion of all other workers with lung cancer (possibly age-adjusted). The appropriate-ness of proportional methodology depends heavily on the homogeneity of the reference group; in this case all workers who are not spray painters. Age-adjustment can be performed as appropriate.

CALCULATION AND ASSESSMENT OF SURVIVAL RATES

Survival-rate calculations in the hospital setting were described in Chapter 17 and elsewhere.[189-192] The observed survival rate is the proportion of persons in a defined population who remain alive during a specified time interval. The beginning of the surveillance period is usually defined by a particular event, such as cancer diagnosis, exposure to a carcinogen, or the beginning of treatment. The surveillance period generally ends at death, although the same methods can be used to evaluate other endpoints, such as cancer recurrence.

Several forms of survival analysis are described in Chapter 17, including the direct method and the life-table (actuarial, cohort) method; often referred to as observed survival rates. The direct observed survival method requires that all subjects be available for survival throughout the complete interval of interest. The life-table observed survival method allows including subjects who may have been lost to follow-up, or may be alive after several years of observation. Survival rates can be expressed as a ratio such as 0.917, or as a percent, 91.7%.

The relative survival rate is "the ratio of the observed survival rate in the study population to the expected survival rate in the subset of the general population with the same characteristics as the study population."[189] The relative survival rate is the observed survival rate, adjusted because some of the subjects can be expected to die from other causes of death than that under study. Age-sex-race/ethnic specific life table probability are generally used to calculate this adjustment. Thus a five-year observed survival rate for breast cancer summarizes how many of the observed breast cancer patients can be expected to die from all causes of death. The five-year relative survival rate of the breast cancer patients is the percent that will die from breast cancer alone. Observed and relative survival rates can differ materially and clarity of definition when presenting data is important.

The cancer survival rate is also sometimes confused with the cancer mortality rate, which is the rate at which persons in the general population die

Table 34-13
Standard US Populations, 1970 and 2000

Age Group	1970	2000
0-4	84,416	69,135
5-9	98,204	72,533
10-14	102,304	73,032
15-19	93,845	72,169
20-24	80,S61	66,478
25-29	66,320	64,529
30-34	56,249	71,044
35-39	54,656	80,762
40-44	58,958	81,851
45-49	59,622	72,118
50-54	54,643	62,716
55-59	49,077	48,454
60-64	42,403	38,793
65-69	34,406	34,264
70-74	26,789	31,733
75-79	18,871	26,999
80-84	11,241	17,842
85+	7,435	15,508
	1,000,000	1,000,000

of cancer during the time period of interest. The mortality rate provides a measure of the risk of death attributable to a disease in a population, whereas the survival rate is determined by following a specific group of people with the disease until death. The survival rate is interpreted as the risk of dying among people who have the disease. Hospitals calculate survival rates for their patients, but if such rates are desired for an entire population, they must be calculated by central registries.

USES OF CANCER REGISTRY DATA

Cancer registries are a rich source of information for a wide variety of surveillance and other important public heath purposes.[193-198] There are several categories into which these uses can be summarized, but no rubric seems completely inclusive.

Cancer Case Statistics:

Population-based cancer registries provide the baseline information defining the burden of new (incident) cancers in the US, in states and other catchment areas. Multihospital central registries that are not also population-based provide similar baseline information for hospital cohorts.[10] Surveillance includes what types of cancers are being diagnosed (patient age, gender and race/ethnicity) and where diagnosed are described. Frequency estimates the prevalence of patients from the incident counts. Several of the standard setters provide population-based statistics, including the International Agency for Research on Cancer, NAACCR, SEER and the American Cancer Society.[14,21,199-202]

Incidence/Prevalence Surveillance (Descriptive Epidemiology)

In addition to these frequencies counts (statistics), central registries provide incidence rates by age group, gender and race/ethnicity. A comparative analysis of such rates is often referred to as descriptive epidemiology.[203-214] Essentially all population-based registries annually publish a report of case frequencies and incidence rates. Depending on the analytic resources of each central registry, a broad range of incidence and prevalence surveillance including time trends is maintained. In some cases analysts of central registry data also perform corresponding mortality surveillance, with the data for

such efforts coming from health department death statistics not central registries.

Patterns of disease occurrence can be studied to identify groups who are experiencing different rates of cancer than others. These comparisons are used to generate hypotheses to explain rate differences and causes, which may lead to analytical studies to test these hypotheses or to develop cancer control programs to reduce the risk in the high-risk groups.

Examples of descriptive data include documentation of the higher rate of prostate cancer in African-American men as compared to white men, lower lung cancer rates in Utah (with a large Mormon population that does not smoke cigarettes) than the rest of the United States, and the rapid rise in diagnosed breast cancer beginning in the 1980s (due to increased use of mammography). One of the most interesting examples has been the comparison of cancer rates in immigrants, between their native and host countries. These studies have shown that many cancers increase or decrease in immigrants to reflect the rates in the host countries. For example, breast cancer rates in Japanese women are low, but they increase in Japanese women immigrating to the United States.

In addition to the basic case frequencies and incidence, central cancer registries can also provide baseline information about the distribution of cancer by stage of disease. For example, areas of high and low early diagnosis of cancer can be determined. For example, the degree of late diagnosis of breast and cervical cancer, and where such cases are being diagnosed.

Cancer Cluster Surveillance:

Reported cancer clusters can become of great public and media concern. Neighborhood groups, real estate interests, industry groups, occupation groups, school groups, and a variety of other interest groups periodically become strongly interested in one or another reported cancer hot spots. In many cases, analysis of clusters along with surveillance of incidence trends are the twin pillars of the original cancer registry justification and funding. That's why the registry was started. Analysis of clusters in time and space is a difficult and demanding task.[215-218] Presentation of this information to the interested parties can also be demanding and time intensive. Essential to cancer cluster analysis is that all cases be included with accurate diagnostic criteria and dates of diagnosis. The population-based central registry is the only available source of such information.[5-7]

Cancer Mapping:

An important element among the tools of cancer surveillance is cancer mapping. The pictorial presentation of color-coded data is an intuitively clear method of analyzing and presenting spatial information. For example, color-coded county maps may be used to show early versus advanced stage diagnosis of breast cancer.

Geographic Information Systems (GIS):

GIS offer interesting potential for analysis of cancer and population-related data.[219-221] Although cancer mapping has long been used in cancer epidemiology, the GIS offer more sophisticated tools than county mapping and color-coding.

Ecologic or Correlation Studies:

Another common form of cancer surveillance is to study whether cancer incidence or mortality rates in a population are correlated with some other factor measured in the population, for example, dietary fat. If incidence is the measure of interest, then the population-based registry is the source of these data. These measures show the amount of change in the factor of interest as the cancer rate changes. One way this can be demonstrated is to plot cancer rates for different countries on the vertical axis of a graph and the corresponding factor of interest for each country on the horizontal axis.[222-223]

A correlation statistic can be calculated, 1.0 indicating perfect correlation and 0.0 indicating no correlation. For example, when colon cancer rates and dietary fat consumed for many countries are plotted, there is a very high correlation between these factors. One limitation of these studies is that they may show that variables are correlated, but there is no way to determine whether one variable causes the other. In fact, they may only be correlated because both are caused by another, unknown, factor. So these studies are only suggestive, but they have been important in creating etiologic hypotheses that can be tested using methods that can determine causality.

Case Control Studies:

In these studies, cases of cancer are compared with similar people from the same population who do not have cancer (serving as the control group) for past exposures that may be related to the disease. These exposures are usually measured by respondent's answers to questionnaires or from historical records (such as health records).[24] If the cancer cases have had more exposure to the variables than the controls, then it can be inferred that exposure to that variable increases one's odds or risk of having the cancer. The cancer registry is important in identifying the cases to be included in these studies, if they are to be representative of all cases.

The registry also facilitates case control studies by providing data that can be included in the analysis such as stage, treatment, and demographic characteristics. It can be seen that case-control studies start with the cases and matching controls, and look backward in time at possible risk factors. This retrospective approach can be efficient and cost-effective.

Cohort Studies:

This type of study begins with identification of a group, or cohort, of individuals who may be disease free. Risks or exposures of interest are then measured and the people are followed to see who gets the disease. The exposures of those with and those without the disease are compared, and if they are excessive in the diseased group, it can be inferred that this exposure may be an important factor in the etiology of the disease.[224,225] In cohort studies in which the disease of interest is cancer, central cancer registries are often used to determine the disease outcome by linking the cohort members to all the cases in the registry. Here, too, the registry can provide data on the patients to be included in the analyses. If the registry includes follow-up as part of their operation, they can also add information on survival status and cause of death. This prospective following of originally well subpopulations may take place over years and be costly, but it allows analysis of all possible health outcomes not just the predefined disease as in case-control studies. Thus, the famous Framingham, Massachusetts cohort study could uncover the unsuspected relationship of heart disease to smoking as well as the suspected relationship to lung cancer.

One type of cohort study is the retrospective cohort. In these studies the cohort is defined today to be some point in the past. For example, we can decide now to study all employees who were employed at a particular nuclear facility on January 1, 1970. The registry is asked to link those early cohort members to today's registry files to determine who has developed the disease. Rates of the disease in the cohort are then often compared to an expected rate. The latter is determined from registry data for the entire population. Examples of these studies include linkages to rosters of occupational groups as identified from employment or union records, college students, and professional societies. These studies are now possible as a result of computers and the linkage programs that have been developed.

Genetic Studies:

In recent years some progress has been made in identifying genes that may be related to different cancers. Consequently, there is a need to identify high-risk families that can be studied and related to the general population. Central registries are increasingly being asked to help identify these families.[226-229] This is done by identifying cancer cases of interest, after which they are contacted to obtain a family history. Families of interest may then be asked to complete more detailed questionnaires, to give blood, and to allow access to pathologic material. In these studies, a family history registry is really being created. Many central registries are in the best position to carry out these tasks, and the family registry becomes an extension of the cancer registry. Sometimes the registry can be linked to an existing database to facilitate genetic research. An important example of this is the work being done with the Utah Cancer Registry. This registry has been linked to the Mormon genealogy database, from which the heritability of cancer has been described.

Basic Science Studies:

Basic science research may look at the mechanisms by which cells become cancerous or metastatic, identify markers for early detection or progression, or identify new methods of screening, treatment, and palliative care. Population-based data have often been used to develop leads for basic science work. An example is the observation that cervical cancer occurred more frequently in some populations, and that it might be sexually transmitted. This eventually led basic scientists to look for the human papilloma virus. Population data can also be used to look, in a general way, at the outcome of different treatments or screening procedures, although they cannot replace the randomized, controlled, clinical trial.

Patterns of Care Surveillance (Clinical Studies).

The central registry can be used to measure treatment in different geographic areas, different types of hospitals (teaching hospitals, county hospitals, HMO hospitals), or different sub-populations. These general assessments can suggest areas where professional education may be appropriate. The National Cancer Data Base and other Commission on Cancer projects have performed patterns of care studies in large multihospital series for decades.[25-26,230-234] Hospital registrars use the aggregate data to evaluate their hospital against composite hospital data in terms of types of cancer seen, patient characteristics, cancer characteristics, treatment, survival and other factors.

If a central registry has set up an RCA system, it can be adapted to identify patients that may be eligible for clinical trials.

Survival Surveillance:

Survival rates are considered a primary measure of the cancer burden. They measure the deadly cost of cancer, and time trends can be used to assess progress in early diagnosis and/or better treatment.[21-22] In the same way that incidence surveillance can be maintained with regard to various demographic and other risk factors of the cases, the same comparative surveillance can be maintained for survival. For example, which anatomic stage of disease group survives best? Is there any difference between stages? Which ethnic/racial group survives best? Which treatment group survives best?

Cancer Control:

Cancer control includes six program types: primary prevention; screening; early diagnosis; treatment; rehabilitation; and palliative care.[235-238] In all of these types, it is striking to note the implications for central registries. Without registries, how will we know which types of people (male, female; older, younger; black, white; which geographic areas; and so on) are at greatest risk for certain types of cancer or have late diagnosis or poor survival? If we do not know how often each type of cancer occurs in a specific population, how do we know where to focus our efforts and prioritize the use of our limited cancer control resources? How will we know that cancer control efforts had any effect, if we do not know how often the disease was diagnosed or treated, or what the survival was before and after the intervention efforts? How can we determine whether cases are found earlier if we do not know their stage at diagnosis before and after any intervention?

Thus, we see that central registries are an integral part of the cancer control process. Cancer registries not only provide data for prioritizing our limited cancer control resources to high-risk groups and geographic areas but also provide the mechanism to evaluate cancer control activities.

HISTORY OF US CENTRAL CANCER REGISTRIES

The initiation of registration of populations with cancer was a slow process, with many false starts.[239-240] In some instances, the early population-based efforts are closely intertwined with hospital registration, each one facilitating the other.

1920s:

A first, but unsuccessful, cancer census took place in London in 1728. It was not until 1900, however, that many researchers and citizens demanded statistics about the disease. Attempts were made to collect these statistics by physician questionnaires, but poor reporting led to many failures. The oldest known example of a modern successful registry is in Hamburg, Germany, where in 1929 a follow-up patient care service was instituted in the local health department.[240]

The activities of the American College of Surgeons (ACOS) in promoting cancer registries also goes back to the 1920s when the organization started a bone cancer registry by asking its members to submit information on living cases with that cancer.[72,246] This was followed by the CoC effort later in the 1920s by collections of cases of cancer of the cervix, breast, mouth and tongue, colon and thyroid.

The Massachusetts Cancer Registry began in 1926 in the State Health Department, centered in an abandoned state hospital, and was designed to establish cancer clinics throughout the state under the direction of Dr. Herbert Lombard.[242] Early in the data collection process, Lombard and his staff reported on the relationship of cancer to population density and a higher cancer rate in foreign born Americans and their children than in native born Americans with native grandparents. They also published one of the first studies linking oral cancer and the use of tobacco.

The registry did not report all cases of cancer in the state but did report and follow cases in the major hospitals. By 1953, 20 hospitals maintained state-aided cancer clinics. They offered multi-disciplinary diagnostic consultative services for referred cancer patients.

Following Dr. Lombard's retirement in 1959, the Massachusetts state cancer registry lost its funding. There was a brief resurgence of interest in the early 1960s when the NCI funded the program to assist in obtaining data for its End Result Program. Attempts were made to fund a cancer registry in Boston in the late 1960s but this initiative also failed through lack of state funding. The registry was reorganized in 1982 and now claims coverage of an estimated 95% of cancer patients in the state.

1930s:

In 1930 the Commission on Cancer developed standards for hospital cancer clinics and by 1937 there were 240 approved cancer clinics.

The first truly population-based registry in the United States was the Connecticut Tumor Registry, which was founded in 1941 but registered cases back to 1935.[243,244] This registry has been in continuous operation since then and is now part of the SEER program.

The Connecticut Cancer Registry was started when a group of New Haven physicians began compiling data, which showed a steady increase in the cancer rates in New Haven. They proceeded to form cancer clinics in their hospitals and maintain uniform records. From these beginnings, the State Medical Society formed a Tumor Study Committee to coordinate cancer control activity in the State, and this body was instrumental in getting state legislation passed which created a Division of Cancer and other Chronic Diseases in 1935. In 1941, the tumor registry began operating statewide with a team from the Division visiting each hospital and abstracting all cancer records for the period 1935 to 1940. Subsequently the tumor clinic registrar, trained by the state team, continued abstracting and sending abstracts of cancer cases to the central cancer registry. It is the oldest continuous state cancer registry in the United States and has served as a model for other state registries. The Connecticut Tumor Registry first published incidence data in 1947, and every year thereafter.

New York State's interest in cancer control goes back to the late nineteenth century, when Dr. Roswell Park received a grant from the State Legislature to set up a state pathology laboratory in Buffalo. The Roswell Park Memorial Hospital, a 300 bed state cancer research hospital developed from these beginning.[245]

A Division of Cancer Control was established in 1931 at the Institute. Cancer was made a reportable disease in 1939 in New York State, exclusive of New York City, and transferred operations to the State Health Department in Albany. Its function was expanded from public education to training, nursing and laboratory resources and research. Cancer reporting started in 1940 with the endorsement of the Medical Society of the State of New York. The State Registry has been a source for a number of research projects. Under the direction of Dr. Peter Greenwald, studies on the clustering of Hodgkin's disease cases and a number of surveillance studies were instituted.

The earliest attempt in the United States to estimate cancer incidence for the entire country was in 1937. Since cancer was not a reportable disease nationally, the National Cancer Institute performed a study of a sample of the cases in 1937 to determine the incidence of cancer. This was referred to as the Ten Cities Cancer Survey.[246] Under the direction of Harold F. Dorn, the survey was conducted over a period of three years, 1937-1939, in a convenience sample of ten areas, mostly urban, comprising about ten percent of the country's population.

Reports were obtained from every hospital and from all but two percent of the physicians. It is estimated that only 8.5% of the cases were reported by death certificates only. The data from the study was used for estimating the incidence of cancer for the whole country and for observing variations by site, age, race and region of the country. It served as a baseline for evaluating cancer trends in subsequent national cancer surveys. And it taught much about the techniques to use and pitfalls to avoid in achieving complete registration in cancer surveys.

1940s:

In 1948-1949, the NCI conducted its 2nd National Cancer Incidence Survey in the same 10 areas surveyed in 1937-39.[247] This survey was expanded to include analysis not only of age, sex and race but also by marital status and income class and by stage of disease and histologic type of cancer. Another section of the survey showed trends by site since the first survey.

The American Cancer Society (ACS) realized the need for registering cancer cases in the late 1940s and started giving assistance to hospital, regional and state registries. Requests came from hospital administrators, county and state medical societies.

In California cancer registration in hospitals started in 1949 when the California Tumor Registry in the State Health Department was founded.[248] In that year abstracting of cases in hospitals began going back to 1942. Over the next 14 years, many more hospitals were added so that by 1956, 53 hospitals had cancer registries.

1950s:

A manual for hospital cancer programs was prepared by the CoC in 1954, including a section on methods for reporting end results. In 1956 the requirements were amended to specify that an approved cancer program must have a cancer registry.

Personnel from the American Cancer Society helped found cancer registries in Iowa and Puerto Rico in the early 1950s, which remain viable today. They also started registries in Alabama, Kentucky, and Michigan (Calhoun County). Some of the registries failed through lack of continuing funding but were reinstituted at a later date.

The data from the Connecticut Cancer Registry was integrated with data from eleven other cancer centers to become part of the End Results Group of the National Cancer Institute's in 1956. The End Results Group issued four reports in the 1950s and 1960s. These reports were attempts to present survival figures on newly diagnosed cases from a number of state cancer registries and large hospital cancer registries in different parts of the country. The reports showed survival rates by age, sex, race and stage by site of cancer for different time periods of diagnosis going back to the 1940s. While these data did not comprise a random sample of all cancer cases in the country, they were the major source for tracking national survival rates by site and time period.

The Utah Cancer Registry was founded in 1966 by Charles R. Smart, M.D., an early advocate of cancer registries and their computerization.[249] The Utah Registry was established by the incorporation of several hospital cancer registries into a central registry, and with the cooperation of the remaining hospitals in the state. The primary purposes of the Registry were to provide service to hospitals and physicians, to provide a mechanism to stimulate frequent physician examinations of patients for recurrent or secondary malignancies, and to serve as an educational resource for physicians treating cancer patients.

1960s:

Another survey, the Third National Cancer Survey (TNCS) was conducted by the NCI in 1969 to 1971, with some different geographic areas added.[250] This was planned as a three-year survey around a census year in seven metropolitan areas and two entire states. A three-year survey was planned to get adequate incidence data on rare sites and to expand the coverage on rural areas of the country. Seven of the ten cities included in the 1937 and 1947 surveys were also in the TNCS for trend analyses. The entire states of Iowa and Colorado were in the survey, and the Minneapolis-St. Paul metropolitan area was added. The Commonwealth of Puerto Rico also participated in the survey. In addition to analyses by demographic variables, site, histologic diagnosis, and stage of disease, the survey included questions on a 10% sample of cases in regard to treatment, duration of hospitalization, cost of medical care, and the economic impact on the family. In addition to the all sites survey, a special survey on skin cancer was conducted in four of the ten areas.

The survey compiled over 180,000 new cases over the three-year period with 90.1% microscopically confirmed. In the earlier two surveys about 74% were microscopically confirmed. Only 2.1% of the diagnosed cases were by death certificate only.

The primary purpose of these surveys was to obtain morbidity, mortality, and prevalence data. Patients were not followed for outcome. Because patients could not be followed for survival from surveys conducted every ten years, and because of the cost of setting up registries every ten years, the Third National Cancer Survey in 1969-1971 was the last of its kind.

1970s:

In the early years of the Connecticut Registry's operations, compliance by physicians and hospitals in the state to furnish basic data and follow-up data was voluntary. Cancer became a reportable disease by law in 1971 and in 1973 the law was extended to apply to private pathology laboratories.[244] The NCRA was chartered in 1974.

By 1972, new CoC standards stated that approved hospital cancer programs in hospitals with 300 or more cancer patients annually must have full facilities and personnel, an active cancer registry and ongoing research in cancer. Activities by the College expanded in the late 1970s and 1980s to provide expert help in setting up cancer registries in hospitals, and to provide expert assistance in design of forms and coding and technical assistance with computer operations.

Regional population based registries were formed in Los Angeles County in 1972 and the San Francisco-Oakland Bay Area (SFO) in 1973. The primary purpose of, and funding for the Los Angeles County registry was provided to facilitate population-based analytic epidemiologic studies. In 1973, the Utah Registry also began epidemiologic studies of the Utah population. The Utah Cancer Registry covers a low-risk population, with low levels of overall cancer incidence.

In 1973, the Surveillance, Epidemiology, and End Results (SEER) Program was started by the National Cancer Institute and has continued until now.[26] The program is designed to give annual reports on cancer incidence, mortality and survival from areas comprising about ten percent of the population of the United States.[251] The areas in the 1973 survey included the entire states of Connecticut, Iowa, New Mexico, Utah and Hawaii, and the metropolitan areas of Atlanta, Detroit, Seattle and San Francisco-Oakland. Data from Puerto Rico are also collected but published separately.

A fifth report from the End Results Group was published in 1976 and included data from two state cancer registries and two hospital registries.[22] Comparison of overall five-year relative survival rates in whites showed an increase from 39% in cases diagnosed in 1950-1959 to 41% in 1967-1973. Among blacks the increase was from 29% to 32%. Survival rates, as published by the NCI, thereafter were obtained from data collected in the SEER Program.

Interest in central cancer registries grew with the start of the SEER program in 1973, which gave continuing financial assistance to the existing cancer registries in its program. By 1977, there were 20 state cancer registries, and by 1979, 797 hospital cancer programs had been approved by the CoC.[64]

1980s:

In 1980, the NCI published data on five-year survival rates from the same four registries as their 1976 report for 1960-1963 and 1970-1973.[21] The report showed a statistically significant increase in five-year survival rates in the latter period in 17 of 35 sites in males and 26 of 35 sites in females.

In the 1980s, some additional state governments decided to fund central cancer registries. Seven additional registries began between 1980 and 1984 and ten additional started between 1985 and 1989.

In addition to SFO and LA, other California regional registries were organized between 1984 and 1988, and in 1988 a statewide cancer reporting system was started. In 1983 The NCRA started a credentialing process for cancer registrars (CTR).

In 1987, cancer control leaders formed the American Association of Central Cancer Registries (AACCR). The founding sponsors of the organization include the National Cancer Institute, the American Cancer Society, the National Tumor Registrars Association (now known as the National Cancer Registrars Association), the American College of Surgeons, and the American Association of Cancer Institutes. The purpose of the organization is the development and application of cancer registration and morbidity survey techniques to the conduct of cancer control programs. Its goals are to provide technical assistance to central cancer registries; to collect and publish combined cancer data from eligible members on a periodic basis; and to hold periodic scientific meetings for its members.

In 1995, the name was changed to NAACCR to formalize the inclusion of Canada (first as AACCR then NAACCR) By the 1980s, statewide registries were operating in 37 states, DC, Puerto Rico and Virgin Islands.

1990s:

An important event which led to further development of state registries was the passage of the US Cancer Registries Amendment Act in 1992, which allocated money to fund registries in all states. This program is administered by the Centers for Disease Control and Prevention (CDC).[6] In 1995, funds were allocated to 42 states and territories and the District of Columbia, representing 93% of the US population. It was recognized that it would be several years before all of these registries would be population-based and reporting all cases.

NAACCR published data set and data transfer standards for cancer registries. Later in 1995, NAACCR published incidence data from 48 central registries in the United States and Canada."

Table 34-14
Timeline of US Central Cancer Registry History

1926	Pilot Massachusetts Registry
1935	Reference date for Connecticut Registry
1937-39	Ten Cities Cancer Survey
1939	New York law making cancer reportable (excluding New York City)
1941	Connecticut Registry started.
1948-49	Second National Cancer Survey
1949	California Tumor Registry started.
1950s	Registries started in Alabama, Iowa, Kentucky, Puerto Rico, and Michigan (Calhoun County)
1954:	CoC published manual for hospital cancer programs.
1956	End Results Group started.
1966	Utah Registry started.
1969-71	Third National Cancer Survey
1971	Connecticut law making cancer reportable by hospitals
1972	Los Angeles County Registry started.
1973	SEER Program started.
1973	Connecticut law making cancer reportable by independent pathology laboratories
1973	San Francisco-Oakland Registry started.
1974	NCRA formed
1977	Twenty state registries exist.
1979	797 CoC-approved hospital cancer programs
1983	CTR credentialing began.
1987	NAACCR formed.
1989	Thirty-seven state registries exist.
1994	Standardized data set established by NAACCR Uniform Data Standards Committee (UDS)
1996	Standardized edits established by NAACCR UDS.
1998	First NAACCR Incidence Report
1992	US Cancer Registries Amendment Act passed.
1995	First SEER Incidence Report
1993	NPCR started.
1997	NAACCR registry certification program started.

Additional registries are added each year as more of them become population-based and are able to identify at least 95% of the cases in their areas.[20]

By 1993, there were more than 1300 hospitals with CoC approved cancer programs.[252]

In 1997, NAACCR instituted a program to annually review and certify that a registry's data is complete, accurate, and timely. Silver or Gold recognition is awarded based on increasing levels of quality excellence.

2000s:

As of 2000, the NPCR program was providing funding for 45 states, 3 territories, and the District of Columbia. Forty-three of these grants are to enhance current statewide registries, and two are to plan new registries. Funds for the remaining five states are provided by the SEER program.

Much progress has been made in central cancer registries in the United States since the first attempt in Massachusetts in 1927. Most states now have registries and legislation requiring cancer reporting. Many registries also share data on patients diagnosed in one area who reside in another. What has not changed, however, is the reliance central registries have on hospital registries. In fact, in this country central registries grew out of hospital registries, and most still rely on them to identify and report the bulk of the cancer cases. It continues to be essential for these two types of registries to work together to help each other accomplish their goals of reducing the incidence, morbidity, and mortality of cancer.

SUMMARY

The central registry, because of its comprehensive coverage, is an essential tool in community-based and other research. To some extent, the data may be underutilized. This is often due to limited funds. Yet, the registry is essential for many types of research and should be utilized. As expressed by Greenwald et al., "We think that any registry—hospital, local, regional, or national—must devote at least as much resources, time, and talent to its use for research and control purposes as it does to data acquisition, computerization, and publication of annual reports. Otherwise, it is doubtful that the registry investment is being optimally utilized."[235]

Much of the information for this chapter is derived from the earlier textbook on Central Cancer Registries[1] and the faculty members of the accompanying NAACCR Short Course.[171] The writings and teaching materials of the course were used extensively. We are indebted to the authors and faculty for their description of many ideas and concepts, including Toshi Abe; Tim Aldrich; Donald F. Austin; Judy Boone; Susan Capron; Darlene Dale; Dennis Deapen; Rosemary Dibble; Jim Enders; Jack Flannery; Gilbert H. Friedell, MD; Lawrence Garfinkel; Marc T. Goodman; Barry Gordon; Susan Galloway Hilsenbeck; Holly L. Howe; Suzanna S. Hoyler; Carol H. Johnson; Betsy Kohler; Jill MacKinnon; Kathleen McKeen; Lilia O'Connor; Steve Peace; Mary Potts; Walter Price; Jennifer Seiffert; Charles R. Smart; Sue Watkins; Dee West; Lynne R. Wilkens; and John L. Young. Our special thanks to Tom C. Tucker, our partner in these efforts.

STUDY QUESTIONS

True or False?

1. Central (population-based) registries report all cases diagnosed in a specified population at risk, and they are the source for calculation of incidence rates.

2. One of the affiliations that central registries have found most useful is with private insurance companies so that patient names can be disseminated.

3. Because cancer cases are reported to central registries from many hospitals, casefinding is not that important, because each case will almost certainly be reported by someone.

4. Many central registries are not computerized because such automation has proven too time-consuming, expensive and difficult.

REFERENCES

1. MacLennan R, Muir C, Steinitz R, Winkler A. Cancer Registration and Its Techniques. Lyons, France: IARC Scientific Publications; 1978: No. 21.

2. Jensen OM, Parkin DM, MacLennan R, Muir CS, Skeet RG. Cancer Registration Principles and Methods. Lyons, France: IARC; 1991. IARC Scientific Publication No. 95.

3. Menck, HR, and Smart CR, eds. Central Cancer Registries: Design, Management and Use. Langhorne, Penn: Harwood Academic Publishers; 1994.

4. Menck HR, West D. Central cancer registries. In Hutchinson CL, Roffers SD, Fritz AG, eds. *Cancer Registry Management Principles & Practice*. Dubuque, Iowa: Kendall/Hunt Publishing Company; 1997.

5. McKeen KM, Davidson ANM. The Surveillance, Epidemiology and End Results Program: Cancer Registry Management Principles & Practice (eds CL Hutchinson, SD Roffers, AG Fritz). Dubuque, Iowa: Kendall/Hunt Publishing Company; 1997.

6. Hutton MD, Simpson LD, Miller, DS, Weir HK, McDavid, K, Hall, HI. Progress toward nationwide cancer surveillance: An evaluation of the National Program of Cancer Registries, 1994-1999. *J of Registry Management:* 2001. 28(3):113-120.

7. Howe HL. Population-based cancer registries in the united states. In Howe HL, et al, eds. *Cancer Incidence in North America, 1988-1990.* Springfield, Ill: American Association of Central Cancer Registries; April 1994:VI 1-10. Available at *http://www.naaccr.org.*

8. ELM National Oncology Data Base. Rockville, Md: ELM Services Inc.; 1988.

9. Liss JM. "The MRS National Data Set 1989," part 1: "Description and Overview." *Medical Registry Reports.* 1991; 5:1-5, Hackensack, NJ: Medical Registry Services, Inc.

10. Eberle C, Fremgen A, Wynn G. The National Cancer Data Base. In Hutchinson CL, Roffers SD, Fritz AG, eds. *Cancer Registry Management Principles and Practice.* Dubuque, Iowa: Kendall/Hunt Publishing Company; 1997.

11. Dorn R. *Federal Registries.* In Hutchinson CL, Roffers SD, Fritz AG, eds. *Cancer Registry Management Principles and Practice.* Dubuque, Iowa: Kendall/Hunt Publishing Company; 1997.

12. Automated Central Tumor Registry (ACTUR). *Defense Enrollment Eligibility Reporting System. Users Manual.* UM1006EL R2. Washington, DC: The Assistant Secretary of Defense for Health Affairs and the Assistant Secretary of Defense for Force Management and Personnel; 1992.

13. Parkin DM, Sanghvi: Cancer registration in developing countries, In Jensen OM, Parkin DM, MacLennan R, Muir CS, Skeet RG, eds. *Cancer Registration Principles and Methods.* Lyons, France: IARC Scientific Publication No. 95.

14. IARC/IACR. *Cancer Incidence in Five Continents.* Lyons, France: International Agency for Research on Cancer; 1993:Vol 6. IARC Publication No. 120.

15. Roffers SD. Cancer Registries in Other Countries. In Hutchinson CL, Roffers SD, Fritz AG, eds. *Cancer Registry Management Principles and Practice.* Dubuque, Iowa: Kendall/Hunt Publishing Company; 1997.

16. Health and Welfare Canada. *The Making of the Canadian Cancer Registry: Cancer Incidence in Canada and Its Regions 1969 to 1988.* Bureau of Chronic Disease Epidemiology, Laboratory Centre for Disease Control, Health and Welfare Canada, Ottawa, K1A 0L2.

17. Skeet RG. Manual and computerized cancer registries. In Jensen OM, Parkin DM, MacLennan, Muir CS, Skeet RG, eds. *Cancer Registration Principles and Methods:* Lyons, France: IARC; 1991, IARC Scientific Publication No. 95.

18. Young JL, Jensen OM, Parkin DM, MacLennan R, Muir CS, Skeet RG, eds. The hospital cancer registry. In *Cancer Registration Principles and Methods:* Lyons, France: IARC; 1991. IARC Scientific Publication No. 95.

19. Austin DF. Types of registries: goals and objectives. In Menck HR, Smart CR, eds. *Central- Cancer Registries: Design, Management and Use.* Langhorne, Penn: Harwood Academic Publishers; 1994: 1-11.

20. Clive RE, Miller DS. Introduction to cancer registries. In Hutchinson CL, Roffers SD, Fritz AG, eds. *Cancer Registry Management Principles and Practice.* Dubuque, Iowa: Kendall/Hunt Publishing Company; 1997.

21. Kosary CL, Ries LAG, Miller BA, et al. *SEER Cancer Statistics Review, 1973-1992: tables and graphs.* Bethesda, Md: National Cancer Institute, National Institutes of Health; 1995. NIH Publication No. 96-2789.

22. Myers MH, Ries LA. Cancer patient survival rates: SEER program results for 10 years of follow-up. *CA Cancer J Clin.* 1989; 39(1): 21-32.

23. Parkin DM, Hakulinen. Analysis of Survival, in Cancer Registration Principles and Methods: In Jensen OM, Parkin DM, MacLennan R, Muir CS, Skeet RG, eds. Lyons, France: IARC; 1991. IARC Scientific Publication No. 95.

24. Deapen D, Berglund LC, Bernstein LC, Ross RK. *Cancer in Los Angeles County: A Bibliography 1972-2000.* Cancer Surveillance Program, University of Southern California School of Medicine; 2001.

25. Guinan P, Stewart AK, Fremgen AM, Menck HR. Patterns of care for metastatic carcinoma of the prostate gland: results of the American College of Surgeons' patient care evaluation study. *Prostate Cancer and Prostatic Diseases.* 1998; 1: 315-320.

26. Janes RH, Niederhuber JE, Chmiel JS, etc. National patterns of care for pancreatic cancer: results of a survey by the Commission on Cancer. *Annals of Surgery.* 1996; 223: 261-272.

27. Steele GD, Osteen RT, Winchester DP, Murphy GP, Menck HR. Clinical Highlights from the National Cancer Data Base: 1994. *CA Jrl for Clinicians.* 1994; 44: 71-80.

28. ACS Cancer Facts and Figures. Atlanta, Ga: American Cancer Society.

29. Hisserich JC, Martin SP, Henderson BE. An areawide cancer reporting network. *Publ Health Rep.* 1975; 90:15-17.

30. Deapen D, Menck HR, Ervin IL, Leventhal M, Niland JC. Experience in developing e-path cancer reporting for rapid case ascertainment. *J Registry Management.* 2002;29:2, 44-51.

31. Jensen OM, Whelan S: Planning a cancer registry. In Jensen OM, Parkin DM, MacLennan, Muir CS, Skeet RG, eds. *Cancer Registration Principles and Methods.* Lyons, France: IARC; 1991. IARC Scientific Publication No. 95.

32. Watkins S, MacKinnon J, Price W. Legislation, affiliation and governance. In Menck HR, Smart CR, eds. *Central Cancer Registries: Design, Management and Use.* Langhorne, Penn: Harwood Academic Publishers; 1994:13-18.

33. Fisher R, Haenlein M. Legislative authorizations for cancer registries. In. *State Cancer Legislative Database Update.* Bethesda, Md: National Cancer Institute, National Institutes of Health; 1991.

34. CDC. State Cancer Registries: Status of Authorization Legislation and Enabling Regulations-United States. *MMWR.* October 1993. 43:71-75.

35. CDC: Cancer Legislative Information. Available at: *http://www.cdc.gov/cancer/ legislat.htm.*

36. Bates PM. Proactive, productive, and progressive: new legislation helps keep the "pro" in cancer registries. *For the Record.* May 20, 2002.

37. CDC: A Sample of resources for Legislators and Others Making Decisions Related to Public Health and Cancer. Available at *http://www.cdc.gov/legislation/ legislativeresources.htm.*

38. Fritz A, Roffers S. *Marketing Cancer Information and Services.* National Cancer Registrars Association. Available at *http://www.ncra-usa.org.*

39. Desler MS. Interfacing with organizations. In Hutchinson CL, Roffers SD, Fritz AG, eds. *Cancer Registry Management Principles and Practice.* Dubuque, Iowa: Kendall/Hunt Publishing Company; 1997.

40. Watkins S, MacKinnon J, Price W. Budgets and staffing. In Menck HR, Smart CR eds. *Central Cancer Registries: Design, Management and Use.* Langhorne, Penn: Harwood Academic Publishers; 1994: 111-130.

41. Steban D, Whelan S, Laudico A, Parkin DM. *Manual for Cancer Registry Personnel.* Lyons, France: IARC; 1995. IARC Technical Report No. 10.

42. Ward S, DeCoe BM. Cancer registry personnel: office space, and equipment. In Hutchinson CL, Roffers SD, Fritz AG, eds. *Cancer Registry Management Principles and Practice.* Dubuque, Iowa: Kendall/Hunt Publishing Company; 1997.

43. National Cancer Registrars Association, Inc., American College of Surgeons Commission on Cancer. *Cancer Registry Staffing & Compensation Manual.* Results of a Survey Conducted for the National Cancer Registrars Association. Alexandria, Va, National Cancer Registrars Association; 2001.

44. Joneikis VK. Cancer registry management. In Hutchinson CL, Roffers SD, Fritz AG, eds. *Cancer Registry Management Principles and Practice.* Dubuque, Iowa: Kendall/Hunt Publishing Company; 1997.

45. Phillips K. How much time would a registrar take if a registrar did have time. *Advance.* May 21, 2001.

46. Menck HR, Parkin DM, eds. *Directory of Computer Systems Used in Cancer Registries.* Lyons, France: WHO International Agency for Research on Cancer; 1985.

47. Watkins S. Cancer registry budget. In Hutchinson CL, Roffers SD, Fritz AG, eds. *Cancer Registry management Principles and Practice.* Dubuque, Iowa: Kendall/Hunt Publishing Company; 1997.

48. Muir CS, Demeret E. Cancer Registration: Legal Aspects and Confidentiality. In Jensen OM, Parkin DM, MacLennan R, Muir CS, Skeet RG, eds. *Cancer Registration Principles and Methods.* Lyons, France: IARC; 1991. IARC Scientific Publication No. 95.

49. Coleman MP, Muir CS, Menegoz F. Confidentiality in the cancer registry. *Br J Cancer.* 1992;66:1138-1149.

50. Stiller CA. Cancer registration: its uses in research and confidentiality in the European Community. *J Epidemiol Comm Health.* 1993;47:342-344.

51. Chen VW. The right to know vs. the right to privacy. *J Registry Management.* 1997:125-127.

52. NAACCR. 2002 NAACCR Workshop Report: Data Security and Confidentiality. Springfield, Ill: North American Association of Central Cancer Registries; May 2002: 56. Available at http://www.naaccr.org/workshopreports.html.

53. NAACCR, Policy Statement 99-01: Confidentiality. Available at: *http://www.naaccr.org.*

54. Berry G. HIPAA's Impact on the CTR professional. *Advance.* February 18, 2002.

55. The National Cancer Registrar Association Guide to the Interpretation of the Code of Ethics. In Hutchinson CL, Roffers SD, Fritz AG, eds. *Cancer Registry Management Principles and Practice.* Dubuque, Iowa: Kendall/Hunt Publishing Company; 1997.

56. Coughlin SS, Clutter GC, Hutton M. Ethics in cancer registries. *JRM.* 1999;26, 5-10.

57. Overton P, McCracken KJ. Using the NCRA code of ethics: responsible reporting. *The Connection.* 1997;16.

58. Coughlin SS, Soskolne CL, Goodman KW. *Case Studies in Public Health Ethics.* Washington DC: American Public Health Association; 1997.

59. Levine RJ. The Institutional Review Board. In Coughlin SS, Beauchamp TL, eds. *Ethics and Epidemiology.* New York, NY: Oxford University Press; 1996: 257-273.

60. Johnson C, Phillips JL. Standards for data and data management: In Hutchinson CL, Roffers SD, Fritz AG, eds. *Cancer Registry Management Principles and Practice.* Dubuque, Iowa: Kendall/Hunt Publishing Company; 1997.

61. Gordon B. *Data Set Planning.* In Menck H, Smart C, eds. *Central Cancer Registries: Design, Management and Use.* Langhorne, Penn: Harwood Academic Publishers; 1994.

62. Howe HH. Recommendations for public use files of national cancer data. A report of a workshop held at the Broadmoor, Colorado Springs, Colo, August 25-27, 1997. North American Association of Central Cancer Registries, November 1997.

63. MacLennan R. Items of patient information which may be collected by registries. In Jensen OM, Parkin DM, MacLennan R, Muir CS, Skeet RG, eds. *Cancer Registration Principles and Methods.* Lyons, France: IARC; 1991. IARC Scientific Publication No. 95.

64. Hultstrom D, ed. *NAACCR Standards for Cancer Registries, Volume II: Data Standards and Data Dictionary.* Version 9.1. Springfield, IL: North American Association of Central Cancer Registries, March 2001.

65. Commission on Cancer. *Manual for Cancer Programs.* Chicago, Ill: American College of Surgeons; 1956.

66. SEER Program. *The Seer Program Code Manual,* rev. ed. Bethesda, Md: National Cancer Institute; 1992.

67. Shambaugh, E. Comparability of cancer data. *Proceedings of Central Registry Workshop, December 7 and 8, 1979.* Chicago, Ill: American College of Surgeons.

68. Commission on Cancer American College of Surgeons. *Facility Oncology Registry Data Standards* (FORDS). Chicago, Ill: American College of Surgeons; 2002.

69. SEER. *The SEER Program Code Manual,* 3rd ed. Baltimore, Md: National Institutes of Health; 1998. NIH Publication No. 98-2313.

70. NAACCR. Abe JT, Seiffert JE, eds. *Standards for Cancer Registries Volume I: Data Exchange Standards and Record Description.* Version 9.0.

71. Clive R. *Major Standard Setters for Central Registries.* Course materials for the NAACCR Shortcourse, at menckh@aol.com.

72. Codman EA. The improper Bostonian. *ACOS Bulletin.* January 1999. Volume 84, Number 1.

73. Brennan M, Clive R, Winchester D. The CoC: Its roots and its destiny. *ACOS Bulletin.* 1994; 79(6) 14.

74. Blankenship C, Moore M, Opaluch GM, Sylvester J. The American College of Surgeons Commission on Cancer and the Approvals Program: In Hutchinson CL, Roffers SD, Fritz AG, eds. *Cancer Registry Management Principles and Practice.* Dubuque, Iowa: Kendall/Hunt Publishing Company; 1997.

75. Greene F, Morrow M, Sylvester J. New initiatives underway at the ACoS Commission on Cancer. *Oncology Issues.* October 2000; 22-23.

76. Morrow M, Sylvester J. The cancer program of the American College of Surgeons. *Current Problems in Cancer.* 2001; 25(2):98-112.

77. Menck HR, Blankenship C, Fremgen AM. The National Cancer Data Base and Physician Network. *Topics Health Inform Manage.* 1997; 17:45-59.

78. Sylvester J, Blankenship C, Carter A, Douglas L, Stewart A. Quality Control: The American College of Surgeons Commission on Cancer Standards, National Cancer Data Base, and Cancer Liaison Program. *Journal of Registry Management.* 2000; 27(2): 68-74.

79. McGinnis L. The Field Liaison Program: why bother? *ACOS Bulletin.* 1983; 68(9): 22.

80. Jessup JM, Menck HR, Winchester DP, Hundahl SA, Murphy GP. The National Cancer Data Base Report on Patterns of Hospital Reporting. *Cancer.* 1996; 78:1829-37.

81. Menck HR, Bland KI, Scott-Conner CEH, Eyre H, Murphy GP, Winchester DP. Regional Diversity and Breadth of the National Cancer Data Base. *Cancer.* 1998; 83: 2649-58.

82. AJCC Cancer Staging Manual, 5th ed., American Joint Committee on Cancer, Irvin D. Fleming, et al, eds. Lippincott-Raven; 1997.

83. Hutchinson CL, Roffers SD, Fritz AG. Cancer Registry Management Principles & Practice, Dubuque, Iowa: Kendall/Hunt Publishing Company; 1997.

84. Seiffert J, Young JL: The North American Association of Central Cancer Registries. In Hutchinson CL, Roffers SD, Fritz AG, eds. *Cancer Registry Management Principles and Practice.* Dubuque, Iowa: Kendall/Hunt Publishing Company; 1997.

85. Swan J, Wingo P, Clive R, et al. Cancer surveillance in the US: Can we have a national system? *Cancer.* October 1, 1998; 83(7).

86. World Health Organization. *International Classification of Disease for Oncology,* 1st ed. Geneva, Switzerland: World Health Organization, 1976.

87. World Health Organization. *International Classification of Diseases for Oncology,* 2nd ed. Geneva, Switzerland: World Health Organization; 1990.

88. World Health Organization. *International Classification of diseases for Oncology,* 3rd ed. U.S. Interim Version 2000 (ICD-O-3). Geneva, Switzerland: World Health Organization, 2000.

89. Douglas LL. Collaborative stage: An update. *JRM.* 2001; 28(4);196-203.

90. Facility Oncology Registry Data Standards (FORDS). *Standards of the Commission on Cancer. Volume II.* Chicago, Ill: American College of Surgeons Commission on Cancer; 2002.

91. NAACCR. *Consensus Standards for Cancer Registries.* Supplement to NAACCR Volume II, Chapter 6. Pathology Laboratory Electronic Reporting Requirements. Data Items, Formatting, Recommendations Version 1.1; September 2000.

92. NAACCR. *Standards for Cancer Registries., Volume III: Standards for Cancer Registries Completeness, Quality, Analysis, and Management of Data.* NAACCR; 1994.

93. Tucker T, Howe H, Kohler B, Fulton JP. *Adapting the HL-7 Standard for Cancer Registry Work.* Available at: *http://www.naaccr.org.*

94. Health Level Seven (HL-7), at *http://www.hl7.org.*

95. Toal S, Lezin N. Working Toward Implementation of HL7 in NAACCR Information Technology Standards: Meeting Summary Report. Available at *http://www.cdc.gov/cancer/npcr/npcrpdfs/hl7mtg8.pdf*

96. SEER Program. Book 2 Cancer Characteristics and Selection of Cases (1991). NIH Publication No. 92-993. Available at *http://seer.cancer.gov/publications/onlinepubs/pubs.html.*

97. Surawicz T, McCarthy BJ, Jukich PJ, Davis FG. The accuracy and completeness of primary brain and central nervous system tumor data: results from the Central Brain Tumor Registry of the United States. *J of Registry Management.* 2000; 27(2):51-55.

98. Jean-Baptiste R, Gebhard IK, eds. Procedure Guidelines for Cancer Registries, Series IV. Cancer Case Ascertainment. NAACCR; February 2002.

99. Seiffert J, Hoyler SS, McKeen K, Potts M. Casefinding, abstracting, and death clearance. In Menck HR, Smart CR eds. Central Cancer Registries.- Design, Management and Use. Langhorne, Penn: Harwood Academic Publishers; 1994, 35-64.

100. Potts M, Hafterson J, Wacker FF, Serbent J: Case ascertainment. In Hutchinson CL, Roffers SD, Fritz AG, eds. *Cancer Registry Management Principles and Practice.* Dubuque, Iowa: Kendall/Hunt Publishing Company; 1997.

101. Powell J. Data sources and reporting. In Jensen OM, Parkin DM, MacLennan R, Muir CS, Skeet RG, eds. *Cancer Registration Principles and Methods.* Lyons, France: IARC; 1991. IARC Scientific Publication No. 95.

102. Menck HR. E-path reporting: electronic casefinding. *J Registry Management.* 2002;29:2, 37-38.

103. Dale D, Golabek JK, Chong N. The impact of E-path technology on the Ontario Cancer Registry operations. *JRM.* 2002;27(2):52-56.

104. Aldinger WL, Rydzewski S. Early experiences with E-path reporting in Pennsylvania: non-hospital sources. *JRM.* 2002;27(2):39-43.

105. Phillips JL, Menck HR: Computerization. In Menck H, Smart C, eds. *Central Cancer Registries: Design, Management and Use.* Chur, Switzerland, Harwood Academic Publishers; 1994.

106. Menck HR. Selecting your cancer registry software. *Oncology Issues.* 2002;17:32-34.

107. NAACCR Procedure Guidelines for Cancer Registries, Series II. Calculating the DCO Rate, June 2000.

108. NAACCR. *Death Clearance Procedures for Central Registries.* CD Training Module. Available at at: *http://www.naaccr.org.*

109. Fulton JP, Wingo P, Jamison M, Roffers S, Howe HL, Chen VW. *Exploring the Effects of Death Certificate Follow-Back on Cancer Registration.* Available at *http://www.naaccr.org.*

110. Johnson CH, Hutchinson CL. General principles of abstracting and cancer registry files. In Hutchinson CL, Roffers SD, Fritz AG, eds. *Cancer Registry Management Principles and Practice.* Dubuque, Iowa: Kendall/Hunt Publishing Company; 1997.

111. LeTendre DC, Rosemary D, Riddle S, Creech CM. *Where did they really live? Resolving discrepancies in address at diagnosis. J of Registry Management.* 2000; 27(2):57-58.

112. Dolecek TA, Lawhun G, Vann S, Snodgrass JL, Stewart SL. *Hispanic identification in the Illinois State Cancer Registry. J of Registry Management.* 2000; 27(2):43-50.

113. Berry G. Collecting race and ethnicity data in the Registry. *Advance.* December 17, 2001.

114. NAACCR. *Cancer Registry Management Reports* (NAACCR Instructional Module for Cancer Registries). J. Seiffert, North American Association of Central Cancer Registries; 1998.

115. Coleman MP, Bieber CA. CANREG: Cancer registration software for microcomputers. In Jensen OM, Parkin DM, MacLenna R, Muir CS, Skeet RG, eds. *Cancer Registration Principles and Methods.* Lyons, France: 1991; IARC Scientific Publication No. 95.

116. Williamson TJ, McKelvey LW. Computer principles. In Hutchinson CL, Roffers SD, Fritz AG, eds.

Cancer Registry Management Principles and Practice. Dubuque, Iowa: Kendall/Hunt Publishing Company; 1997.

117. Rocky Mountain Cancer Data Systems—Research Park, 420 Chipeta Way, Suite 120, Salt Lake City, UT 84108. (801) 581-4307. *http://rmcds6.med.utah.edu.*

118. Cancer Patient Data Management System, Kentucky Cancer Registry, 2365 Harrodsburg Road, Lexington, KY 40536-3381. (859) 219-0773. *www.kcr.uky.edu.*

119. Registry Plus™—Centers for Disease Control and Prevention. www.registryplus.org.

120. Précis-Central Central Registry Data Management System IMPAC, Medical Systems Inc., 100 W. Evelyn Avenue, Mountain View, CA 94041. (650) 623-8800. *www.impac.com.*

121. C/NET Solutions, 1936 University Ave., Suite 112, Berkeley, CA 94704-1024. (800) 366-2638 *www.askcnet.org.*

122. CansurFacs Cancer Management System, PRE-MIER Cancer Registry System, *Précis-Hospital Registry Management System,* IMPAC Medical Systems Inc., 100 W. Evelyn Avenue, Mountain View, CA 94041. (650) 623-8800. *www.impac.com.*

123. C/NExT—C/NET Solutions, 1936 University Ave., Suite 112, Berkeley, CA 94704-1024. (800) 366-2638. *www.askcnet.org.*

124. Electronic Registry Services - 270 Northland Blvd, Suite 111, Cincinnati, OH 45246. (800) 824-9020. *www.ers-can.com.*

125. IMPATH Cancer Registry (formerly Medical Registry Services)—One University Plaza, Hackensack, NJ 07601. (201) 487-2266. *www.medregistry.com.*

126. Oncolog, Inc.—1665 Liberty Street SE, P.O. Box 2226, Salem, OR 97308. (800) 345-6626. *www.oncolog.com.*

127. Van Holten V: Editing for consistency of data items. In Jensen OM, Parkin DM, MacLenna R, Muir CS, Skeet RG, eds. *Cancer Registration Principles and Methods.* Lyons, France: IARC; 1991. IARC Scientific Publication No. 95.

128. NAACCR. *Volume IV: Standard Data Edits, Standards for Cancer Registries.* Available at: *http://www.naaccr.org.*

129. Commission on Cancer American College of Surgeons. *Standards of the Commission on Cancer, Volume III: Data Edits.* Available at *http://www.facs.org/dept/cancer/index.html.*

130. Capron S. *NAACCR Call for Data 2000 Instructions.* Available at: *http://www.naaccr.org.*

131. NAACCR. New Instructions for Using Metafiles and GenEDITS. Available at *http://www.naaccr.org.*

132. NAACCR Edits metafile (NAACCR9B, computer program), 2002. Available at *http://www.naaccr.org/standards/edits.html.*

133. NAACCR Edits Changes, NAACCR9/9A/9B (spreadsheet), 2002. Available at *http://www.naaccr.org/standards/edits.html.*

134. Correa C. *Using EDITS to Improve Data Quality.* Available at: *http://naaccr.org.*

135. SEER Edit Documentation. Bethesda, Md: SEER Program, National Cancer Institute; 1993.

136. SEER Publications. Available at *http://www.seer.cancer.gov,* including ICD-O-2 to 3* and ICD-O-3 to 2, ICD-9 to ICD-10, ICD-10 to ICD-9, ICD-O-2 to ICD-9, ICD-O-2 to ICD-10, ICD-O-1 to ICD-O-2, ICD-0-2 to ICD-9-(CM), ICD-0-2 to ICD-10.

137. Clark PM, Gomez EG. Details on demand: consumers, cancer information, and the Internet. *Clinical J of Oncology Nursing.* 2001; 5;1: 19-24.

138. Fritz, AG. Just trying to keep up: journal scanning services. *J of Registry Management* . 2000; 27(1):25-26.

139. Wiggins I, ed.. Using Geographic Information Systems Technology in the Collection, Analyses and Presentation of Cancer Registry Data: A Handbook to Basic Practices. Springfield, Ill: NAACCR, October 2002.

140. Thomas B. *Generalized Record Linkage System.* Available at: *http://www.naaccr.org.*

141. Borges HT, Watkins J, Stafford R, Biggar RJ. Linkage of selected AIDS and cancer registries in the United States. *J of Registry Management.* 2001; 28(2):89-92.

142. Cooksley C, Hwang L, Ford CC. HIV and cancer: Community-based analysis of trends and registry linkage. *J of Registry Management.* 2001; 28(2):82-88.

143. SEER Stat 4.2, and SEER Prep 1.9. Available at *http://seer.cancer.gov.*

144. SEER Joinpoint Regression Program. Available at *http://seer.cancer.gov.*

145. Kim HJ, Fay MP, Feuer EJ, Midthune DN. Permutation Tests for Joinpoint Regression with Applications to Cancer Rates. *Stat Med.* 2000;19:335-351.

146. Skeet RG. Quality and quality control. In. Jensen OM, Parkin DM, MacLennan R, Muir CS, Skeet RG, eds. *Cancer Registration Principles and Methods.* Lyons, France: IARC; 1991. IARC Scientific Publication No. 95.

147. Hilsenbeck SG: Quality control in central cancer registries. In Menck H, Smart C, eds. *Design, Management and Use.* Langhorn, Penn: Harwood Academic Publishers; 1994:131-78.

148. Parkin DM, Chen VW, Ferlay J, Galceran J, Storm HH, Whelan SL, eds. *Comparability and Quality Control in Cancer Registration* rev. 1996. Lyons, France: IARC Technical Report No. 19.

149. Ross F, Roffers SD. Quality control of cancer registry data. In Hutchinson CL, Roffers DS, Fritz AG, eds. *Cancer Registry Management Principles and Practice.* Dubuque, Iowa: Kendall/Hunt Publishing Company; 1997.

150. Roffers SD. Demystifying total quality management. *The Abstract.* September 1992; 19:1.

151. Gavin C. Improving Quality: Guide to Effective Programs. Meisenheimer. Aspen Publishers; 1992.

152. Fritz AG. The SEER Program's commitment to data quality. *J of Registry Management.* 2001; 28(1):35-44.

153. Berry G. Navigating the Gray Areas of Registry Data. *Advance.* November 19, 2001.

154. Hall HI, Gerlach KA, Miller DS. Methods of quality management. *J Reg JRM.* 2002:29; 72-77.

155. Izquierdo JN, Schoenbach VJ. The potential and limitations of data from population-based state cancer registries. *J of Registry Management.* 2000; 27(4).

156. Malnar K, Phillips JL, Fritz AG et al. Quality of oncology data: findings from the Commission on Cancer PCE Study. *J of Registry Management.* 2001; 28(1):24-34.

157. Gross L. The nuts and bolts of quality control in the cancer registry. *Advance.* February 18, 2002.

158. Roffers, S.D. Case completeness and data quality assessments in central cancer registries and their relevance to cancer control. In Howe HL, et al., eds. *Cancer Incidence in North America, 1988-1990.* Sacramento, Calif: American Association of Central Cancer Registries; 1994:V1-7. Available at: *http://www.naaccr.org.*

159. Fulton JP, Wingo P, Jamison M, Roffers SD, Howe HL, Chen VW. Exploring the effects of death certificate follow-back on cancer registration. In Howe L, ed. *Cancer Incidence in North America, 1988-1992.* Sacramento, Calif: North American Association of Central Cancer Registries; April 1996: Available at *http://www.naaccr.org.*

160. Fulton JP, Howe HL. Evaluating the incidence-mortality ratios in estimating completeness of cancer registration. In Howe HL, et al. eds. *Cancer Incidence in North America, 1988-1991.* Sacramento, Calif: North American Association of Central Cancer Registries; 1995:Sec VI:1-9. Available at *http://www.naaccr.org.*

161. Tucker TC, Howe HL. Measuring the quality of population-based cancer registries: the NAACCR perspective. *JRM.* 2001; 28(1):41-5.

162. NAACCR Standard to Assess the Completeness of Case Ascertainment. NAACCR Newsletter, Nov 1996. Available at *http://www.naaccr.org.*

163. Dale D, Chong N. Moving from Baseline to Certification. Available at *http://www.naaccr.org.*

164. Howe H. *Using the Feedback from Registry Certification.* Available at *http://www.naaccr.org.*

165. Tucker TC. *Registry Certification.* Available at: *http://www.naaccr.org.*

166. Hotes J, Howe HL, Wu XC, Correa C. *Hurdles in Achieving Registry Certification, 1995-1997.* Available at *http://www.naaccr.org.*

167. SEER Program. Self Instructional Manuals for Tumor Registrars, Book 1 through 8. Bethesda, Md: SEER Program, National Cancer Institute.

168. SEER Program. *Principles of Oncology for Cancer Registry Professionals.* National Cancer Institute.

169. SEER PROGRAM. *Principles and Practice of Cancer Registration, Surveillance, and Control Training Program.* Rockville, Md. National Cancer Institute.

170. Cancer Registration and Surveillance Training Modules. Available at *http://www.training.seer.cancer.gov.*

171. NAACCR Short Course. Central Cancer Registries: Design, Management and Use—The short course given annually at the NAACCR meeting.

172. University of Southern California Cancer Surveillance Program, Cancer Registrar Training Program. Available at *http://www.ncra-org/training.html.*

173. University of Pittsburgh in Pennsylvania, Health Information Systems Major. Available at *http://www.him.upmc.edu.*

174. Northeastern University, Boston, Ma. Available at *a.collins@nunet.neu.edu.*

175. Santa Barbara City College. Available at *http://online.sbcc.net.*

176. Programs at Emory University. Available at *http://cancer.sph.emory.edu.*

177. Cancer Registry Training Program, Commission on Cancer, American College of Surgeons. Available at *http://www.facs.org/dept/cancer.*

178. CTR Corner. Available at *http://www.facs.org/dept/cancer/index.html.*

179. NAACCR Standards for Cancer Registries Query Database [on-line].

180. West DW, Flannery J, Dibble R. Central cancer registries: follow-up. In Menck HR, Smart CR, eds. *Central Cancer Registries: Design, Management and Use.* Langhorne, PA: Harwood Academic Publishers, 1994;188-91.

181. Ashley P, Gress D, Towarnicj C. Monitoring patient outcome: follow-up. In Hutchinson CL, Roffers SD,

Fritz AG, eds. *Cancer Registry Management Principles and Practice.* Dubuque, Iowa: Kendall/Hunt Publishing Company; 1997.

182. Dorn HF. Methods of analysis for follow-up studies. *Human Biology.* 1950; 22: 238-48.

183. NCRA Follow-up Resources. Available at *http://www.ncra-usa.org/links.html#follow.*

184. Boyle P, Parkin DM. Statistical methods for registries. In Jensen OM, Parkin DM, MacLennan R, Muir CS, Skeet RG, eds. *Cancer Registration Principles and Methods.* Lyons, France: IARC; 1991. IARC Scientific Publication No. 95.

185. Goodman MT, Wilkens LR. Calculation and assessment of incidence rates. In Menck HR, Smart CR, eds. *Central Cancer Registries: Design, Management and Use.* Langhorne, Penn: Harwood Academic Publishers, 1994; 195-231.

186. California Cancer Registry. *Cancer Incidence and Mortality in California by Detailed Race/Ethnicity, 1988-1992.* April 1995;27 (191).

187. Surawicz TA, Kupelian VA, Davis FG. Changes in age-adjusted disease incidence using the Year 2000 standard population: an example using Central Brain Tumor Registry of the United States data. *J of Registry Management.* 2001; 28(2):61-64.

188. Decoufle P, Thomas PL, Pickle LW. Comparisons of the proportionate mortality ratio and standardized mortality risk measures. *Am J Epidem.* 1980;111:263-268.

189. Wilkens LR, Goodman MT. Calculation and assessment of survival rates. In Menck HR, Smart CR. eds. *Central Cancer Registries: Design, Management and Use.* Langhorne, Penn: Harwood Academic Publishers, 1994; 233-57.

190. AJCC. Cancer Survival Analysis. In AJCC Cancer Staging Manual. 5th ed. Philadelphia, Penn: Lippincott-Raven Publishers; 1997.

191. AJCC. Reporting of Cancer Survival and End Results. In AJCC Staging of Cancer. 4th ed. Philadelphia, Penn: Lippincott-Raven Publishers; 1992.

192. Shambaugh EM, Young JL, Zippin C, et al. Book 7: *Statistics and Epidemiology for Cancer Registries.* U.S. Department of Health and Human Resources, Public Health Service, National Institutes of Health, NIH Publication No. 94-3766, 1994.

193. Austin, DF. Cancer registries: A tool in epidemiology. In Lillienfeld AM, ed. *Reviews in Cancer Epidemiology, vol. 2.* New York, NY: Elsevier North-Holland; 1983.

194. Aldrich T. Research uses of central cancer registries. In Menck HR, Smart CR, eds. *Central Cancer Registries: Design, Management and Use.* Langhorne, Penn: Harwood Academic Publishers, 1994; 296-97.

195. Hoyler SS, Malnar K. Data utilization. In Hutchinson CL, Roffers SD, Fritz AG, eds. *Cancer Registry Management Principles and Practice.* Dubuque, Iowa: Kendall/Hunt Publishing Company; 1997.

196. Jensen OM, Storm HH. Reporting of results. In Jensen OM, Parkin DM, MacLennan R, Muir CS, Skeet RG, eds. *Cancer Registration Principles and Methods.* Lyons, France: IARC; 1991. IARC Scientific Publication No. 95.

197. Wingo PA, Parkin DM, Eyre HJ. Measuring the occurrence of cancer: impact and statistics. In Lenhard R, Brady L, Osteen R, Gansler T, eds. *Clinical Oncology,* 3rd ed. American Cancer Society; Atlanta, Georgia.

198. Hatzell T, Aldrich TE, Cates W, Shin E. Public health surveillance. In Novick LF, Mayes GP, eds. *Public Health Administration: Principals for Population-Based Management.* Gaithersburg, Md: Aspen Publishers; 2000.

199. Parkin DM, Aslan AA. *Cancer Occurrence in Developing Countries.* Lyons, France: IARC; 1986. IARC Scientific Publication No. 75.

200. Howe HL, Chen VW, Hotes J, Wu XC, Correa C, eds. *Cancer in North America, 1994-1998, Volume One: Incidence.* Springfield, Ill: North American Association of Central Cancer Registries; April 2001.

201. Howe HL, Chen VW, Hotes J, Wu XC, Correa C, eds. *Cancer in North America, 1994-1998, Volume Two: Mortality.* Springfield, Ill: North American Association of Central Cancer Registries, April 2001.

202. Cancer Facts and Figures. Atlanta, Ga: American Cancer Society National Headquarters; 1998.

203. Harras A, ed. *Cancer Rates and Risks,* 4th ed. NIH Publication No. 96-691. May 1996.

204. Aldrich T. Statistics and epidemiology: In Hutchinson CL, Roffers SD, Fritz AG, eds. *Cancer Registry Management Principles and Practice.* Dubuque, Iowa: Kendall/Hunt Publishing Company; 1997.

205. Howe HL, Wingo PA, Thun MJ, et al. Annual report to the nation on the status of cancer (1973 through 1998), featuring cancers with increasing trends. *JNCI.* 2001;93:824-842.

206. SEER Program. Racial/Ethnic Patterns of Cancer in the United States 1988-1992, SEER.

207. SEER Program. *Cancer Incidence and Survival among Children and Adolescents: United States SEER Program 1975-1995.*

208. SEER Program. Prostate Cancer Trends 1973-1995. SEER

209. Histology of Cancer—Incidence and Prognosis (Cancer January 1, 1995 - Vol. 75, No. 1), SEER.

210. Menck HR, Mills PK, Menck-Taylor JC. Time trends and metropolitan clustering of AIDS-related cancer: cancer registry-based surveillance. *J of Registry Management.* 2001; 28(2):70-76.

211. West M, Lynch CF, Wagner DM. Descriptive epidemiology of head and neck cancer in Iowa, 1973-1998. *J of Registry Management.* 2001: 28(4).

212. Menck HR, Casagrande JC, Henderson BE. Industrial air pollution. Possible effect on lung cancer. *Science.* 1974; 183: 210-12.

213. Perkins CI, Morris CR, Wright WE, Young JL Jr. Cancer incidence and mortality. In *California by Detailed Race/Ethnicity, 1988 to 1992.* Sacramento, Calif.: State of California, Department of Health Services; 1995.

214. Fulton JP, et al. Urbanization in cancer incidence, United States, 1988-1992. In Howe HL ed. *Cancer Incidence in North America, 1989-1993; Vol 1.* Sacramento, Calif: North American Association of Central Cancer Registries; 1997:VI1-VI9.

215. Thacker SB. Time-space clusters: the public health dilemma. *Health and Environment Digest.* 1989; 3:4-5.

216. CDC. CDC: guidelines for investigating clusters of health events. *Morbidity and Mortality Weekly Report.* 1990; 39(RR-1 1):1-23.

217. CDC. Guidelines for investigating disease clusters. *MMWR* 1990; 39(RR-11)1-23.

218. Heath CW, Hasterlik RJ. Leukemia among children in a suburban community, 1963. *CA Cancer J Clin.* 1990; 40:27-50.

219. Croner CM, Sperling J, Broome FR. Geographic Information Systems (GIS):New Perspectives in Understanding Human Health and Environmental Relationships. *Statistics in Medicine.* 1996; 15:1961-88.

220. Clarke KC, McLafferty SL, Tempalski BJ. On epidemiology and geographic information systems: a review and discussion of future directions. *Emerging Infectious Diseases.* 1996; 2(2):85-92.

221. Aldrich TE, Andrews KW, Liboff AR. Brain cancer risk and EMF: assessing the geomagnetic component. *Archives of Env. Health.* 2001; 56(4):314-19.

222. Aldrich TE, Griffin JR. Environmental Epidemiology and Risk Assessment. New York, NY: Van Norstrand Reinhold; 1993.

223. Houk VN., Thacker SB. Registries: one way to assess environmental hazards. *Health and Environment Digest.* 1987; 1:5-6.

224. Horn-Ross PL, Hoggatt KJ, West DW, et al. Recent diet and breast cancer risk: the California Teachers Study. *Cancer Causes Control.* 2002; 13:407-415.

225. Lew EA, Garfinkel L. Mortaliity at ages 75 and older in the Cancer Prevention Study (CPS I). *CA Cancer J Clin.* 1990; 40(4):210-224.

226. Williams R. Clinical screening and genetic testing project of high-risk African-American breast cancer families. *J of Registry Management.* 2001; 28(3):151-153.

227. Friedman DL. Multiple cancer familial syndromes. *J of Registry Management.* 2001; 28(3):139-145.

228. Harrison B. Genetic testing and counseling for predisposition to cancer. *J of Registry Management.* 2001; 28(3):146-150.

229. Ballinger L. Hereditary cancer susceptibility. *J of Registry Management.* 2001; 28(3):134-138.

230. Steele GD, Winchester DP, Menck HR, Murphy GP. National Cancer Data Base *Annual Review of Cancer Patient Care 1992.* Atlanta, Ga: American Cancer Society; 1992.

231. Spath P. Cancer Patient Care Evaluation Guide. Chicago, Ill: American College of Surgeons;

232. Wingo PA, Luke E, O'Brien K, et al. Population-based patterns of care studies: collaboration among state cancer registries, the American College of Surgeons, and the American Cancer Society. *J of Registry Management.* 2001; 28(1):5-16.

233. Osteen RT, Steele GD, Menck HR, Winchester DP: *Regional Differences in Surgical Management of Breast Cancer, CA.* 1992; 42: 3943.

234. Steele GD, Winchester DP, Menck HR. The National Cancer Data Base: a mechanism for assessment of patient care. *Cancer.* 1994; 73: 499-504.

235. Greenwald P, Sondik EJ, Young JL Jr. Emerging roles for cancer registries in cancer control. *Yale Journal of Biological Medicine.* 1986; 59:561-66.

236. Parkin DM, Wagner G, Muir CS. *The Role of the Registry in Cancer Control.* Summit, NJ. IARC; 1985,1989.

237. Friedell GH, Tucker TC. Central cancer registries: prevention and control. In Menck HR, Smart CR eds. *Central Cancer Registries: Design, Management and Use.* Langhorne, PA: Harwood Academic Publishers; 1994: 296-97.

238. Armstrong BK. The role of the cancer registry in cancer control. *Cancer Causes and Control.* 1992; 3:569-79.

239. Garfinkel, L. History of US central cancer registries. In Menck HR, Smart CR, eds. *Central Cancer Registries: Design, Management and Use.* Langhorne, Penn: Harwood Academic Publishers, 1994; 303-309.

240. Wagner G. History of cancer registration. In Jensen 0M, Parkin DM, MacLennan R, et al., eds. *Cancer Registration Principles and Methods.* IARC Scientific Publications No. 95. Lyons, France: WHO International Agency for Research on Cancer; 1991: 3-6.

241. Stephenson GW. The Commission on Cancer. a historical review. *Bull Amer Coll Surg.* Sept. 713, 1979.

242. US Dept of Health Education and Welfare. *A History of Cancer Control in the United States 1946-71.* Book 2, DHEW Publication No (NIH) 78-1518, Washington DC.

243. Flannery JT, Janerich DT. The Connecticut Tumor Registry: yesterday, today and tomorrow. *Conn Med.* 1985; 11: 709712.

244. Griswold MH, Wilder CS, Cutler SJ, Pollack ES. *Cancer in Connecticut 1935-51.* Hartford, Conn: Conn State Dept of Health; 1955.

245. Ferber B, Handy VH, Gerhardt PR, Solomon M. *Cancer in New York State, Exclusive of New York City, 1941-1960.* A Review of Incidence Mortality, Probability and Survivorship. Albany, NY. N.Y. State Dept of Health; 1962.

246. Dorn HF. *Illness from Cancer in the United States.* Washington DC: US Govt Printing Office; 1944.

247. Dorn HF, Cutler SJ. *Morbidity from Cancer in the United States, Publ Health Monogr 56.* Washington DC, US Dept of Health Education and Welfare; 1959.

248. California Tumor Registry. *Cancer Registration and Survival in California.* Berkeley, Calif: Calif State Dept of Health: 1963.

249. Smart CR. Cooperative tumor registry. *Rocky Mt Med J.* 1968;65(11):27.

250. Biometry Branch, National Cancer Institute. *Third National Cancer Survey: Incidence Data, Monogr 41.* Bethesda, Md: 1975. National Cancer Institute. DHEW Publ No. (NIH) 75787.

251. Surveillance Programs, Division of Cancer Prevention and Control. *Cancer Statistics Review 1973-1986.* Bethesda, Md: National Cancer Institute, 1989. NIH Publ No. 89-2789.

252. Commission on Cancer. *Data Acquisition Manual.* Chicago, Ill: American College of Surgeons; 1988.

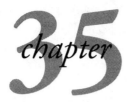

CANCER REGISTRIES IN OTHER COUNTRIES

Herman R. Menck
MBA, CDP

INTRODUCTION

The US cancer registry professional can better understand US registries by contrasting them with registries in other countries, and the differing approaches taken to cancer registration in these other countries. Such a comparative assessment better defines what US registries have chosen to do, and not do.

Differences in Other Countries

In many cases, differences between US registries and other registries are the logical result of somewhat, or in some cases markedly, different medical conditions and attitudes existing in these other host countries.[1-2] These differences include both advantages and disadvantages and are summarized in Table 35-1.

The Commission on Cancer of the American College of Surgeons (CoC) role is paramount to both US hospital-based and population-based registration.[3-7] The CoC Approvals Program causes some 2000 hospitals to fund their own clinically oriented registries. These hospital-based registries then provide in turn to the US population-based programs a majority of the national cancer case information at little or no cost. These hospital-based registries provide the initial core of data that enables national US cancer surveillance.

In other countries, the absence of a hospital Approvals Program largely shifts the cost burden of case ascertainment and reporting to the budget of the population-based registries. This generally requires a more significant governmental commitment to national cancer surveillance.

The hospital-based programs in the US play an additional role in influencing physician attitudes toward cancer registration, in creating a professional cadre of some 3,000 cancer registrars, fostering interest in patient follow-up, disease staging, and registry software.

In some other countries there not only is not a network of hospital-based cancer registries, but in some developing countries there is a general lack of basic health services.[2]

Some countries lack complete and timely age, and sex-specific census information, which provides the necessary denominator for incidence rate calculations. Conversely, some countries have a methodological advantage over the US because they encourage or allow the use of a universal patient identifier.[8] This not only facilitates cancer registration, but improves prospects for a life-long follow-up and integrated vital status and medical record history.

Basic Cancer Surveillance

There is a basic underlying interest in most countries to monitor the burden of cancer amongst their peoples. This sustains a high level of cancer registration internationally. Besides the US, nearly 200 central registries are known to have population-based cancer surveillance. Cancer registration in other countries has been previously described.[9-13] A measure of this interest is seen in International publications such as *Cancer Incidence in Five Continents,*[14-22] and other special reports.[23-25] This basic type of cancer surveillance centered on population data has also been previously described.[26-27]

Some countries study the expression of cancer in different subpopulations within their country. For example, the high risk to nasopharyngeal cancer among Chinese males has been studied to better understand this disease.[28] Manifold risk to nasopharyngeal cancer in Chinese compared to other men may provide clues to the causal network of this disease. Resolving high risk factors in Chinese can be of help not only to these males, but also potentially to all other men and women.

Comparative International Research and Surveillance Potential

In addition to basic cancer surveillance within each country itself, registration in other countries has been facilitated by an interest in international comparisons, and migrant analyses. There is interest in studying populations in countries with significantly different life styles, and different genetic backgrounds.

International Comparisons: For example, the incidence of stomach cancer in different countries and populations is studied for patterns of difference, possibly related to nutritional, or other causes. Risk levels for the different countries are compared. Both subpopulations at low risk and high risk are of etiologic interest.

There is great interest in studying cancer incidence in developing countries.[29-35] A major thrust for the International Association of cancer Registries of the International Agency for Research On Cancer (IARC/IACR) is to perform cancer surveillance

Table 35-1

Differences in Registry Conditions in Other Countries

Medical mileau
- Lack of, or low level of, basic health services
- Different medical care delivery systems
- Absence of the CoC Approvals Program
- Different physician attitudes toward cancer registration
- Different physician attitudes toward privacy/confidentiality
- Source and Level of government support provided (from little to a lot)
- Lack of census (demographic) data

Registry infrastructure
- Lack of (appropriate) trained registry personnel
- Lack of adequate follow-up system
- Lack of data processing facilities

Population attitudes/characteristics
- Different population attitudes toward (public) health
- Different population attitudes toward privacy/confidentiality
- Diversity of lifestyles and ethnic factors
- Allow use of universal patient identifier (e.g. Social Security number)

Table 35-2

Examples of Ethnic/National Surveillance Comparisons Using Popualion-Based Cancer Registry Data[23]

Ethnic Group	Registry
Japanese	Osaka, Hawaii, San Francisco, Los Angeles
Chinese	Shanghai, Hong Kong, Singapore, Hawaii, San Francisco, Los Angeles
Filipino	Manila, Hawaii, Los Angeles
Malay	Singapore
Indian	Singapore, Fiji
Latin-American	Cali, Columbia, Lima, Peru, San Francisco, Los Angeles
Alaska native	Alaska
Black	San Francisco, Los Angeles
European	New Caledonia, New South Wales, New Zealand, Hawaii, British Columbia, Seattle, San Francisco, Los Angeles

there. The seminal event in this effort of other registries in other countries registries is the periodic publication of "Cancer in Five Continents," now in its eighth edition. Other publications have overviewed international cancer incidence comparisons, including one based on Pacific basin Registries which is summarized in Table 35-2.

Migrant Studies

Migrant: The rationale for this form of surveillance, which is a special case of international comparison, is to contrast the incidence of cancer in a defined ethnic or national subpopulation of interest in their base country and in one or several countries of migration.[35-38]

For example, just as it was of interest to better understand the high risk of nasopharyngeal cancer among Chinese males in China, it is also important

to understand how that risk may change among first and succeeding generations of Chinese males immigrants to other countries.

These migrant studies can normally be accomplished with traditional incidence rate surveillance. In addition the use of proportional methodologies can extend surveillance capabilities to populations with complete case ascertainment, but incomplete census data. Thus you can have complete population-based cancer case data, and it can be used without denominators. Extensive comparisons among varied ethnicities and nationalities have been made.[39]

EARLY HISTORY OF CANCER REGISTRATION IN OTHER COUNTRIES

Despite country-to-country differences, cancer registration and surveillance is truly international. The oldest form of citizen "registration" of any type were early censuses. First there was a population census. Later a census of cancer patients was taken. This effort then later led to what we now describe as cancer registries.

The earliest censuses of cancer patients were performed in Europe in the 1890s and before.[40-41]

Table 35-3

Earliest Censuses of Cancer Patients[43]

Year	Country
1900	Germany
1900	Holland
1902	Spain
1904	Portugal
1904	Hungary
1905	Sweden
1905	Denmark
1905	Iceland

These are summarized in Table 35-3. This early cancer registry effort predates cancer registration in the US by three decades. The first known population-based cancer registration effort was based on a mail questionnaire sent to the physicians of Hamburg, Germany.[42] At approximately the same time, a registry in the Netherlands sponsored a similar effort (Table 35-3).

These early cancer censuses led to the formation of long lasting cancer registries in many countries (Table 35-4). To put these dates in perspective with North American registry history, the first US population-based registry was formed in 1936 in Connecticut.[44-45] This was followed by the first "national" US survey in 1937-1939,[46-47] and the first Canadian registry in Saskatchewan in 1944.[48]

Roffers[13] has noted the important role of a European meeting in the 1940s. "The worldwide establishment of today's cancer registries is a result of activities at a conference in Copenhagen, Denmark, in 1946. Participants in this conference were leaders in the field of cancer control. They emphasized the need for setting up improved and internationally comparable morbidity statistics, using uniform nomenclature and classification, as well as an ideal standard population. Toward this goal, participants at that conference recommended the worldwide establishment of epidemiological cancer registries."

"The World Health Organization accepted these recommendations . . . These beginnings led to the establishment of nearly 100 epidemiological cancer registries throughout the world by 1975."

The IARC/IACR was established in 1966. By the mid 1990's, the organization included nearly

Table 35-4

Early Continuing Cancer Registries in Other Countries[40]

Year	Country
1929	Germany (Hamburg)
1942	Denmark
1943	Belgium
1944	Canada Saskatchewan
1945	England and Wales
1948	New Zealand
1948	USSR
1950	Yugoslavia Slovenia
1952	Hungary
1952	Norway
1953	German Democratic Republik
1953	The Netherlands
1954	Iceland
1958	Sweden
1959	Japan Miyahi
1960	Isreal
1960	Spain Zaragonza

400 members from approximately 100 countries. Annual scientific meetings are held.

USES OF CANCER REGISTRATION IN OTHER COUNTRIES

Usage among registries of other countries covers a full range of activities including descriptive studies, analytic studies, patient care-oriented studies, survival analysis, public health and population screening programs.[12] Similarities with US registry usage is prevalent.

Descriptive studies: The type of statistics provided by registries usually closely follows local interest. Subpopulations of special interest are identified. Special exposures and time trend are noted.

Analytic studies: Registries provide population-based rosters for enrollment in analytic studies, notably including case-control studies. Record linkage of cancer rosters with exposure data bases are sometimes processed.

Survival analysis is common among registries of other countries. Some international comparisons have been made, leading to studies to better understand underlying reasons for international differences.[49]

Public health planning: Registry data from other countries is commonly used to estimate the magnitude of the local cancer burden. These provide a data baseline for resource planning and management.

CURRENT STATUS OF CANCER REGISTRATION IN OTHER COUNTRIES

Population-based cancer registries throughout the globe are burgeoning. It is now much rarer for a country not to have such a central registry, than to have one. This includes many developing countries. Building on work of others, such as Doll,[14] Wagner,[40] Muir,[19] and others, Parkin and associates[22] have recently broadened the scope of coverage of Cancer in Five Continents to include 186 registries, reporting on 214 populations from 57 countries (Table 35-5). It would be difficult to exaggerate the importance of this IARC/IACR effort.

Other country registries exist than are included in Cancer in five Continents. Data submitted from 49 registries were not accepted for publication in Volume VIII.[22]

Table 35-5
List of Other Countries Represented by Registries in Cancer Incidence in Five Continents, Volume VIII.[22]

Country	Registries	Populations

- *Africa:* Algeria, La Reunion, The Gambia, Mali, Uganda, Zimbabwe
- *Central and South America:* Argentina, Brazil, Columbia, Costa Rica, Cuba, Ecuador, La Martinue, Puerto Rico, Uraguay
- *North America:* Canada
- *Asia:* China, India, Isreal, Japan, Korea, Kuwait, Oman, Pakistan, Philippines, Singapore, Thailand, Viet Nam
- *Europe:* Austria, Belarus, Belgium, Croatia, Czech Republic, Denmark, Estonia, Finland, France, Germany, Iceland, Ireland, Italy, Latvia, Lithuania, Malta, The Netherlands, Norway, Poland, Portugal, Russia, Slovakia, Slovenia, Spain, Sweden, Switzerland, United Kingdom, Yugoslavia,
- *Oceania:* Australia, New Zealand

DIFFERENCES IN THE ADMINISTRATION AND OPERATION

The basic operation of registries from other countries have been previously described. (1-2, 11-22) There is of course great commonality of function between US registries and registries from other countries. Mutual factors of interest include advisory committees, population (census) determinations, legal aspects, confidentiality, security, space planning, funding, personnel (staff size, qualifications, training), equipment, document control, computerization, data set design (standards), casefinding, case consolidation (record linkage), abstracting, coding and classification, quality control (completeness, accuracy, data edits), and follow-up, statistical methods, survival analysis, and reporting of results (uses of data) occur in most registries.

Despite this commonality in virtually every function somewhat different methods and tools have been employed, and some noteworthy differences exist. In *Cancer Incidence in Five Continents,* a brief description of each registry is given, including a definition of the registration area, reference date, rationale and hosting organization, legal justification, sources of information, casefinding methodology, key personnel, and uses of the data.

The most international progress on standardization has been made in factors relating to merging and consolidation of the data. This progress includes rules for population estimation, data set design, classification and coding. In the US the dominant standard setters have historically been the CoC and the SEER Program. In registries from other countries, the IARC/IACR has established the baseline standards. Because US registries also contribute to the IARC/IACR publications, they also pay attention to IARC/IACR standards. Important differences do exist regarding rules for counting multiple primaries.

A detailed comparison of country to country methodology is not included here, however a brief description of several registry's methods and procedures is instructive. Almost all central registries start with basic computing, and enhance automation as they mature, and as funding allows. Menck and Parkin reviewed the status of central registry computerization in the 1980's based on a IARC/IACR survey.[50] Widespread use of main frame and minicomputer systems were reported. Beyond computing, the other important procedural difference often includes the degree to which active versus passive registration methodologies are used.

Great Britain: The Thames Cancer Registry, a leader in Europe, uses procedures very similar to many central registries in the US.[51] Operation of the registry is based on a sophisticated on-line computer system. Record linkage, coding of data, and data edits are computerized. Some treatment is included in the patient data set, and death certificates are checked, and passive follow-up is performed.

Philippines: In the Rizal Cancer Registry in the early 1990s, procedures were less computerized[52] including: 1) master patient index utilizing index cards, 2) manual editing, 3) paper case finding lists from hospitals, and 4) manual checking for duplicate reports. Cases were abstracted to paper, which were then coded and keypunched. Updating records included updating the manual accession register, and master patient index card.

Since that time registry operations have been increasingly managed using the IARC/IACR CAN-REG software. During the 1980s, Mr Menck, serving as a consultant to the IARC/IACR, installed early test versions of CANREG in the Philippines, and Shanghai. This early CANREG version was based on the menu-driven microcomputer system coded in BASIC under DOS by Dr. Charles R. Smart of the CoC. Later, Mr. Bieber of the IACR visited Mr Menck in Los Angeles, and familiarized himself with the original system design. Upon return to France, Mr Bieber redesigned and modernized the system, and the IARC/IACR has maintained it since then. It is made available to registries to facilitate collection and collation of data for *Cancer Incidence in Five Continents,* and has made data from developing countries available that otherwise could not have been included. The IARC/IACR states: "CANREG was designed specifically for cancer registries. . . . CANREG can be installed on systems costing as little as $6000." CANREG is a manifestation of the vision and long range planning of Dr Max Parkin of the IARC/IACR.

Most registries in other countries are frequently used for surveillance purposes, and not necessarily clinically focused. Therefore, their two most important quality considerations often include completeness of case ascertainment and accuracy of population-at-risk estimates.

In some countries, more passive casefinding is followed relying to a larger extent on death certifi-cate monitoring for cancer cases. This results in a somewhat higher reported percentage of cases reported by death certificate only, and higher ratios of mortality to incidence.[53]

Over time, the legal underpinnings and privacy concerns of central registries in other countries have ranged from a reluctance to have cancer reporting in Germany as late as the 1980s, to legal authorization and use of universal patient identifiers in Scandinavia.

The sources of case information and casefinding procedures for most central registries are described in *Cancer Incidence in Five Continents.* There is strong international similarity. Several quality control measures, regarding completeness of reporting, are given. Included by primary site, are the percentage of incident cases that are pathologically confirmed; the percentage that were reported by death certificate only, and the ratio of the mortality rate to the incidence rate expressed as a percentage.

SUMMARY

In summary, population-based registries from other countries have much in common with US population-based registries, and provide a rich source of comparison data. Some registries in developing countries are early in the development and evolution of their computerization efforts, and in casefinding.

This chapter builds on the writing of Steve Roffers in the first edition. His authorship, and activity in International Registries is gratefully acknowledged.

STUDY QUESTIONS

1. What is the role of the IARC/IACR in population-based cancer registration?
2. What is the CANREG system?
3. What broad-based publication of cancer incidence is published every few years?

REFERENCES

1. Parkin DM. Cancer registration in developing countries. In: Cancer Registration Principles and Methods: Jensen OM, Parkin DM, MacLennan R, Muir CS, Skeet RG, eds. Lyons, France: IARC; 1991. IARC Scientific Publication No. 95.

2. Olweny CLM. The role of cancer registration in developing countries. In: Parkin DM, Wagner G, Muir CS, eds. *The Role of the Registry in Cancer Control.* Lyons, France, 1985. IARC Scientific Publications N. 66.

3. Brennan M, Clive R, Winchester D. The CoC: its roots and its destiny. *AcoS Bulletin.* 1994; 79(6): 14.

4. Young JL. The hospital-based cancer registry. In: *Cancer Registration Principles and Methods:* Jensen OM, Parkin DM, MacLennan R, Muir CS, Skeet RG, eds. Lyons, France: IARC; 1991. IARC Scientific Publication No. 95.

5. Blankenship C, Moore M, Opaluch GM, Sylvester J. The American College of Surgeons Commission on Cancer and the Approvals Program. In: *Cancer Registry Management Principles and Practice* Hutchinson CL, Roffers SD, Fritz AG, eds. Dubuque, Iowa: Kendall/Hunt Publishing Company, 1997.

6. Stephenson GW. The Commission on Cancer. A historical review. *Bull Amer Coll Surg.* Sept: 7-13, 1979.

7. Menck HR, Bland KI, Scott-Conner CEH, Eyre H, Murphy GP, Winchester DP. Regional diversity and breadth of the National Cancer Data Base. *Cancer.* 1998; 83: 2649-58.

8. Sturm HH. Appendix 3(a) The Danish Cancer Registry, a self-reporting national cancer registration system with elements of active data collection. In: *Cancer Registration Principles and Methods:* Jenson OM, Parkin DM, MacLennan R, Muir CS, Skeet RG, eds. Lyons, France: IARC; 1991. IARC Scientific Publication No. 95.

9. Knoweldon J, Mork T, Phillips AJ. *The Registry in Cancer Control.* Geneva, Switzerland: UICC; 1970.

10. Clemmesen J. Statistical studies in the aetiology of malignant neoplasms. *Acta Pathol Microbiol Scand.* 1965; 1, Suppl 247.

11. MacLennan R, Muir C, Steinitz R, Winkler A. Cancer Registration and Its Techniques. Lyons, France. IARC; 1978.

12. Jensen OM, Parkin DM, MacLennan R, Muir CS, Skeet RG. *Cancer Registration Principles and Methods.* Lyons, France: IARC; 1991. IARC Scientific Publication No. 95.

13. Roffers SD. Cancer registries in other countries. In: *Cancer Registry Management Principles and Practice* (Hutchinson CL, Roffers SD, Fritz AG, eds.) Dubuque, Iowa: Kendall/Hunt Publishing Company; 1997.

14. Doll R, Payne P, Waterhouse JAH. *Cancer Incidence in Five Continents,* Vol 1. Geneva, UICC: Berlin. Springer, 1966.

15. Doll R, Muir C, Waterhouse JAH. *Cancer Incidence in Five Continents,* Vol II, Berlin Heidelberg; New York, Spring; 1970.

16. Doll R. Cancer in five continents. *Proc R Soc Med.* 1972:65, 49-55.

17. Waterhouse JAH, Muir CS, Correa P, Powell J. *Cancer Incidence in Five Continents.* Vol III, Lyons, France: International Agency for Research on Cancer; 1976. IARC Scientific Publications No. 15.

18. Waterhouse JAH, Muir CS, Shanmugraratnam K, Powell J. *Cancer Incidence in Five Continents.* Vol IV, Lyons, France: International Agency for Research on Cancer; 1982.

19. Muir CS, Waterhouse JAH, Mack TM, Powell J, Whelan S. *Cancer Incidence in Five Continents.* Vol V; 1987.

20. Parkin DM, Muir CS, Whelen SI, Gao YT, Ferlay J, Powell J. *Cancer Incidence in Five Continents,* Vol VI. Lyons, France: International Agency for Research on Cancer; 1992. IARC Publication No. 120.

21. Parkin DM, Whelan SL, Ferlay J, Raymond L, Young J. *Cancer Incidence in Five Continents,* Vol VII; 1997.

22. Parkin DM, Whelan SL, Ferlay J, Teppo L, Thomas DB. *Cancer Incidence in Five Continents,* Vol VIII. Lyons, France: International Agency for Research on Cancer; 2002. IARC Publication No. 155.

23. Menck HR, Henderson BE. Cancer incidence rates in the Pacific Basin. *Natl Cancer Inst Monogr.* 1979; 53: 119-124.

24. Menck HR, Henderson BE. Cancer incidence patterns in the Pacific Basin. *Natl Cancer Inst Monogr.* 1982; 62:101-109.

25. Menck HR, Henderson BE: Cancer Incidence in the Pacific Basin. *Natl Cancer Monogr.* 1985; 70.

26. Parkin DM, Wagner G, Muir CS. *The Role of the Registry in Cancer Control.* Lyons, France: 1985. IARC Scientific Publications N. 66.

27. Armstrong BK. The role of the Cancer Registry in cancer control. *Cancer Causes and Control.* 1992; 3: 569-79.

28. Yu MC, Ho JHC, Henderson BE, Armstrong RW. Epidemiology of Nasopharyngeal Carcinoma in Malaysia and Hong Kong. In: *National Cancer Institute Monograph 69,* December 1985, Fourth Symposium on Epidemiology and Cancer Registries in the Pacific Basin. Bethesda, Md: US Dept. of Health and Human Services. NIH Publication No. 85-2768.

29. Correa P, Haenszel W, Tannenbaum S. Epidemiology of Gastric Carcinoma: Review and Future Prospects.

30. Third Symposium on Epidemiology and Cancer Registries in the Pacific Basin. *Natl Cancer Inst Monogr;* 1982.

31. Li Hun-Yoo. Investigation of geographic patterns of cancer mortality in China. *Natl Cancer Inst Monogr.* 1982.

32. Li CC, Yu MC, Henderson BE. Some epidemiologic observations of nasopharyngeal carcinoma in Guangdong People's Republic of China. *Natl Cancer Inst Monogr.* 1982.

33. Fujimoto I, Hanai A, Sakagami F. Cancer registries in Japan: Activities and incidence data. *Natl Cancer Inst Monogr.* 1977; 47: 7-15.

34. Lee HP, Shanmugaratnam K. Cancer incidence in Singapore: 1973-77. *Natl Cancer Inst Monogr.* 1982.

35. Atkinson L, Clezy JK, Reay-Young PS. *The Epidemiology of Cancer in Papua New Guinea.* Erskineville, New South Wales: Star Printery; 1974.

36. Munoz N, Correa P, Cuello C. Histologic types of gastric carcinoma in high- and low-risk areas. *Int J Cancer.* 1968; 3:809-818.

37. Wynder EL, Kmet J, Dungal N. An epidemiologic investigation of gastric cancer. *Cancer.* 1963; 16:1451-1496.

38. Haenszel W, Kurihara M, Locke FB. Stomach cancer in Japan. *J Natl cancer Inst.* 1976; 56:265-274.

39. Decoufle P, Thomas PL, Pickle LW. Comparisons of the proportionate mortality ratio and standardized mortality risk measures. *Am J Epidem.* 1980; 111:263-268.

40. Wagner G. Cancer Registration: Historical Aspects. In: Parkin DM, Wagner G, Muir CS. *The Role of the Registry in Cancer Control.* Lyons, France: 1985; 3-12. IARC Scientific Publications N. 66.

41. Wagner G. History of cancer registration. In: Jensen OM, Parkin DM, Maclennan R, et al., eds. *Cancer Registration Principles and Methods.* Lyons, France: WHO International Agency for Research on Cancer; 1991: 3-6. IARC Scientific Publications No. 95.

42. Katz A. Die Notwendifkeit Einer Sammelstatistik Uber Krebskerkungen. *Dtsch Med Wcchk.* 1899; 25:260-261, 277.

43. Lasch CH. Krebskankenstatistik. Beginin and Ausicht. *Z Krebsforsch* 1940; 50:245-298.

44. Griswold MH, Wilder CS, Cutler SJ, Pollack ES. *Cancer in Connecticut 1935-51.* Hartford, Conn: Conn State Dept of Health, 1955.

45. Connelly RR, Campbell PC, Eisenberg H. Central Registry of Cancer Cases in Connecticut. *Publ Health Rep.* 1968; 83:5: 386-396.

46. Dom HF. *Illness from Cancer in the United States.* Washington, DC: US Govt Printing Office; 1944.

47. Dorn HF, Cutler SJ: Morbidity from cancer in the United States. *Publ Health Monogr 56.* Washington DC: US Dept of Health Education and Welfare; 1959.

48. *The Making of the Canadian Cancer Registry: Cancer Incidence in Canada and Its Regions 1969 to 1988.* Bureau of Chronic Disease Epidemiology, Laboratory Centre for Disease Control, Health and Welfare Canada, Ottawa, K1A 0L2.

49. Berrino F, Sant M, Verdecchia A, Capocaccia R, Hakulinen T, Esteve J. Survival of Cancer Patients in Europe, The EUROCARE Study. Oxford Press.

50. Menck HR, Parkin DM. *Directory of Computer Systems Used in Cancer Registries.* Lyons, France: WHO International Agency for Research On Cancer: 1985.

51. Skeet RG. The Thames Cancer Registry. In: Jensen OM, Parkin DM, MacLennan R, Muir CS, Skeet RG, eds. *Cancer Registration Principles and Methods.* Lyons, France: IARC; 1991. IARC Scientific Publication No. 95.

52. Laudico AV, Esteban D. The Department of Health—Rizal Cancer Registry. In: Jensen OM, Parkin DM, MacLennan R, Muir CS, Skeet RG, eds. *Cancer Registration Principles and Methods.* Lyons, France: IARC; 1991. IARC Scientific Publication No. 95.

53. Coleman MP, Bieber CA. CANREG: Cancer registration software for microcomputers. In: Jensen OM, Parkin DM, MacLennan R, Muir CS, Skeet RG, eds. *Cancer Registration Principles and Methods.* Lyons, France: IARC; 1991. IARC Scientific Publication No. 95.

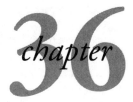

36
chapter

OTHER HEALTH REGISTRIES

Ryan Intlekofer
RN, CTR

INTRODUCTION

The history of health registries dates back at least as far as the late sixteenth century when weekly *Bills of Mortality* were published in England tabulating deaths by causes. The usefulness of this type of written tabulation through study became more evident over time and in the early 1900's the first modern case registries to study cancer were initiated.

By definition, registries are a structured system developed for the collection, storage, distribution, and analysis of a select segment of health data on individuals. The main reasons for establishing health registries are: the collection of information on individuals with a particular disease process or condition, risk factor, genetic disorder, or prior exposure to substances. Many health registries are also used for monitoring therapies and outcomes.

Technological advancements have allowed for a greater number and more diverse population of registries to develop and flourish. The utilization of current electronic technology and informatics can produce seemingly instant results when compared to earlier systems.

Information collected and maintained in high quality registries provides an essential benefit to public health surveillance and medicine in several different ways. The information gathered in registries can give an accurate assessment of the enormity of a problem, and can determine the incidence of disease as well as evaluate trends and survivorship. Registry data may be useful in identification of individuals at high risk of developing certain diseases and in monitoring the delivery of services to them. These data might be used to investigate hypothesis, and if confirmed, other investigative or preventative measures can be employed. Registries are also a rich source of potential donors, such as those registered in the National Bone Marrow Registry, whose efforts match suitable recipients and registered donors.

Registries may be population-based, hospital-, or facility-based, or have a special purpose. The data collected may be prospective, retrospective, or concurrent. These criteria are established at the inception of any registry and may include a combination of these items, based on individual needs. Although these registries have clearly different objectives, all have standard elements.

STANDARD ELEMENTS

All registries must have established criteria for inclusion or exclusion of individuals. All have developed a select set of data items to collect. Health Registries characteristically focus efforts on a particular disease, a group of similar diseases, exposures, or treatments. As examples, Table 36-1 compares five different registries. Each registry has defined the types of cases to be included and has established a list of data items collected. Table 36-2 lists some common data items collected.

Data on individuals are collected from multiple sources. They may include vital statistics, physician records, hospital records and reports, and outpatient diagnostic or treatment centers. In some registries, case ascertainment may also include review of likely sources, for example, a review of all birth records at a facility to find possible birth defects.

Registries are developed to address a specified area of need and may include cases based on geographic area, diagnostic setting, frequency, incidence, prevalence or other criteria determined at the establishment of the registry.

REGISTRY TYPES AND DATA COLLECTION

Population based registries assess data collected within a defined geographic area or region, county, or state. Hospital- or facility-based registries assess data collected within that hospital or facility. Special purpose registries collect data on specific treatments, devices, or specific disease process. These may be short- or long-term in nature, and may be very specific in type of data collected.

Prospective registries are maintained to monitor a disease's incidence or process for a specified length of time. They require that the cases entered into the study be clinically free of disease at the time of admission into the database. Risk factors are assessed and individuals followed and monitored for indication of the development of disease.

One example of this type of registry is the Agricultural Health Study. This is a long-term study of agricultural exposures and chronic disease (especially cancer) among commercial or private pesticide applicators (and their spouses, if married) in Iowa and North Carolina. Individuals enrolled in the

Table 36-1
Data Item Correlation Chart

Data Item	Type of Registry				
	Cancer	AIDS	Cardiac	Diabetes	Trauma
Patient Demographics					
Name	✓	✓	✓	✓	✓
Race/Ethnicity	✓	✓	✓	✓	✓
Sex	✓	✓	✓	✓	✓
DOB/Age	✓	✓	✓	✓	✓
Address	✓	✓	✓	✓	✓
Unique patient number (ssn)	✓	✓	✓	✓	✓
Past Medical History					
Previous applicable diagnosis	✓	✓	✓	✓	na
Risk factors	✓	✓	✓	✓	na
Case (Disease) Identification					
Class of case	✓	✓	na	na	na
Date of diagnosis/surgery	✓	✓	✓	✓	✓
Disease coding	ICD-O	ICD-9	ICD-9, DRG	ICD-9, DRG	ICD-9
Surgery	treatment	therapy	✓	na	✓
Date of admission	✓	✓	✓	na	✓
Date of discharge	✓	✓	✓	na	✓
Length of stay	computable	computable	✓	na	✓
Diagnosis procedures	✓	✓	✓	na	✓
Severity of disease	✓	✓	✓	na	✓
First course of treatment	✓	✓	✓	✓	✓
Follow-Up Information					
Date of contact	✓	✓	✓	na	na
Patient condition at follow-up	✓	✓	✓	na	na
Disease condition at follow-up	✓	✓	✓	na	na
Additional treatment	✓	✓	✓	na	na
Other					
Physicians	✓	✓	✓	na	na

study are linked annually to mortality and cancer registry incidence databases in both states, and mortality data is being obtained every other year from the National Death Index.[1] With the focus limited to persons in Iowa and North Carolina, the Agricultural Health Study is also an example of a population based registry.

Retrospective registries collect information on a specific population with a definitive diagnosis of disease. These registries may include any and all diag-

nostic data, stage of disease at diagnosis, and disease progression. They may also include information on treatment modalities employed and outcome. A familiar example of this type of registry is the cancer registry. Others are diabetes and AIDS registries.

Concurrent registries contain ongoing clinical research and evaluate specific events, procedures, or new treatments. These registries include those involved in clinical trials (refer to chapter on Clinical Trials for detailed information). Another example of

Table 36-2

Common Data Elements to Consider Including in a Registry Database

Data Elements	Examples
Case identification	Study number
	Accession number
	Health record number
	Device number (e.g., implant)
Patient identifier	Social security number
	Date of birth
Demographics	Address
	Gender
	Race/ethnicity
	Occupation
	Religion
Diagnosis element	Anatomic site
	Morphology
	Test value or result
	Diagnostic laboratory tests
	Radiology tests
Therapy/treatment	Chemotherapy
	Implant
Extent of disease	Stage
	Scores
	Severity
Disease status	No evidence of disease
	Never disease-free
	Recurrence
	Metastatic
Vital status	Alive
	Dead
Outcome assessment	Follow-up
	Survival analysis
	Quality of life

this type of registry is a trauma registry. Trauma registries evaluate an event, motor vehicle crash, or traumatic injury. These registries provide a detailed review of injury. This information is valuable in determining needs assessment for rehabilitative efforts and used to develop safer products.

DATA STANDARDS

Appropriate care must be taken to assure that standards are set and maintained (refer to chapter on standards for data management). Only by maintaining high standards, can registries produce valuable data to assist researchers in public health and medicine. To do this, registries must have appropriate written policies and procedures covering all aspects of operations. Codes and data standards must be developed and quality control activities established to ensure provision of consistent, timely, and accurate data. These registries and the data collected must meet scientific and clinical review standards. Most are governed by an internal Institutional Review Board (IRB) or external IRB that monitor human subject research, special committees or federal and state regulation and as such must be able to withstand intense scrutiny and inspection. Policies governing reporting and dissemination of data also must be established. Access to, storage, and use of data must be clearly defined and confidentiality of subjects strictly maintained.

FUNDING AND MANAGEMENT OF REGISTRIES

Registries are funded and managed by many different entities. These are listed below with one representative example given for each.

1) The Federal Government: One example is the National Exposure Registry, operated by the Agency for Toxic Substances and Disease Registries (ATSDR) is designed to identify and enroll persons who may have been exposed to a hazardous environmental substance and provide follow up monitoring of these persons.
2) State Governments: Registries of persons diagnosed with sexually transmitted diseases or other specific infectious diseases.
3) Universities: The Surveillance, Epidemiology, and End Results (SEER) cancer registries. They are supported by funds from the Federal government (NCI).
4) Groups or individual hospitals: Registries including persons diagnosed or treated at the individual facilities. This could include individuals with rare disease types, or to isolate specific treatments.
5) Nonprofit organizations: the United States Eye Injury Registry—a nonprofit organization sponsored by the Helen Keller Eye Research Foundation.
6) Private groups: Transplant registries.

Funding sources may change after the registry is established. A nationally funded registry may be closed after a period of time, but an individual state or region may decide the registry is of continued benefit and will continue to support it with local funding.

A few examples of different types of registries are listed in Table 36-3.

Table 36-3

Registry Name	Description
Acyclovir/Valacyclovir in Pregnancy Registry	This registry was designed to assess the outcome of pregnancies exposed to acyclovir or valacyclovir for potential birth defects from exposure to these drugs. Studies were completed in 1999.
Immunization Registries	Monitors population for completeness of vaccination coverage within a community and identify subgroups who may need targeted interventions.
Agency for Toxic Substances and Disease	Reports findings to Congress for public health implications.
Alzheimer's Disease Registry	Includes the review of staging the severity of the disease and dementia.
Auto-Immune Deficiency Syndrome (AIDS) Registry	Requires that the diagnosis be made by meeting the Centers for Disease Control (CDC) criteria for AIDS.
Cardiac Registry	Developed to compile data for analyzing clinical results in standards of care. Items include risk assessment, patency of vessels, measurements of time of procedures, complications and outcomes. Within cardiac registries, there may be multiple types, including catheterization registries and open heart surgery registries. The focus of these registries is to quantify the effect of the procedures on the patient's outcome. Many items can be studied from these data. Assessments include new drugs, devices, and techniques. From these results, standards of care are reviewed and appropriate changes may be instituted.
Central Registries for Child Abuse and Neglect	Each state is mandated by law to provide a reporting system to collect information on reported abuse and neglect. These registries serve a valuable function by identifying subpopulations at risk and quantifying that risk relative to the general population.
Congenital Birth Defects Registry	Tracks the occurrence of birth defects, and provides information to health agencies. Investigates causes and clusters of birth defects, and is used to provide improved treatment, professional and public education.
Connective Tissue Disease Registry	Determines the frequency of CTD by registering incidence. The goal is the establishment of standardized population based registries that can identify the etiology and preventive measures.
Diabetes Registry	Compares mortality rates. Also includes prevention and the role of diabetes care as well as the contribution of the disease to adverse outcomes.
Insulin Dependant Diabetes Mellitis (IDDM) Registries	There are over 20 IDDM registries in the US and throughout the world. In the US, these registries are frequently supported by federal funds. The purpose is to determine incidence of IDDM in defined populations, and to enroll people in case control studies and other research projects. Case finding procedures use hospital and other medical records to identify cases for inclusion.

(continued)

Table 36-3
(continued)

Registry Name	Description
Diethystilbestrol Registry	The National Institutes of Health (NIH) undertakes longitudinal studies on the long-term health effects of DES exposures.
Huntington's Disease Registry	Maintains a repository of HD information for researchers and families.
International Bone Marrow Transplant Registry	Reviews relative risks of treatment related mortality and treatment failures. Also determines if outcomes are different in small or large treatment centers.
The United States Eye Injury Registry	A nonprofit organization sponsored by the Helen Keller Eye Research Foundation; is a federation of state eye registries that use a standardized form to obtain voluntary data on eye injuries and to obtain 6 month follow-up information. The primary purpose is to provide prospective population-based data to improve prevention and control of eye injuries.
International Breast Implant Registry	Registry for women with breast implants. Independent of manufacturers and funded by fees and donations. Provides women with up to date information on their transplants and notifies them if important safety information is announced regarding the implant. Women enrolled may also record symptoms related to their implants.
International Cooperative Pulmonary Embolism Registry	Tracks patients who have experienced pulmonary embolism. The mortality rate and rate of recurrent pulmonary embolism are recorded two weeks and three months after the first occurrence. This registry is the largest such project dedicated to understanding pulmonary embolism.
International Implant Registry	Established in 1988, provides notification services to patients with medical devices such as pacemakers, heart valves, prosthetic limbs, and orthopedic joints.
International Retinoblastoma Registry	Registers and monitors families with a retinoblastoma patient.
National Deaf Registry	A resource for hereditary deafness research.
Temporal Bone Registry	Established to encourage individuals with ear disorders to pledge their temporal bones at death to scientific research. This registry also provides professional and public education.
National Familial Brain Cancer Registry	Documents the occurrence of primary brain cancers as a familial disorder and evaluates this malignancy. Initially, family screening and review of health records, pathology reviews and phone interviews were done. Plans were for epidemiologic, cytogenic and molecular-biologic studies to follow.
National Genetic Registry	Collects information on genetic services throughout the United States.
National Infectious Diseases Registry	Under direction of the Centers for Disease Control and Prevention (CDC), this registry collects hospital infection rates. Includes review of hospital and microbiology reports.
National Registry of Myocardial Infarction	Reviews the effectiveness of hospital programs to reduce the time to treatment for myocardial infarction and for continuous quality improvement surveillance.

Table 36-3
(continued)

Registry Name	Description
National Registry for Supported Angioplasty	Collects data on patients undergoing supported angioplasty.
North American Malignant Hyperthermia (MH) Registry	Collects information on susceptibility and risk factors to help determine specificity of guidelines for MH.
Organ Transplant Registry	Supports both clinical and research requirements of a transplant program.
Spinal Cord Injury Registry	Surveillance system for sentinel injuries at the state and national level. Gathers information for injury prevention methods and planning for services. Evaluates the efficacy of treatment and monitors outcomes.
Twin Registry	Includes quantitative twin data on monozygotic and dizygotic pairs.
Trauma Registry	Requires that trauma be diagnosed and assessed as a Level I trauma. The goal is to provide information to decrease morbidity and mortality.
United Network for Organ Sharing (UNOS) Registry	Under contract with the US Department of Health and Human Services, administers the Organ Procurement and Transplantation Network. Operates and maintains the list of patients waiting for solid organ transplants.
Rare Disease Registries	There are numerous rare disease registries in operation for conducting research and to act as a resource for those affected by rare diseases.

SUMMARY

The contribution made by health registries to public health and to medical and scientific research can only be realized by obtaining and maintaining exacting data and by ensuring these data are fully analyzed and utilized. The importance of this contribution cannot be denied.

The knowledge, skills, and abilities cancer registrars possess through their education and training are easily converted for use in these other registries. Registrars are the backbone of any registry and their skills make the difference in the quality and value of the data collected.

STUDY QUESTIONS

1. Identify and describe three types of registries.
2. List five data elements that could be included in a registry.
3. List three possible benefits of a registry.
4. Describe why data standards are important for all registries.
5. List three sources of funding for registries.

RESOURCES

Subject	Organization
AIDS	Centers for Disease Control (CDC)
Birth	Iowa Birth Defects Registry, March of Dimes
Cancer	American Joint Committee on Cancer
	Commission on Cancer of the American College of Surgeons
	National Cancer Institute
	National Cancer Registrars Association
	International Association of Cancer Registries
	North American Association of Central Cancer Registries

Cardiac   American College of Thoracic
                   Surgeons
               American College of Cardiology
               Society of Thoracic Surgeons
               Canadian Cardiovascular Society
Diabetes   American Diabetes Association
Transplant   North American Transplant
                   Organization
               United Network for Organ Sharing
Trauma   Association for the Advancement of
                   Automotive Medicine
               Committee on Trauma, American
                   College of Surgeons
               American Trauma Society

REFERENCES

1. *Cancer in Iowa 2002.* The State Health Registry of
   Iowa, University of Iowa.

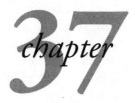

chapter 37

NETWORKING WITH ORGANIZATIONS

Marilyn S. Desler
CTR

INTRODUCTION

The National Cancer Registrars Association held its first meeting in 1974, over 40 years after the advent of registries. Since 1974, the profession of the cancer registrar has undergone tremendous changes, not the least the change from manual data collection to computerization. Data collection is more sophisticated, technical, and clinical in nature. Quality assessment and patient care evaluation activities can comprise a large part of a registrar's job. Registrars manage a database, operate sophisticated software programs, produce professional reports with graphics, and conduct clinical studies.

Registrars work in hospital-based, state, central, or regional registries. They may travel to different locations, acting as circuit riders for those institutions or patient care facilities that do not have a registry but have an obligation to report to a specific entity. Job opportunities now include quality management, customer support for software programs, and cancer program management. Hospitals eager to meet specific standards and prove they are providing excellent care to their cancer patients must monitor that care against specific criteria. Experienced cancer registrars provide an invaluable service to institutions in this manner.

Cancer program management entails staffing and coordinating cancer committees, tumor boards, and cancer registries, publishing annual reports, analyzing data and study findings, and presenting them in an easy-to-understand format. Cancer program managers are responsible for maintaining cancer program approval by the Commission on Cancer (CoC) of the American College of Surgeons. The cancer program manager is also an active participant in cancer program surveys. Cancer registry software companies hire registrars as support personnel, providing yet another opportunity in the profession and creating a strong selling point for these vendors. Many registrars find themselves traveling across the nation in these roles.

Professional survival in the cancer registry field is dependent on exposure to new ideas and standards, education, and networking. The best way to achieve any of these goals is through networking. *Merriam Webster's Collegiate Dictionary* defines interface as "the means by which interactions or communication is achieved."' In other words, interaction and communication can enhance the profession.

The dictionary defines networking as "the exchange of information or services among individuals, groups, or institutions."[1] The most important word in this definition is *exchange*. In order for an organization to meet the needs of its users, there must be a dialogue between them. The members become resources for each other. Knowledge of the associations or organizations that meet certain needs and provide accessibility to different resources is imperative. In today's world of information management, it is more necessary than ever that registrars not only be informed of, but also use, all available resources.

Cancer data management is beset with many rules, standards, and requirements from many different groups. The success of accurate data collection relates to the professional's ongoing education and exposure to networking. A cancer registrar must know what is available to them to achieve these goals and then avail themselves of those options. To be successful in any field, one must know as much as they can about all aspects of the profession. Cutting through the maize of acronyms can be of great benefit.

REVIEW OF RESOURCES

Many benefits can be reaped from affiliation with professional organizations, which provide the following:

- A means of networking
- A source of knowledge
- References
- Education

Listed below are two examples of associations from which cancer registrars can obtain valuable resources:

- **American Cancer Society (ACS)**
  The ACS can provide educational material for the registrar as well as the general public. An excellent resource manual is their *Textbook of Clinical Oncology.* The bimonthly publication *CA-A Cancer Journal for Clinicians* can also be obtained from them.
- **National Cancer Registrars Association (NCRA)**
  This is an organization of cancer registry professionals. Membership benefits include a quarterly journal and newsletter, training books,

information on training workshops and the annual conference, and discounts for membership activities. The annual conference provides an excellent opportunity to meet and network with colleagues from across the nation and around the world.

Registrars in turn can help these organizations. Many of these groups exist because people volunteer their time and expertise to enhance them. The ACS has a salaried staff, but the heart of the organization is its volunteers. The NCRA is a group whose members volunteer their time and talents to maintain the association's mission of educating the membership. The National Cancer Data Base (NCDB) would be unable to reach its goal of gathering national data if hospital registries did not provide information.

Registrars can be a valuable resource to many organizations. Interaction benefits both the registrar and the organization. Sharing is important for everyone involved in the fight against cancer.

ACRONYMS

The definition of *acronym* is "a word formed from the first (or first few) letters of a series of words,"[1] as in NCRA—the National Cancer Registrars Association.

Acronyms have been popular in the business world for years. Unfortunately, individuals who have not been in a particular field for long may have trouble deciphering the acronyms in common use in that field. Tables 37-1 through 37-3 provide a guide to acronyms in the field of cancer registries.[2-11]

Table 37-1

Guide to Acronyms in the General Healthcare and Cancer Registry Field

Acronym	Name	Description and Contact Information
AACR	American Association for Cancer Research	Association to foster cancer research. Publishes *Cancer Research* (semimonthly). 215/440-9300. www.aacr.org
ACCC	Association of Community Cancer Centers	Association of institutions and individuals involved in providing cancer care in the community. They seek to improve the quality of care available to cancer patients. Publishes *Oncology Issues.* 301/984-9496 www.accr-cancer.org
ACE	Association of Cancer Executives	Professional organization for administrators of cancer programs. 708/719-1ACE
ACoS	American College of Surgeons	Voluntary, scientific, and educational institution organized to improve the care of the surgical patient. Sponsors the Commission on Cancer (*See* CoC). 312/664-4050. www.facs.org
ACoSOG	American College of Surgeons Oncology Group	Founded by NCI to perform prospective, randomized trials to evaluate surgical therapies in the management of solid malignant tumors. www.acosog.org
ACS	American Cancer Society	Voluntary organization with divisions nationwide that provide education, research, and services to cancer patients and families. Publishes many educational resources available for use in the registry, such as *Cancer Manual* 8th ed.; *Textbook of Clinical Oncology;* and *CA-A Cancer Journal for Clinicians.* 1-800/ACS-2345. www.cancer.org

Table 37-1
(continued)

Acronym	Name	Description and Contact Information
ACTG	AIDS Clinical Trials Group	Federal government-administered program of the NIH AIDS researchers. Coordinates testing of experimental drugs used in AIDS treatment. 301/496-8210.
AFIP	Armed Forces Institute of Pathology	Many pathologists use AFIP as a consultant for confirmation of diagnoses. 202/576-2904. Group of healthcare institutions and individuals interested in providing better health services. 312/280-6000. www.afip.org
AHA	American Hospital Association	Association of physicians that provides an overall informational base for its members and the public. 312/464-4818. www.aha.org
AHIMA	American Health Information Management Association	Organization of health information management professionals (ARTs, RRAs). 312/787-2672. www.ahima.org *RHIT* (Registered Health Information Technician)— Credentials awarded by AHIMA to individuals who pass a national exam that evaluates their expertise in the management of health information. Available to those who complete a two-year course in health information management. *RHIA* (Registered Health Information Administrator)— Credential awarded by AHIMA to individuals who pass a national exam that evaluates their expertise in the management of health information. Available to those who complete a four-year college curriculum in health information management.
AIDS	Autoimmune Deficiency Syndrome	Syndrome that results from a vitally induced, progressive depletion of cell-mediated immunity.
AJCC	American Joint Committee on Cancer	Multidisciplinary body that includes representatives from six national organizations. It guides development and use of the TNM prognostic system. Publishes and maintains the *Manual for Staging of Cancer*. 312/664-4050. www.cancerstaging.org/
AMA	American Medical Association	Association of physicians that provides an overall informational base for its members and the public. 312/464-4818. www.ama-assn.org
AMFAR	American Foundation for AIDS Research	Foundation that raises funds to support research on AIDS. Formed by merger of AIDS Medical Foundation and National AIDS Research Foundation. 213/857-5900. www.amfar.org
APON	Association of Pediatric Oncology Nurses	Group of pediatric oncology nurses that holds an annual conference. It provides a certification for pediatric oncology nurses. 708/966-3723. www.apon.org

Table 37-1

(continued)

Acronym	Name	Description and Contact Information
ASCO	American Society of Clinical Oncology	Association of physicians and paramedical personnel who have a predominant interest in the diagnosis and total care of cancer patients. Publishes journal of *Clinical Oncology.* 312/644-0828. www.asco.org
ASH	American Society of Hematology	Association of physicians and paramedical personnel who have a predominant interest in the diagnosis and total care of cancer patients. Publishes journal of *Clinical Oncology.* 312/644-0828. www.hematology.org
ASPHO	American Society of Pediatric Hematology/Oncology	Society consisting of physicians interested in pediatric oncology. An annual conference is held in the fall. 310/668-3850. www.aspho.org
ATLL	Adult T-cell leukemia and lymphoma	Diseases to which HTLV-I and HTLV-II have now been shown to be causally linked.
CALGB	Cancer and Leukemia Group B	National group conducting clinical trials for cancer patients. www.calgb.org
CAP	College of American Pathologists	Association of pathologists that provides pathology codes used by healthcare professionals. 708/446-8800. www.cap.org
CC	Cancer Care (formerly National Cancer Foundation [NCF])	Promotes and assists in the development of services to cancer patients and their families. 212/221-3300.
CDC	Centers for Disease Control and Prevention	Federal agency charged with protecting public health and providing leadership and direction in the prevention and control of disease. 404/639-3286. www.cdc.gov
CIS	Cancer Information Service	Funded by NCI, staffed with trained counselors providing information about cancer causes, prevention, detection, diagnosis, rehabilitation, and research. 1-800/4-CANCER. http://cis.nih.gov
CoC	Commission on Cancer	Multidisciplinary body of the ACoS that strives to reduce the morbidity and mortality caused by cancer through prevention monitoring and reporting of care, standard setting, and education. It has a cornerstone approvals program, which conducts voluntary surveys of cancer programs in a variety of settings. Publishes *Standards of the Commission on Cancer, vol. 1: Cancer Program Standards,* and vol. II: *Facility Oncology Registry Data Standards (FORDS); Perspective on Quality; Annual Review of Patient Care; Patient Care Evaluation,* books 1 and 2; and the newsletter *News from the Commission on Cancer.* 312/664-4050. www.facs.org/dept/cancer/index.html

Table 37-1
(continued)

Acronym	Name	Description and Contact Information
COG	Childrens Oncology Group	COG was formed by the merger of the four national pediatric cancer research organizations: the Children's Cancer Group, the Intergroup Rhabdomyosarcoma Study Group, the National Wilms Tumor Study Group, and the Pediatric Oncology Group. Nearly 90% of the children with cancer in North America now have access to the state-of-the-art care of the physician-researchers of the Children's Oncology Group (COG). Member-institutions are located in almost every state and province, at over 235 prestigious medical centers.
CTR	Certified Tumor Registrar	Credential earned by individuals who pass a national examination by NBCR that evaluates knowledge of cancer registry professionals. 913/438-NCRA or 913/599-4994.
ECOG	Eastern Cooperative Oncology Group	National group that conducts clinical trials for cancer patients. www.ecog.org
EDITS	Exchangeable-edits, Data-dictionary, and Information Translation Standard	Standard sponsored by the CDC that optimizes software to coordinate standards for creating and exchanging data. 770/488-4783.
FAB	French-American-British	FAB system for leukemias which provided a system for the classification of lymphoid and myeloid leukemia and myelodysplasia.
FIPS	Facility Information Profile System	Collaboration between CoC and ACS to provide information to the public on the cancer experience of individual facilities.
FORDS	Facility Oncology Registry Data Standards	Data standards for cancer data collection developed by the CoC.
GOG	Gynecological Oncology Group	National group that conducts clinical trials for women with gynecological cancers. 215/854-0770.
HEDIS	Health Employer Data Information Set	Total scoring system for quality in HMOs.
HIPAA	Health Insurance Portability and Accountability Act of 1996	The Centers for Medicare and Medicaid Services (CMS) is responsible for implementing various unrelated provisions of HIPAA, and HIPAA may mean different things to different people. One portion addresses the security and privacy of health data.
HIV	Human immunodeficiency virus	Retrovirus of the lentivirus group known as human immunodeficiency virus type 1, or HIV-I, subsequently referred to as HIV.
HMO	Health maintenance organization	A managed care group that provides healthcare for its subscribers.
HTLV	Human T-cell leukemia virus, types I and II	Viruses that have now been shown to be causally linked to ATLL in transforming T-cell tropic retroviruses distantly related to HIV.

Table 37-1
(continued)

Acronym	Name	Description and Contact Information
IACR	International Association of Cancer Registries	Association of central cancer registries that holds annual conferences in different locations around the world. Oll 33 72738485, FAX Oll 33 72738575 (France). www-dep.iarc.fr/iacr.htm
IARC	International Agency for Research on Cancer	Agency established in 1965 by the World Health Assembly and independently financed within the framework of the World Health Organization. Headquarters in Lyon, France. Conducts research concentrating on the epidemiology of cancer and the study of potential carcinogens in the human environment. The agency also conducts a program for the education and training of personnel for cancer research. The IARC was given the responsibility by WHO for the neoplasm chapter of ICD-10 and revision of ICD-0. Publishes a variety of documents including *International Incidence of Childhood Cancer.* Oll 33 72738485, FAX Oll 33 72738575 (France). www.iarc.fr
ICD-0	*International Classification of Diseases*	System for coding neoplasms by topography for *Oncology* and morphology, published by WHO, that is used by cancer registrars. It is an extension of the neoplasm section of the International Classification of Diseases 9th revision (ICD-9) and is identical to the morphology field for neoplasms in SNOMED.
IPA	Independent Physician Association	A group of physicians who provide care for managed care groups.
IRB	Institutional Review Board	Institutions engaged in research are required to provide evidence that an independent peer review mechanism is in place and is commensurate with national standards. Patients participating in trials must give their informed consent, and the research projects must be approved by a human-subjects review committee-the IRB.
JCAHO	Joint Commission on Accreditation of Healthcare Organizations	Independent professional organization that evaluates and accredits health care organizations. JCAHO has established indicators for monitoring cancer patient care. It publishes *Perspectives.* 708/916-5600. www.jcaho.org
KS	Kaposi's sarcoma	Rare vascular tumor arising from the mid-dermis. The form of KS associated with the AIDS outbreak is sometimes referred to as epidemic KS or AIDS/KS. Very rarely, KS occurs in people with AIDS who are not homosexual or bisexual males.
MOTNAC	*Manual of Tumor Nomenclature and Coding*	Original coding manual published by the ACS. The morphology section of ICD-O includes a one-digit expansion of the MOTNAC morphology. MOTNAC has been replaced by *ICD-O.*

Table 37-1
(continued)

Acronym	Name	Description and Contact Information
NAACCR	North American Association of Central Cancer Registries (formerly AACCR)	Organization of central cancer registries and organizations in related fields that works toward a uniform, standardized national cancer data set. Publishes *Standards for Cancer Registries, vol. 1: Data Exchange Standards and Record Description* (for programmers); vol. 11: *Data Standards and Data Dictionary* (for registries); vol. III: *Standards for Completeness, Quality, Analysis, and Management of Data* (for central registries); and vol. IV. Standard Data Edits. 916/737-4070. www.naaccr.org
NAC	National AIDS Clearinghouse	CDC clearinghouse that collects, analyzes, and disseminates information on HIV and AIDS. 1-800/458-5231.
NCDB	National Cancer Data Base	Joint project of the ACoS and the ACS. Data are obtained from hospital-based registries for analysis and publication in aggregate form for use in comparison studies. Publishes *Annual Review of Patient Care.* 312/664-4050 Research-based institution sponsored by NIH that funds outside research activities and develops its own research in the prevention and control of cancer. Publishes *Annual Cancer Statistics Review.* 301/496-8510. www.facs.org/dept/cancer/ncdb/index.html
NCI	National Cancer Institute	Research-based institution sponsored by NIH which funds outside research activities and develops its own research in the prevention and control of cancer. Publishes *Annual Cancer Statistics Review.* 301-496-8510. www.seer.ims.nci.nih.gov
NCRA	National Cancer Registrars Association	Professional association for persons interested in the cancer registry field. Publishes the quarterly journal *The Journal of Registry Management;* the quarterly newsletter *The Connection;* and other educational materials. Sponsors annual conference and regional workshops. 913/438-NCRA. http://ncra-usa.org
NCQA	National Committee for Quality Assurance	Accepted accreditation body for Managed Care Organizations (as JCAHO is to hospitals). 202/628-5788.
NIH	National Institutes of Health	Principal biomedical research agency of the federal government. One major component is the National Cancer Institute (NCI). www.nih.gov
NOCA	National Organization for Competency Assurance	Organization that conducts an annual workshop to help boards organize and develop rules for certification exams. 202/857-1165. www.noca.org
NPCR	National Program of Cancer Registries	Nationwide program that supports the establishment or enhancement of cancer registries in states and territories of the United States. Funded via the Cancer Registries Amendment Act and administered by the CDC. 404/488-4783. www.cdc.gov/cancer/nprcr

Table 37-1
(continued)

Acronym	Name	Description and Contact Information
NSABP	National Surgical Adjuvant Breast and Bowel Project	Supported by NCI, NSABP conducts clinical trials to address therapy and biology of primary breast and colon cancer. Headquarters in Pittsburgh, Pennsylvania. 412/383-1400. www.nsapb.pitt.edu
ONS	Oncology Nursing Society	Association of oncology nurses that holds an annual conference, usually in May. Provides certification for oncology nurses. 412/921-7373. www.ons.org
PCP	Pneumocystis carinii pneumonia	Disease for which the etiologic agent is a parasite that is activated with HIV infection. In early 1981, a new epidemic of KS and PCP was first reported in young men of homosexual or bisexual orientation-the beginning of AIDS.
PDQ	Physician Data Query	Up-to-date comprehensive cancer treatment database, provided by NCI that is vailable to physicians and allied health personnel.
PPO	Preferred Provider Organization	A managed care group.
QM	Quality Management	Tool used by many businesses to monitor the service given to their customers and to identify opportunities to improve.
REAL	Revised European-American Lymphoma	REAL Classification (6) for non-Hodgkin Lymphoma.
RTOG	Radiation Therapy Oncology Group	Group of clinical radiation therapy investigative centers that conduct cooperative clinical trials and studies to improve the care of patients with cancer. 215/574-3150.
SEER	Surveillance, Epidemiology, and End Results	Program sponsored by NCI that provides data compiled from population-based registries. Publishes *SEER Self-Instructional Manuals for Tumor Registrars,* and *Summary Staging Guide.* 301/496-8510. http://seer.cancer.gov
SNOMED	Systematized Nomenclature of Medicine	Revision of SNOP developed by CAP, sharing morphology with the ICD-O. SNOMED's topography is different from ICD-O.
SNOP	Systematized Nomenclature of Pathology	Original coding system of morphology and topography codes published by CAP.
SOCRA	Society of Clinical Research Associates	Professional association for individuals and organizations involved in clinical trials. Conducts certification exam for clinical research associates. 1-800-SOCRA92.
SSG	Summary Staging Guide	Site-specific staging schemes devised by SEER.
SWOG	Southwest Oncology Group	National group that conducts clinical trials for cancer patients. 210/677-8808. www.swog.org

Table 37-1
(continued)

Acronym	Name	Description and Contact Information
TNM	T=Tumor size or extension N=Regional nodal involvement M=Metastatic involvement	Staging scheme of the AJCC cancer staging.
UICC	(Union Internationale Contre le Cancer) International Union Against Cancer	Organization of voluntary national groups, organizations, committees, institutions, governmental agencies, and so on that internationally promotes a campaign against cancer through research and therapeutic and preventive resources. Publishes TNM *Classification of Malignant Tumours*. Based in Geneva, Switzerland. Oll 42 22 320 1811. www3.uicc.org
WHO	World Health Organization	International organization that recognizes the fundamental right of all people to receive healthcare. Publishes the world-standard diagnosis coding systems *ICD-9, ICD-10* and ICD-O. For cancer-related information: Oll 33 72738485, FAX Oll 33 72738575 (Switzerland). http://mim.nih.gov/english/funding/who.html

SUMMARY

The cancer registrar's future is unlimited. A registrar can grow professionally as far as he or she can envision. One known factor in an individual's survival and growth in the profession is involvement with peers. Extending horizons strengthens professional positions. Other local registrars can provide guidance through their own knowledge and experience. Professional organizations provide not only social opportunities but also opportunities for growth and education.

STUDY QUESTIONS

1. What term describes the exchange of information between individuals or groups?
2. How do registrars find out what resources are available to meet their needs?
3. How can registrars serve as resources to others?
4. What institute is a major component of the NIH?

REFERENCES

1. *Merriam Webster's Collegiate Dictionary, 10th ed.* Springfield, Mass: Merriam-Webster, Inc.; 1993.
2. Watkins S. *Tumor Registry Management,* 2nd ed. Tumor Registrars Association of California; 1986.
3. Menck HR, Seiffert JE, eds. *Standards for Cancer Registries,* vol. II: *Data Standards and Data Dictionary.* Sacramento, Calif: American Association of Central Cancer Registries; 1994.
4. *Standards for Cancer Programs,* rev. ed. Rockville, Md: Association of Community Cancer Centers; 1993.
5. Percy C, Van Holten V, Muir Cm eds. *International Classification of Diseases for Oncology (ICD-O),* 2nd ed. Geneva, Switzerland: World Health Organization; 1990.
6. *Standards of the Commission on Cancer,* vol. 1: *Cancer Program Standards.* Chicago, Ill: American College of Surgeons; 1996.
7. Girard ML, Peterson TH. *The United States Government Manual, Office of the Federal Register, National Archives and Records Administration.* Lanham, Md: Bernan Press; 1993/94.
8. Schwartz CA, Turner RL eds. *Encyclopedia of Associations,* 29th ed., vol. 1, Part 2, Section 8: "National Organizations of the US"; and vol. 1, part 3, "Name and Keyword Index." Detroit, Mich: 1995.
9. Beahrs OH, Henson DE, Hutter RVP, et al., eds. *Manual for Staging of Cancer,* 4th ed. Philadelphia, Penn: J. B. Lippincott; 1992.
10. Holleb AI, Fink DJ, Murphy GP. *American Cancer Society Textbook of Clinical Oncology.* Atlanta, Ga: American Cancer Society; 1991.

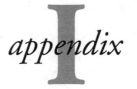

appendix

THE NATIONAL CANCER REGISTRARS ASSOCIATION GUIDE TO THE INTERPRETATION OF THE CODE OF ETHICS

The National Cancer Registrars Association

GUIDE TO THE INTERPRETATION OF THE CODE OF ETHICS
(Established 1986, Revised 1995, Revised 2002)

Preamble

The cancer registrar is concerned with the development, use, and maintenance of hospital-based, centralized, or special purpose cancer programs that meet the needs of physicians, administrators, and planners; protect the patients' rights to privacy; and comply with ethical and legal requirements of the healthcare delivery system. To provide members of the Association and other registry professionals with definitive and binding guidelines of conduct, the National Cancer Registrars Association, Inc., adopted the following Code of Ethics, outlining principles of personal and professional conduct.

I. GENERAL

A. Conduct myself in the practice of the cancer registry profession so as to bring honor and dignity to myself, the cancer registry profession, and the Association.

GUIDES

1. The cancer registrar shall maintain high standards of conduct, integrity, and fairness in all professional actions and decisions to establish and sustain an irreproachable, professional reputation. Examples:

   a. Make judgments and decisions without personal bias or prejudice.

   b. Give primary consideration in all decisions as to the affect actions may have on a patient's health and welfare.

2. Business on behalf of the employer should be conducted honestly and ethically, declining favors that will influence any decisions, and avoiding commercialization of one's position.

3. A member has the obligation to refrain from commenting disparagingly, without justifications, about the professional work of another member.

4. Evaluation of performance of another registrar should be done fairly and with objectivity. Examples:

   a. Never let personal prejudice influence the type of evaluation or reference given.

   b. Offer only job-related, solicited information.

5. The cancer registrar shall use professional titles and degrees as earned and consistent with the dignity of the profession. A certified tumor registrar should use the letters CTR.

6. The cancer registrar shall not exert undue pressure in obtaining employment/clients.[1] Advertising should contain only the registrar's name, degree(s), address, telephone and fax numbers, nature of services offered, and professional memberships. If requested, a resume and list of references may be furnished. Qualifications listed should be those for which supporting evidence (e.g., employment history) is available.

7. Distribution of announcements concerning the formal organization and availability of cancer registry consultant services is ethical. Repeated distribution of unsolicited announcements is unethical. Any distribution should be in keeping with the practice of other health-related professionals in the community.

---

[1]Client: a person, entity, or organization who engages the professional advice or services of another.

8. Use of business cards and letterhead stationery is acceptable but should not promote a commercial endeavor that may lower public esteem for the profession. The NCRA logo or address may not be used in this context.

9. A member has the obligation to recognize appropriately the contributions of fellow members and co-workers to advance cancer registry practice. Publications should give credit where due to one's peers.

10. A member has the right to speak out against policies espoused by the Association, however, representing one's own view as that of the Association or the majority of the members is unethical.

B. Uphold the doctrine of confidentiality and the individual's right to privacy in the disclosure of personally identifiable medical and social information.

GUIDES

1. The patient has a right to feel confident that all identifiable information about him/her possessed by the cancer registry will be kept confidential unless he/she waives the privilege, or release of the information is compelled by statute, regulations, or other legal means.

2. Use and release of identifiable and non-identifiable information shall be according to the established institutional policies. Example:

   Providing lists of patients' names for marketing research or other commercial use is not a proper function of a health institution and such lists should not be released by a cancer registrar without approval of the chief executive officer.

3. Every effort must be made to ensure that the computerization of cancer registry information is accomplished in a manner that protects the confidentiality of patient information. Example:

   Actively participate in establishing controls to protect the patient's privacy when processing information electronically.

C. Cooperate with other health professions and organizations to promote the quality of healthcare programs and the advancement of medical care, ensuring respect and consideration for the responsibility and the dignity of medical and other health professions.

GUIDES

1. Cooperation with other professions and entities engaged in or supportive of health services is an essential factor in the cancer registry profession's greater aim of improving health services and supporting research relevant to the advancement of medical care. Examples:

   a. Accept the right of other health professions to have purpose in their occupation and attempt to understand the thinking and work patterns of professional groups whose primary interest may be different from yours.

   b. Treat all members of the medical and component professional staff with equal respect and due recognition of the status, privilege, and authority belonging to their respective professions.

   c. Refrain from making decisions or expressing opinions for which you are not qualified.

   d. Assist the medical staff and/or institution in working with other professional groups or entities engaged in utilization review and patient care evaluation, continuing education for professional staff, health services planning, clinical studies, proposed legislation or regulations affecting medical and statistical record systems, and like activities.

2. Courtesy, respect, and cooperation should govern the relationships of fellow cancer registrars. Examples:

    a. Recognize that consultants and co-workers may have differing opinions regarding certain proposals or recommendations. Do not allow such differences to lead to utterances or actions inconsistent with the professional stature and dignity of a colleague.

    b. Do not place loyalty above duty by protecting a fellow cancer registrar who is guilty of unfair or unethical practices. Questions of conduct should be referred to the Ethics Committee for review and evaluation.

II. JOB ORIENTATION

A. Recognize the source of the authority and powers delegated to me and conscientiously discharge the duties and responsibilities thus entrusted.

GUIDES

1. It is the cancer registrar's duty to give loyal service and competently carry out the responsibilities of the position. Accepting a position for which one is inadequately prepared, or vacating a position without responsibility vested in the position or with the policies of the institution, is unethical.

2. The cancer registrar shall always responsibly carry out the duties entrusted to him/her, including:

    a. Rendering a truthful accounting of the status of the work over which one has responsibility.

    b. Assisting the medical staff and other health professional staff in programs related to cancer patient care, cancer education, research, and committee activities in accordance with assigned responsibilities.

    c. Resorting to the special knowledge, skill, or experience of fellow professionals for referral, counsel, guidance, or consultation when one lacks in some detail the capability required to serve an employer.

3. For the protection of the employer/client and cancer registrar (including consultants and part-time supervisors), an agreement[2] should specify responsibilities, functions, objectives, and terms of service to be fulfilled.

4. Relationships with cancer registry and other institutional personnel should be characterized by courtesy and respect. When serving as a consultant, part-time supervisor, or official surveyor/observer, one's responsibility and authority for seeking and obtaining certain information, files, and statistical data should be tempered with respect for another individual's tenable position and the institution's good name in the community.

5. The cancer registrar, including consultants and other advisors, should maintain personal integrity and should not hesitate to advise the employer/client if, in the professional judgment of the registrar, the facility is in danger of errors of commission or omission.

B. Preserve and secure cancer registry records, the information contained therein, and the appropriate secondary records in my custody in accordance with professional management practices, employers' policies, and existing legal provisions.

---

[2]Agreement (Contract): an understanding, preferably in writing, between consultant and client which spells out responsibilities, functions, objectives, and terms of the relationship including financial arrangements and charges.

GUIDES

1. The cancer registrar shall always support and uphold the professional standards that would produce complete, accurate, and timely information to meet the health and related needs of the patient.

2. The cancer registrar shall not participate in any improper preparation, alteration, or suppression of medical/health records or official minutes duly maintained as part of the operation of the health institution.[3]

C. Preserve the confidential nature of professional determinations made by official committees of health and health-service organizations.

GUIDE

The cancer registrar shall abstain from discussing observations, comments, or findings concerning the practice of individuals that result from committee activities (such as medical audit findings, individual patient care, professional standards review recommendations or information obtained from any other source) with anyone except the appropriate institutional authority.

D. Disclose to no one but proper authorities any evidence of conduct or practice observed or revealed in medical reports that suggests possible violation of established rules and regulations of the employer or professional practice.

GUIDE

The cancer registrar shall exercise discretion when releasing or discussing sensitive information acquired during employment or fulfillment of contracted services which concerns the administrative conduct or professional practices within the health institution. Examples:

a. Disclose only to proper authorities the conduct or practices believed to be violating the institution's internal policies and rules.

b. Disclose to proper regulatory or law enforcement agencies the conduct or practices believed to be illegal only when, after informing the health institution, no corrective action has been enacted.

III. COMPENSATION

A. Place service before material gain and strive always to provide services as needed to achieve quality healthcare and treatment for all who are ill with cancer or other neoplasms.

GUIDE

The cancer registrar shall place primary importance on providing a high standard of professional service; financial considerations are secondary to this objective.

B. Accept compensation only for services rendered to, or negotiated with, the health institution.

GUIDES

1. A cancer registrar shall accept neither anything of value from a third party provider of services nor products to the health institution when that third party is functioning for the health institution.

2. Unless openly engaged in placement bureau service, the cancer registrar shall refuse to accept finder and referral fees. The cancer registrar shall refuse acceptance or an offer to divide cancer registrar service fees with another party who is not a partner in or an associate of a medical consultant group.

---

[3]Institution: a public or private organization of facilities and/or staff established to ensure continuity of program; a legally established agency or corporation.

3. The cancer registrar should avoid conflict of interest by providing full disclosure to the employer or client of any interest in a provider of services or products.

IV. PROFESSIONALISM

A. Represent truthfully and accurately professional credentials, education, and experience in any official transaction or notice, including other positions and duality of interests.

GUIDES

1. Misrepresentation of one's professional qualifications, employment, and interests reflects adversely on the profession and on oneself, and lowers public esteem for the profession.

2. A statement of any other positions of duality of interest in the health or health-related fields, both remunerative or non-remunerative in nature, should be made available on request of the employer. Examples of duality of interest are outside consultation services, committee appointments, advisory positions, elected office, business enterprise interests, and the like.

3. Credentials, professional education, and experience are to be stated truthfully and accurately in any official transaction with NCRA or any other professional association, any employer or prospective employer, and any program coordinator or publisher.

4. Those documents that authenticate registration, accreditation, academic achievements, and membership status in recognized professional organizations may be displayed. Displays that imply qualifications not possessed are unethical.

B. The cancer registrar shall strive to increase the profession's body of systematic knowledge and individual competency through continued self-improvement and application of current advancements to the conduct of cancer registry practices.

GUIDES

1. The achievements and preservation of professional status are accomplished through the mastery of cancer registry activities competently applied and the continual striving for the application of new knowledge and increased skills. Examples:

    a. Acquire information by reading pertinent literature.

    b. Attend workshops, institutes, and other continuing education programs.

    c. Examine and scrutinize functions performed as a cancer registrar for purpose of self-evaluation in carrying out professional duties.

2. Advancements in the knowledge and practice of cancer registry administration emerge through participating in studies and projects related to the principles and practices underlying its activities. Examples:

    a. Promote and/or participate in advancing the development, maintenance, use, and preservation of cancer registry practices.

    b. Foresee subjects necessary in current and future training of cancer registrars.

3. The cancer registrar shall share information regarding changes in practice with fellow cancer registrars to increase professional knowledge and skills in accordance with the mission of the Association. The cancer registrar shall exercise care to distinguish the sharing of such information from the promotion of products or services of the employer or favorite commercial firm.

4. The cancer registrar should provide for professional growth and development of those under his/her supervision.

C. Participate in developing and strengthening professional manpower and appropriately represent the profession in public.

GUIDE

The future of the profession is dependent upon the affirmative and responsible activities of members to recruit and train fellow cancer registrars. Examples:

   a. Encourage and assist in the recruitment of students for professional training, while the need exists.

   b. Help the student and new cancer registrar to participate in activities and services for their continued development as cancer registrars.

   c. Use your special skills and knowledge to enhance the status and productivity of professional colleagues through participation in continuing education programs and publication of scholarly papers.

   d. Promote understanding of, respect for, and interest in the profession within one's community.

V. ASSOCIATION

A. Discharge honorably the responsibility of any Association position to which I am appointed or elected.

GUIDE

The Association has a dual responsibility: safeguarding the members of the profession and promoting the services to be rendered by the professional to the health field. These two functions should be borne in mind in any deliberation undertaken by members, committees, officers, or delegates of the Association. Examples:

   a. Discharge one's obligation to the profession with integrity, discretion, and by one's best endeavors in representing the Association.

   b. Perform conscientiously the duties of any Association office to which elected or the assignments of any committee to which appointed.

   c. Resign one's office or assignment if unforeseen circumstances prevent one from carrying out the responsibilities of an office or committee after the acceptance of the post.

   d. Preserve the confidentiality of any privileged information obtained as a member of the Executive Board or of a committee or other empaneled group, including information about qualifying examinations gained while serving the National Cancer Registrars Association, Inc.

B. Uphold the standards of the profession by reporting to the Ethics Committee of this Association any breach of this code of ethics by fellow members of the profession.

GUIDES

   1. Any evidence of illegal, unfair, or incompetent practice or unethical conduct by fellow members or persons credentialed by this Association should be reported to the Ethics Committee of the National Cancer Registrars Association, Inc.

      a. Transmit all referrals in writing, accompanied by supportive evidence of the unethical behavior or alleged violation.

      b. Do not shield an individual guilty of unfair or unethical practices.

   2. Judgments of unethical behavior and recommendations for sanctions are the responsibility of the Ethics Committee rather than of individuals.

C. Acknowledge that a finding of guilt of a violation of the Code of Ethics will render me ineligible to be nominated for or elected to an office in the association.

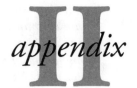

QUESTIONS
AND ANSWERS

CHAPTER 1: INTRODUCTION TO CANCER REGISTRIES

1. What is the ultimate goal of cancer registration?
   Answer: The ultimate goal of cancer registration is to prevent and control cancer, including the improvement of cancer patient care.

2. List three methods of quality control of registry data.
   Answer: Methods of quality control of the registry data include computerized edit checks, visual review, chart comparison, cross-abstracting, and editing at the state and national levels of the individual registry and the merged data.

3. What organizations have led the way in registrar education?
   Answer: The three national organizations that have led the way in the education and training of cancer registrars are the SEER program, the CoC, and the National Cancer Registrars Association (NCRA).

4. What are the major milestones of the National Cancer Registrars Association?
   Answer: The major milestones of the National Cancer Registrars Association are the development of educational standards, a formal certification program, mandatory continuing education, a code of ethics, and regional and annual national educational programs for cancer registrars.

5. List four ongoing issues in cancer registration.
   Answer: Ongoing issues in cancer registration include continually honing the base of knowledge due to medical and technological advances, the scope and shape of the data requirements, staging and coding due to changing medical technology and science, implementation of new standards, financial pressures of healthcare facilities and providers, recognition and compensation, being responsive to demands of multiple individuals and organizations, and backlogs in cancer registry abstracting and follow-up.

CHAPTER 2: THE NATIONAL CANCER REGISTRARS ASSOCIATION, INC.

1. List five of NCRA's committees.
   Answer: NCRA's committees include Annual Conference Program Committee, Awards, Continuing Education, Continuing Education Program Recognition, Communications, Education, Ethics, Finance, Formal Education, Governance Planning and Evaluation Committee, Legislative, Membership, Nominating, Public Relations, and Website.

2. Identify two different features the *Journal of Registry Management* provides the membership.
   Answer: The Journal of Registry Management provides the membership with registry management and scientific articles, and the Continuing Education Quiz.

3. What requirements must be met before a person is allowed to take the certification exam?
   Answer: Eligibility requirements that must be met to take the certification exam include a combination of experience in the cancer registry field and educational background.

4. What five goals were identified in the strategic planning process?
   Answer: The five goals identified in the strategic planning process were education, administration, certification, communication, and advocacy.

CHAPTER 3: THE NATIONAL PROGRAM OF CANCER REGISTRIES

1. What is the goal of the National Program of Cancer Registries (NPCR)?
   Answer: The goal of the NPCR is to build state and national capacities to monitor the burden of cancer including the disparity among various subgroups in the population, provide data for research, evaluate cancer control activities, and plan for future healthcare needs.

2. List three programs of NPCR.
   Answer: The program standards for NPCR are legislative authority, data content and format, completeness, timeliness, quality, annual report, and data use.

3. How is high quality data achieved for NPCR goals?
   Answer: High quality data is achieved through compliance of funded registries with established data quality standards, periodic external audits, and the evaluation of the quality of data that state

registries submit annually to the NPCR—CSS with feedback by NPCR staff members.

4. What publication is coauthored by CDC and NCI in collaboration with NAACCR?
   Answer: The publication that is coauthored by CDC and NCI in collaboration with NAACCR is the United States Cancer Statistics.

CHAPTER 4: HEALTH INFORMATION PRIVACY AND SECURITY

1. Why is there a need to protect confidential information?
   Answer: Refer to the section titled Introduction.

2. What is the Health Insurance Portability and Accountability Act (HIPAA)?
   Answer: Refer to the section titled Current Drivers of Privacy and Security Protection—HIPAA.

3. Who owns the patient medical record?
   Answer: Refer to section titled Individual Right of Control.

4. What steps must be established in order to safeguard confidential information?
   Answer: Refer to the section titled Physical Safeguards.

5. Name the four areas of access for electronic information that must be analyzed for protection of confidential information.
   Answer: Refer to the section titled Technical Security Mechanisms.

CHAPTER 5: LEGAL AND ETHICAL ASPECTS OF CANCER DATA

1. The National Cancer Act of 1971 led to the establishment of what organization? For what purpose?
   Answer: The National Cancer Act of 1971 led to the establishment of the Surveillance, Epidemiology, and End Results (SEER) Program of the National Cancer Institute. The National Cancer Act of 1971 mandated the collection, analysis, and dissemination of data for use in the prevention, diagnosis, and treatment of cancer.

2. Public Law 102-515, the Cancer Registries Amendment Act, established what program? For what purpose?
   Answer: Public Law 102-515, the Cancer Registries Amendment Act, established the National Program of Cancer Registries (NPCR). The NPCR gives authority to the Center of Disease Control and Prevention to provide funds to states and territories to enhance existing population-based cancer registries; to plan and implement registries where they do not exist; to develop model legislation and regulations for states to enhance viability of registry operations; to set standards for completeness, timeliness, and quality; and to provide training.

3. Define the term *confidential data* and explain its importance in cancer registry operations.
   Answer: Confidential is defined as "told in trust, imparted in secret; entrusted with private or secret matters." Cancer registries contain cancer data, data that are highly confidential. One of the most important responsibilities of cancer registry professionals is to safeguard the confidentiality of cancer patient information.

4. List three inappropriate releases of cancer registry data.
   Answer: Three inappropriate releases of cancer registry data include the following: businesses using cancer registry data to market a product to cancer patients, healthcare institutions trying to recruit new patients, and insurance companies or employers trying to determine the medical status of a patient.

5. List three measures used for data security.
   Answer: Three measures used for data security include the following: locks and alarms should be installed to control access to the registry; fireproof, lockable file cabinets should be considered for filing hard-copy abstracts, computer printouts, and other reports; computer back-ups should be stored off-site in a secured, structurally fit safe.

CHAPTER 6: CANCER REGISTRY PERSONNEL, OFFICE SPACE, AND EQUIPMENT

1. How can registrars project the number of cases that will be accessioned into the registry over a year?
   Answer: Refer to the section titled Establishing the Caseload.

2. How is the staffing required for abstracting registry cases calculated?
   Answer: See Table 6-1, Performing a Time-and-Motion Study for Abstracting.

3. List the factors that affect the number of staff required for follow-up.
   Answer: See Table 6-2, Factors Affecting Staffing for Follow-Up.

4. What is the most important key factor in meeting today's standards in office design?
   Answer: See Table 6-4, Factors to Consider in Planning the Registry Office.

CHAPTER 7: CANCER REGISTRY BUDGET

1. Identify and describe two budget objectives.
   Answer: Refer to Table 7-2, Budget Objectives.

2. Define fixed, variable, and semivariable cost components of budgets.
   Answer: Refer to Table 7-3, Budget Terms.

3. Contrast direct and indirect costs.
   Answer: Refer to Table 7-3, Budget Terms.

4. Describe the five steps of the budget cycle.
   Answer: Refer to Table 7-4, Five Steps of the Budget Cycle.

5. Name and describe one of the three types of budgets presented in the chapter.
   Answer: Refer to Table 7-1, Types of Budgets.

CHAPTER 8: CANCER REGISTRY MANAGEMENT

1. List the uses of registry data.
   Answer: Refer to the section titled Cancer Registry Planning.

2. Identify and describe at least six areas of responsibility that position descriptions should address.
   Answer: Refer to Table 8-1, Details to Be Included in Position Descriptions.

3. What are the benefits of delegating shared cancer registry responsibilities?
   Answer: Varying staff responsibilities allows the supervisor to achieve goals while providing staff

with the opportunity to expand their knowledge and skills.

4. List eight of the items that should be included in the policy and procedure manual.
   Answer: Refer to Table 8-2, The Cancer Registry Procedure Manual Includes, But is Not Limited To.

5. List the conditions under which a registry's reference date can be changed.
   Answer: Refer to Table 8-4, Reasons for Possible Change of Reference Date.

CHAPTER 9: THE AMERICAN COLLEGE OF SURGEONS COMMISSION ON CANCER

1. What is the goal of the Commission on Cancer?
   Answer: The goal of the Commission on Cancer is to reduce the morbidity and mortality of cancer through education, standard setting, and the monitoring of quality care.

2. How many CoC-approved cancer programs are there in the US?
   Answer: At present, there are more than 1,400 CoC-approved cancer programs in the United States and Puerto Rico.

3. *The Cancer Program Standards, 2004* focus on eight areas of evaluation. List five.
   Answer: Refer to Table 9-2, Cancer Program Standards: Eight Areas of Evaluation.

4. List a benefit of cancer program approval.
   Answer: Ensures that the structure and processes necessary for quality cancer care are in place.

5. What are the three eligibility requirements that must be met before a cancer program can be considered for survey?
   Answer: Refer to Table 9-3, Requirements for a Cancer Program to Be Considered for Approval.

6. Give an example of a new CoC cancer program standard.
   Answer: Examples of new standards include the requirement that case abstracting is performed or supervised by a Certified Tumor Registrar (CTR); as of 2005, programs are required to implement the use of a staging form in the medical record to document staging by the managing physician; cases

submitted to the NCDB for the most recent accession year requested meet the established quality criteria included in the annual Call for Data.

7. What percentage of newly diagnosed cancer patients are accessioned annually into the NCDB?

   Answer: Currently, the NCDB collects data on approximately 70% of all incident cancer diagnoses annually, and includes detailed information on over 13 million cancer patients in the US representing 60 different cancer sites.

8. Name an activity of the Disease Site Teams (DSTs).

   Answer: The Disease Site Teams (DSTs) assess the quality of cancer care by conducting research using NCDB resources, developing focused studies, collaborating with national agencies in cancer care initiatives, designing educational interventions, and evaluating quality of cancer registry data.

9. For what purpose(s) do CoC-approved cancer programs use the NCDB Hospital Comparison Benchmark Reports?

   Answer: The Hospital Comparison Benchmark Reports are used as a tool to evaluate and compare the cancer care delivered to patients diagnosed and/or treated at a facility.

10. What are the specific duties of the cancer liaison physician?

    Answer: These physicians serve as the link between the CoC and hospitals with approved cancer programs or those hospitals that are working toward approval. The liaison physician is required to: have a strong commitment to the success of the cancer program and the quality of care provided to patients with cancer, be an active member of the cancer committee, participate in cancer conferences, and have an interest in working with and volunteering for the local American Cancer Society on cancer control initiatives.

CHAPTER 10: CANCER PROGRAM SURVEY AND APPROVAL PROCESS OF THE AMERICAN COLLEGE OF SURGEONS COMMISSION ON CANCER

1. Outline the responsibilities of the key contact for survey preparation.

   Answer: Refer to Table 10-1, Responsibilities of the Key Contact.

2. Describe three uses for the SAR.

   Answer: The SAR provides a summary of demographic information, resources, and services; and description of annual cancer program activity for the facility.

3. Discuss three reasons to involve all members of the cancer program team in the on-site visit.

   Answer: Involvement of all members of the cancer program team is essential to help the surveyor understanding the program organization, strengths, and opportunities for improvement. All team members are encouraged to describe their achievements and challenges, as well as plans and goals for their area of responsibility.

4. Identify four ways that a facility can market its approved program.

   Answer: Following the survey, the CoC-approved program is provided with a press kit and free marketing materials that can be used to promote the facility cancer program. Information describing the facility's CoC-approval status can be shared with facility staff and the community by placing notices or advertisements in local newspapers, magazines, reports, or brochures, or posting information in the facility intranet or website.

CHAPTER 11: JOINT COMMISSION ON ACCREDITATION OF HEALTHCARE ORGANIZATIONS (JCAHO)

1. Describe Total Quality Management (TQM).

   Answer: The short answer is that TQM is an organizational environment in which 100% quality is pursued. Refer to the section titled Performance Improvement for further details.

2. What is the uninterrupted process of evaluating outcomes and the processes to achieve the goals of Total Quality Management?

   Answer: The uninterrupted process of evaluating outcomes and the processes to achieve the goals of TQM are included in the cycle for continuous performance improvement. The cycle is design, measurement, assessment, and improvement (or innovation). Refer to the section titled Framework for Improving Performance for further details.

3. What indicates that priorities for improvement have been communicated to the staff throughout

the organization with a framework provided for reaching goals?

Answer: The Indicator Measurement System (IMSystem) provides hospitals with internal and external benchmarking capabilities. Refer to the section titled The Indicator Measurement System (IMSystem) for further details.

4. What do critical pathways define?

Answer: Critical pathways define the optimal sequence and timing of functions performed by physicians, nurses, and other staff for a particular diagnosis. Refer to the section titled Framework for Improving Performance for further details.

CHAPTER 12: CASE ASCERTAINMENT

1. Describe the activities involved in the case ascertainment cycle.

Answer: See Table 12-1, Case Ascertainment Cycle.

2. What factors should be considered in identifying the type of case ascertainment sources to be used by the registry?

Answer: Refer to the section titled Identifying Source Documents.

3. Describe the difference between active and passive case ascertainment.

Answer: Refer to the section titled Determining Reporting Methods.

4. What is a suspense file?

Answer: Refer to the first paragraph of the section titled Linking Identified Cases.

5. What are the benefits of maintaining a history file of nonreportable cases?

Answer: The primary benefit of maintaining a history file of nonreportable cases is to prevent repeated pulling and review of the same health record. See the section titled Linking Identified Cases.

CHAPTER 13: RAPID CASE ASCERTAINMENT

1. Why is rapid case ascertainment important?

Answer: The goal of rapid case ascertainment is to support and facilitate epidemiologic and clinical research by providing the rapid identification of cases eligible for studies requiring case identification shortly after diagnosis. For malignancies associated with high morbidity or mortality, such as lung, pancreatic, or ovarian cancer, it is particularly important to identify cases immediately after diagnosis so as not to lose the ability to interview patients directly.

2. Describe how rapid case ascertainment occurs.

Answer: Rapid case identification is achieved in one of two ways: central registry personnel traveling into the field to collect cases for specific studies, or automated reporting of filtered pathology reports directly to the central registry. The path or other report is screened for mention of cancer and collected within 6 weeks of the initial date of diagnosis, or sooner. Some central registries utilize a two-phase reporting requirement wherein an initial report containing patient demographics, tumor site, and histology is sent by the reporting facility to the central registry within 6 weeks of the initial date of diagnosis.

Many central registries have rapid case ascertainment (RCA) units that are available on an adhoc basis to perform case finding for special studies. These RCA staff can collect data that may fall outside the confines of the standard central registry abstract as required by individual researchers such as specimen numbers, first language spoken by the patient or date of next clinic appointment.

New technology in the area of electronic pathology reporting has led to an increased interest and use of this method for overall central registry casefinding and rapid case ascertainment for special studies.

3. Describe the costs involved with rapid case ascertainment.

Answer: The cost of the rapid case methods varies greatly. The two-phase system is relatively inexpensive in that a small amount of data is being gathered and reported through an existing mechanism, namely hospital to central registry. The establishment and maintenance of an RCA unit bears a significant ongoing cost in that trained personnel are needed to perform accurate case review. The process of reviewing numerous pathology reports to find those meeting stringent eligibility requirements can be time consuming and labor intensive. Electronic pathology reporting systems bear a substantial up-front cost in personnel, software, and equipment.

CHAPTER 14: STANDARDS FOR DATA AND DATA MANAGEMENT

1. Define the term *standard*.
   Answer: Standards are rules set by authority.

2. List three functions of shared standards.
   Answer: Shared standards ensure clarity of communication, protect the integrity of data when they are pooled or compared across multiple sources, and focus attention on key aspects of cancer care or cancer control.

3. In one or two sentences, describe the role of each of the following organizations for cancer registry standards:
   a. American Cancer Society (ACS)
   b. American Joint Committee on Cancer (AJCC)
   c. Commission on Cancer (CoC)
   d. National Cancer Registrars Association (NCRA)
   e. National Program of Cancer Registries (NPCR)
   f. North American Association of Central Cancer Registries (NAACCR)
   g. Surveillance, Epidemiology, and End Results (SEER)
   h. World Health Organization (WHO)
   Answer: Refer to the section titled The Standard Setters.

CHAPTER 15: CODING OF NEOPLASMS

1. Name the current coding books used in the United States for (a) coding mortality and (b) coding neoplasms for cancer registries.
   Answer to (a): International Classification of Diseases, 9th revision, Clinical Modification (IDC-9-CM).
   Answer to (b): International Classification of Disease for Oncology, 3rd edition (ICD-O-3).

2. Describe at least two differences between ICD and ICD-O.
   Answer: Refer to the section titled History of Coding Neoplasms for the many differences.

3. The complete code for a neoplasm contains ten characters. What are the principal parts of the code and what do they represent?
   Answer: Refer to the section titled Basics of Coding Neoplasms.

4. What is the most important concern in coding neoplasms?
   Answer: Refer to the first three sentences of the Summary section.

5. Name three organizations that have helped to develop the topography and morphology codes used to code neoplasms.
   Answer: The American Cancer Society, the College of American Pathologists, and the World Health Organization are three organizations that have helped to develop the topography and morphology codes used to code neoplasms.

CHAPTER 16: EXTENT OF DISEASE AND CANCER STAGING

1. Define staging.
   Answer: A short definition for staging is the grouping of cases into broad categories based on extent of disease.

2. List three uses of staging information.
   Answer: Refer to the section titled Purposes of Staging.

3. Why do staging schemes change?
   Answer: Staging schemes change because of the continuing investigation of cancer—the more that is learned, the more our references may have to be adopted and changed.

4. Describe two ways that cancer cells can metastasize to other parts of the body.
   Answer: Refer to the section titled The Disease Process of Cancer.

5. How do the clinical and pathologic staging bases differ in the American Joint Committee on Cancer staging system?
   Answer: Refer to the section titled American Joint Committee on Cancer (AJCC) Staging System.

6. What is the CS System and what issues does it resolve?
   Answer: Refer to the section titled Collaborative Staging.

CHAPTER 17: CANCER TREATMENT

1. What is the purpose of a biopsy?
   Answers: Refer to the section titled Diagnostic Surgery for descriptions of the different kinds of biopsies.

2. Why is chemotherapy combined with surgery?
   Answers: Most patients receive both surgery and adjuvant treatment because approximately 70% have micrometastases when they are diagnosed. Chemotherapy is a systemic method of cancer control that is effective in destroying those micrometastases. Because surgery can remove the bulk or almost the entire cancerous tumor and chemotherapy can kill the micrometastases, this combination is highly effective in evoking a "cure."

3. Describe stereotactic radiosurgery.
   Answers: Sterotactic radiosurgery involves focusing a radiation beam on a small area and delivering very high doses of radiation. Delivering a very high dose to a focused, small area destroys the cancerous tissue and preserves more of the normal tissue in the surrounding area.

4. What is the definition of cancer treatment?
   Answers: Refer to the section titled Introduction.

5. Describe endocrine treatment and give an example.
   Answers: Refer to the section titled Hormone Therapy.

CHAPTER 18: CLINICAL TRIALS

1. Define a clinical trial. How does it differ from a clinical study and a protocol?
   Answer: Refer to the last paragraph of the section titled Introduction.

2. Define the term *institutional review board*. What is the main purpose of this group?
   Answer: Refer to the section titled The Institutional Review Board, Definition and Purpose.

3. What is informed consent? Why is it important?
   Answer: Refer to the section titled Informed Consent.

4. Describe one of the three phases of a clinical trial.
   Answer: Refer to the section titled Clinical Trial Phases.

5. Why is *The Belmont Report* considered important to researchers? List the three principles stated in this report.
   Answer: Refer to the section titled Ethics.

CHAPTER 19: GENERAL PRINCIPLES OF ABSTRACTING AND CANCER REGISTRY FILES

1. List common sections of the cancer registry abstract.
   Answer: See Table 19-1, Common Sections in a Cancer Registry Abstract.

2. What diagnostic tests can be used to find the tumor size or staging information.
   Answer: Refer to the section titled Stage of Disease at Diagnosis.

3. What determines the data set that will be collected by the cancer registry?
   Answer: Refer to the sections titled Introduction and Data Standards.

4. What is the significance of a sequence number?
   Answer: Refer to the section titled Sequence Number.

5. Where would the registrar find most of the patient identification information?
   Answer: Refer to the section titled Patient Identification.

6. How is the first course of treatment time period determined?
   Answer: Refer to the section titled First Course of Treatment.

7. List two files commonly required for cancer registries?
   Answer: Refer to the sections Patient Index and Accession Register.

CHAPTER 20: MONITORING PATIENT OUTCOME: FOLLOW-UP

1. What is the primary purpose of follow-up?
   Answer: See the first sentence of the section titled Introduction.

2. What is the required rate (percentage) for follow-up in programs approved by the Commission on Cancer of the American College of Surgeons?

   Answer: Approved programs must meet or exceed the target rate of 80% for all analytic reportable patients from the cancer registry reference date, and 90% follow-up rate is maintained for all analytic reportable patients diagnosed within the last five years, or from the cancer registry reference date, whichever is shorter.

3. After what time period are cases considered delinquent if no contact has been made?

   Answer: A case is considered delinquent if no contact has been made within 15 months after the date of last contact. Refer to the section titled Requirements of the Commission on Cancer.

4. List three types of patients that are not required to be followed in programs approved by the Commission on Cancer of the American College of Surgeons.

   Answer: See Table 20-1, Types of Reportable Cases Excluded from Calculations of CoC Follow-Up Rates for Approved Cancer Programs.

5. Explain the benefit of providing patients with cancer registry brochures.

   Answer: Refer to the section titled Cancer Registry Brochures.

CHAPTER 21: QUALITY CONTROL OF CANCER REGISTRY DATA

1. Give two examples of acceptance sampling used for cancer registry data.

   Answer: Refer to the section titled Basic Methods.

2. Describe three examples of computerized data edit checks.

   Answer: See Table 21-1, Examples of Computerized Data Edit Checks.

3. Describe three methods of monitoring completeness.

   Answer: Refer to the section titled Case Completeness.

4. Name three prerequisites for quality control of data in a cancer registry.

   Answer: Refer to the section titled Requirements.

5. Describe two methods of monitoring timely cancer reporting.

   Answer: Refer to the section titled Timelines.

CHAPTER 22: COMPUTER PRINCIPLES

1. What is a bit? What is the difference between a bit, a byte, and a word?

   Answer: A bit, which comes from binary digit, is the smallest unit of data storage, and is represented by either 0 or 1. Usually data is comprised of groups of eight bits, called a byte. A byte can signify numbers from 0 to 255. To represent numbers larger than 255, groups of bytes are assembled together. Programmers call a group of two bytes a word (16 bits).

2. A workstation and a server are both types of computers. How are they used? How are they similar to one another? Different from one another?

   Answer: A computer set up for a single user comprises a basic workstation. Frequently multiple computers are grouped together in a network. In a network often the data is maintained in a central location, usually on a microcomputer with a large reservoir of memory. This computer is called a server. Several workstations are attached to the server, which lets the workstations access those data simultaneously. The network must maintain appropriate rules of operation such as record locking. The network just described is said to have file server architecture, or client/server architecture. In the client/server configuration, the system takes a much more active role in management of the data than in the file server system.

3. What is the purpose of backups? Discuss the relative benefits and drawbacks of each type of backup media presented in this chapter.

   Answer: The purpose of backup is to provide an electronic copy of the registry files so that backup can be used to cost effectively and completely restore a registry in the event of a software, hardware, or other catastrophe. Several methods/media of backup can be considered, including floppy disks, magnetic tape, disk (hard) drive, CD-ROM, DVD, and mirroring.

   Floppy disks are a cheap and straight-forward method of backup. Many users are experienced with floppies. They suffer from limited capacity (1.44 megabytes per floppy) and therefore often require multiple diskette follow-up, which can be error-prone and labor intensive.

Magnetic Tape: Tape backup systems have evolved rapidly in terms of increased capacity and improved reliability, although they are still relatively slow. To compensate for this, most tape systems now come with software that allows the user to schedule tape backup to activate at night or at some other time when the computer system is not in use.

One disadvantage of tape systems is that the integrity of the backup can't be tested until the entire backup is restored from tape to a hard drive, requiring more regular testing. Some registries have considered the cost of the blank backup tapes a disadvantage.

Hard drive methods are probably one of the most under-utilized yet time- and cost-efficient backup options. The costs can be more than offset by the time saved by a registrar. The concept is simple. For nightly backups, a registrar simply copies the entire registry from its home hard drive to a designated directory on another. In general, backup to another hard drive has several advantages over backup to a floppy disk or tape. It is many times faster than the two other backup alternatives, and, most importantly, a registrar can test the integrity of the backup very easily. Removable, or detached hard drives (or backpacks), can be easily taken to a remote storage location, and are relatively inexpensive.

Plummeting prices have made the CD-ROM an attractive alternative. One can easily make a resilient and reliable backup of even the largest registry to a medium that is compact and can be stored indefinitely.

Another type of reliable backup for the registry is the DVD-ROM. The DVD specification supports disks with capacities from 4.7GB to 17GB and access rates of 600KBps to 1.3 MBps.

Disk duplexing and disk mirroring can supplement other backup methods, but does not replace the need for periodic backup to a separate device.

4. What are computer viruses? How can a registrar protect against them?

Answer: A virus is a computer program designed with certain special characteristics that enable it to damage or destroy the contents of a computer hard drive or floppy disk. Protection against the threat of viruses should include the following considerations: a backup program with copies held for at least two or three months; use of a virus protection software package, with regular updates; minimization of the contact the registry computer system has with outside files; verification that the IT department of the registry's hosting organization has a regular program of virus prevention; avoiding booting the registry system with a floppy diskette instead of the hard drive.

CHAPTER 23: DATABASE MANAGEMENT SYSTEMS

1. What distinguishes two-tier from three-tier client server architecture? Which do you think would be more appropriate in a cancer registry setting?
   Answer: In a two-tier arrangement, the user system interface is located in the user's desktop and the database management services are in a server that is a more powerful machine that services many clients. Processing management is split between the user system interface and the database server.

   A two-tier arrangement is a good solution when the number of users is small. When the number of users increases, performance will deteriorate. Three-tier architecture emerged to overcome these limitations. In three-tier architecture, a middle tier is added between the user system interface and the database server. This middle tier can perform a variety of functions, from queuing, application execution, or database staging.

2. What is the purpose of consolidation? How is consolidation assisted by a registry's data management system?
   Answer: Cancer registry data collection is complicated because frequently parts of the data are received from different sources at different points in time. These various parts or records must be merged together, or consolidated. Consolidation typically requires the use of special software designed to match records of information about the

same patient. Records can be matched by comparing personal identifying data items from each record in an attempt to determine whether two or more records pertain to the same person. Matches can be made deterministically or probabilistically. Matching may be conducted by comparing one record against the entire database. Typically, record consolidation is highly dependent on registry computerization, and specifically data base management consolidation techniques.

CHAPTER 24: SNOMED CLINICAL TERMS®: MODERN TERMINOLOGY FOR USE IN CANCER REGISTRIES

1. What are the two types of relationships found between SNOMED CT concepts?

   Answer: The two types of relationships are the "IS-A" relationship that connects concepts in a single hierarchy, and the "Attribute" relationship that connects concepts in different hierarchies. The IS-A relationship is also known as a "super type-subtype" relationship or a "parent-child" relationship.

2. What is a concept in SNOMED CT?

   Answer: Concepts are the most basic components in SNOMED CT. For example "Hairy cell leukemia" is a concept. In SNOMED CT, concepts are abstract entities. Concepts also can have multiple levels of "granularity"(specificity) and are organized into hierarchies. Each concept has a unique numerical "Concept Identifier." The concept identifiers are meaningless numbers and imply no hierarchical information. This is intentional so that a concept may be organized into more than one hierarchy. For example, the morphology concept Hairy cell leukemia has the concept identifier 54087003.

3. Why are the morphologic terms such as malignant neoplasms contained in the Body Structure hierarchy and not the Clinical Finding hierarchy?

   Answer: It's a matter of definition. The Body Structure hierarchy is defined as including concepts of normal and abnormal anatomical structures used to specify the locations of diseases and procedures. Morphologic abnormality is included under Body Structure hierarchy and not the Disease hierarchy because structural changes on a cellular level in disease and abnormal development are being described in relation to its body structure. Since pathology reports are based on histologic characteristics and changes on the cellular level, the Neoplasm concepts, which are morphologic, are included in this hierarchy. Key concepts in the pathology report of a cancer patient are derived from this hierarchy. The topography codes ("C" codes of ICD-O 3) are found in this hierarchy. Body structure also includes abnormal body structures such as Morphologic abnormality concepts (the so-called "M" codes).

4. What will the agreement between the CAP and the NLM mean for cancer registries in terms of SNOMED CT use?

   Answer: This agreement (license) will allow cancer registries to obtain the core content of SNOMED CT without charge.

CHAPTER 25: STATISTICS AND EPIDEMIOLOGY

1. What type of data is stage-at-diagnosis?
   A. nominal
   B. ordinal
   C. interval/ratio
   D. continuous
   Answer: B. ordinal

2. Which of these estimates of risk is characteristic of the case-control study design?
   A. chi-square
   B. relative risk
   C. SMR
   D. odds ratio
   Answer: D. odds ratio

3. The enormous technological advance in population-based surveillance due to the emergence of GIS represents what sort of implications for cancer registry data reporting?
   A. studies over time
   B. mapping of cases to study "place" effects
   C. studies of treatment outcomes with gastric studies
   D. international studies of cancer among migrants
   Answer: B. mapping of cases to study "place" effects

4. Registrars may encounter which form of a cohort study in a hospital-based setting?
   A. screening for breast cancer
   B. a case-control study for a rare cancer
   C. a historical cohort for occupational exposure
   D. a clinical trial for a new medication
   Answer: D. a clinical trial for a new medication

5. Incidence differs from prevalence because it
   A. includes new and active cases, at a point in time.
   B. includes living and deceased cases of disease at a point in time.
   C. is based on morbidity only, not fatal cases over a period of time.
   D. includes only new cases of disease, over a period of time.
   Answer: D. includes only new cases of disease, over a period of time.

6. The epidemiologist's triad of causation is represented by these three components:
   A. agent, host, environment
   B. person, place, and time
   C. observe, hypothesize, test
   D. primary, secondary, tertiary prevention
   Answer: A. agent, host, environment

7. If you are told to produce a frequency polygon showing the decline in annual mortality from cancer over the last ten years, how will you recognize the correct figure made by your computer program?
   A. It will be a line chart.
   B. It will have bars extending from the left axis.
   C. It will have bars extending from the abscissa.
   D. It will have incidence rates on the x-axis.
   Answer: A. It will be a line chart.

8. Using tests in parallel to increase the effectiveness of screening for disease means
   A. using one test, then another, and a person must fail all of them.
   B. using more than one test, and a person must fail the majority.
   C. increasing the prevalence by selecting a high-risk population.
   D. using one test, then testing those who are "positive" with a second test.
   Answer: D. using one test, then testing those who are "positive" with a second test.

9. This study design features randomization, and all of the subjects have disease.
   A. clinical trial
   B. community trial
   C. case-control study
   D. historical cohort study
   Answer: A. clinical trial

10. Some times the change in the coding scheme for disease (e.g., with death certificates or hospital records) leads to a systematic error in assigning people to disease categories. This is:
    A. a form of misclassification bias.
    B. a form of selection bias.
    C. differential for exposed versus non-exposed persons.
    D. damn stupid, and plain, bad luck for the investigator.
    Answer: A. a form of misclassification bias.

11. Presuming that you wish to compare the rate of lung cancer to annual cigarette sales, by county, in your state, which statistical test would you perform for a simple measure of the agreement between these two values, while also limiting the impact of the extreme values that might be found for rates in some of the smaller population counties?
    A. Pearson's Correlation Coefficient
    B. Spearman's Correlation Coefficient
    C. linear regression
    D. logistic regression
    Answer: B. Spearman's Correlation Coefficient

12. *In situ* fraction of cancer is considered a "national chronic disease indicator" for progress with cancer control. If you wanted to compare the proportion of breast cancer cases diagnosed at the *in situ* stage for your county to that of the state, to assess the need for (or benefit from) local screening activity, what statistical test would you apply with the observed and expected cases?
    A. the t-test
    B. Wilcoxson sign-rank test
    C. 1.96 standard deviations
    D. chi-squared test, one degree of freedom
    Answer: D. chi-squared test, one degree of freedom

13. In developing a research protocol, which of the following is NOT a critical consideration?
    A. Internal Review Board [IRB] review of the study protocol
    B. protection of privacy for case data
    C. additional time it will take for completing paperwork for the study
    D. description of the consideration for informed consent or its waiver
    Answer: C. additional time it will take for completing paperwork for the study.

14. In testing two survival rates for their difference, it is common to compare median survival, e.g., the curves of cumulative survival reach 50%. Which is the appropriate test for assessing the statistical significance of these two values when making such a comparison?
    A. Z—test
    B. t—test
    C. chi-squared
    D. correlation coefficient
    Answer: B. t-test

15. If you were asked to find the "expected" cancer cases for a particular county, you might call an epidemiologist or statistician for assistance. To request the appropriate calculation, what sort of "standardization" would you request?
    A. age-standardization
    B. directly standardized rates
    C. joinpoint analysis
    D. indirect standardization
    Answer: D. indirect standardization

16. Many states present their cancer in percentiles, e.g., quartiles, or quarters of the county-specific rates. National statistics often use deciles (10%) fractions for their county-level mortality maps. For a state with 100 counties, what would a cancer incidence map with shading by quintiles mean?
    A. Ten percent of the counties would be shown as "High."
    B. Twenty percent of counties would be shaded as "Very Low."
    C. Five of the counties would be shown as "High."
    D. You cannot tell without the state rate and standard deviation.
    Answer: B. Twenty percent of counties would be shaded as "Very Low."

17. As cancer mortality rates are dropping in the United States, which is the best explanation of this pattern?
    A. Deaths occurring later in life reduce the age-adjusted rates.
    B. Deaths occurring earlier in life reduce the age-adjusted rates.
    C. More minority populations reduce the cumulative rates.
    D. Incidence rates are rising so there is a greater prevalence of cancer.
    Answer: A. Deaths occurring later in life reduce the age-adjusted rates.

18. Assume the national cancer incidence rate for lung cancer is 65.5/100,000 (standard error = 2.34); the state rate is 97.6/100,000 (standard error = 3.74) and your county rate was 102.4/100,000 (standard error = 5.42). You want to do a **one-tailed** test at the $p < 0.05$ level of significance, of the evidence for your county being statistically significantly higher than these other two referent groups. How many standard error units would you use for your comparison?
    A. 1.96 cumulative area remaining under the curve = 0.025
    B. 0.05 cumulative area remaining under the curve = 0.495
    C. 1.282 cumulative area remaining under the curve = 0.10
    D. 1.645 cumulative area remaining under the curve = 0.05
    Answer: D. 1.645 cumulative area remaining under the curve = 0.05

CHAPTER 26: REPORT GENERATION

1. What is the first step in selecting the data to be included in a report?
   Answer: See Table 26-1, Overview of Report-Writing Steps.

2. Name three sources of information about cancer that a registrar should review as examples of report generation.
   Answer: To remain constantly aware of data issues, registrars should become familiar with studies of cancer data across the nation. These are published by state or regional central registries, the National Cancer Institute's SEER Program, the CoC's National Cancer Data Base, the American Cancer

Society, the North American Association of Central Cancer Registries, and other scientific sources.

3. What are four influences of hospital-specific case mix on data analysis?

   Answer: Refer to the section titled Data Analysis and Interpretation.

4. Titles of tables and charts should answer what four questions?

   Answer: Titles should tell who is represented by the data, what items are being shown, where the data were generated, and what time period the data cover.

5. Give three features of a comparative database that may affect whether it may be suitable for your benchmarking purposes.

   Answer: Age, geographic setting, socioeconomic status, culture, etc.

6. What is the most important key to effective technical writing?

   Answer: The guiding principle of report writing can be summarized by what is known as the KISS Principle - Keep It Short and Simple. For further details refer to the section titled Written Communication Skills.

CHAPTER 27: DATA UTILIZATION

1. What data elements should be used in a report to an administrator who is doing research on the possibility of starting a community mobile mammography unit?

   Answer: See Table 27-1, Summary of Oncology Data and Uses. Starting a community mobile mammography unit includes facility usage, community programs, and cancer control, so those three columns in Table 27-1 would be applicable.

2. What type of report should be given to the medical staff if they are anticipating the recruitment of a pediatric oncologist?

   Answer: A physician referrals and usage report would be useful. Also, Table 27-1 can be useful in determining the oncology data that should be addressed in such a report (especially the columns Facility Usage, Referral Patterns, and Clinical Care) for the recruitment of a pediatric oncologist.

3. What data items are needed to link registry data with the financial department?

   Answer: Refer to the section titled Financial Analysis.

4. What data items are needed by an outside researcher who is writing an article on breast cancer in the community?

   Answer: See Table 27-1, Summary of Oncology Data and Uses.

5. What approvals process is necessary to give the researcher the requested data?

   Answer: Refer to the section titled Release of Data.

CHAPTER 28: CANCER PROGRAM ANNUAL REPORTS

1. Name four factors that can affect the budget of an annual report.

   Answer: See Table 18-3; Factors Affecting an Annual Report Budget.

2. In programs approved by the Commission on Cancer, who is responsible for analyzing outcomes that may be included in the annual report?

   Answer: A physician member of the cancer committee provides an overall narrative analysis or critique of the major-site data.

3. Name two databases that can be used to compare registry data in a cancer program annual report.

   Answer: The inclusion of comparison data using the National Cancer Data Base (NCDB) benchmark reports or other national, state, or regional data enhances the facility information.

4. What department or person is usually appointed as the coordinator of the cancer program annual report?

   Answer: The cancer committee often delegates the preparation of the text to an annual report team or subcommittee. The cancer registry staff and one or more physician members of the committee are often appointed to this team or subcommittee. Other members representing departments or areas providing care to the cancer patients as well as a representative from public relations or marketing may be selected.

CHAPTER 29: DEPARTMENT OF DEFENSE AND OTHER FEDERAL REGISTRIES

1. Name three departments of the federal government that have registries.

   Answer: Three departments of the federal government that have registries are all branches of the military establishment, the Department of Veterans Affairs, the National Institutes of Health, and the Indian Health Service.

2. Name the three military service branches.

   Answer: The three military service branches are the US Army, US Air Force, and the US Navy.

3. Name a military-specific data set.

   Answer: Military-specific data sets include branch of service, sponsor SSN, active duty status, exposure to Agent Orange, and participation in Desert Storm.

4. Name five different types of registries.

   Answer: Types of registries include HIV and AIDS, diabetes, spinal cord injuries, prostheses, pacemakers, Agent Orange exposure, radiation exposure, Persian Gulf Syndrome, bone marrow transplantation, organ donor recipients, mammography, cervical screening, benign colon polyps, burn patients, and laryngectomies.

5. What is the acronym for the military tumor registry software program?

   Answer: The acronym for the military tumor registry is ACTUR.

6. What is the main difference between federal registries and their private counterparts?

   Answer: The major difference between federal registries and their private counterparts is in the way the programs are established.

CHAPTER 30: PEDIATRIC CANCERS

1. Identify and describe two factors thought to cause childhood cancers.

   Answer: Genetic and familial factors, viral agents, and ethnic factors are thought to cause various childhood cancers. Refer to the section titled Epidemiology for further details.

2. Adult cancers are mainly of endothelial and epithelial surfaces, adenocarcinoma, and squamous cell carcinoma. What are the common types of childhood cancer?

   Answer: Children more commonly have tumors of mesenchymal, neural, and germ cell origin, such as sarcomas, leukemias, and teratomas. Refer to the section titled Epidemiology for further details.

3. Name the national clinical trial group presently studying childhood cancers in the United States and Canada.

   Answer: The Children's Cancer Group and the Pediatric Oncology Group are two national clinical trial groups that study childhood cancers. Refer to the section titled Pediatric Clinical Trial Groups for further details.

4. When analyzing childhood cancers, what is the major difference between adult and childhood cancers?

   Answer: Refer to the first paragraph of the section titled Analysis of Childhood Cancers.

5. Identify and describe one factor associated with second malignant neoplasms in survivors of childhood cancers.

   Answer: Refer to the section titled Second Malignant Neoplasms.

CHAPTER 31: THE NATIONAL CANCER DATA BASE

1. Name the two groups or bodies that provide the advisory structure for the NCDB and list their respective charges.

   Answer: The Quality Integration Committee (QIC) is the central advisory panel that guides and assists in the prioritization of the work conducted by the National Cancer Data Base staff. The Committee is concerned with, and represents the CoC in matters addressing the progress and direction of research and continuing education as it pertains to improving the care of cancer patients.

   Thirteen Disease Site Teams (DSTs) meet the national demand for ongoing assessment of the quality of cancer care. The purpose of the DSTs is to: 1) conduct research using NCDB resources; 2) develop focused studies; 3) develop educational interventions including program content and rec-ommending speakers; 4) evaluate quality of cancer registry data; and 5) collaborate with other national leaders and agencies in cancer care.

2. What tools does the NCDB employ to evaluate data quality in submitted records?

    Answer: The NCDB EDITS metafile utilizes standardized and nationally accepted data edits and can be accessed using GenEdits, free software available from the Centers for Disease Control. Instructions for using the NCDB metafiles and EDITS software are available on the NCDB web page, the GenEdits software are available from the CDC and NAACCR websites. When data files are received, each case submitted undergoes three par-allel editing processes. Each of these steps employs the same NCDB metafile made available to reg-istries to pre-edit their data transmission file.

3. What is the formal mechanism instituted between the cancer programs and the ACoS to assure compliance with the privacy regulations?

    Answer: The NCDB is committed to ensuring the strictest adherence to the CoC's policies on data confidentiality and has implemented all the appropriate policies, procedures, and information systems to comply with the rules and regulations concerning privacy of patient data under HIPAA and is in compliance with the final regulations released in August 2002. The CoC has entered into a "business associate" (BA) agreement with each approved cancer program and as such func-tions as an organization that performs activities such as quality assurance and improvement or accreditation functions for a covered entity ('160.103).

4. Describe a limited data set.

    Answer: As defined by the HIPAA privacy regula-tions, a limited data set is defined as one which does not include any of the 14 following data ele-ments: name; street address; phone/fax numbers; email addresses; social security number; certificate or license numbers; vehicle identification num-bers; URLs or IP addresses; full face photographs; medical record numbers; health beneficiary num-bers; other account numbers; devise identifiers or serial numbers; and biometric identifiers.

5. The NCDB annual Call for Data requests mul-tiple years of data. Describe what kind of data is

represented in data submitted from "older" years.

Answer: Case records from "older" years are used to update those previously reported and included 5-year, 10-year, and 15-year follow-up information.

6. Name two different methods of survival analysis.

    Answer: Outcomes, or survival analysis, are per-formed by computing observed or relative survival rates, depending upon the focus of the analytic task. Observed survival rates are computed using the actuarial method, compounding survival in one-month intervals from the date of diagnosis, with death from any cause as the recognized end-point.

    Relative survival rates are the ratio of the observed survival rate to the expected survival rate of per-sons of the same sex, age, and racial or ethnic background. Expected survival rates are computed in single-year increments using the most recent life-expectancy tables published by the National Center for Health Statistics. Using this methodol-ogy, the relative survival rates become risk-adjust-ed for the demographic variability in patient populations, and can be calculated in the absence of specific and reliable cause of death information for each patient.

7. Describe two features of the NCDB Hospital Comparison Reports.

    Answer: The Hospital Comparison Benchmark Reports include 1) data on each of the NCDB analytic disease sites; 2) greater user control over the type of cases selected; 3) access to an extensive list of co-variates (including patient insurance sta-tus, an aggregate measure of median family income, tumor behavior, and detailed information on the type of radiation and/or systemic therapy administered as part of the first course of therapy); 4) three report options: show data reported to the NCDB from their own cancer registry, show aggre-gated data, display a comparative report that con-tains data reported from the user's hospital registry along side with aggregated data.

8. For what purposes can a cancer program use benchmarking applications?

    Answer: Benchmarking applications allow hospi-tals to view local, state, regional, or national norms for treatment patterns and outcomes. These reports should enable physicians and registrars at cancer treatment facilities to identify patterns of care in their own institution that differ significantly from patterns in similar institutions or differ from state, regional, or national norms. Such information can be useful for identifying issues for quality improvement studies, a requirement of the CoC Cancer Program Standards 2004 (Standard 8.1). The information may also be useful for planning and marketing purposes.

CHAPTER 32: NORTH AMERICAN ASSOCIATION OF CENTRAL CANCER REGISTRIES, INC.

1. What four membership categories are available for NAACCR?
   Answer: The four membership categories available for NAACCR membership are full, sponsor, sustaining, and individual.

2. Name the members of the Board of Directors that governs NAACCR.
   Answer: The Board includes the President, President-elect, Treasurer, six Representatives-at-Large, one Sponsoring Member Organization representative, and the Executive Director.

3. Name two major groups of activities of NAACCR.
   Answer: The major groups of activities are establishing and maintaining a consensus of standards for data definitions, variable codes, data exchange formats, measures to assess data quality and data presentation; training and educating registry staff; certifying registries that meet national data quality standards for producing accurate cancer statistics; evaluating and publishing data from member registries; and promoting the use of registry data.

CHAPTER 33: THE SURVEILLANCE, EPIDEMIOLOGY, AND END RESULTS PROGRAM

1. What does the acronym SEER stand for?
   Answer: Surveillance, Epidemiology, and End Results (SEER) Program of the National Cancer Institute.

2. On what date did the SEER Program begin case ascertainment?
   Answer: SEER Case ascertainment began on January 1, 1973.

3. What is the SEER follow-up rate for cases in which the patient was less than 20 years of age at the time of diagnosis?
   Answer: The standard for those younger than 65 is 85%. Meeting the standard for the group of patients who were less than 20 years of age at diagnosis has proven to be difficult as this is a more mobile group.

4. Which SEER publications would serve as useful resources for cancer registrars?
   Answer: A variety of SEER educational and training materials, morphologic and extent of disease (stage) references, and operational data standards publications would be useful. These are listed in detail on the SEER website.

5. What is the death certificate only (DCO) rate, after followback, allowable for SEER registries?
   Answer: The SEER DCO standard is 1.5%.

CHAPTER 34: CENTRAL CANCER REGISTRIES

True or False?

1. Central (population-based) registries report all cases diagnosed in a specified population at risk, and they are the source for calculation of incidence rates.
   Answer: True

2. One of the affiliations that central registries have found most useful is with private insurance companies so that patient names can be disseminated.
   Answer: False

3. Because cancer cases are reported to central registries from many hospitals, casefinding is not that important, because each case will almost certainly be reported by someone.
   Answer: False

4. Many central registries are not computerized because such automation has proven too time-consuming, expensive, and difficult.
   Answer: False

5. What is the difference between an observed survival rate and a relative survival rate?
   Answer: The relative survival rate is the ratio of the observed survival rate in the study population to the expected survival rate in the subset of the

general population with the same characteristics as the study population. Thus, the relative survival rate is the observed survival rate, adjusted because some of the subjects can be expected to die from causes of death other than that under study. Age-sex-race/ethnic specific tables life probability are generally used to calculate this adjustment.

CHAPTER 35: CANCER REGISTRIES IN OTHER COUNTRIES

1. What is the role of the IARC/IACR in population-based cancer registration?
    Answer: The IARC/IACR is the international association of central (population-based) cancer registries. A major thrust for IARC/IACR is to perform cancer surveillance in developing countries.

2. What is the CANREG system?
    Answer: CANREG is a computer System for central registries distributed by the IACR/IARC.

3. What broad-based publication of cancer incidence is published every few years?
    Answer: Cancer Incidence in Five Continents now in its eighth edition.

CHAPTER 36: OTHER HEALTH REGISTRIES

1. Identify and describe three types of registries.
    Answer: Refer to Table 36-3.

2. List five data elements that could be included in a registry.
    Answer: Refer to Table 36-2.

3. List three possible benefits of cancer registry.
    Answer: Benefits of registries are the collection of information on individuals with a particular dis-ease process or condition, risk factor, genetic disorder, or prior exposure to substances; monitoring therapies and outcomes; and ongoing clinical research.

4. Describe why data standards are important for all registries.
    Answer: Data standards are important for all registries because by maintaining high standards, registries can produce valuable data to assist researchers in public health and medicine.

5. List three sources of funding for registries.
    Answer: Funding sources include the federal government, state governments, universities, groups or individual hospitals, nonprofit organizations, and private groups.

CHAPTER 37: NETWORKING WITH ORGANIZATIONS

1. What term describes the exchange of information between individuals or groups?
    Answer: Networking is defined as the exchange of information between individuals or groups.

2. How do registrars find out what resources are available to meet their needs?
    Answer: Other local registrars can provide guidance through their own knowledge and experience, and affiliation with professional organizations provide opportunities for growth and education.

3. How can registrars serve as resources to others?
    Answer: Registrars serve as resources for one another by exchanging information with each other.

4. What institute is a major component of the NIH?
    Answer: One major component of the NIH is the National Cancer Institute (NCI).

GLOSSARY OF REGISTRY TERMS

The following terms appear in one or more chapters of this textbook. In many cases, the term is well defined in the text and can be located through the index. In other cases, a definition has been obtained from another source. Most terms are listed under the noun form; a few are listed under the first word in the phrase or a descriptive term. Phrases that include the same term are usually grouped together. Primary terms and cross-references to other terms are shown in ***bold italics.*** A term used a second time in the same definition is abbreviated. *Italics* are used for equivalent terms or subcategories of a term which are not listed independently. The names of publications are shown in SMALL CAPS.

abscissa   see *axis.*

abstract   a summary, abridgment, or abbreviated record that identifies pertinent cancer information about the patient, the disease, the cancer-directed treatment, and the disease process from the time of diagnosis until the patient's death. The *a.* is the basis for all of the registry's functions.

abstracting   the process of collecting and recording pertinent cancer data from a health record. *Concurrent a.* starts when the patient is in the hospital and is usually completed by the time the first course of therapy has begun and the health record is sent for filing.

abstractor   an individual who collects and codes cancer registry data.

acceptance sampling   the inspection and subsequent approval (acceptance) or rejection of a product; for example, computerized *edit checks* for registry data.

accession   to enter a case into a registry and assign it a number. The *a. number* is a unique number assigned to the patient by the registrar, indicating the year in which the patient was first seen at the reporting institution and the sequential order in which the patient was identified by the registry or abstracted into the database. The *a. n.* is used for all additional primaries the patient may develop, regardless of the year in which subsequent reportable tumors occur. The *a. register* is an annual, sequential listing of all reportable cancers and reportable-by-agreement cases included in the registry.

accrue   to enter into a research study.

accuracy   correctness; in registry terms, a true representation on the *abstract* of the facts in the *source document.* See also *consistency, reliability, validity, reproducibility,* and *concordance.*

Acquired Immunodeficiency Syndrome (AIDS)   a usually fatal, viral (human immunodeficiency virus—HIV) disease spread by sexual contact or contact with blood from an infected person, which gradually destroys a person's immune system.

active reporting   see *case finding.*

actuarial method   see *survival calculation.*

adjuvant therapy   a treatment modality given in conjunction with another treatment modality, such as chemotherapy given following surgery or radiation for localized disease, with the intent to destroy *micrometastases.*

administration   the part of a health care facility which deals with day-to-day operations of the facility rather than direct patient care. *A.* usually includes the chief executive officer of the facility, medical staff office, accounting, housekeeping, human resources, and other departments.

Agenda for Change   a program of the *Joint Commission on Accreditation of Healthcare Organizations* which emphasizes *continuous quality improvement* of all facets of health care services. The *A. f. C.* shifted the focus from examining an institution's capabilities to deliver quality care to monitoring their performance in health care delivery and evaluating the actual improvements achieved in their results. *See Chapter 11.*

aggregate data   information about a group of patients, combined without personal identifiers; the opposite of *confidential data. A. d.* is considered nonconfidential because it does not name specific people or facilities.

AJCC staging   see *TNM staging* and *American Joint Committee on Cancer.*

alkylating agent   a chemotherapeutic drug that causes cross-linking of DNA strands, abnormal base pairing, or DNA strand breaks, thus interfering with DNA replication.

allele   one of two or more alternative forms of a gene in the same position on a chromosome.

allocation of resources   decisions made regarding how equipment, personnel, and other components of an operation or service (in other words, resources) are to be used; management of resource consumption.

allowable code check   a type of *edit check* in which the computer reviews a single data element to see that it contains a correct code. For example, allowable codes for the data item "sex" might be 1, 2, and 9; the case would not pass the edit check if this field contained an "F." See also *range check.*

alpha error   see *hypothesis.*

alphafetoprotein (AFP)   a protein made by fetal liver cells (hepatocytes) that serves as a biological marker for hepatoblastoma.

ambiguous terminology a list of commonly used descriptive terms which may or may not indicate tumor involvement; for example, a "probable" metastasis is to be interpreted as tumor involvement, but a "possible" metastasis is not.

ambulatory walking or moving; in other words, not confined to a hospital bed; sometimes referred to as **outpatient.**

American Association of Central Cancer Registries (AACCR) see **North American Association of Central Cancer Registries (NAACCR).**

American Association of Cancer Institutes (AACI) an organization composed of member representatives from U.S. academic cancer treatment institutions; one of the sponsoring organizations of NAACCR.

American Cancer Society (ACS) a national organization founded in 1913, devoted to fundraising for cancer research and disseminating information about cancer treatment to the public; formerly the American Society for the Control of Cancer.

American College of Radiology a professional organization of medical specialists in radiology (diagnostic imaging); among its responsibilities is setting standards for mammography facilities in the United States.

American College of Surgeons (ACoS) a professional organization of surgeons and physicians founded in 1913. In addition to surgical issues, the ACoS has supported cancer and trauma registries and standards for hospitals. *See Chapter 9.*

American Joint Committee on Cancer (AJCC) the parent organization guiding the development of the **TNM staging** system in the United States; formerly the American Joint Committee for Cancer Staging and End Results Reporting.

analytic a category of **class of case** which indicates that the cancer was initially diagnosed and/or treated at a specific health care facility and is eligible for inclusion in that registry's statistical reports of treatment efficacy and survival; the opposite of **nonanalytic.**

ancillary drugs agents that enhance the effects of cancer-directed treatment but which do not directly affect the cancer; for example; colony-stimulating factors improve the speed of repopulating the bone marrow after a cycle of chemotherapy.

Ann Arbor staging a specialized staging system for malignant **lymphoma** (Hodgkin disease and non-Hodgkin lymphoma).

annual report a publication produced on a yearly basis that describes the activities of an organization. A cancer program's **a. r.** also includes statistics on the types of cancers diagnosed and treated at a health care facility.

ANNUAL REVIEW OF PATIENT CARE a yearly publication of the National Cancer Data Base which describes patterns of treatment and provides a benchmark for participating institutions to compare facility data with national aggregate data.

anomaly a marked deviation from normal standard. In anatomic terms, an incorrectly formed or placed organ. A **congenital a.** is one that is present at birth, such as an improperly developed heart valve. A **horseshoe kidney** is a type of **a.** in which both kidneys are united at their lower poles.

ANOVA analysis of variance; a **statistical technique** comparing the means from multiple samples simultaneously; also called *F-test. See Chapter 25.*

antimetabolite a chemotherapeutic agent that replaces natural substances as building blocks in DNA molecules, thereby altering the function of enzymes required for cell metabolism and protein synthesis.

antitumor antibiotics chemotherapy agent **natural products** that prevent nucleic acid synthesis and block DNA translation and ribonucleic acid (RNA) transcription.

approval in registry terms, meeting specific standards for the quality of a **cancer program** and passing a survey by the Commission on Cancer of the **ACoS. Categories of a.** are based on the facility's **caseload,** staff qualifications, available services, and other factors. Categories include NCI-designated, teaching, community, comprehensive community, special, freestanding, integrated, managed care, and affiliate. *See Chapter 9.*

ascertainment see **casefinding.**

Association of Community Cancer Centers (ACCC) an organization of member cancer treatment centers, mostly in health care facilities, whose purpose is to promote quality cancer care in all aspects (including research, prevention, screening, diagnosis, and treatment) for patients with cancer and the community.

astrocytoma　a type of ***glioma*** (brain tumor) noted for its starlike extensions into the surrounding tissue.

at risk　a statistical and epidemiologic term meaning that a person has the chance or opportunity to develop a disease. A person exposed to asbestos is said to be ***a. r.*** to develop ***mesothelioma.***

AUA staging　a specialized staging system for prostate cancer developed by the American Urological Association; sometimes called *Whitmore staging.*

audit　a formalized, retrospective review of patient records to determine quality of care, case completeness, or data quality.

autopsy　the pathologic examination of a dead person; a postmortem examination of a body; also called *necropsy.* An ***a. report*** is the detailed information about organs and structures in the body. Occasionally, the only diagnosis of a cancer is noted at the time of autopsy; ***a. r.***s are used in casefinding.

autopsy staging　in the ***TNM staging*** system, a ***staging basis*** designating that the information used to assign the ***T, N,*** and ***M*** categories was obtained from the postmortem examination of the patient.

axis　the vertical or horizontal scale on a graph. The horizontal scale is the *x-axis* or *abscissa,* which is labeled for categories. The vertical scale is the *y-axis* or *ordinate,* which is labeled with the actual count or value.

backlog　the number of cases yet to be identified and/or abstracted within a specified time; for example, if a registry is expected to abstract 600 cases in six months and has only completed 400, that registry has a ***b.*** of 200 cases.

bar chart　a graphic presentation of information which displays the magnitude of one ***variable*** at various points in time or compares the magnitude of several variables. Types of ***b. c.*** include *stacked columns* or *component columns,* where the length of the column is the sum of the totals in the segments; *paired bar charts,* where the zero point is in the center of the graph and distributions of two variables can be shown at the same time.

basement membrane　a microscopic anatomic structure in most organs which forms the deep boundary of the mucosal surface. Tumor invasion or penetration through the ***b. m.*** indicates that the tumor is no longer ***in situ*** and has become invasive or ***localized.***

behavior　how a tumor acts; for example, benign, malignant (noninvasive or invasive), or metastatic.

bell-shaped curve　see ***kurtosis.***

benchmark　a term borrowed from physics, where marks were actually made on the bench surface to gauge or measure something; to compare a facility's performance or outcomes to another source. ***Internal b.***s measure the facility's results against itself, usually from a previous period of time. ***External b.***s compare the facility's outcomes to another facility's or to aggregate data (a ***reference database***) from a standard-setting organization.

benign　not malignant; not invasive; usually harmless; favorable for recovery.

beta error　see ***hypothesis.***

bias　systematic errors in the analysis of data. The principal sources of bias are *misclassification* (when subjects are assigned to the wrong groups), *selection* (when all of the subjects in a population do not have the same opportunity to be included in a study), and ***confounding.***

biological response modifier (BRM) therapy　see ***immunotherapy.***

biopsy　to remove all or part of a tumor in order to determine a microscopic diagnosis. An ***aspiration b.*** uses a needle to suction into a syringe some fluid, cells or tissue, which are then reviewed under a microscope. An ***excisional b.*** usually removes the entire, or most of, the tumor. An ***incisional b.*** removes only a portion of the tumor with the intent of diagnosis.

biostatistics　see ***statistics.***

blank space　see ***white space.***

blanket permission　in registry terms, a general approval by a facility's medical staff for the registry to contact patients directly (by letter or phone) in order to obtain current ***follow-up*** information.

blood-brain barrier　a mechanism of the vascular system of the brain which filters out or inhibits the flow-through of certain molecules, such as chemotherapy drugs.

Board of Regents the governing body of the *American College of Surgeons.*

bone marrow transplant a type of *immunotherapy* in which a patient is given *myeloablative* doses of chemotherapy in order to destroy all tumor cells, after which bone marrow is returned to the body to restore marrow and immune system function. The types of *b. m. t.* are *autologous* (the bone marrow being restored is that of the patient), *allogenic* (the bone marrow is from another person and has been matched to the patient) or *sysgeneic* (from an identical twin).

borderline a disease process which cannot be determined to be completely benign, yet which does not meet all criteria for malignancy; also described as *uncertain whether benign or malignant.* *B.* cases are not usually *accessioned* into a cancer registry.

brachytherapy a type of *radiation therapy* where the radiation source is placed in direct contact with the tumor, for example, cesium capsules inserted into the uterus for treatment of endometrial cancer.

Breslow's microstaging for malignant melanoma, a quantitative measurement in millimeters of the depth of invasion from the basal lamina of the skin to the greatest depth of tumor penetration.

budget a document listing anticipated costs and income for a particular department or organization. *See Chapter 7.* The *capital b.* is used to plan and purchase major equipment with a life expectancy of two or more years. The *expense b.* includes the allocation of expenditures for personnel, supplies, office equipment, postage, maintenance, and other planned outlays of funds. The *operating b.* includes revenues and expenses. A *program planning b.* is built around identifiable projects that must be accomplished. A *production b.* is a list of expenses anticipated when a document is published, such as size and type of paper, number of copies, binding, and so forth. The *revenue b.* forecasts income from various sources to offset anticipated expenses. A *traditional b.* is based on previous experience and uses forecasting to account for inflation and other variables. A *zero-based b.* is a resource allocation method that requires budget makers to examine every expenditure during each budget period and to justify that expenditure in light of current budget needs.

budgetary control the use of a budget to regulate and guide activities requiring and using resources for the development of new services, expanding or contracting services, increasing revenues, or decreasing operating expenses.

budgeting the process of planning future activities and expressing those plans in a formal manner in terms of cost. *See Chapter 7.*

bypass surgery an operation that creates a passage around a tumor or other lesion, usually performed to relieve symptoms in cancer patients.

calendar year a twelve month period starting January 1 and ending December 31; see also *fiscal year.*

call for data a request for submission of cancer cases to the *National Cancer Data Base* or other aggregate databases.

cancer a cellular tumor exhibiting the characteristics of *invasion* and *metastasis;* a *malignant* tumor. The term *c.* does not by itself indicate where the malignancy arose.

Cancer and Leukemia Group B (CALGB) a *clinical trial group,* formerly the Acute Leukemia Group B, which has developed *protocols* for both adult and childhood cancers. The pediatric section separated from CALGB in 1980 to form the *Pediatric Oncology Group.*

cancer cluster the observation that an unusual number of a specific type of cancer case appears during a certain time period or in residents of a small, well-defined area, such as a street, school district, or in the path of exhaust from a polluting smokestack. These clusters are usually the subject of epidemiologic investigation by a state cancer registry.

cancer committee an organized group of health care professionals (physicians and nonphysicians) which directs the long-range planning and general activities of the cancer services in a health care facility.

cancer conference a meeting of medical professionals to discuss the diagnosis and treatment of patients; sometimes called *tumor board.*

cancer control actions taken to reduce the frequency and impact of cancer; any effort to provide information and procedures to help reduce the financial and medical burden of cancer in a population. C. *c. programs* are specific efforts to reduce the amount or severity of a particular type of cancer; for example, screening activities for prostate, colon, or breast cancer. C. *c. type registries* are operated primarily to support the targeting and evaluation of control programs.

cancer identification   the section of an *abstract* containing data items that describe the disease, such as the primary site, histology, date of initial diagnosis, diagnostic confirmation, stage at diagnosis, and so forth.

CANCER INCIDENCE IN FIVE CONTINENTS   published every five years by the International Agency for Research on Cancer, this book reports cancer incidence and mortality figures of member cancer registries of the International Association of Cancer Registries.

CANCER INCIDENCE IN NORTH AMERICA   an annual publication of the North American Association of Central Cancer Registries which reports age-specific and age-adjusted incidence rates and data quality indicators for registries which meet its standards for completeness and timeliness and submit aggregate data to NAACCR.

Cancer Liaison Physician Program   a grassroots network of physicians designated by the CoC to assist health care facilities in developing their cancer programs.

Cancer Management Course   a physician-oriented program of the *CoC* which presents extensive site-specific information on state-of-the-art cancer diagnosis and treatment.

cancer mortality atlas   a map or series of maps which show mortality rates due to various types of cancers. In most cases, the maps are drawn to the level of county detail.

cancer notification form   see *confidential report of morbidity.*

cancer prevention   efforts to develop methods to stop cancer before it develops; stop-smoking programs are efforts at preventing lung cancer. See also *cancer control.*

cancer program   all of the departments and services in a health care facility involved in diagnosing, treating, and rehabilitating cancer patients. The activities of the *c. p.* are overseen by the *cancer com-

mittee. An approved c. p. is* a facility that has been surveyed and has met the standards of the Commission on Cancer; see also *approval.* The *c. p. manager* is the person responsible for maintaining *c. p. approval* by the Commission on Cancer.

CANCER PROGRAM MANUAL   the Commission on Cancer document used between 1981 and 1995 which defined the guidelines for quality cancer programs; replaced by *Standards of the Commission on Cancer, volume I: Cancer Program Standards.*

CANCER PROGRAM STANDARDS   a publication of the *COC* used between 1996 and 2003 which lists the specific guidelines for evaluating the full spectrum of cancer care in a facility in ten areas; replaced by Commission on Cancer, Cancer Program Standards, 2004.

Cancer Registries Amendment Act   Public Law 102-515, enacted in 1992, which provided funding for establishing or enhancing central cancer registry operations in all states.

cancer registry   a data collection system that assesses the occurrence and characteristics of reportable neoplasms; a data system designed for the collection, management, and analysis of data on persons with the diagnosis of a malignant or neoplastic disease (cancer). Two main types of *c. r.* are *hospital-based* and *population-based.* A *central c. r.* is a registry that collects cancer information from more than one facility and consolidates multiple reports on a single patient into one record. A *multihospital c. r.* is a *c. c. r.* consisting of cases from a group of hospitals and is generally not *population-based.* A *national c. r.* is a central registry that collects information on all residents within a nation and can produce incidence and mortality rates based on a known population. A *regional c. r.* is a central registry that collects information on all residents within a defined geographic area, such as a city, county or counties, a valley, or multiple states. A *special purpose c. r.* is one that collects data on only one type or aspect of cancer, such as ovarian tumors, pediatric malignancies, or leukemia. A *state c. r.* is a central registry that collects information on all residents of a state, regardless of whether they were treated within the state or not. *For a list of countries that maintain central cancer registries, see Chapter 35.*

cancer surveillance   the process of monitoring the *incidence* and *mortality* of cancer.

cancer-directed treatment procedures that destroy, modify, control, or remove primary, regional, or metastatic cancer tissue.

CancerLit a database of cancer literature available from the National Library of Medicine.

carcinogen something that has been shown to cause, or linked with the development of, cancer. *C.*s include the tar in cigarettes, asbestos, and ionizing radiation.

carcinogenesis the start of a cancer; a two-step process (*initiation* and *promotion*) in which a neoplasm becomes a cancer.

carcinoma a *malignant* tumor of *epithelial* origin, in contrast to malignancy of supporting structures (*sarcoma*) or *hematopoietic* structures (*lymphoma* and *leukemia*).

carcinomatosis invasion of many organs of the body at the same time by *metastases*.

case an occurrence of a primary cancer. A patient with two *primary* cancers represents two *c.*s. *C. consolidation* combines data from multiple sources pertaining to the same person or case into a single record containing the most complete information from all sources; also called *record linkage;* commonly a function of a central registry. **C. definition** is the process of establishing the criteria for inclusion and exclusion for *casefinding* reportability.

case ascertainment see *casefinding.*

case-control study a type of epidemiologic research in which cases of cancer are compared with people from the same population who do not have cancer (the control group).

case-sharing agreement a contract between agencies or facilities wherein the parties agree to provide confidential information under carefully controlled circumstances for the purposes of research or patient follow-up.

casefinding the systematic process of identifying all cases of a disease eligible to be included in the registry database for a defined population, such as patients of a hospital or residents of a state. Also called *case ascertainment.* **Active c.** is performed by registry personnel who screen the *source documents* themselves. A *c.* **completeness log** is a list by year and month in which the number of cases identified each month can be compared. *Combination c.* is the use of active

review by the registrar for critical casefinding sources and passive review of other sources as provided by reliable participants in other departments. *Passive c.* is performed by other health care professionals whom the registry relies on to notify the registrar of potentially reportable cases; also called *self-reporting.* See also *rapid case ascertainment.*

caseload the number of records handled by a registry in a period of time, usually the number of new cancer cases annually entered into the registry.

catchment area see *service area.*

category see *tabular list.*

CCH Pediatric Grouping System a specialized way of categorizing childhood cancers and benign conditions by morphology and topography codes to simplify gathering or reporting cases, developed by the Columbus (OH) Children's Hospital.

censor to exclude or remove an observation from a *survival calculation* because the subject was eligible at the beginning of the interval but did not complete the interval.

Centers for Disease Control and Prevention (CDC) a federal agency of the Department of Health and Human Services. In particular, one of the centers of the CDC, the National Center for Chronic Disease Prevention and Health Promotion (NCCDPHP) is responsible for the administration and conduct of the *National Program of Cancer Registries (NPCR)* and other cancer-related programs in the United States.

central cancer registry see *cancer registry. See also Chapter 34.*

certification the process of testing a person to assure that he or she meets established standards of knowledge to perform a specific job. *C.* is often accomplished by means of a standardized test. *C. examination:* the test itself, administered twice per year by the *National Board for the Certification of Registrars.*

Certified Clinical Research Associate (CCRA) the credential awarded to data managers who pass a certification examination testing clinical trials and general oncology knowledge.

Certified Tumor Registrar (CTR) the credentials granted to a person who has passed the cancer registry *certification examination.*

charts 1. visual displays of information, such as line graphs, pie graphs, and bar graphs; see also **graphics.** 2. health care jargon for the patient medical record.

chemotherapy the use of cancer-killing drugs to treat cancer; types of **c.** include **alkylating agents, antimetabolites, antitumor antibiotics,** and **natural products.**

Children's Cancer Group (CCG) an international **clinical trial group** devoted to the treatment of children's cancer that has developed a series of staging systems for various children's malignancies. Its former name was the Children's Cancer Study Group.

Clark's level of invasion for malignant melanoma, a descriptive measurement of tumor involvement of specific layers of the skin.

Class of case a registry term describing whether a case can be included in the statistical analysis of the database and based on where the initial diagnosis and treatment of the patient occurs. The main categories of *c. of c.* are *analytic* and *nonanalytic.*

classification an organized system of names; a way of grouping concepts or cases based on specific criteria that shows relationships among the groups but does not necessarily imply **prognosis.**

classification of subjects the capability of a study to distinguish participants or cases in the study on the basis of various factors (such as exposure and endpoint). For example, if the study asks "do persons with a certain exposure experience a different pattern of disease than do persons without that exposure" or "do people with a specific disease have more of a history of a certain exposure than persons without the disease," the same four groups are described for the study.

clinical indicator a quantitative measure of an aspect of patient care that can be used as a guide to monitor and evaluate the quality and appropriateness of health care delivery.

clinical practice guidelines carefully developed standards of medical practice outlining strategies for patient management that describe a range of acceptable ways to diagnose, manage, or prevent specific diseases and conditions; sometimes referred to as *clinical guidelines.* Often *c. p. g.* are developed by hospitals or by managed care organizations to provide optimal care to their patients.

clinical protocol studies see **clinical trials.**

clinical staging in the **TNM staging** system, a **staging basis** designation that the information used to assign the **T, N,** and **M** categories was obtained before any definitive treatment for the tumor was begun.

clinical study a scientific approach used to evaluate disease prevention, diagnostic techniques, and treatments; see also **clinical trials.**

clinical trials carefully planned scientific studies used to compare one treatment to another. **In-house c. t.** are studies designed by physicians or other staff at an institution and sometimes shared with affiliate members at other institutions. A **c. t.** is a subset of a **clinical study** that evaluates investigational (nonstandard) medications, treatments, and diagnostic or preventive techniques or devices, or a combination of these elements; also called *clinical protocol.* See also **phase.** A **c. t. group** is an organization of researchers that formulates and conducts scientific studies involving specific medical conditions, diseases, or target populations to improve treatment and outcomes; also called *cooperative group.*

CoC see **Commission on Cancer.**

code a symbol or value assigned to a concept; a set of symbols arranged systematically for easy reference. The verb form **to c.** is the process of assigning a symbol or value. **C. categories** are the names or concepts represented by symbols or values, such as race codes or morphology codes; for example, the **c. c.** is "adenocarcinoma" and the code itself is 8140/3.

code of ethics a document or list of guidelines describing appropriate professional behavior.

coding the process used to transpose text into codes; the assignment of a case to a category using standardized rules.

cohort study a type of epidemiologic research in which a group of individuals who are disease-free, but who have a known risk or exposure, are followed for a period of time to see who will develop the disease under study. This is a **prospective** type of research. A **retrospective c. s.** is one in which the cohort has been previously identified and the registry is asked to link cohort members to the registry to determine who has developed the disease.

combination reporting see **casefinding.**

Commission on Cancer (CoC) a division of the **American College of Surgeons** which consists of over 100 representatives from professional organizations involved in cancer control; originally called the Cancer Campaign Committee. The standing committees of the **CoC** are Approvals, Cancer Liaison, Education, Executive, Standards, and National Cancer Data. *See Chapter 9.*

COMMISSION ON CANCER, CANCER PROGRAM STANDARDS, *2004:* a publication of the Commission on Cancer, which lists specific standards and guidelines in eight areas for **cancer program approval.**

Committee on Approvals the segment of the **Commission on Cancer** which administers the activities of the Approvals Program. *See Chapter 9.*

comorbidity the presence of another disease or diseases that affect the management of the disease currently under treatment; for example, diabetes is a **c.** which affects how quickly a patient can heal after surgery.

comparative data see **reference database.**

comparison groups persons representing the general population or background situation used in lieu of a true control group (having no exposure other than that of the study) to be compared to the study group.

completeness the comprehensiveness of the data set collected, the specification of code values (as opposed to blank and unknown code values), and the avoidance of omissions; assurance that all cases in a specific population have been included in the disease registry.

complication an adverse effect or unfavorable result of a procedure or process; for example, infection is a potential **c.** of a surgical procedure.

component columns see **bar chart.**

computer *For all computer-related terminology, please see the separate glossary at the end of Chapter 22.*

computerized axial tomography (CT) a radiographic method of examining the body by creating an image from cross-sectional computerized "slices" of tissue; also called **CAT** *scanning.* The computer calculates the degree of multiple x-ray beams that are not absorbed by all the tissue in its path and creates a computer image showing the geography and characteristics of tissue structures within solid organs.

concordance agreement between abstractors and coders given the same information and coding guidelines; see also **reproducibility.**

confidential private or secret [Webster's New World Dictionary]. C. **data** is information that identifies a specific patient, physician, or facility, and includes the patient's name, address, phone number, or social security number.

confidential morbidity report (CMR) a standardized data collection form required by many central cancer registries to notify the registry of a new case of cancer; also called *cancer notification form.*

confidentiality the concept of maintaining the privacy of personal information obtained in the process of work. A **c. agreement** is a written statement describing a facility's confidentiality policies, which is signed by an employee, contractor, or data requestor who agrees to abide by the policies and protect private information from becoming public. A **c. pledge** is a brief statement in which an employee or contractor agrees to keep patient information private.

confounder a factor that is known to be associated with the occurrence of a medical condition. For example, medical conditions vary by age, race, sex, etc. If not taken into consideration, these factors can interfere with the correct interpretation of study data.

CONNECTION, THE the official quarterly newsletter of **NCRA.**

connective tissue body structures that connect, support, and surround other tissues and organs including muscle, tendon, fat, nerves, fibrous tissue, blood vessels, and lymph vessels. **Sarcomas** arise in **c. t.**

consent form see **informed consent.**

consistency in registry terms, application of abstracting and coding rules or guidelines in the same way for every case.

consultant in registry terms, a technical-level representative of the Commission on Cancer who provides assistance with cancer program problems and registry questions.

contact in registry terms, a person or office that is likely to know the whereabouts and status of a patient for follow-up purposes.

contiguous directly adjacent; continuously adjoining; without lapse or intervening space; used in reference to *regionalized* cancers and extent of disease.

continuing education a requirement for Certified Tumor Registrars to obtain additional knowledge and upgrade their skills in order to maintain their *certification.*

continuous quality improvement (CQI) the uninterrupted process of evaluating *outcomes* and the processes to achieve the goals of *total quality management.*

control list a printout or other document that identifies all patients due for *follow-up* at a given point in time, such as a specific month and year. The *c. l.* is compared to the hospital admission and outpatient records to identify and update cases which have been seen at the facility since the *date of last contact.*

cooperative group see *clinical trial group.*

correlation the statistical analysis of the variation between two variables that is related to their dependence on one another. The value of the *c.* is the *rho statistic.* The two principal types of *c.* are *Pearson's* and *Spearman's. See Chapter 25.*

correlational study a type of epidemiologic research in which rates of cancer or mortality are analyzed against some other factor measured in the population, such as dietary fat or amount of sunlight; also called *ecologic study.*

costs the expenses incurred in running a business. *See Chapter 7.* *Direct c.* are those that originate in and are directly charged against a department's budget, such as personnel expenses. *Fixed c.* are those that tend to remain unchanged over a period of time even when the volume of activity changes, such as equipment leasing. *Indirect c.* are those that are general in nature and benefit several departments or services, such as electricity, building maintenance, and Human Resource services. *Semivariable c.* are those that increase or decrease with changes in activity but are directly proportional to changes in operative volume. *Variable c.* are those that change in response to changes in the volume of activity, such as staffing and supplies.

cover sheet the registration form or patient information portion of a health record; includes the patient's name and address, contact information, insurance information, and other data items useful for matching and following the case.

critical pathway a description of key elements in the process of care that should be accomplished in order to achieve maximum quality at minimum cost. The *c. p.* defines the optimal sequence and timing of functions performed by physicians, nurses, and other staff for a particular diagnosis.

cross-classifying a process, usually computerized, in which records are sorted in a variety of ways in order to identify any anomalies in the data; for example, comparing age with site in order to identify any cancers that would be unusual for a particular age group.

curative with the intent to remove all cancer so that it will not return.

CURRENT PROCEDURAL TERMINOLOGY (**CPT**) a coding book for operations, tests, and other health care services.

customer a *marketing* term meaning any person who makes use of a product or service. In registry terms, a *c.* is anyone who requests data from the registry.

cycle in chemotherapy terminology, the administration of one phase of a planned sequence of chemotherapy. Several *c.*s may be part of a planned *regimen.*

cytogenetic pertaining to chromosomes, the cellular constituents of heredity.

cytology the microscopic review of cells in body fluids obtained from aspirations, washings, scrapings, and smears; usually a function of the pathology department. The *c. report* is the documentation of the microscopic examination of cells in body fluids and their diagnosis.

data a fact, statement, or specific piece of information. In statistical terms, there are four types of *d.: qualitative* (classifying into related groups), which is subcategorized as *nominal* (naming, such as race or gender) and *ordinal* (ranked or placed into an order, such as stage of disease) and *quantitative* (actual values or measures), which is subcategorized as *interval* (measures or amounts based on an arbitrary starting point, such as body temperature) and *ratio* (measures or amounts based on a scale on which zero means there is none, such as tumor size or age).

DATA ACQUISITION MANUAL **(DAM)** the standardized registry data definitions and collection instructions published by the Commission on Cancer used in approved cancer programs between 1986 and 1995.

data edit report a listing of the failed or reviewable *edit checks* for a database.

data element a fact, category of information, or specific item of information; also called a *field*. See also *data set*. Sex, race, name, and primary site are examples of *d. e.*s.

data manager a specialist in collecting cancer information for *clinical trials* and maintaining the paperwork required by federal guidelines; also called *clinical research associate*.

data security measures taken to protect confidential information about patients in any form (electronic, paper, or film) from unauthorized viewing, including locked cabinets and rooms, encrypted files, and passwords.

data set a list of *data elements* that must be collected to meet the minimal needs of a group's goals, often with an additional list of elements that are recommended for the most effective operation. An *optional d.s.* is the nonrequired items that enhance registry reporting and analysis; also called *supplemental data set*. A *required d.s.* is the minimum set of information mandated by an organization.

data utilization the process of analyzing collected cancer data and converting it into information about treatment, survival, and other factors affecting cancer patients.

date of first recurrence the point (month, day, and year) a cancer reappears after a *disease-free* interval.

date of initial diagnosis the first time (month, day, and year) that a recognized medical practitioner says there is cancer (either clinically or pathologically).

date of last contact the most recent point in time (month, day, and year) that a patient's health status is known.

death certificate only (DCO) a case that has been reported to a central registry through the state's vital statistics office based on a cancer diagnosis on the death certificate. The ratio of *d. c. o.* cases to incident cases in a period can be used as a measure of casefinding completeness in the central registry. *D. c. o.* cases are those that remain after *follow-back* procedures have been completed.

death clearance the process of linking death certificates from a state's vital statistics office with registry records in order to obtain death data for previously registered cancer cases. See also *follow-back*.

debulking the surgical removal of as much tumor as possible, with or without total removal of the primary tumor, so that adjuvant therapy will be more effective; also called *cytoreductive surgery*.

dedicated intended for a specific purpose. A *d.* oncology nursing unit treats only cancer patients.

definitive treatment see *cancer-directed*.

degrees of freedom a statistical term that describes the number of individual values that are free to vary once the sum and the number of observations are specified; used for calculating *variance*.

delinquent a *follow-up* status indicating that there has been no contact with the patient for more than fifteen months since the *date of last contact*.

demography, demographics the statistical and quantitative study of characteristics of human populations. *Demographics* are those data elements that describe the patient, physical environment, and geographic location.

Department of Health and Human Services (DHHS) the part of the executive branch of the federal government that is the principal agency for protecting the health of all Americans and providing essential human services. The *National Cancer Institute*, the *Centers for Disease Control and Prevention*, and the Food and Drug Administration are all parts of DHHS.

designed studies optimizing a system by investigating the current level of quality through a formalized plan and analysis; for example, a reabstracting study to evaluate the accuracy and completeness of the original abstracting and coding.

diagnosis the identification of the nature and extent of a tumor or other condition. The *admitting d.* is a tentative or working diagnosis that distinguishes whether the cancer diagnosis was made prior to admission or whether the diagnosis was unknown at the time of admission. The *d. index* is a listing, usually computerized, of patients discharged from the hospital, organized by disease or diagnosis code (usually *ICD-9-CM*), usually prepared by the Health Information Department.

Diagnosis Related Grouping (DRG) a method of grouping illnesses to determine the cost of treatment and the reimbursement rate paid by Medicare or Medicaid. Originally the approach involved coding with ICD-9-CM and grouping by homogeneous costs, using major diagnosis, length of stay, secondary diagnosis, surgical procedure, age, and type of services required. DRGs, in short, put the burden of responsibility on hospitals to closely monitor a patient's length of stay and the services provided.

differentiation how much or how little a tumor resembles the normal tissue from which it arose; also called ***grade***. *D.* is often categorized as well differentiated (closely resembling normal cells), moderately differentiated, poorly differentiated, or undifferentiated (having no resemblance to normal cells; anaplastic).

direct extension a term used in ***staging*** to indicate ***contiguous*** growth of tumor from the primary into an adjacent organ or surrounding tissue.

disclosure divulging information about a patient under appropriate circumstances, such as by written authorization of the patient; see also ***release of information.***

discontinuous tumors which are not connected; tumors in more than one area with normal tissue between them; often a sign of metastasic disease.

disease index see ***diagnosis index.***

disease-free having no clinical evidence of active cancer.

disseminated in registry terms, a tumor that has spread throughout the body. Some tumors, such as leukemias, are *d.* at diagnosis; others become *d.* as the result of ***metastasis.***

distant a category of the ***summary staging*** system in which there is tumor at sites in the body remote from the organ of origin; tumor cells may have arrived at the *d.* site by traveling in the lymphatic system or the vascular system (***hematogenous***), by floating to the surface of another organ in the fluid of a body cavity (***implantation***), or by direct growth through an organ adjacent to the primary.

distribution the dispersal or variation of a series of values for a variable; see ***frequency distribution. Normal d.:*** see ***kurtosis.***

DNA deoxyribonucleic acid, the carrier of genetic information for all living organisms.

double-blind study a clinical research experiment in which the agent being tested or its action is not known to the patient or the investigator.

Dukes' staging a specialized staging system for cancers of the rectum and colon, initially described in 1929 by Dr. C. E. Dukes. Several modifications of *D. s.* have been published by different researchers and these are frequently referred as *D. s.*

early stage a cancer diagnosed when it is minimally invasive and more easily treated than if it were found at an advanced stage. Early stage cancers are potentially more curable than ***late stage*** tumors.

ecologic study see ***correlational study.***

ectoderm the outermost of the three cell layers in a developing embryo; the origin of epidermal tissues such as the skin, nails, hair, nervous system, and external sense organs.

edit check computerized comparison of data fields for logic and accuracy in any of several ways: ***allowable code checks, range checks, interitem checks, interrecord checks,*** and ***interdatabase checks.***

editing reviewing the information on a case for logic, consistency, and possible errors.

educational standards a list of criteria describing the minimum knowledge required to perform a specific job. ***NCRA*** has published *e. s.* for cancer registrars.

efficacy the power to produce a desired effect; effectiveness.

eligible case a record meeting the criteria for inclusion in a registry; also described as ***reportable.***

end results the evaluation of cancer therapy through the analysis of patient survival after treatment.

End Results Program a federal program between 1956 and 1972 consisting of hospitals affiliated with medical schools across the country that monitored the survival of hospitalized cancer patients; predecessor of the ***SEER Program.***

endocrine therapy see ***hormone therapy.***

endoscopy the use of a fiberoptic instrument to visually examine passages (such as the colon) or the inside of hollow organs (such as the bladder) or viscera (such as the contents of the abdomen). Procedures are usually described by the organ they inspect, such as bronchoscopy (bronchus of lung), or gastroscopy (stomach).

endpoint the health consequence of some **exposure**, usually an undesirable health event such as the occurrence of disease or death but occasionally a beneficial event such as recovery from an illness or healing of a wound. To view the exposure-endpoint relationship as being a cause-and-effect sequence is unrealistic in epidemiology. Exposure-endpoint associations imply a risk relationship, not certain causation.

enzyme one of many complex proteins that are produced by living cells and catalyze specific biochemical reactions in the human body. *Topoisomerase* is a DNA repair *e.*

EOD the 10-digit anatomic coding system developed by the SEER Program to describe **extent of disease,** incorporating three digits for tumor size, two digits for extension of tumor, one digit for lymph node involvement, and two digits each for the number of regional lymph nodes pathologically examined and involved by tumor.

epidemiology literally, the study of epidemics; a branch of medical science concerned with studying the patterns of incidence, distribution, and control of disease in human populations; the basic science of public health. The basic attributes of *e.* study are evaluating person, place, and time in relation to the disease.

epidemiological reasoning a three-step sequence used in the study of disease: (1) determination of an association between an **exposure** and an **endpoint**; (2) formulation of a biologic inference (in other words, a **hypothesis**) about that relationship; and (3) testing of the hypothesis.

epithelial pertaining to the covering (epithelium) of internal or external surfaces of the body. *E.* cells include **squamous, columnar,** and **transitional** types.

error see **hypothesis**.

error of omission incorrect information as a result of the unavailability of correct information; for example, a tumor size marked as unknown because the correct tumor size was in a pathology report that was misfiled.

ethics moral philosophy pertaining to acceptable professional behavior in circumstances where actions may be interpreted as questionable. **Biomedical e.** deals with moral decisions in medicine. **E. issues** concern human experimentation (see **clinical trials**) and issues of life and death.

etiology the cause of an event, usually a disease. **E.** is also the general name for the study of causes of disease.

experimental therapy treatment that has not been approved by the Food and Drug Administration of the federal government, usually involving clinical research trials of prospective new chemotherapy drugs. See also **investigational.**

exposure an ambient environmental factor (such as air pollution), a factor in the individual's environment (such as smoking or diet), or a personal characteristic (such as age, race, or sex) considered to be a precedent factor associated with a likelihood of one's experiencing some health event or endpoint. A person with such an *e.* is said to be **at risk.**

extent of disease the detailed description of how far a cancer has spread from the primary site at the time of diagnosis; a type of classification based on human anatomy that pertains to cancer spread in an individual case.

extramural research federally funded research conducted by investigators at nonfederal institutions such as universities and teaching hospitals; the opposite of **intramural research.**

F-test see **ANOVA**.

FAB (French-American-British) classification a specialized morphological categorization of acute lymphocytic and acute myelogenous leukemias.

FACILITY ONCOLOGY REGISTRY DATA STANDARDS (FORDS): a 2002 publication of the Commission on Cancer (CoC), which details the CoC-required data set and codes, data collection rules, and other information necessary to accurately abstract and manage cancer cases.

FIGO the French acronym for the International Federation of Gynecology and Obstetrics; the major international proponent of staging systems for gynecologic cancers.

final diagnosis   see *pathology report.*

first course of therapy, first course of treatment medical care that is planned or given at the time of initial diagnosis when it has the greatest chance of eliminating the cancer; also called *initial treatment.*

fiscal year   a financial term indicating a twelve-month period which does not necessarily coincide with a calendar year. For example, a *f. y.* may run from July 1 of a given year to June 30 of the following year.

Fisher's exact test   see *nonparametric statistics* and *Chapter 25.*

flag   in registry and computer terms, a data field that indicates a special status; for example, an incomplete case or a data field requiring an *override.*

flow cytometry   a series of clinical tests to measure and describe the cellular and DNA activity of a tumor.

follow   in registry terms, to maintain annual contact with a patient or his or her physician in order to monitor the patient's health following a diagnosis of cancer. See *follow-up.*

follow-back   reviewing a patient's medical history to ascertain if a case reported first by a death certificate ever had that cancer diagnosed at any other source while the patient was alive.

follow-up   an organized system of long-term surveillance of patients; the activities involved in monitoring patients after discharge; the process of obtaining annually updated information regarding a patient's health status to ensure continued medical surveillance. *Active f.* refers to someone, usually a physician or cancer registrar, initiating direct contact with patients to encourage them to see their physician. *F. data* in an *abstract* include those fields useful for tracking the patient after he or she has left the hospital, including the name, address, telephone number, and relationship of a relative, friend, or neighbor who is most likely to know how to locate the patient. *F. letters* are written requests for information on a patient's health status which can be addressed to a physician, the patient, or a *contact.* The *f. rate* is a calculation of the percentage of patients who have current information (within fifteen months) on their health status; the target rate is 90 percent successful *f. F. staff* are the individual(s) in a registry who conduct all patient tracking activi-

ties. *Passive f.* refers to methods that do not require contact with hospitals, physicians, or patients, in order to determine the patient's vital status, such as linkage with voter registration records or driver's license lists.

Framework for Improving Performance   a part of the joint Commission's *Agenda for Change;* describes specific objectives for ascertaining quality of care.

freestanding   a diagnosing or treatment facility (which may or may not be affiliated with or owned by a hospital) which maintains its own patient records. Usually *f.* facilities are in a separate building, such as a surgery or radiation oncology center, and have their own management structure.

frequency   how many observations of a variable have a certain value. The *absolute f.* is the raw number of observations having a certain value. The *cumulative f.* is the percentage of observations having a specific value or less than that value. The *relative f.* is the proportion or percentage of observations that have a specific value.

frequency distribution   a visual depiction of the pattern of occurrence over the range of values for a variable. Common *f. d.*s are the *histogram* and *frequency polygon.* See also *kurtosis* and *skew.*

frequency polygon   a type of *histogram* in which a line connects the top midpoint of each bar; sometimes called an *area chart.*

friable   prone to crumbling or breaking. A *f.* tumor can fall apart when grasped by an instrument.

frozen section   a pathologic examination technique where part of a biopsy specimen is quickly frozen, sliced thinly, and microscopically examined to determine the presence or absence of cancer cells.

full-time employee (FTE)   a person who works forty hours per week or the equivalent; for example, two people each working twenty hours per week would be the equivalent of one FTE.

genetic study   a type of epidemiologic research in which patients and their families are evaluated for the presence of genes which may cause or contribute to the development of cancer.

geocoding   the assignment of a census tract code to the patient's residence at diagnosis.

germ cell tumor a neoplasm that arises from cells that develop into sperm or eggs or cells that resemble those that give rise to sperm or eggs.

glioma a type of tumor arising from the supporting or glial cells of the brain, including **astrocytoma,** oligodendroglioma, and ganglioglioma.

global pricing agreement a written contract that provides a single reimbursement fee for a service, regardless of how costly the treatment is for an individual patient.

grade how much or how little a tumor resembles the normal tissue from which it arose; the aggressiveness of a tumor; also called **differentiation. G.** is also the description or name of the sixth digit of the **ICD-O** morphology code.

grand rounds an educational meeting of medical professionals.

Grants Administration see **Office of Sponsored Research.**

graphics the various ways to present data in pictures or visual detail, including such methods as a **table, bar chart,** or **line graph;** also called **charts.**

gross description see **pathology report.**

growth fraction the number of cells undergoing division at any one time; see also **s-phase.**

gynecologic pertaining to women's health and female reproductive organs.

health care reform the process of reviewing and adjusting patient management patterns and services in order to reduce costs.

health information management department the part of a health care facility that gathers, analyzes, and stores the medical documents for each patient, insuring completeness and coding and indexing the records for future reference; also called **health record department.**

health record the detailed medical information maintained on a patient; also called **chart.**

hematogenous blood-borne; referring to tumor cells which have been carried through the bloodstream to a distant site where they were filtered out and began to grow.

hematopoietic pertaining to the tissues that generate blood components, such as the blood marrow and stem cells.

heterozygosity having different **alleles** at a given locus in a chromosome.

histogram a graphic presentation of information which displays the magnitude of a continuous variable.

histologically confirmed a diagnosis made on the basis of a microscopic examination of tissue.

histology the study of the microscopic structure of tissue.

history the portion of the health record that provides the background of the current illness, including type and duration of symptoms, exposures, and other information that might affect the diagnosis.

history file a list of nonreportable cases which have been identified by the registry but not included in the registry database. Usually the reason for not accessioning the case is that it was diagnosed prior to the registry's **reference date.**

hormone a natural substance produced by the body that controls reproduction, growth, or metabolism in organs distant from where the hormones are produced. **H. therapy** can be the use of surgery, radiation therapy, or drugs to interfere with hormone production, thereby preventing or delaying recurrence of the cancer; also called *hormone manipulation* or *endocrine therapy.* **H. replacement therapy** is the administration of a drug or hormone to restore normal levels of a needed hormone after removal of a gland that produces hormones.

horseshoe kidney see **anomaly.**

hospice an inpatient or outpatient program of nursing and supportive care for terminal patients.

hospital-based a registry that collects information on all patients who use the services of a hospital or health care facility.

host performance scale a classification system describing a patient's **quality of life.** The *Karnofsky scale* and the *Eastern Cooperative Oncology Group (ECOG) scale* are two types of **h. p. s.** that record the physical status of the patient.

hypothesis in statistics, a scientific observation or statement which is to be proven or disproven by research and testing. The **alternative h.** is a statement that there is a real difference between two groups for example, as a result of a different type of treatment. The **null h.** is a statement that there is no difference between the two measurements being compared. Two types of errors can occur when a *h.* is tested: *type I* or *alpha error* occurs when the *n. h.* is true when the statistical test finds that it is false, and *type II* or *beta error* occurs when the *n. h.* is false but it is accepted as true.

ICD (International Classification of Diseases) see ***International Statistical Classification.*** Various editions of this disease coding system include ICD, 1965 revision (ICD-8); ICD, adapted for use in the United States 1967 (ICDA-8); the Hospital Adaption of ICD (HICDA); ICD, ninth revision (ICD-9) and ICD, ninth revision—Clinical Modification (ICD-9-CM).

ICD-O　　see ***International Classification of Diseases for Oncology.***

ill-defined site　　in registry terms, a cancer that originated in an area of the body that cannot be precisely described or coded to a single organ, such as the arm (a general term) or the abdomen (composed of many organs).

immunotherapy　　treatment that boosts, directs or restores the body's normal immune system and enhances the body's own ability to fight the cancer; also called *biological response modifier therapy.*

implantation　　a tumor which has begun to grow on the surface of an organ because tumor cells floated from a primary site in the fluid (ascites) of a body cavity and settled on the surface of another organ.

in situ　　French for "in place"; a tumor confined to the organ of origin without invasion; a tumor that fulfills all microscopic criteria for malignancy except invasion of the organ's ***basement membrane;*** malignant tumor which has not begun to invade; also described as *intraepithelial, noninvasive,* or *noninfiltrating.*

in-depth report　　part of an ***annual report*** in which information on one or more types of cancer is presented in detail; one of the required content items for approval of the annual report by the Commission on Cancer.

incidence　　how many times something occurs; for example, the number of times new cancer is diagnosed in a defined population during a defined period of time such as a year. A new occurrence of a cancer is called an *incident case.* See also ***rate. I. ratio***—see ***relative risk.***

informed consent　　the description of a scientific study and its procedures, written in nontechnical language, which is explained to, and must be understood and voluntarily signed by the patient, parent, or guardian before he or she is accepted into a ***clinical trial.***

infratentorial　　see ***tentorium cerebelli.***

infusion　　the administration of chemotherapy over an extended period of time by mixing the drug with a diluting solution and letting it flow into a blood vessel or body cavity. ***Hepatic artery i.*** is the insertion of a catheter into the hepatic artery in order to deliver a concentrated dose of chemotherapy to the liver. The ***i. center*** is the part of a health care facility that administers chemotherapy to inpatients or outpatients.

initial treatment　　see ***first course of therapy.***

initiation　　the transformation of a normal cell to one that has the potential for malignant growth; one of the two steps of ***carcinogenesis.***

inpatient　　a person spending at least one night in a health care facility in order to be diagnosed or treated.

institutional review board (IRB)　　a committee in a health care facility whose membership, composition, purpose, and functions are specified by federal law and whose purpose is to provide a complete and adequate review of human research activities commonly conducted by the institution and to protect the rights (confidentiality and ethical issues) of all human subjects participating in scientific research.

interdatabase check　　a type of ***edit check*** in which the computer checks two or more databases for consistency. For example, if the cancer registry shows that a patient has lung cancer, the hospital billing record should also show a diagnosis of lung cancer.

interdisciplinary　　coordinated activity between various health specialists. Cancer treatment frequently involves *i.* communication, interaction, and planning among nurses, surgeons, and radiation or medical oncologists.

intergroup　　cooperative studies conducted by more than one ***clinical trial group*** in order to ***accrue*** larger numbers of patients from a wider geographical area into a study. For example, the CCG and POG combine efforts to study diseases such as the ***I.*** Rhabdomyosarcoma Study Group.

interitem check a type of *edit check* in which the computer compares two or more data elements for logic. For example, an *i.* edit might check the fields "Primary Site" and "Sex"; this edit would fail if the primary site was prostate and sex was female.

International Agency for Research on Cancer (IARC) an independently financed organization within the framework of the World Health Organization, based in Lyon, France, dedicated to worldwide research on the epidemiology of cancer and the study of potential carcinogens in the human environment; affiliated with the *International Association of Cancer Registries.*

International Association of Cancer Registries (IACR) an organization based in Lyon, France, created in 1965, and consisting of member population-based registries throughout the world. The purposes of IACR include improving the quality of data on cancer incidence and mortality and comparability between registries by standardizing methods of registration, definitions, and coding and to disseminate information on the multiple uses of cancer registry data in epidemiologic research and the planning and evaluation of cancer prevention and therapy; affiliated with the *International Agency for Research on Cancer.*

INTERNATIONAL CLASSIFICATION OF DISEASES FOR ONCOLOGY **(ICD-O)** the worldwide standard coding system for cancer diagnoses, now in its second edition. *See Chapter 15.*

INTERNATIONAL STATISTICAL CLASSIFICATION OF DISEASES AND RELATED HEALTH PROBLEMS, TENTH REVISION **(ICD-10)** the most recent edition of the coding system used worldwide for assigning morbidity and mortality codes to health records and death certificates. For names of predecessors, see *ICD.*

International Union Against Cancer the name in English of the French-named Union Internationale Contre le Cancer **(UICC)**, the international organization which promotes the use of the *TNM staging* system worldwide; also referred to in English as the UICC.

interrecord check a type of *edit check* in which the computer checks multiple records for consistency. For example, the same patient cannot be coded as "alive" on one primary and coded as "dead" on another primary.

interval see *data.*

intervention an action is taken in an attempt to effect a change. For example, publicity about the availability of mammography in a non-English-speaking community is an *i.* which can be studied or evaluated to determine its success in reducing the number of late-stage cancers diagnosed in that community.

intramural research federally funded research conducted at the *National Institutes of Health* Clinical Center in Bethesda, Maryland; the opposite of *extramural research.*

intramuscular injection of a drug or chemotherapy agent into a muscle.

intraperitoneal injection of a drug or chemotherapy agent into the peritoneal cavity.

intrathecal injection of a drug or chemotherapy agent into the cerebrospinal fluid surrounding the brain and spinal cord in order to reach tumor cells in the brain or spine with an agent that cannot cross the *blood-brain barrier.*

intravenous administration of a drug or chemotherapy agent by injecting it directly into the bloodstream through a vein.

intussusception the telescoping of the large bowel or small intestine upon itself, sometimes caused by a tumor mass in the bowel wall.

investigational a technique, drug, or treatment that is being evaluated by means of a scientific or research study. *I.* **drugs** have not yet been approved by the Food and Drug Administration for general use, but can be used in a *clinical trial.*

involved in registry terms, considered to contain or be affected by cancer.

job description see *position description.*

Joint Commission on Accreditation of Healthcare Organizations (JCAHO) the agency which establishes and oversees quality standards for hospitals and psychiatric, long-term care, and certain other health facilities in the United States; formerly the joint Commission on Accreditation of Hospitals. *See Chapter 11.*

JOURNAL OF REGISTRY MANAGEMENT the official quarterly journal of *NCRA* which publishes scientific articles on registry science.

Kaplan-Meier calculation   see *survival calculation.*

Kruskal-Wallis test   see *nonparametric statistics* and *Chapter 25.*

kurtosis   the statistical description of the spread or dispersal of values along a range of data. Types of *k.* include *platykurtosis* (flatter and wider than a normal distribution), *leptokurtosis* (higher and narrower than a normal distribution), and *mesokurtosis* (the normal distribution or *bell-shaped curve*).

Langerhans cell histiocytosis (LCH)   a condition consisting of a proliferation of histiocytes, eosinophils, and lymphocytes.

latency   the interval from the start of a disease until it is clinically detected. The *l.* period for most cancers is believed to be ten to twenty years.

late stage   a cancer that has spread beyond anatomic boundaries and that can no longer be treated with localized surgery or radiation therapy.

legal   pertaining to the law. In registry terms, usually pertaining to the *release of information* about a patient. *L. aspects* of policies imply circumstances pertaining to regulations of administrative agencies, common law, and statutory law.

legislative mandate   in registry terms, a law, regulation, or other governmental ruling empowering a central registry to establish and maintain a mechanism for cancer data collection and related surveillance activities. A *l. m.* can include funding, confidentiality policies, and penalties for not reporting eligible cases to the central registry.

leptokurtosis   see *kurtosis.*

leukemia   the presence in the blood of malignant cells which developed in the bone marrow.

leukocoria   a white spot on the eye indicative of possible *retinoblastoma.*

life-table method   see *survival rate.*

line graph   a graphic presentation of information showing a trend over time by displaying an increment of time on the *x*-axis and the amount, frequency, or percentage on the *y*-axis.

list   a graphic display of information about a single variable in text format.

localized   a category of the *summary staging* system in which the tumor is confined to the organ of origin without extension beyond the primary organ.

longevity   the length of time a registry has been established, based on the *reference date.*

lost to follow-up   a case for which all *contacts* for *follow-up* have been exhausted without successfully obtaining current information on the patient's health status at a point in time more than fifteen months after the *date of last contact;* see also *delinquent.*

lymphadenopathy   enlargement of lymph nodes, but not necessarily indicating tumor involvement.

lymphoma   malignancy of lymphoid tissues, in other words, those tissues and organs that produce and store cells that fight infection and disease; subdivided into *Hodgkin disease* and *nonHodgkin lymphoma.* *Burkitt l.* is a rapidly growing tumor first described by Dr. Dennis Burkitt in Africa; African Burkitt is characterized by massive cervical node and jaw involvement; American Burkitt has a more disseminated presentation with an abdominal mass and malignant peritoneal and pleural effusions.

M   in the *TNM staging* system, the element that describes the presence or absence of distant metastases.

magnetic resonance imaging (MRI)   a diagnostic technique that uses strong magnetic fields that take advantage of cellular properties to define internal structures.

malignancy   an invasive, uncontrolled growth of cells capable of invading surrounding structures and producing a *metastasis.*

managed care   the process of monitoring patient treatment in order to maximize quality and minimize cost. *M. c. organizations* are groups of health care providers whose purpose is to deliver quality medical services in the most cost-effective means possible in an attempt to reduce health care costs.

management   in registry terms, how the patient is diagnosed, treated, and followed; sometimes called *case management.*

manager   the individual in a registry who handles administrative and staffing issues and supervises others in the registry.

Manchester (UK) Children's Tumour Registry classification   a specialized scheme for the classification of cancer in children, divided into twelve main diagnostic groups containing several subclassifications.

Mann-Whitney U test   see *nonparametric statistics* and *Chapter 25.*

manual   by hand; in registry terms, not involving a computer program. A *tickler file* is a *m.* follow-up system.

MANUAL FOR TUMOR NOMENCLATURE AND CODING (MOTNAC)   the earliest publication providing topography and morphology codes for cancer diagnosis, first published by the American Cancer Society in 1951.

margin   in medical terms, the edge of a surgical resection or the rim of normal tissue surrounding a tumor; usually referred to as normal, clear, or uninvolved if there is no evidence of tumor at the edge. In business terms, *m.* is the profit and loss incurred as a result of an activity. A registry can perform this type of margin study on a cancer service (such as mammography screening) if it has access to a patient's financial records.

market-share studies   analysis of *referral patterns* and *treatment patterns* together with other information to determine a facility's or organization's market share (proportion of "available" business activity). For example, *m. s.* could determine that a hospital was treating a smaller proportion of all of the breast cancer cases in a city because of competition from a newly opened facility.

marketing   the process of informing others of the usefulness of a service or product. *M.* is a combination of publicity and customer education about the service or product. For example, a cancer registry markets its data (a product) to make its *customers* aware of the services it offers.

master patient index (MPI) file   the alphabetized, computerized list or card file that includes every patient, alive and dead, that has been accessioned into the registry since the *reference date;* also called *patient index.*

matching   a design strategy used in epidemiology to make the study groups as comparable as possible. For example, if the study groups are made to be comparable with respect to age, any difference between them cannot be due to the influence of age. *M.* can be for the whole study group or for individuals. Individual *m.* may be one-to-one or many-to-one, which means that more than one comparison person is selected for each study subject.

matting   in registry terms, the lumping together of lymph nodes into a single mass, usually the result of tumor growth between the nodes.

mean   the average of a series of numbers.

measures of central tendency   statistical calculations that describe how alike the values in a range of numbers are; a collective term for *mean, median,* and *mode.*

median   the midpoint or middle value in a series of numbers.

MEDLINE   a database of indexed medical literature available through the National Library of Medicine.

medulloblastoma   a radiosensitive tumor of undifferentiated neuroepithelial cells arising in the cerebellum.

mesenchymal   pertaining to the mesenchyme; the diffuse network of cells forming the embryonic mesoderm and giving rise to the blood and blood vessels, the lymphatic system, and cells of the reticuloendothelial system.

mesokurtosis   see *kurtosis.*

metastasis, metastases (plural form)   any tumor spread to a part of the body away from the primary. See also *distant spread. Drop m.* is a specific type of tumor spread into the spinal cord and cauda equina from the brain.

microinvasion   tumor extension through the *basement membrane* (a histological landmark in an organ), visible only through the microscope; an indication that the tumor is invasive and no longer *in situ.*

micrometastases   secondary tumors that are not visible to the unaided eye. *M.* can grow and develop into distant recurrences if they are not treated and destroyed by systemic therapy.

microscopic confirmation   diagnoses that include hematology, cytology, and tissue examinations.

microscopic description   the part of the *pathology report* that describes what the pathologist diagnoses with the aid of a microscope.

mitosis   that part of the cell cycle in which the cell is actively dividing.

mode   one of the measures of central tendency which describes the most frequently occurring value in a series of numbers. *Bimodal* means that a range of numbers has two most-common values.

morbidity a **complication** or other effect of disease, such as impaired organ function as a result of a surgical procedure.

morphology the science of structure and form without regard to function; the name of the **ICD-O** code describing the specific type of tumor.

morphology groupings ranges or categories of **ICD-O** histology codes; usually used for aggregate reporting or data analysis of related types of cancer.

mortality death.

multicentric, multifocal in registry terms, the presence of more than one area of tumor in an organ or tissue.

multidisciplinary consisting of representatives from many health specialties; for example, surgery, pathology, radiology, medical oncology, and radiation oncology. The **COC** requires that the **cancer committee** be **m.**

multihospital registry see **central cancer registry.**

multiple primaries the situation in which a patient has more than one cancer; see also *primary.*

myeloablative lethal to bone marrow cells, usually referring to a drug or radiation administered prior to a **bone marrow transplant.**

myelodysplastic syndrome a unique preleukemic state in which the bone marrow shows progressive deterioration in red blood cell production, platelet formation, and white blood cell maturation.

N in the **TNM staging** system, the element that describes the presence or absence of tumor in regional lymph nodes.

National Board for Certification of Registrars (NBCR) an independent organization responsible for developing and administering the **certification examination** for cancer registrars.

National Cancer Act of 1971 a federal law that mandated the collection, analysis, and dissemination of data for use in the prevention, diagnosis, and treatment of cancer; the legal authorization for the establishment of the **SEER Program** of the **National Cancer Institute.**

National Cancer Data Base (NCDB) a clinically-oriented electronic database of cancer cases submitted to the Commission on Cancer by approved cancer programs in the United States, which can be used as a **reference database** to compare the management of cancer patients in one facility or region with similar patients in other regions or nationally. *See Chapters 9 and 31.*

National Cancer Data Committee the committee that oversees the **National Cancer Data Base** and patient care evaluations; see *Commission on Cancer.*

National Cancer Institute (NCI) one of the twenty-four institutes of the **National Institutes of Health (NIH),** established under the earlier "National Cancer Act" (of 1937) as the federal government's principal agency for cancer research and training. The National Cancer Act of 1971 broadened the scope and responsibilities of the NCI, and legislative amendments have maintained the NCI's authorities and responsibilities and added new information dissemination mandates as well as a requirement to assess the incorporation of state-of-the-art cancer treatments into clinical practice. NCI is the governmental agency which houses the **SEER Program.**

National Cancer Registrars Association (NCRA) a professional organization composed of cancer data specialists, whose purpose is to promote the education and professional development of cancer registrars and cancer registries; formerly the **National Tumor Registrars Association.**

National Center for Health Statistics a federal center of the **Centers for Disease Control and Prevention** which provides population and mortality data that are used by the SEER Program and others to derive cancer incidence, mortality, and survival rates.

National Institutes of Health (NIH) originally established in 1887 and now composed of twenty-four separate institutes, centers, and divisions, the **NIH** is one of eight health agencies of the Public Health Service which, in turn, is part of the U.S. Department of Health and Human Services. **NIH** is federally mandated and funded to support and conduct biomedical research.

National Program of Cancer Registries (NPCR) a federally funded program, operated by the **Centers for Disease Control and Prevention** (CDC), to assist state central cancer registries to meet minimum standards for completeness, timeliness, and data quality. NPCR was funded by the **Cancer Registries Amendment Act.**

National Wilms' Tumor Study Group an *intergroup study* of the treatment of patients with Wilms' tumor with a goal of developing more effective treatments for children with Wilms' tumor, as well as looking for the causes of this cancer.

natural product a chemotherapeutic agent that is derived from a plant or other organism rather than a chemical compound; *n. p.*s include *antitumor antibiotics, plant alkaloids* and *enzymes.*

necropsy see *autopsy.*

neoplasm a new growth; the term *n.* itself does not carry any association of being *benign* or *malignant.*

nephroblastoma see *Wilms' tumor.*

nesting combining two study designs to get the best of both choices, more data more quickly and at lower cost.

neuroblastoma a tumor of childhood arising from immature nerve cells in the neural crest ectoderm.

neuropeptides chains of protein building blocks that act on nerve cells.

nomenclature a system of names; an organized way of naming things.

nominal see *data.*

nonanalytic a category of *class of case* which indicates that the case was referred to the reporting facility for recurrence or subsequent therapy after the cancer was initially diagnosed and treated at another facility; the opposite of *analytic.* A *n.* case is generally not included in statistical reports of treatment and survival, but may be included in administrative reports.

non-cancer-directed procedures which do not attempt to modify, control, remove, or destroy cancer tissue; for example, bypass surgery, radiation to a single tender area of bone metastases, or removal of a painful primary or metastasis tumor mass.

noncontiguous see *discontinuous.*

noninfiltrating, noninvasive see *in situ.*

nonparametric statistics various statistical techniques which can be used for small numbers of subjects or severely skewed distributions, including the *Kruskal-Wallis test, Mann-Whitney U test, Fisher's exact test,* and the *Wilcoxon signed rank test. See Chapter 25.*

nonreportable not meeting the criteria for inclusion into a registry; see *reportable.* For example, a malignant diagnosis identified in the disease index may not be supported by the medical record itself (in other words, miscoded), rendering the case *n.*

North American Association of Central Cancer Registries (NAACCR) an organization of member cancer registries established in 1987, whose purpose is to promote standardized data collection, quality, and consistency of central cancer registry operations, and exchange of information among population-based central cancer registries in North America. *See Chapter 32.* This organization was formerly known as the *American Association of Central Cancer Registries (AACCR).*

nuclear medicine a medical specialty or department of a health care facility which uses *radioactive isotopes* to diagnose and treat patients.

objective(s) the measurable ends to which a person or organization strives; for example, one *o.* for a cancer registry is to maintain a 90 percent successful follow-up rate.

Office of Sponsored Research a federally required office in any institution involved in research that serves as a liaison or clearinghouse for communications between the facility and the *clinical trial group,* DHHS, or other organizations that grant funds for research, as well as controlling and coordinating the funding of research activities; also called *Grants Administration.*

oncology the study of cancer as a disease process; the study of tumors.

oncology indicators specific *outcomes measures* designed to assess the quality of cancer care in an institution; see also *clinical indicator.* An example of an *o.i.* for lung cancer is "the number of unresectable tumors determined at thoracotomy."

operations manual in a registry, the specific instructions for initiating and terminating the computerized cancer registry program, including instructions for completing routine tasks, backup and data loss prevention procedures, and descriptions of edit checks and potential problems and their resolution, and a disaster recovery plan.

operative report a summary of pertinent observations noted during the course of a surgical procedure dictated by the surgeon; also called a *surgery report.*

The *o. r.* is useful to the registry because it contains detailed information about the location of the tumor and any extension, nodal involvement, or metastasis spread which was not biopsied or resected.

optional data   see *data set. O. d.* includes financial data (insurance payer information as well as charges and reimbursements), laboratory studies, service utilization, and other items of specific interest to the facility collecting them.

oral   administration of drugs or chemotherapeutic agents by mouth (swallowing them) so that the drug can be absorbed through the gastrointestinal tract into the bloodstream.

ordinal   see *data.*

ordinate   see *axis.*

other cancer-directed therapy   a category of treatment that includes cancer treatments whose action or efficacy has not been clearly defined, such as *experimental therapy, unproven therapy,* and *double-blind studies.*

outcome   the result of an interaction between a patient and the health care system, usually the results of a study. Examples of measurable *o.*s include *survival, patient satisfaction,* and time to recurrence. *O. measurement* is the process of analyzing whether a plan executes what it is capable of doing and, when it does, what the results are. *O. measures* are statistical statements that describe the expected results; for example, one *o. m.* for breast cancer is "the proportion of all breast cancers of known stage diagnosed at an in situ stage."

outpatient   a person treated without having to occupy a bed overnight at a health care facility. An *o. clinic* is a facility, usually affiliated with a hospital, where patients are examined and treated but they do not stay overnight. Also called *ambulatory clinic.*

override   to indicate that a data edit advising a possible inconsistency has been reviewed and the information is correct.

p-value   the result of a statistical test indicating the probability that this statistic is the result of a random observation.

paired bar chart   see *bar chart.*

palliative   intended to relieve symptoms or make the patient more comfortable; action taken to maximize the well-being of patients who cannot be cured. *P. treatment* is considered *non-cancer-directed* treatment.

Pap smear   a type of cytology examination used for the detection of abnormal cervical cells; named for its developer, Dr. George Papanicolaou.

parameter   a specific datum or characteristic; an aspect or criterion being studied; for example, an analysis of survival in white females with breast cancer includes three *p.*s—race, sex, and primary site.

passive reporting   see *casefinding.*

pathologic staging   in the *TNM staging* system, a *staging basis* designating that the information used to assign the T, N, and M categories included the resection of the primary tumor and, for most primary sites, the removal and examination of regional lymph nodes, in addition to the clinical examinations and diagnostic tests.

pathologist   a physician specializing in the microscopic diagnosis of disease.

pathology   the scientific study of the nature of disease, its causes, processes, development, and consequences, especially through the microscopic examination of tissues and cells. The *p. department* is the section of a health care facility responsible for microscopic analysis of tissues and body fluids.

pathology report   the written description of the microscopic examination of a tissue. The *gross description* reports the physical characteristics of the tissue: size, color, and abnormalities visible with the unaided eye. The *microscopic description* reports the cellular characteristics aided by the use *of a microscope:* what cells are involved, the behavior, and the aggressiveness or grade of any abnormality. The *final diagnosis* is a summary of the findings and indicates the pathologist's impression of what was found in concise terms.

patient brochure   a publication describing the services of the cancer registry, designed for patient education.

patient identification   a part of the *abstract* containing data items that identify a specific person, such as a patient's name, address, social security number, health record number, sex, date of birth, race, and so forth.

patient index   see *master patient index file.*

patient log   a listing of the patients treated in a specific department such as radiation or medical oncology; useful for casefinding.

patient privacy   the right of a patient to have his/her medical and other information protected from dissemination to unauthorized persons or agencies.

patient satisfaction   a way of measuring the success of a health care encounter by analyzing the answers to questions asked of the person who received services or treatment.

PDQ (Physician Data Query)   a database of current cancer treatment and protocol information available through the National Cancer Institute.

Pearson's correlation   see *correlation* and *Chapter 25.*

Pediatric Oncology Group (POG)   a pediatric *clinical trial group,* composed of the former pediatric sections of SWOG and CALGB, that has developed a series of staging systems for various children's malignancies.

peer review   monitoring of the activities of medical professionals by other professionals with the same level of knowledge; usually the monitoring of physicians by other physicians.

performance evaluation   a review of the accomplishments and effectiveness of an individual in handling a job. *P. e.*s are conducted by a supervisor in order to help an employee improve job skills.

performance improvement plan   documentation of a health care facility's strategy to make its services more effective; part of a JCAHO survey.

performance measurement system   an interrelated set of outcomes measures, process measures, or both, that supports internal comparisons of an organization's performance over time and external comparisons of performance among organizations at comparable times [Joint Commission definition].

person-year   a statistical calculation in which the number of cases in the population is multiplied by the years *at risk;* used to express a *rate* over a period of time. For study designs where subjects are followed through time, each person contributes a *p.* for each year of participation; for example, a group of 100 persons studied from January 1, 1990 to December 31, 1999 (10 years) contributes 1,000 *p.* to the study (10 years times 100 persons).

phase   one of the series of steps necessary to complete a *clinical trial. P. I* (Phase One) clinical trials test the initial safety of new drugs, devices, treatment modalities, or combinations of these elements. *P. II* (Phase Two) clinical trials focus on dose responses, frequency of drug dosage, and other areas of safety, as well as drug efficacy; also called *pivotal trials. P. III* (Phase Three) clinical trials compare the research drug, method, or device with current standard treatment. *P. IV* (Phase Four) clinical trials provide additional details regarding a drug's safety and efficacy.

physical examination   the careful inspection of the body looking for signs of disease. For cancer patients, the *p. e.* can yield information on the size and location of the tumor, involved lymph nodes, organ enlargement, or other abnormalities resulting from the disease process.

pictorial chart   a graphic presentation of information which uses symbols to display volume or magnitude. Maps and anatomic drawings are also considered *p. c.*s.

pie chart   a graphic presentation of information which displays the relationship of parts to a whole in circular format.

piggy-backing   a research term where one test or procedure is used for two purposes in order to lower costs for a scientific study; for example, using a blood test that diagnosed a leukemia as the required blood test for a study.

pivotal trial   see *phase.*

plant alkaloids   a chemotherapy agent of *natural products* derived from specific types of growing plants, which interfere with cell division by inhibiting *mitosis.*

platykurtosis   see *kurtosis.*

ploidy   the number of sets of chromosomes in a cell.

PNET (primitive or peripheral neuroectodermal tumor)   a tumor of the embryonal neural cells arising in the central nervous system or soft tissues.

population   in statistical terms, the individuals who make up a certain category defined for scientific study. In demographic terms, the residents of a specified area.

population-based a *central cancer registry* that collects information on all residents of a defined geographic area with a known census. *P.* registries are the only type of registry that allows the calculation of incidence and mortality rates. The two types of *p.* registries are *incidence-only* and *multipurpose,* which combine incidence reporting with patient care, end results, and various other research and cancer control activities.

position description a document delineating all of the responsibilities and other requirements of a named work activity, such as cancer registry abstractor; also called *job description.*

positive predictive value in *screening,* the percentage of all persons tested for a disease who are actually found to have the disease.

power in statistical terms, the effectiveness of a sample to represent the population of which it is a subset.

practice parameters carefully developed guidelines for treating a patient with a specific diagnosis, usually describing the minimum or maximum circumstances for administering that treatment.

prevalence how many cases of a particular disease there are in a population at a given point in time. *P.* is a combination of *incident cases* and cases which have been diagnosed and treated in previous years.

primary the organ of origin of a cancer; see also *site.* A *new p.* is one which has been diagnosed as separate and not related to a previous cancer. A *subsequent p.* is any distinct cancer diagnosed after the first one and not related to it. These concepts are synonymous; a cancer is usually called a *n. p.* during the diagnosis and treatment phase and a *s. p.* when referred to retrospectively. A patient with more than one *p.* is said to have *multiple primaries.* An *unknown p.* is a cancer that was first diagnosed from a metastasis site and whose point of origin cannot be determined.

primary prevention a type of *cancer control* effort intended to reduce the exposure to agents causing cancer or to reduce genetic predisposition to a cancer; preventing the occurrence of disease through occupational, environmental, and regulatory controls and lifestyle and behavior modification. See also *secondary prevention.*

primary site table graphic presentation (usually a table of rows and columns) describing the number and characteristics of cases of various types of cancers in the cancer program *annual report;* a way to display a registry's *site distribution* information.

principal investigator (PI) in a health care facility, the leader of research activities who is responsible for conducting the studies designed by the *clinical trial group.*

procedure manual a document that describes in detail how each function or component of an activity is conducted; for example, a *p. m.* should describe each step in the case ascertainment process, whom to contact, and what to do with the information that is gathered.

process controls statistical methods to measure the state of a procedure or function and trigger a review when the result exceeds established limits; for example, monitoring timeliness of reporting in a registry.

product line in hospitals, a group of diagnoses or services which are managed (administratively and financially) as a unit. For example, obstetrical, orthopedic, and oncology services can be considered separate product lines because their patients are usually mutually exclusive. Radiation therapy and chemotherapy might be considered separate *p. l.*s or included under a more general umbrella of oncology services. The *oncology p. l.* may also include nursing units, the *infusion center,* rehabilitation, and other services directly related to the treatment of cancer.

product moment calculation see *survival calculation.*

productivity standards quantifiable guidelines for performing a specific task; for example, stating that on average, an experienced employee in a facility can complete eight abstracts per day uninterrupted by other tasks. *P. s.* are used to measure employee achievement at the time of *performance evaluation* or salary review,

prognosis, prognostic the anticipated outcome of a procedure or status in terms of *survival* or *quality of life;* for example, early stage cancers usually have a good prognosis, meaning that a patient will live a reasonable length of time. *Prognostic* pertains to the factors which help to assess that outcome; for example, the number of involved axillary lymph nodes is a prognostic factor for breast cancer.

progress notes the part of the health information record which summarizes diagnostic findings on a daily basis, usually handwritten by the health professionals taking care of the patient.

progression of disease the advancement of the cancer to other organs despite treatment. Unlike **recurrence,** there is not a **disease-free** interval before **p. o. d.** begins.

promotion causing a cell to grow rapidly and to metastasize as a result of uncontrolled growth; one of the two steps in **carcinogenesis.**

prophylaxis, prophylactic the use of a specific action to prevent disease; for example, radiation to the central nervous system to prevent brain metastases from lung cancer.

proportion a mathematical representation showing the relation of a part to the whole; the elements that make up the numerator (upper part of a fraction) are a subset of the elements that make up the denominator (lower part of a fraction).

prospective study looking forward from the exposure to the later occurrence of disease or injury. A **p. s.** begins collection of cases at the present time for a specific period, such as a year; also called **cohort study.**

protocol a detailed description of the study question, the plan for conducting the study, and assurances about the process of conducting a **clinical trial** or other research study.

Public Law 102-515 The Cancer Registries Amendment Act, law number 515 of the 102nd Congress of the United States, which established the **National Program of Cancer Registries (NPCR).**

qualitative see **data.**

quality fitness for use; excellence. In registry terms, assurance that the information collected is accurate, complete, and usable for analysis. **Q. assurance** is the ongoing objective assessment of important aspects of patient care and the correction of identified problems. **Q. control,** in general terms, is a carefully planned set of activities by which database managers monitor current quality and take appropriate remedial action to positively affect future quality, maximizing correct reporting and characterizing the reporting process in measurable terms. Specifically, **q. c.** is the process of checking data for accuracy and timeliness.

Q. improvement is the process of reviewing various facets of a job or project in order to determine what factors about it can be made better.

quality of life those factors reflecting a patient's general status, not just cancer-related disabilities; an important concern in treating a patient and returning him or her to a fully functional life. Also called **quality of survival.**

quantitative see **data.**

radiation oncology department that section of a health care facility which treats patients using beam radiation (**teletherapy**) or **brachytherapy;** also called the **radiation therapy** department.

radiation therapy cancer-directed treatment by radioactivity which kills cells by damaging *DNA,* thereby affecting the ability of the cell to divide. **R. t.** is treatment using invisible, high-energy rays emitted by radiation sources which can be at a distance from the tumor (**teletherapy**) or close to it (**brachytherapy**).

radioactive isotopes natural substances (elements) that emit radiation (invisible rays) which can be used for cancer diagnosis and treatment. **R. i.**s can be attached to small molecules and given intravenously. The **r. i.** is attracted to a particular type of tissue, such as thyroid, and concentrates there, providing lethal doses of radiation to cancer cells.

radiocurable the ability to administer a sufficient dosage of radiation therapy to completely kill the tumor and cure the patient without excessively damaging the normal tissue surrounding the tumor.

radiographic study see **x-ray.**

radiosensitive responding to **radiation therapy.**

random sample a method of statistical selection in which every individual in the **population** has an equal and independent chance of being chosen for study.

randomization the assignment to a **treatment arm** of a **clinical trial** by chance, in order to eliminate statistical bias and assure valid results to the study.

range checks computerized **edit checks** which test that a code is within the scope of acceptable codes; for example, a code 7 would fail a **r. c.** if the code structure only included the values 1 through 5. See also **allowable code check.**

rapid case ascertainment   special **casefinding** procedures which allow early or preliminary reporting of certain types of cases in order to get notification of eligible study subjects to researchers.

rate   the measurement of change in a variable over a period of time. An **age-specific r.** is calculated for cases within a range of age at diagnosis, for example, under fifty years. The cancer **mortality r.** is the measurement of how many persons in the general population die of cancer during the time period of interest. A **crude r.** is calculated for an entire population. The **incidence r.** measures the frequency at which people at risk develop a disease over a specified time period. An **age-adjusted i. r.** minimizes the effects of differences in age distributions across time or in different study groups by using standardized population tables to allow comparison of rates in populations that have different age distributions. The **annual i. r.** is the incidence rate calculated for a one-year period. A **site-specific r.** is calculated for a particular cancer primary, such as lung or breast. A **specific r.** is one calculated for a subgroup of the population. See also **survival rate.**

ratio   a fraction formed of two independent measures, where the numerator is not a subset of the denominator. See also **data.**

reabstracting study   a formal procedure conducted to check the accuracy of data in the cancer registry against the **source document(s).**

recoding study   a quality control mechanism in which source documents are reviewed and assigned codes by a second abstractor in order to evaluate the accuracy of the data in the registry.

record linkage   combining information from several sources on the same patient, usually by means of computerized matching programs. See also **case consolidation.**

recurrence   the return of a cancer that was not previously clinically apparent symptomatic, usually at a site distant from the primary (**metastasis**). **Local r.** is a return of the primary tumor itself. **Regional r.** is return of the tumor in an area beyond the limits of the original organ. **Distant r.** is **disseminated,** or in an area remote from the original tumor.

recurrent staging   in the **TNM staging** system, a **staging basis** designating that the patient had been previously treated for this cancer, but was **disease-**

free for a period of time before developing a **recurrence** and that the information used to assign the T, N and M categories was based on the recurrence, not the original cancer.

reference database   a compilation of information which can be used as a comparison, or **benchmark;** also called *comparative data.*

reference date   the starting date established for a registry, usually January 1 of a given year, after which all cases diagnosed or treated at the facility, regardless of **date of initial diagnosis,** must be entered into the registry.

referral patterns   information on why physicians treat their patients at specific facilities or why patients choose to use the services of a specific facility.

regimen   a combination of chemotherapy drugs administered in a planned sequence in order to act at different points in the cell cycle. A **r.** may consist of several **cycles** of chemotherapy.

regional lymph nodes   those lymph nodes which are the first level of lymphatic drainage from an organ; **r. l. n.**s can usually be removed as part of the **cancer-directed treatment.**

regionalized   a category of the **summary staging** system in which the tumor involves more than the organ of origin by means of **direct extension** or spread to regional lymph nodes.

Registered Health Information Administrator (RHIA)   the credentials given to health information management professionals who pass a test which establishes management-level knowledge of health information management department operations.

Registered Health Information Technician (RHIT)   the credentials awarded to health information management professionals who pass a test which establishes baseline knowledge about health information management department operations.

registry   see also **cancer registry;** a comprehensive health information system designed for the collection, analysis, and dissemination of a specific set of health data; a database that identifies and enumerates every instance of a reportable disease in a defined population. A **concurrent r.** collects data on cases that meet specified criteria on an ongoing basis. A **prospective r.** collects data on a specific population with no clinical evidence of the disease at the time of entry into the database, and based on defined study criteria, monitors the disease's incidence or natural history for a specified length of time. A *retrospective r.* collects data on a previously identified specific population meeting a specified criterion such as an established diagnosis of a particular disease. A *special purpose r.* collects data on cases with a specified criterion, disease process, population, or device. *For a list of many types of disease registries, see Chapter 36.*

REGISTRY OPERATIONS AND DATA STANDARDS **(ROADS)** a publication, volume II of *Cancer Program Standards* of the COC used between 1996 and 2002, which details the COC-required data set and codes.

rehabilitation the process of returning a patient to normal or near-normal function after treatment.

relapse the return of a cancer after a clinically disease-free interval. The term *r.* is usually used to describe the return of a leukemia, lymphoma, or other hematopoietic malignancy, rather than the return of a carcinoma; see also *recurrence.*

relative risk a measure of disease frequency in which a comparison is made between a measure that is *expected* (a point of reference such as the general population) and a measure that is *observed* (found to have the disease or condition being studied); also called the *incidence ratio.*

release of information the sharing of facts about a patient; also called *disclosure. R. of i.* can be authorized (intentional) or unauthorized (deliberate or unintentional).

reliability the agreement of different coders using the same information and coding guidelines; see also *reproducibility.*

remission complete or partial disappearance of the signs and symptoms of disease in response to treatment; the period in which a disease is under control.

reportable meeting the criteria for inclusion in a registry. The *r. list* identifies all diagnoses and types of cases to be included in the cancer registry database and should also specify which diagnoses are *nonreportable. R.-by-agreement* cases are those *benign* or *borderline* disease processes which a facility's cancer committee has decided should be collected because they are of local interest.

reproducibility in registry terms, the ability of another person to replicate the same codes given the same information and coding guidelines; also referred to as *reliability.*

required data see *data set.*

research protocol see *protocol.*

resection the removal of tissue from the body, usually an organ and its regional lymph nodes. A *surgical r.* removes a tumor with margins of normal tissue with the intent to remove the entire tumor. A *total r.* removes the primary tumor, surrounding tissue, and regional nodes.

residual tumor the amount of primary cancer remaining after the most definitive *resection.*

resource consumption see *allocation of resources.*

retinoblastoma a tumor that is the most common primary eye malignancy in children.

retrospective study looking back to the exposure history after the disease or injury has occurred; for example, cases already in a registry database which meet specific criteria for analysis. In many instances, the cancer registry identifies cases to be included from its files and the researcher then collects any information not available in the database.

rhabdomyosarcoma a common soft-tissue malignancy of muscle origin.

rho statistic see *correlation.*

risk the relationship between the health experience observed for a study group and what would have been expected on the basis of the *comparison group's* health experience. When this value is expressed as a ratio (risk = observed/expected), it is a measure of the strength of association that exists between an *exposure* and an *endpoint.* It may be shown as a decimal fraction (for example, 1.5) or multiplied by 100 to give a percentage (150 percent). *R.* may imply either an adverse (> 1.0) or a beneficial (< 1.0) relationship; no risk is shown by a value of 1.0.

s-phase the point in the cell cycle when cells are actively synthesizing *DNA*; in *flow cytometry* it is the percentage of cells in active DNA synthesis.

salvage therapy treatment given after the failure of *first course of therapy* in order to prolong survival or to improve quality of life; a second attempt to cure the patient; see also *subsequent treatment.*

sample   in statistical terms, a subset of a **population.**

sampling   the process of selecting data to represent the population being studied. Types of **s.** include *simple,* **random,** *convenience,* and *stratified.*

sarcoma   tumor arising in the supporting structures of the body (bone, muscle, connective tissue). A **s.** does not have a basement membrane and cannot be described or staged as **in situ.** *Ewing's s.* is a particular type of childhood tumor that can arise either in bone (osseous) or in soft tissue (extraosseous). **Soft-tissue s.** is a term for any tumor of **mesenchymal** origin arising in nonskeletal **connective tissue,** such as muscles, tendons, and blood vessels.

scan   a visual report or image of a body part created by computerized tomography, magnetic resonance imaging, or tracing the absorption of a radioactive isotope.

screening   a search for occult, undetected, or early stage disease in a population in order to determine the prevalence of a disease.

second course of treatment   see **subsequent treatment.**

secondary prevention   efforts to deter a disease from incapacitating or threatening the life of a patient after the disease has occurred; the type of disease prevention practiced by conventional medicine.

section   see **tabular list.**

SEER Program   see **Surveillance, Epidemiology, and End Results Program.**

self-reporting   see **casefinding.**

sensitivity   in **screening,** the search for people with a particular disease. See also **specificity.**

sequence number   a unique identifier for each separate primary for a patient which describes the chronology of diagnoses, allowing the registry to identify patients who have **multiple primaries.** The **s. n.** indicates the number of primary cancers the patient has had in his or her lifetime, not just the number of primary cancers included in the reporting registry. The **s. n.** is numeric for cancers, alphabetic for benign or borderline tumors.

service area   the geographic region from which patients come to a health care facility; the region from which a hospital chooses to attract patients; also called *catchment area.*

site   in registry terms, where a cancer is growing in the body. The **primary s.** is the organ of origin; where the cancer started in the body; also called the *topographic s.* A **metastasic s.** is where the cancer has spread to; also called a **metastasis. S. distribution—** see **primary site table.**

site visit   formal inspection by members of a **clinical trial group** of a facility that participates in clinical trials to assure that the facility meets all standards for research and documentation.

site-specific   pertaining to a particular primary cancer; for example, **s.** surgery codes are individualized to each type of cancer (breast, colon, lung, etc.).

skew   the shape of a frequency distribution that is not symmetrical. When the longer tail of a curve trails to the left, it is called *left-skewed* or *negatively skewed.* When the longer tail of the curve trails to the right, it is called *right-skewed* or *positively skewed.*

SNOMED   see *SYSTEMATIZED NOMENCLATURE OF MEDICINE*

Society of Clinical Research Associates (SoCRA)   a professional organization of *data managers* and other health care professionals involved in clinical trials.

source documents   the medical records, disease indices, patient lists, pathology reports, or other original records from which **reportable** cases can be identified and cancer information can be abstracted.

Southwest Oncology Group (SWOG)   formerly the Southwest Cancer Study Group, a **clinical trial group** established in 1956. Now strictly for adult tumors, the pediatric section separated in 1980 to form the **Pediatric Oncology Group.**

Spearman's correlation   see **correlation** and *Chapter 25.*

specificity   in **screening,** the search for persons who do not have the disease under study. See also **sensitivity.**

stacked columns   see **bar chart.**

stage grouping   in the **TNM staging** system, the process of assigning a general category (**I, II, III,** and so forth) conveying disease progression and **prognosis** information for a specific case, based on specific criteria.

stage, stage of disease   categories describing how far a cancer has spread, usually at the time of diagnosis.

The *s. o. d.* is that part of the *abstract* containing the data items that identify cancer spread and confirm and support the assigned *s*. See also *staging*.

staging   a common language developed by medical professionals to communicate information about a disease to others. *S.* usually conveys anatomic *extent of disease* or *prognostic* information about an individual case; a shorthand method of describing disease. Also, the grouping of cases into broad categories based on extent of disease. *S.* usually refers to groups of cases with the same characteristics.

staging basis   in the *TNM staging* system, the point of evaluation; the time at which information on the tumor is collected. See also *clinical staging, pathologic staging, autopsy staging,* and *recurrent staging.*

staging laparotomy   a careful operative exploration of the abdomen to rule out occult abdominal disease and accurately determine the stage of disease; used to stage Hodgkin disease.

standard deviation   the measure of variation about the mean, or average, in a series of numbers.

standardization   in registry terms, the use of uniform guidelines that describe data elements and their codes and how those codes are applied, assuring that cases from registries adhering to those standards are coded by the same rules and edited and updated according to the same guidelines.

standard(s)   guidelines that indicate the optimum achievement level for a particular function or activity; for example, the *s.* for case abstracting is to have the abstract completed within six months of the patient's first discharge from the health care facility. *Data s.* are guidelines that provide uniformity of definitions and code structures for data elements and consistent use of codes. *S. of care* are carefully developed guidelines for the treatment of patients with a specific condition, such as *critical pathways* and *practice parameters.*

STANDARDS OF THE COMMISSION ON CANCER   a multiple volume publication of the Commission on Cancer used between 1996 and 2003 which provides specific guidelines for *cancer program approval.* See *Cancer Program Standards* and *Registry Operations and Data Standards.*

statistical techniques   using information gained from a sample, which is a subset of a larger group, in order to make statements about the *population* of interest; mathematical methods used to help distinguish between a true association and one that results from chance. *See Chapter 25.* Statistical techniques include *hypothesis testing,* the *z-test* (which measures the difference between an observation and the sample mean), *t-test* (which compares one distribution with another to determine whether they represent two different distributions or populations), the *chi-squared test* (which assesses variability about an expected value), *ANOVA* (analysis of variance or the *F-test*), *multivariable regression, correlation,* and *nonparametric statistics.*

statistics   a branch of mathematics dealing with the collection, analysis, interpretation, and presentation of masses of numerical data. *Biostatistics* are mathematical analyses having to do with living organisms, such as survival analyses for cancer patients.

stem cell transplant   a type of *bone marrow transplant* in which stem cells (the immature cells from which all blood cells develop) are obtained from the bloodstream and then used to restore the bone marrow.

stereotactic   approached from more than one direction, usually two. *S. radiosurgery* involves focusing radiation beams on a small area and delivering very high doses of *radiation therapy.*

steroid   a type of *hormone therapy* which is specifically toxic to lymphoid malignancies. *S.*s are also used to alter immune system response and the reaction of cancer cells to chemotherapy, thereby improving treatment response.

subcategory   see *tabular list.*

subclassification   see *tabular list.*

subcutaneous   injection of a drug or chemotherapy agent under the skin.

subsequent primary   see *primary.*

subsequent treatment   any additional therapy administered after the failure of the first course of therapy, due either to progression of disease or the lack of response to initial treatment.

summary staging   a system of describing the anatomic spread of cancer in broad or general terms: *localized, regionalized,* and *distant;* sometimes called *general staging. S. s.* was originally developed in California, was later adopted by the SEER Program, and was last updated in 2001.

supervisor   any individual directly responsible for overseeing daily operations of a program, department, or its staff.

SUPPLEMENT ON THE TUMOR REGISTRY   the Commission on Cancer document used between 1981 and 1986 which provided standardized guidelines and coding mechanisms for cancer data; replaced by the *Data Acquisition Manual (DAM)* (1986–1996) and later by **Standards of the Commission on Cancer, volume II: Registry Operations and Data Standards (ROADS) (1996–2002).** The Facility Oncology Registry Data Standards (FORDS) is the current CoC-required data set and coding manual used to collect accurate data and manage cancer cases.

supplemental data   see *data set.*

supportive care   treatment that enhances the patient's quality of life but does not directly affect the cancer, such as administering drugs to improve appetite or reduce brain swelling.

supratentorial   see *tentorium cerebelli.*

surgery   most often includes the removal of tissue from the body; see also *resection. Cytoreductive s.* removes as much gross disease as possible in order to improve the efficacy of adjuvant treatment; also called *debulking. Diagnostic s.* identifies the histologic type of cancer and estimates the stage of disease but leaves gross tumor in the body; see also *biopsy. Function-preserving s.* is treatment to remove as much tumor as possible without affecting mobility or activity level; for example, a wide excision of a rhabdomyosarcoma of the arm is a more *f. s.* than amputation. *Palliative s.* attempts to reduce pain or correct functional abnormalities in order to improve quality of life, but it does not modify, control, remove, or destroy cancer tissue. *Preventive s.* is intended to avoid the development of cancer by removing a diseased organ before it becomes malignant. *Reconstructive s.* restores the function or appearance of organs or tissues that were either removed or changed by cancer-directed treatment. *Tissue-sparing s.* is an attempt to remove all tumor from an organ while maintaining the organ's form and structure. An example of *t. s.* is lumpectomy for breast cancer.

surgery report   see *operative report.*

Surveillance, Epidemiology and End Results (SEER) Program of the National Cancer Institute a federally funded consortium of population-based cancer registries representing approximately 14 percent of the U.S. population, established by the **National Cancer Act of 1971** to collect and publish information on cancer incidence, mortality, survival and trends over time from selected geographic areas in the United States. *See Chapter 33.* **SEER Program** participants were selected primarily for their ability to operate and maintain a population-based cancer reporting system and for their epidemiologically significant population subgroups.

survey   in registry terms, a detailed review of a cancer program comparing it to established standards for availability of services, patient management, and dissemination of cancer information.

Survey Application Record (SAR):   a Commission on Cancer (CoC) web-enabled cancer program *Survey Application Record (SAR)* that is a primary source of cancer program information, and provides a summary of facility demographic information, resources, services, and description of annual cancer program activity of the cancer program. Information recorded in the SAR is used by both the CoC surveyor(s) and CoC staff to evaluate and rate the program's compliance with the CoC standards at the time of cancer program survey.

survival   how long a patient has lived since diagnosis or some other beginning point. See also *survival calculation.* In general terms, the probability of living a given length of time (such as five-year survival) based on the characteristics of a group of patients. The *s. curve* is the graphed series of *s.* calculations at intervals. The *s. rate* is a calculated number or percentage reflecting the proportion of persons in a defined population who remain alive during a specified time interval. *Adjusted s.* calculations take into account whether the patient died of cancer. *Cumulative s.* is the dependency of the later time periods on the earlier survival rates, for example, third interval survival is a proportion of the patients living through the second interval, which is a proportion of patients who lived through the first interval. *Observed s.* calculations include all patients regardless of their cause of death. *Relative s.* calculations factor in the survival rate of a similar population without the characteristic (such as cancer) in question.

survival calculation   a mathematical formula for determining the survival rate at a set of intervals. The *direct method* requires that all subjects be available for survival throughout the complete interval of interest; in other words, all patients would have to be diagnosed at least five years ago in order to calculate a 5-year survival by this method. The *life-table method* creates a series of calculations based on the number of patients who die and who are withdrawn alive during an interval (usually a year or month); also called the *actuarial* or *cohort method* of calculating survival. The life table method takes the data for the time that a subject has survived and uses them for analysis as long as possible. The *Kaplan-Meier* or *product moment* calculation is a variation of the life table method in which the *s.c.* is made each time a patient dies, rather than at the end of an interval.

survivor's day a public event, usually sponsored by a health care facility, which honors patients who have successfully fought and survived cancer.

survivorship function the shape of a survival curve, based on individual survival rates at various points in time; also called the *survival function.*

suspense in registry terms, awaiting further action. The *s. file* or *s. list* is an inventory or document identifying potentially reportable cases which have not been abstracted; a list of cases which have been ascertained but not yet completed. A *s. case* is a reportable disease awaiting completion and entry into the registry database.

syndrome a group of symptoms or characteristics which appear together and identify a specific disease. For example, *superior vena cava s.* consists of venous engorgement, hepatic enlargement, and edema resulting from lymphatic or metastatic disease obstruction of the superior vena cava.

synthesis the part of the cell cycle in which DNA is replicated as the cell prepares to divide.

SYSTEMATIZED NOMENCLATURE OF HUMAN AND VETERINARY MEDICINE (SNOMED International) the most recent edition of SNOMED, incorporating codes for all medical and veterinary diagnoses, procedures, etiologies, and other descriptors of disease, published by the College of American Pathologists.

SYSTEMATIZED NOMENCLATURE OF MEDICINE (SNOMED) a comprehensive coding system for all medical diagnoses and conditions, published by the College of American Pathologists.

SYSTEMATIZED NOMENCLATURE OF PATHOLOGY (SNOP) a 1965 publication of the College of American Pathologists which provided codes for most tissue diagnoses, including cancer morphology; replaced by SNOMED.

systemic throughout the body; pertaining to or reaching all organs. Chemotherapy is *s.* treatment because it circulates throughout the body in the bloodstream and reaches all organs.

T in the *TNM staging* system, the element that designates the size and invasiveness of the primary tumor.

table a graphic display or arrangement of information into rows and columns comparing more than one variable in order to summarize and present detail that would be cumbersome in narrative form.

tabular list a listing or table of items in numerical order; in registry terms, the sequential list of topography and morphology codes in ICD-O or the numeric list of diagnoses in ICD-9. The divisions of the tabular list in ICD-9-CM are *chapter* (major disease concept), *section* (usually site-specific disease groupings within a range of three-digit codes), *category* (a specific three-digit code number), *subcategory* (further definition of the category at the decimal or fourth digit level) and *subclassification* (the fifth-digit detail of the code).

telemedicine the practice of medicine, usually the process of diagnosing and recommending treatment, at a distance from the patient. Videoconferencing, television linkage, and computer imaging allow a patient in a rural area to be reviewed by physicians at a major referral facility without either the patient or the physician having to travel a great distance.

teleprocessing the linkage of computers via telephone lines in order to transfer data or access the files of a central computer from a second, remote computer.

teletherapy a type of *radiation therapy* where the radiation source is at a distance from the tumor, which is treated by a focused beam of radiation; also called *beam radiation* or *external beam radiation.*

tentorium cerebelli a flap of meninges that separates the posterior fossa from the cerebral hemisphere. *Infratentorial* tumors are those that arise in the cerebellum or brain stem; *supratentorial* tumors are those that arise in the forebrain or cerebrum.

teratogen an agent (chemical or other factor) causing physical defects in a developing embryo.

therapy   see *treatment. Induction t.* attempts to induce or achieve remission or reduction in bone marrow blasts after a diagnosis of leukemia. *Consolidation t.* is a more intensified treatment intended to cure the patient. *Maintenance t.* is the continuation of therapy as part of the initial treatment after evidence that the cancer is in remission; also called *continuation treatment. Prophylactic t.* is given to certain cancer patients in an effort to prevent central nervous system disease.

Third National Cancer Survey   a federally funded program between 1969 and 1971 which monitored the incidence and prevalence of cancer in the United States by surveying certain population areas covering about 10 percent of the population; a predecessor of the *SEER Program.*

tickler   in registry terms, a reminder. A *t. card,* also called a *follow-up card,* contains patient identifiers, contact information, and the date of last contact. It is used to remind the registrar to obtain follow-up on the patient at a twelve-month interval after the last contact date. A *dual t. file* is a card file containing two sets of monthly guides. The card for a case which has been successfully followed is moved from the current year to the appropriate month for the following year. The *t. file* is the *manual* equivalent of the *control list.*

time-and-motion study   an analysis of work activity that involves measuring how long a task takes to accomplish and how much physical activity is involved (for example, sorting, moving, organizing, and filing patient records).

timeliness   the degree to which various stages of the registration process occur on schedule; assurance that all cases have been included in a disease registry within a specified period of time, for example, within six or twelve months after diagnosis.

TNM staging   a method of describing how far a cancer has spread from its point of origin in terms of the tumor (T), involved regional lymph nodes (N), and distant metastases (M), plus a *stage grouping* and a *staging basis;* also called *AJCC staging.*

topography   in registry terms, the name of an anatomic site and its related code.

toxicity   the negative effect of a cancer treatment on normal tissue. Adriamycin is an anticancer drug which has a side-effect of cardiac *t.*

TQM   total quality management; the process of quality; quality from start to finish. A corporation-wide belief that everyone in the organization is responsible for assuring that every step or activity of the organization is subjected to improvement in the level of excellence; also called TQI or total quality improvement. See also *continuous quality improvement.*

treatment   the attempt to cure a cancer or relieve symptoms of a cancer by various methods such as surgery, radiation therapy, chemotherapy, hormone therapy, or immunotherapy. Also called *therapy. Cancer-directed t.* is an attempt to modify, control, remove, or destroy the cancer; also called *definitive treatment. Non-cancer-directed t.* is that which diagnoses the cancer or relieves symptoms, but does not attempt to cure the cancer. A *t. arm* is one of the therapy options being studied in a *clinical trial. T. patterns* are the therapy options for curing cancer; some types of cancer can be treated in a variety of ways and it is important to know which method results in the best survival and other outcomes. A *t. plan* is the therapy decision(s) determined by a physician for an individual patient based on a number of disease-specific and patient-specific factors.

trend   an increase or decrease in a *variable* over time.

Triad Clinical Cancer Control Program   a cooperative arrangement among Cancer Liaison Physicians, American Cancer Society divisions and units, and members of the National Cancer Registrars Association to identify issues, develop strategies, implement programs, and evaluate the effects of these activities on cancer control at state and local levels.

triad of disease   an epidemiologic concept that disease can be prevented by eliminating any one of the three elements (triad) necessary for a disease to occur: the *agent* (the actual biologic cause of the disease process), *host* (a person who is at risk for or susceptible to contracting the disease), or *environment* (the place where the agent and the host encounter each other).

tumor   a swelling or mass; a new growth of tissue or cells.

tumor board   a meeting of medical professionals where the diagnosis and treatment of patients is discussed; see also *cancer conference.*

tumor marker   a substance in the blood or other human tissue that can assist in determining the presence or absence of cancer. *Alphafetoprotein* is a type of *t. m.*

type I error, type II error   see *hypothesis.*

UICC   see *International Union Against Cancer.*

uncertain malignancy   see *borderline.*

Uniform Data Standards (UDS) Committee   a standing committee of NAACCR charged with compiling and resolving issues in coding, editing, and data exchange standards among NAACCR member organizations.

unproven therapy   treatment of cancer by means of drugs or other methods which have not been shown to be effective according to the American Cancer Society.

utilization review   the assessment of all hospital admissions for their appropriateness and medical necessity, as well as for *allocation of resources.*

validity   in registry terms, assessment of whether a specific piece of information in the registry is true or correct when compared to the *source document* from which it was taken.

variable   a category of information; for example, race and sex are two demographic *v.s.*

variance   the dispersal of observations about a *measure of central tendency.*

viscera   plural of viscus; internal organs.

visual review   the process of editing an abstract by visually comparing data fields; a supplementary quality control procedure to computerized edit checking.

vital status   whether a patient is alive or dead.

War on Cancer   President Richard Nixon's phrase describing increased efforts to reduce the morbidity and mortality of cancer, established by the *National Cancer Act of 1971.*

white space   the unprinted margin around a table or text; part of the graphic design of a report; also called *blank space.*

Wilcoxon signed rank test   see *nonparametric statistics* and *Chapter 25.*

Wilms' tumor   an embryonal malignancy (*nephroblastoma*) that almost always arises in the kidney.

withdrawn alive   a term used in *survival calculation* which means that a patient has been excluded (*censored*) from the life table calculation without dying. For example, a disease-free patient diagnosed two years ago would be *w. a.* at twenty-four months in a life table, even though the survival was calculated to five years.

World Health Organization (WHO)   an international agency of the United Nations responsible for health matters in many countries; for registries, the sponsor and publisher of the *International Statistical Classification of Diseases and Related Health Problems* and the *International Classification of Diseases for Oncology.*

written authorization   a paper signed by the patient which permits a facility to release information about him/her to another person or facility for the purpose of research, continuation of care, or administrative planning.

x-axis   see *axis.*

x-ray   the common name for a roentgenogram or radiologic examination of an organ made by sending a beam of radiation through the organ to expose a special type of photographic film, which then provides an image of the organ for diagnosis; also called *radiographic study.*

y-axis   see *axis.*

INDEX

INDEX

543

Database(s)
  adaptability of, 214
  comparison between, 310–11
  before computers, 232
  data comparison and, 308–11
  data elements for inclusion, 460
  database models, 232
  DBMS and, 232–33
  evolution of, 232
  hierarchical models, 232–33
  of hospital registries, 350–52
  Mormon genealogy database, 434
  multiple, 239
  relational models, 233, 234
  of SEER Program, 309, 364
Database administrators, 236, 237
Database management systems (DBMS),
    231–40, 241
  characteristics of, 236–37
  computing environments, 234–36
  databases and, 232–33
  future directions, 238–40
  generally, 234
  glossary of terms, 240–41
  record linkage in, 237–38, 239, 240
  support of consolidation, 237
Database models, 232
Datalinks Web application (CoC), 377,
    378
Date of last contact, 195, 196
Daumas-Duport et al classification of
    gliomas, 353
DBMS. See Database management
    systems
DCO (Death Certificate Only) rates,
    399–400, 418
De-identified information, 36–37
De-identified results, 37
Death certificate follow-back, 418, 426
Death Certificate Only (DCO) rates,
    399–400, 418, 426
Death clearance, 413, 418
Declaration of Helsinki (1964), 169
DEERS (Defense Eligibility and
    Enrollment Reporting System)
    program, 421
Defense Eligibility and Enrollment
    Reporting System (DEERS)
    program, 341, 421
Definitive therapy, 311
Degrees of freedom, 267
Delinquent patients, 186–87, 196
Deming, W. Edwards, 102
Demographics
  patient demographics, 326, 397,
    414–15
  See also Geographic analysis
Department of Defense (DoD), 340–41,
    405

Department of Health and Human
    Services (HHS), 29, 169–70,
    172–73
Department of Motor Vehicles (DMV)
    records, 423, 428
Department of Veterans Affairs, U.S.,
    340, 405
Descriptions (SNOMED), 250–51
Descriptive data, 432
Descriptive studies, foreign, 452
Designed studies, 200, 426
Deterministic match, 237
Device, 224
DHHS. See Department of Health and
    Human Services
Diagnosis
  confirmation of, 415
  patient data utilization and, 326
  stage of disease at, 182–83
  by surgery or biopsy, 158–59
  use of diagnostic information, 326
Diagnosis Related Grouping (DRG)
    codes, 317
Digestive sites, 310
Direct (random) access, 224, 228
Direct method of survival analysis, 278
Disaster planning, 38–40
Discharge summaries, 149
Disciplinary action procedures, 39
Disclosure accounting, 35
Disease frequency, 281–82
Disease indices, 111, 112, 116
Disease site, reporting by, 379, 380–81
Disease Site Teams (DSTs), 376, 377, 384
Disease triad, 280
Disk drives, 224–25
Disk duplexing, 216, 225
Disk operating system (DOS), 225, 226
Disk optimizing, 225
Disposal of records, 35
Distant node metastasis, 150
Distributions
  frequency distributions, 263–64
  in statistics, describing, 264–66
DMV (Department of Motor Vehicles)
    records, 423, 428
Documentation, 94, 96
DoD (Department of Defense), 340–41,
    405
Domain, 233
Dorn, Harold F., 436
DOS (disk operating system), 225, 226
DOS prompt, 225
DRG (Diagnosis Related Grouping)
    codes, 317
Drug accountability, 173
Drug Amendments Act of 1962, 169
Drugs
  in chemotherapy. See
    Chemotherapeutic agents

clinical trials of. See Clinical trials
treatment with. See Cancer treatment;
    Chemotherapy
DSTs (Disease Site Teams), 376, 377,
    384
Dual tickler file, 195–96
Dukes staging system, 153
"Dumbbell" tumor, 355
Duplicate reports, 423, 426
Duty of care, 30
DVD-ROM disks, 217, 225

E

E-path reporting, 118, 119, 413, 417–18
EBV (Epstein-Barr virus), 349, 354
Ecological studies, 433
EDI (electronic data interchange),
    422–23
Edit checking
  computerized, 211, 225, 227, 425
  data quality control and, 201–2, 425
  edit check warning, 212
Edit reports (NCDB), 378–79
EDITS software, 21, 425
Educational programs, 399
  ACoS Division of Education, 86–87
  cancer registrar education, 4–6, 123
  of CoC, 86–87
  continuing education, 56–57
  of NAACCR, 391–92, 427
  by NPCR, 21, 25
  professional education, 322
  public education, 322, 324, 400
  quality control of, 427
Effective number exposed, 278, 279
Electronic data interchange (EDI),
    422–23
Electronic medical record (EMR), 246
Electronic pathology reporting (E-path),
    118, 119, 413, 417–18
Ellsworth, Reese, 361
Employees. See Personnel
EMR (electronic medical record), 246
Enabling legislation, for registries, 405
Encryption, 37, 43, 55
End Results Group (NCI), 396, 436,
    437
End Results Program, 2, 435
Endocrine therapy, 164
Endoscopic retrograde
    colangiopancreatogram (ERCP), 147
Endoscopy, 146–47
Endpoint, 292
England (Gr. Britain)
  Bills of Mortality, 2, 458
  Manchester Children's Tumour
    Registry, 364
  terminology, 246
  Thames Cancer Registry, 454

Revenue, 70
Revenue budgets, 66
Rhabdomyosarcoma (RMS), 344, 345, 356–57
Rho statistic, 277
Right of review, 35
Risk, 292
Risk measurement, 282
Rizal Cancer Registry, 454
RMS. *See* Rhabdomyosarcoma
Royal College of Physicians, 132

S

Sample, statistical, 262, 292
SAR (Survey Application Record), 83, 92, 93, 94, 378
Sarcomas
  bone sarcomas, 350, 358–59
  Ewing sarcoma group, 357–58
  Kaposi's sarcoma, 165, 357
  non-RMS sarcoma, 350, 356
  rhabdomyosarcoma, 344, 345, 356–57
  soft tissue sarcomas, 356–57
  spread of, 345
Screen (of monitor), 228
Screening
  in epidemiology, 285–86
  mass screening for pediatric cancers, 356
Search Term List (NAACCR), 118
Second-generation languages (2GL), 227, 228
Second malignant neoplasms (SMN), 348–49, 361
Second National Cancer Survey, 396, 436
Secondary prevention, 280
Sector, 228
Secular trends, 291
Security, 37–43
  defined, 32
  designing for, 52
  HIPAA provisions, 54
  issues for central registries, 408–9
  operational policies and procedures, 37–40, 186
  physical safeguards, 40–41
  responsibility for, 237
  sufficiency of, 36
  technical mechanisms, 42–43
Security and Electronic Signature Standard, 29
Security standard (HIPAA draft), 47–49
SEER. *See* Surveillance, Epidemiology, and End Results Program (SEER)
SEER *Cancer Statistics Review,* 309, 398
SEER Program Code Manual, 415
SEER *Summary Staging Manual 2000,* 180
SEER*Prep, 392, 424

SEER*Stat, 392, 401, 424
Selection bias, 284–85
SEM (standard error of the mean), 273
Sensitivity screening, 285
Sentinel health events (SHEs), 289, 290
Sequence number, 182
Serial access, 228
Server, 214, 228
SHEs (sentinel health events), 289, 290
Signed authorizations, 34, 55
SIR (Standardized Incidence of Mortality Ratio; SMR), 284
Site distribution, 326
Six Sigma program, 200
Skewed distributions, 265, 266
Skin cancers, 288–89, 310
Smart, Charles R., 388, 436, 454
SMN (second malignant neoplasms), 348–49, 361
SMR (Standardized Incidence of Mortality Ratio; SIR), 284
SNODO *(Standard Nomenclature of Diseases and Operations),* 132
SNOMED. *See Systematized Nomenclature of Medicine*
SNOMED Reference Terminology (SNOMED RT), 135, 246
SNOP (Systematized Nomenclature of Pathology), 123, 133, 246, 248
Social context hierarchy, 254
Social Security Death Index, 189
Society of Clinical Research Associates (SoCRA), 174
Society of Surgical Oncology (SSO), 174
Socioeconomic measures, 379
SoCRA (Society of Clinical Research Associates), 174
Soft tissue sarcomas, 356–57
Software, 4, 22, 228, 234
  CCH Pediatric Grouping System in, 364
  completeness edits, 212, 221
  computerized registries, 195
  costs of, 219
  custom output programs, 424
  data coding, 211
  data entry, 211
  data management tools, 392
  for e-path reporting, 418
  edit checking, 211, 225, 227, 425
  format edits, 211–12, 224
  geocoding programs, 423
  graphics packages, 303
  inter-field edits, 212, 225
  inter-record edits, 212, 225, 237
  intra-record edits, 237
  query system, 213, 228
  registry requirements and, 210–13
  saving "suspense" cases, 181

spreadsheets, 312
standardizing edits, 212–13
statistics software, 213–14
vendors, 213
word processing programs, 311–12
See also specific software packages
Software development, 21–22, 422
Sondik, Edward, 388
Soundex, 237
Source documents, 110, 111, 114
Source of cases. *See* Casefinding
Sources of information, 190, 332, 458
Southwest Oncology Group (SWOG), 362
Spearman's correlation, 277
Special concept hierarchy, 254
Specificity screening, 285
Specimen hierarchy, 253
Spreadsheet software, 312
SQL (structured query language), 213, 215–16, 228, 233
SSO (Society of Surgical Oncology), 174
Stacked columns, in bar charts, 304, 305
Staffing of registries. *See* Personnel
Stage distribution, 326
Stage of disease, 182–83
Staging and scales hierarchy, 254
Staging systems, 149–54, 311
  AJCC system, 149, 151–52, 382, 384
  AUA system, 153
  CCG system, 356
  Chang staging classification, 353–54
  collaborative staging, 152–53
  Collaborative Staging System, 152–53, 382
  colon and rectum staging, 153
  Evans Staging System, 356
  gynecologic staging, 153
  lymphoma staging, 153–54
  melanoma staging, 153–54
  for pediatric cancers, 363
  prostate staging, 153, 154
  requirements for, 149
  SEER extent of disease coding, 149, 151, 154
  Summary Stage System, 412
  summary staging, 149–51
  TNM system, 88, 123, 151–52, 183, 254, 256–57, 259, 357
Standard deviation, 267, 268
Standard error of the mean (SEM), 273
Standard Nomenclature of Diseases and Operations (SNODO), 132
Standard setters for statistics, 122–25, 410, 413, 432, 453
Standardization
  of data. *See* Data standardization
  of edits, software and, 212–13
  of performance measures, 106

Technical security mechanisms, 42–43

Technical writing, 312

Technology
  policies and procedures for, 38
  rapid casefinding and, 118, 119
  security mechanisms, 42–43

Telecommunication, 215

Telephone follow-up, 189

Teletherapy, 159–60

"Ten Cities Study" (NCI), 396, 410, 436

Teratogens, 347

Terminology
  ambiguous, 414
  CPT4 codes, 317
  SNOMED. *See Systematized Nomenclature of Medicine*
  SNOMED International, 135
  SNOMED RT, 135, 246
  statistical, 262–70

Tertiary prevention, 280

Test-case studies, 204–5

Testing in parallel, 285

Testing in series, 285

Tests of significance, 267, 269–70

Textbook of Clinical Oncology (ACS), 466

Thames Cancer Registry, 454

Third National Cancer Survey (TNCS), 396, 410, 437

Thoracoscopy, 146

Three-dimensional conformal radiation therapy (3D-CRT), 159–60

Three-tier architecture, 235–36

3D-CRT (three-dimensional conformal radiation therapy), 159–60

Tickler file, 195–96

Time-and-motion studies, 60, 61

Time frame for abstracting, 181

Timeliness of data, 207, 400, 416

Title/title page of annual report, 331

T.J. Hooper, et al v. Northern Barge Corp., et al, 30

TNCS (Third National Cancer Survey), 396, 410, 437

TNM (tumor-node-metastasis) cancer staging system, 88, 123, 151–52, 183, 254, 256–57, 259, 357

Topography codes, 248

Topoisomerase inhibitors, 349

Total Quality Management (TQM), 102

Traditional budget, 66

Training and education. *See* Educational programs

"Treatment only" abstract, 420

Tumor markers, 147

Tumor-node-metastasis (TNM) cancer staging system, 88, 123, 151–52, 183, 254, 256–57, 259, 357

Tuples (records), 233

"Two-sided hypothesis," 276

Two-tier architecture, 235

2GL (second-generation languages), 227, 228

Type I (alpha) error, 271, 272

Type II (beta) error, 271, 272

U

UDSC (Uniform Data Standards Committee), 124–25, 409, 410

UICC (International Union Against Cancer), 123, 152, 153, 257, 411

UND-STS (undifferentiated sarcomas), 356–57

Undifferentiated sarcomas (UND-STS), 356–57

Uniform Data Standards Committee (UDSC), 124–25, 409, 410

Union International Contre le Cancer (UICC), 123, 152, 153, 257, 411

United States Cancer Statistics, 20, 22

United States Eye Injury Registry, 460

Universal patient identifier, 450

US Census Bureau, 340, 415

User authentication, 43

User interface, 234–35

Utah Cancer Registry, 434, 436–37

Uterine cancer, 288

V

Variance, 267

Vendor/business associate control, 39

Veterans Administration, 340, 405

Viral agents, 349

Virus protection, 43

Virus signature, 219, 228

Viruses (computer), 218–19, 228

Visitor control, 40–41

Visual review, 201, 425

Volatility, 228

W

Washington Hospital Center (WHC), 316

WHC (Washington Hospital Center), 316

WHO. *See* World Health Organization

Wilcoxon Signed Rank Test, 277

Wilms tumor, 344, 347, 357–58

Windows, 224, 226, 228

Wireless devices, control of, 41

Withdrawn alive subjects, 278

Within-record edits, 237

Wittes, Robert, 362

Word, 220, 228

Word processing software, 311–12

Work space planning and design, 61–63

Workbook for Staging of Cancer (NCRA), 152

Workstation design, 214–16
  necessary skills, 215
  networking concepts, 214–15
  remote operation, 215
  structured query language, 213, 215–16, 228

Workstations, 228

World Health Organization (WHO), 247–48, 342, 353, 452
  coding of neoplasms, 132, 133, 136
  data standards, 123, 214, 256, 410
  disease staging concept, 144
  ICD-O coding system. *See* International Classification of Diseases for Oncology
  on value of cancer registries, 245

Written communication skills, 311–12

X

X-rays, 145

Z

Z table, 269

Z-test, 270–71, 272

Zero-based budget, 66